Essential Imaging in Rheumatology

John O'Neill
Editor

Essential Imaging in Rheumatology

Springer

Editor
John O'Neill, MB, BAO, BCh, MRCPI, MSc, FRCR
Diagnostic Imaging
McMaster University/St Joseph's Healthcare
Hamilton, ON
Canada

ISBN 978-1-4939-1672-6 ISBN 978-1-4939-1673-3 (eBook)
DOI 10.1007/978-1-4939-1673-3
Springer New York Heidelberg Dordrecht London

Library of Congress Control Number: 2014955607

Printed on acid-free paper

Springer is part of Springer Science+Business Media (www.springer.com)

To My Amazing Alva, Sam, Sophie & Allie

Believe, Always Believe.

To My Wonderful Mum, Paddy, Michael & Tom

Thank you.

Preface

Essential Imaging in Rheumatology has been many years in the making. The original concept was to provide an easy reference text for the rapidly advancing imaging armamentarium in modern rheumatology. No one group was isolated; we wanted everyone, from the medical student looking at a hand radiograph for the first time to the clinical radiologist or rheumatologist, to derive benefit. As the concept evolved, and with the close interaction of my rheumatology colleagues, we decided to embark on a different approach and develop the book with input from both radiologists and rheumatologists, as neither exists separately in real life, so as to serve the needs of all.

In Part I, we provide an overview of available imaging modalities and essential background information. Chapter 1 presents an introduction to the different imaging modalities available to rheumatologists. It describes an assessment technique known as *JABS* (*joint*, *alignment*, *bone*, *soft tissue*), which I use in teaching my residents and fellows. I hope readers find that this method is a useful approach to the evaluation of a potentially unnerving radiograph of an erosive arthropathy. Chapter 2 incorporates a brief review of the clinical approach to the rheumatology patient. The imaging of normal musculoskeletal anatomy and pathology is discussed in Chapter 3. It is a unique chapter in that all relevant pathologies of a particular system are reviewed together to provide readers with a more global perspective of pathology and a differential diagnosis. Chapter 4 offers a review of image-guided musculoskeletal interventions.

Part II reviews pathologies as separate entities, with dedicated chapters on disorders such as rheumatoid arthritis, connective tissue disease, osteoarthritis, osteonecrosis, infection-related arthritis, soft-tissue calcification, and bone and synovial tumors. Each chapter commences with a clinical overview and common clinical presentations, an understanding of which aids the radiologist in providing an appropriate differential diagnosis and the optimal follow-up studies if required. This discussion is in turn followed by a more detailed review of all imaging modalities for the different stages of presentation where appropriate. We hope this format allows the radiologist and rheumatologist to understand the clinical and imaging components respectively.

The apps entitled "Essential Imaging in Arthritis – The Hand," "Essential Imaging in Arthritis – Spondyoarthropathy," and "Essential Imaging in Arthritis – Clinical and Imaging Presentations," which are based on this book, are expected to be available by 2016 through the App Store℠ and Google Play™ store.

Hamilton, ON, Canada

John O'Neill, MB, BAO, BCh, MRCPI, MSc, FRCR

Acknowledgments

We would like to extend our deep gratitude to all who have made this endeavor possible. Thank you to Janet Foltin and Joni Fraser from Springer. Thank you to all the authors without whom this book would not have been possible. Thank you to those who supplied additional images and help in tracking those down, Brenda Johnson, Naveen Parasu, and Mohamed Helal (GE). Thank you to my fellows and residents, current and past, in radiology and rheumatology, for starting the fire to write this book in the first place.

Contents

Contributors

Jonathan D. Adachi, MD, FRCPC Professor, Department of Medicine, McMaster University, St. Joseph's Healthcare, Hamilton, ON, Canada

Raja S. Bobba, MD, MSc Assistant Professor, Department of Medicine, McMaster University, Hamilton, ON, Canada

Raj Carmona, MBBS, FRCPC Assistant Professor, Department of Medicine, McMaster University, Hamilton, ON, Canada

Alfred Cividino, MD, FRCPC Director, Division of Rheumatology, Department of Medicine, McMaster University, Hamilton, ON, Canada

Sanjay Dixit, MBBS, MS, MD, ABIM, FRCPC Assistant Clinical Professor, Department of Medicine and Rheumatology, McMaster University, Hamilton, ON, Canada

Leilani Famorca, MD Division of Rheumatology, McMaster University, Cambridge, ON, Canada

Nader A. Khalidi, MD, FRCP(C) Program Director, Division of Rheumatology, McMaster University, Hamilton, ON, Canada

Maggie J. Larche, MBChB, MRCP (UK), PhD Associate Professor, Division of Rheumatology, Department of Medicine, McMaster University, Hamilton, ON, Canada

Arthur N. Lau, MD, FRCPC Clinical Scholar, Division of Rheumatology, McMaster University, Hamilton, ON, Canada

Kimberly J. Legault, MD, FRCPC Division of Rheumatology, Department of Medicine, McMaster University, Hamilton, ON, Canada

John O'Neill, MB, BAO, BCh, MRCPI, MSc, FRCR Associate Professor, Musculoskeletal Imaging, Diagnostic Imaging, McMaster University/St Joseph's Healthcare, Hamilton, ON, Canada

Viktoria Pavlova, MD, FRCPC Assistant Clinical Professor, Division of Rheumatology, Department of Medicine, McMaster University, Ancaster, ON, Canada

Part I

Introduction

1 Introduction to Imaging

John O'Neill

The armamentarium of imaging modalities available to the rheumatologist has significantly expanded in the last decade. This is particularly true for MRI and ultrasound, which are now part of the standard imaging algorithm in many rheumatological diseases. The rheumatologist and the radiologist require a clear understanding of these pathologies and their variable imaging appearances. However to correctly interpret an image, one needs a basic understanding of how the image is acquired and how changes in acquisition may impact interpretation. This requires a basic understanding of imaging physics. The following is an overview of available imaging modalities in MSK imaging including image aquisition and interpretation.

Radiography

Physics

Plain film radiography is the backbone of imaging with a significant proportion of patient imaging beginning with an X-ray. X-rays are *ionizing radiation* and form part of the electromagnetic spectrum: visible light, infrared rays, and radio waves are some other forms. X-rays have a short wavelength and hence have greater energy allowing for greater penetration of the human body. *X-rays*, like many other great discoveries, were accidentally discovered more than a century ago by Wilhelm Conrad Roentgen. On the evening of November 8, 1895, while researching cathode ray tubes in a darkened room, he noted fluorescence on a paper plate covered on one side with fluorescent material. Because he did not know the type of radiation causing this effect, he called it X-ray. Soon after, he produced the first radiograph, his wife's hand. This caused a revolution in medicine; for the first time, we could noninvasively see inside the human body. Initially radiographs were used to assess the skeleton, as bone due to its density readily stopped the transmission of X-rays. This progressed soon after to assessment of soft tissues, in particular the chest. In 1905, the first book on chest radiography was published.

X-rays are produced inside a vacuum tube where a filament is heated to several thousand degrees centigrade creating a source of free electrons (Fig. 1.1). An electric current is then passed between a cathode (negative) and anode (positive) causing acceleration of the free electrons across the tube, which then impact the anode at high energy. On impact, X-rays are generated when these free electrons give up some of their energy on interacting with the orbital electrons

J. O'Neill, MB, BAO, BCh, MRCPI, MSc, FRCR
Associate Professor, Musculoskeletal Imaging, Diagnostic Imaging, McMaster University/St Joseph's Healthcare, Hamilton, ON L8N4A6, Canada
e-mail: joneill2@me.com

J. O'Neill (ed.), *Essential Imaging in Rheumatology*,
DOI 10.1007/978-1-4939-1673-3_1,

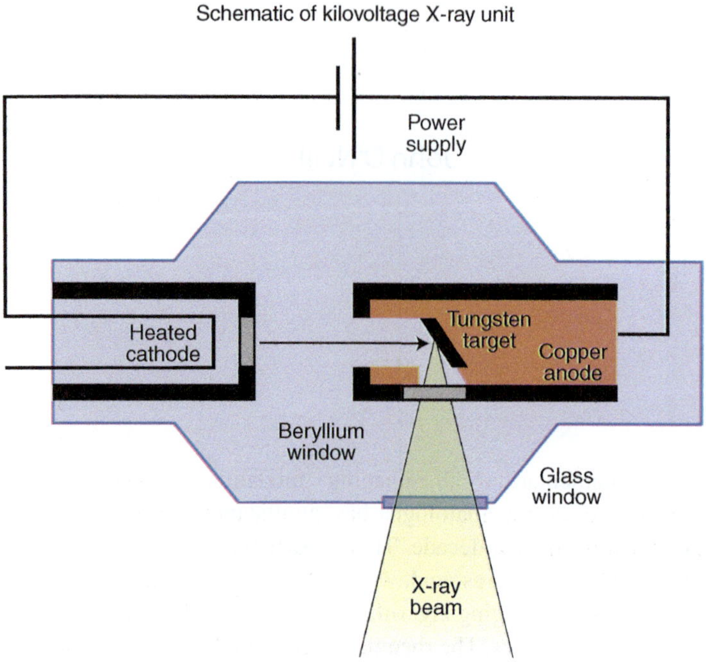

Fig. 1.1 Illustration X-ray production

or nucleus of an atom. The output of the X-ray tube is determined by several factors including the mAs and kVp. Milliampere, mA, is a measure of current, and X-ray production increases linearly with increasing mA. kVp, peak kilovolts, is a measurement of the voltage X-ray tube. The maximum energy of emitted X-rays increases with increasing kVp. The energy of X-rays is measured in electron volts. The beam of X-rays is filtered to remove lower energy rays, and the beam is also collimated so only the area of interest is exposed to the primary beam. Both filtering and collimation reduce radiation dose.

X-rays are attenuated as they pass through the human body; in general the denser the material, the greater the attenuation. The attenuated beam emerges from the body and passes onto a detector, which allows interpretation of the beam. There are several types of detectors including *X-ray film*, which is sensitive to radiation and light. Upon detection a chemical reaction occurs. The more radiodense the material, the greater the attenuation of the X-ray beam. Bone attenuates more than soft tissue and appears radiodense (white) on a radiograph. Tissues that do not diminish X-rays are radiolucent or darker on a radiograph. Examples, in decreasing order of radiodensity (white to black), are bone, soft tissue, fat, and air (Fig. 1.2).

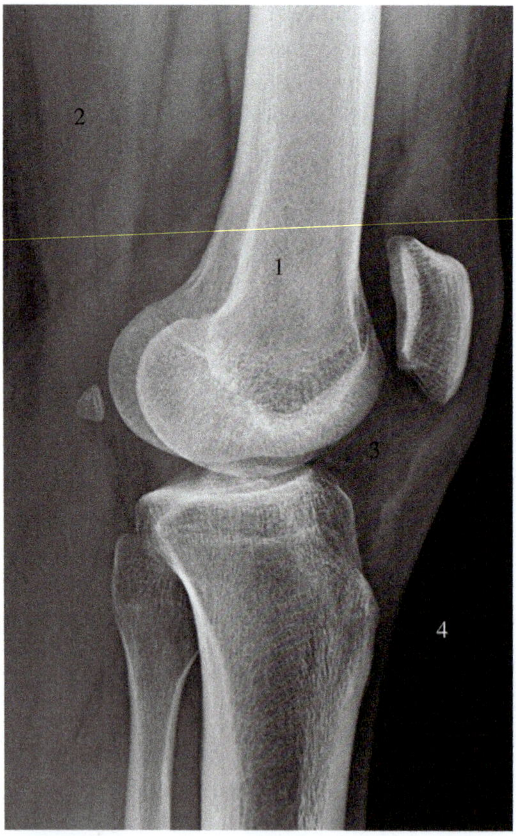

Fig. 1.2 Lateral knee radiograph demonstrating attenuation of X-rays by tissues in decreasing order, *1* bone, *2* soft tissues, *3* fat, *4* air (the greater the attenuation, the whiter the tissue on radiograph)

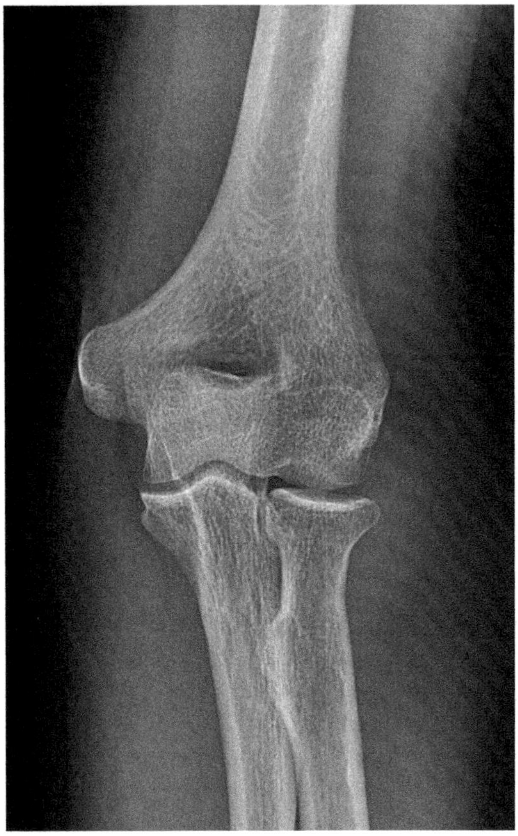

Fig. 1.3 Left elbow radiograph, AP projection

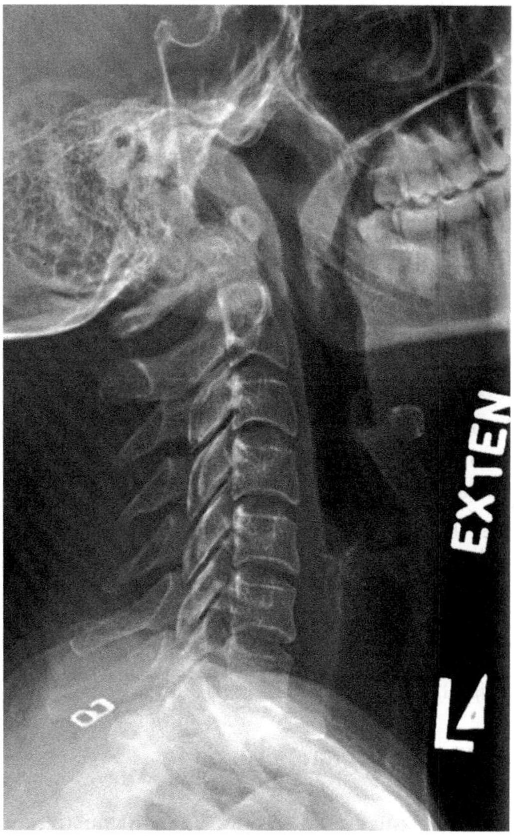

Fig. 1.4 Left (*L*) lateral radiograph, cervical spine in extension (*exten*)

With the advent of the digital age, *digital radiography*, DR, was developed whereby X-rays strike a flat panel detector that in turn converts the signals generated into digital information and creates an image on a computer screen. These allow for a "filmless environment" as images are displayed on monitors. Images can be viewed immediately, have a wider dynamic range, and can be manipulated after being captured. *Computed radiography*, CR, has similar attributes to DR but uses an imaging plate in a cassette, which is then scanned after exposure, converted to an electronic signal, and digitized.

Projections

The two commonest projections are AP and PA. In AP, anterior to posterior, X-rays pass first through the anterior soft tissues, exiting posteriorly to reach the detector; most bone radiographs are acquired as AP projections (Fig. 1.3). The opposite is true for PA projection. Lateral and oblique projections are named with respect to the side closest to the detector. Erect, supine, and standing views indicate the position of the patient (Fig. 1.4).

Image Analysis and Interpretation

Radiographic images should be assessed from multiple perspectives. There are multiple points of reference on the radiograph that should be reviewed before the image is assessed. First, confirm the correct patient was imaged. Rarely the wrong image is assigned to a patient folder; this may be difficult to detect unless the image is not compatible with the clinical picture, e.g., wrong sex, bone, age, etc. Check the image date and time. Depending on the selected format in PACS, the most recent image may be on the left or right of the screen. Confirm that the correct side/part of the body was imaged and was completely imaged, e.g., inadequate inspiration on chest X-ray (CXR). Check for any additional information on the radiograph, e.g., supine, standing, etc.

Image quality may be affected by multiple technical factors. Patient motion causes blurring of the image. Larger patients have more tissue for the X-ray beam to transverse, and if correct technical factors are not chosen, the beam becomes more attenuated, e.g., lower thoracic spine not visualized behind the heart on a CXR. Patient rotation may obscure normal anatomy. Structures furthest from the detector will suffer from magnification and are less sharp. This is most obvious in assessing the cardiopericardial silhouette on a chest radiograph. The heart lies anteriorly and thus is close to the detector on a PA projection, and size can be adequately assessed. However on the AP radiograph, the heart is farther from the detector, is magnified, and is less sharp in outline.

JABS (Joint, Alignment, Bone, Soft Tissue)

Radiographic assessment in rheumatology requires a thorough review with an organized approach. There are many different approaches, and most radiologists have their own although similar method of assessment. In the hand, for example, there are multiple joints to review on three projections: AP, lateral, and oblique. The *JABS* technique was developed for the rheumatology patient: *joint*, *alignment*, *bone*, *soft tissue*.

Joints

Joints are assessed initially. I advise all radiology and rheumatology trainees to take 10 s initially to review the radiograph as a whole to get a global perspective with respect to the extent and severity of disease. It is sometimes easier to have a radiograph with obvious pathology rather than a normal study as the latter often requires a second assessment to exclude occult pathology. If you can identify pathology, then this is where you will start your assessment. It is important to remember that you do not and should not provide an immediate diagnosis. You need to first describe the pathology. By describing the pathology, you may describe changes that help you make the diagnosis which may be different from your initial impression, e.g., erosion with overhanging edge suggests gout. If no pathology is apparent or after you have described the obvious pathology, then you can perform a systematic review at this point using *JABS*.

In the rheumatology patient, the dominant pathology is usually centered at the joint; hence, the *joint* is where we will commence. We will want to compare similar joints at the same time; hence, we review the DIP joints together, the PIP joints, etc. This will allow us to identify subtle changes. Assess the joint space: is it maintained uniformly or is it widened (joint effusion/synovial thickening) or narrowed (cartilage loss)? Assess the subchondral bone: is there any increase sclerosis or cyst formation? Review the cortical margin: are there any focal cortical defects to suggest an erosion? If there is an erosion, assess its size and percentage involvement with respect to the head of the involved bone and use the additional views. Where is the erosion, central (e.g., erosive OA, psoriatic arthritis), marginal/periarticular (e.g., rheumatoid arthritis), or juxta-articular or even remote from the joint (e.g., gout)? Marginal erosions occur in the "bare area," outer margin joints close to capsular attachment where there is no protective articular cartilage covering and where pannus can directly erode the underlying bone, e.g., rheumatoid arthritis. Does the erosion have a sclerotic margin (may indicate an inactive and healing erosion or be a pressure-type erosion as in gout) or not (active erosion, bone unable to lay down new bone due to active disease)? Is there new bone formation? If so, is it typical of an osteophyte (degenerative disease), an enthesophyte, or a new bone related to seronegative arthropathy? Is there periosteal reaction which would again suggest seronegative disease in the absence of trauma?

Alignment

If there is obvious malalignment, this is where we will start. If none, I will obtain a global overview and then commence my review at the distal radioulnar joint and continue distally to the distal phalanges. If malalignment is identified, confirm if it is joint centered and exclude prior trauma. Describe the direction of the alignment for the distal component: is it ulnar/radial or volar/dorsally deviated? Is there underlying subluxation (joint components maintain at least a partial articulation) or dislocation (no residual articulation)? It is important to review all images as reducible subluxations may only be apparent on oblique or lateral views and are reduced on the PA view; hands are placed flat on the table, but recur in the oblique view, e.g., Jaccound's arthropathy.

Bone

Check bone density. Is it normal, increased (rare), or decreased (osteopenia)? Is it localized or generalized or unilateral or bilateral (if both hands or alternate site available for comparison)? Is there a visible cause, e.g., trauma related or disuse? If localized, is it periarticular? What joints are involved, MCPJs and PIPJs in rheumatoid arthritis? Seronegative arthropathies are not usually associated with periarticular osteopenia. If a single joint is involved, always consider infection in the differential. If generalized, calculate the metacarpal index. The metacarpal index (MCI), the combined cortical mid-metacarpal thickness divided by the outer mid-metacarpal diameter, can be measured for the index finger or as a combined measurement of the second to fourth digits. Values are age related but combined cortical width should be greater than 50 % of the mid-metacarpal. If not, this indicates osteopenia and is discussed in more detail in Chap. 11.

Soft Tissues

I will then finally review the soft tissues. There may be localized or diffuse swelling or thinning of the soft tissues. Soft tissue calcification or vascular calcification may be evident. Check for loss or deviation of the normal soft tissue fat planes. Is there any change in the contour of the skin? These changes usually point to localized soft tissue pathology, e.g., soft tissue swelling on the medial margin of the ulnar styloid process suggests tendinous ECU and/or tenosynovitis of the ECU, commonly seen in rheumatoid arthritis, but may be induced by inflammatory changes within the radiocarpal joint. Is there swelling overlying a joint, e.g., the MCPJ, suggesting a joint effusion? This will alert me to closely review this joint for pathology. Is there generalized swelling of an entire digit, dactylitis? This may suggest infection or seronegative disease such as psoriatic arthropathy. Soft tissue loss particularly distally would suggest scleroderma. Is there soft tissue calcification, and is it within expected location of a tendon, hydroxyapatite depositional disease, or an evidence of calcinosis cutis, e.g., SLE? Soft tissue calcification is reviewed in greater detail in Chap. 16. Vascularar calcification is uncommon and is usually suggestive of chronic renal disease – check for changes of hyperparathyroidism – or diabetes. Exclude soft tissue air, ulcers, and radiodense foreign bodies, all of which may indicate the presence of infection.

Once we have reviewed the radiograph, we need to review any previous studies to assess for interval change. Subtle changes may not be evident on comparison with the most recent exam and only become obvious when distant studies are reviewed; thus, it is paramount to review back to the original available study.

Fluoroscopy

Fluoroscopy allows the real-time visualization of low-intensity X-rays via image intensifier systems. In fluoroscopy the patient is placed between the X-ray source and detector, which remain directly opposite each other (Fig. 1.5). The fluoroscopic unit allows for separate movement of both the patient and the image intensifier. The image is displayed on a monitor in the fluoroscopic

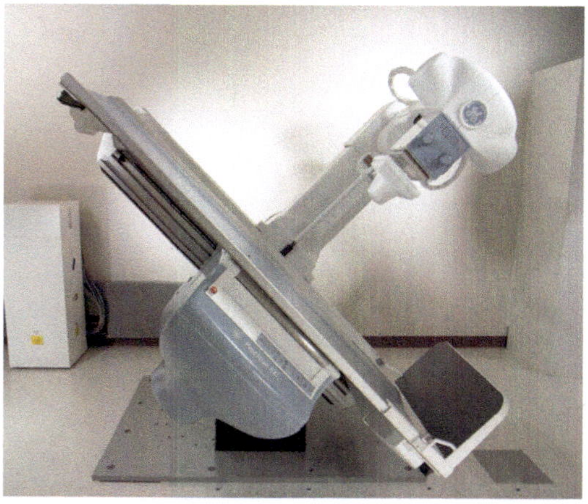

Fig. 1.5 Fluoroscopic unit

room and digitally recorded. Common MSK indications include joint aspirations and injections (Fig. 1.6). Portable fluoroscopy via C-arm units plays an important role in orthopedic surgery as well as many gastrointestinal and urological procedures.

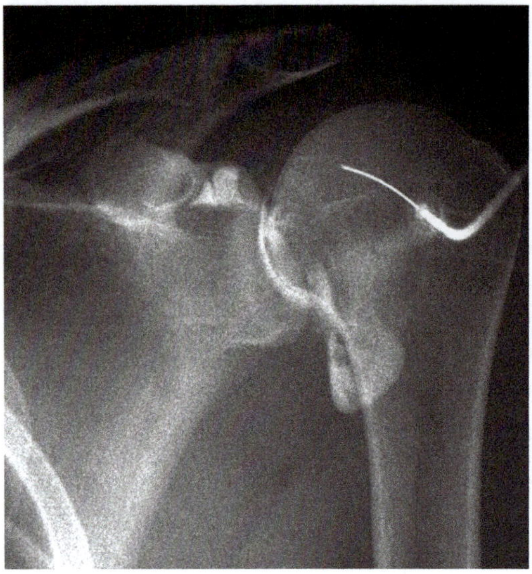

Fig. 1.6 Fluoroscopic image acquired at end fluoroscopically guided shoulder arthrogram procedure

Conventional Tomography

This has gained a lower position on the imaging options with the advent of cross-sectional imaging techniques such as CT and MRI. The X-ray source and detector are moved in a set path during an exposure. Anatomy at a set depth remains in focus, while structures at superficial and deeper levels are blurred. It is rarely used in the radiology department but still maintains a role in dentistry.

Tomosynthesis

This is similar to conventional tomography. However in tomosynthesis only one sweep of the X-ray tube is made during which multiple exposures are taken which can be reconstructed to produce multiple images at different levels (Fig. 1.7). The X-ray tube follows a small rotation angle of <40°. The thickness of each slice can be changed depending on the anatomy of the structure being investigated. There has seen a resurgence of interest in tomosynthesis during the last decade with the availability of flat panel radiographic detectors that would allow low-noise rapid image acquisition without geometric distortion. Initial interest was limited to breast and chest imaging, but recently there has been significant research extension into

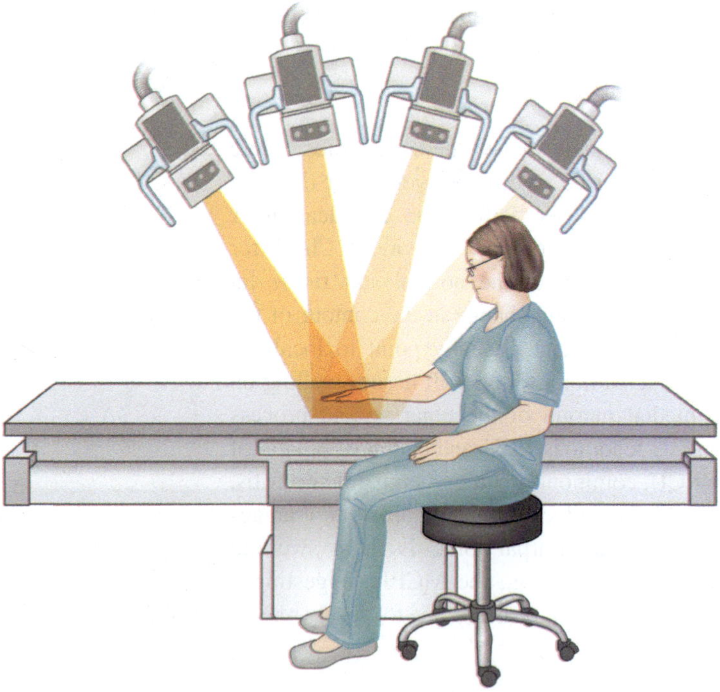

Fig. 1.7 Illustration acquisition tomosynthesis series of hand; note the pathway of the X-ray tube as the images are acquired

musculoskeletal imaging. Recent research, including that at our institution, has demonstrated increased sensitivity and specificity for erosive disease in the hands and wrists (Fig. 1.8). The radiation exposure is low, comparing 30×1 mm slices with two standard radiographs of the hands; the radiation dose is less than three times that of standard radiographs. Tomosynthesis may play a significant role in the future in the detection of erosive disease in rheumatology.

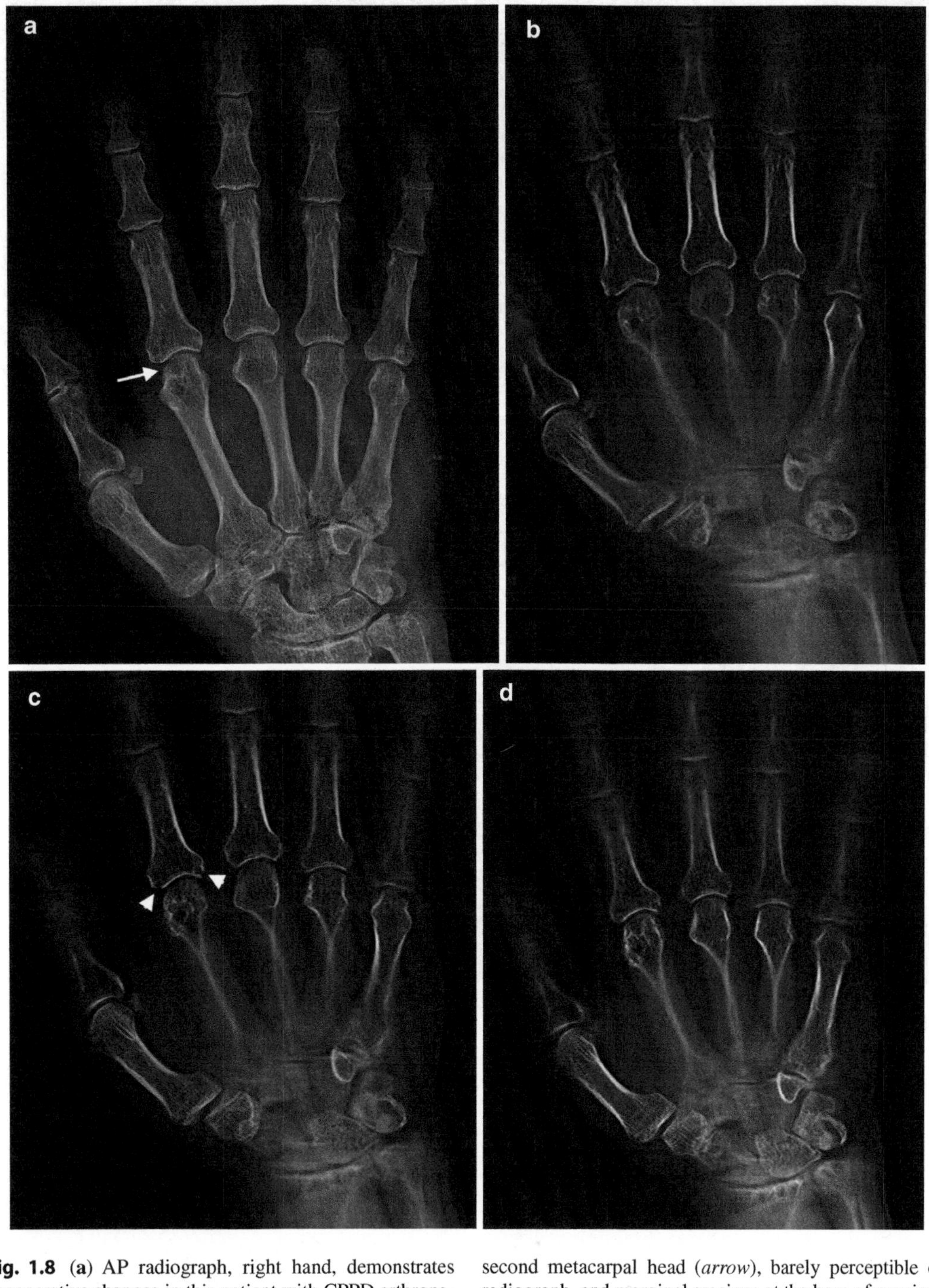

Fig. 1.8 (**a**) AP radiograph, right hand, demonstrates degenerative changes in this patient with CPPD arthropathy and rheumatoid arthritis, no erosions identified; (**b**–**g**) tomosynthesis images demonstrate a subchondral cyst on second metacarpal head (*arrow*), barely perceptible on radiograph, and marginal erosions at the base of proximal phalanx (*arrowheads* on **c**) not seen on AP radiograph

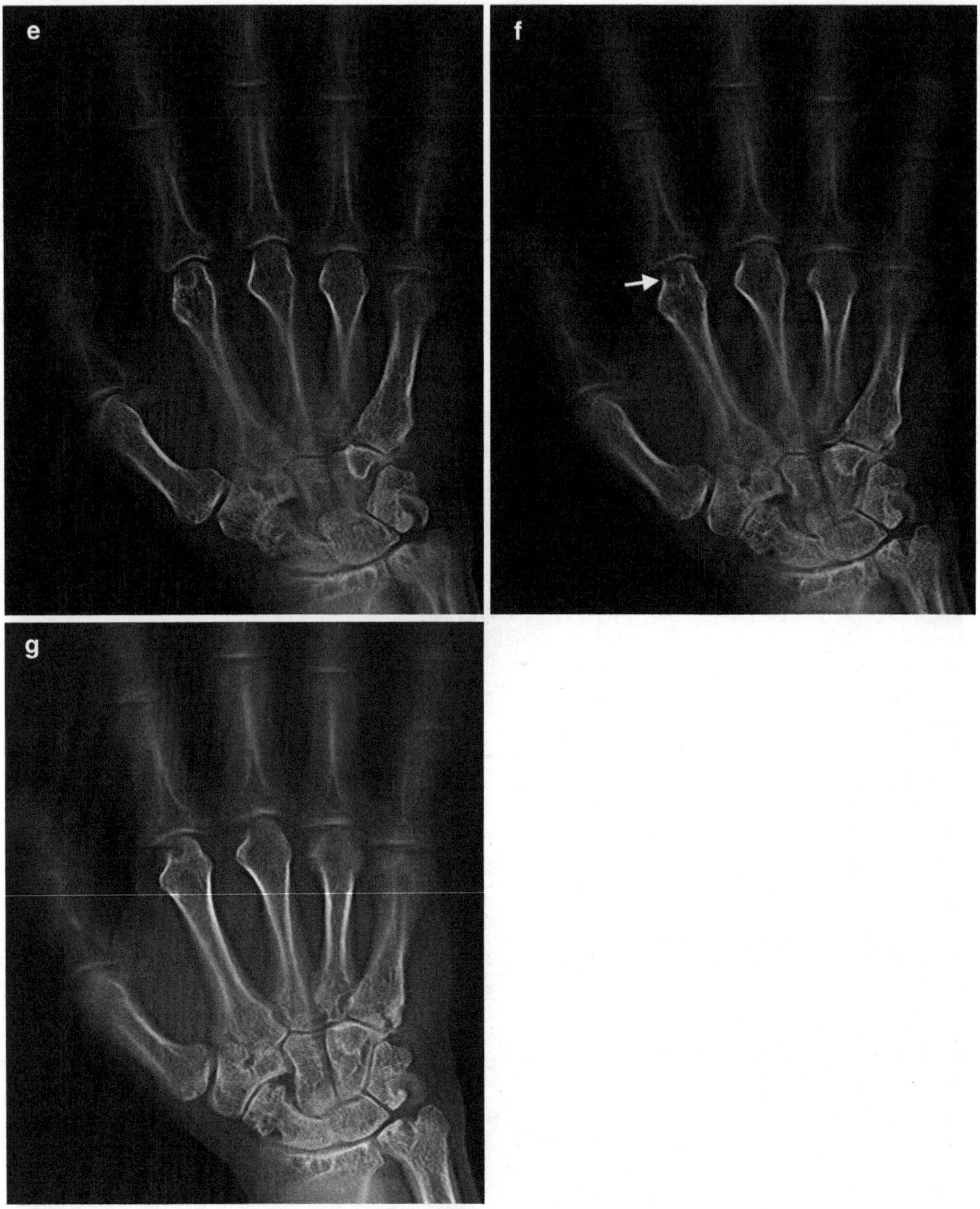

Fig. 1.8 (continued)

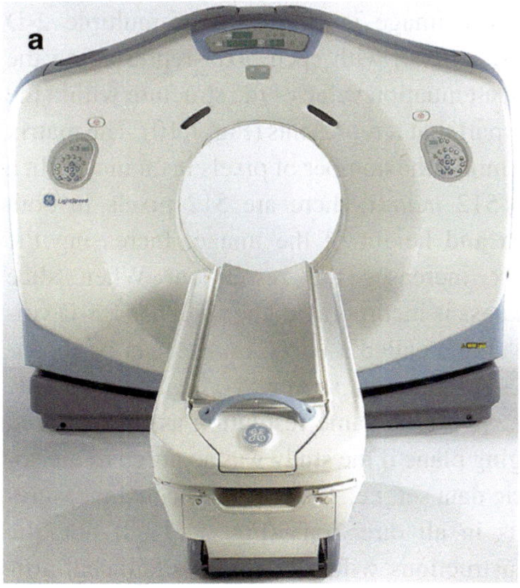

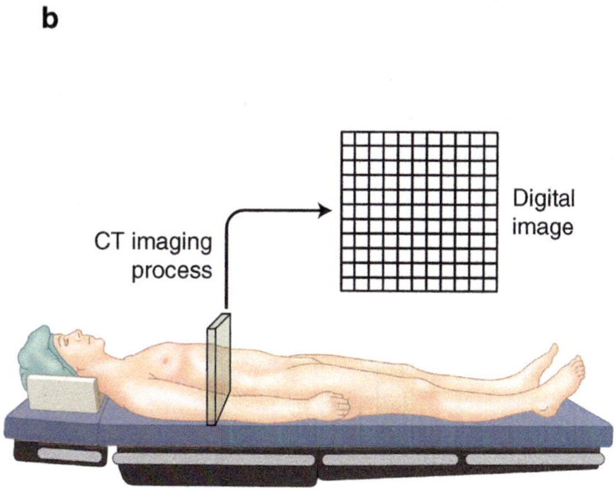

Fig. 1.9 (**a**) CT scanner. (**b**) Illustration of CT image composition

Advantages/Disadvantages

Radiography is an inexpensive, noninvasive low-dose radiation study that is easy to acquire and is readily available. It is usually the first line of imaging in many MSK pathologies offering excellent resolution of bone detail. It can identify calcification within soft tissues that may not be evident on MRI. In rheumatological patients, X-rays can quickly assess multiple joints and help localize pathology for further imaging studies if clinically indicated. In addition, clinicians have most of their experience in imaging with X-rays and their interpretation. Discrimination of soft tissue planes is only possible if there is interposed tissue of different attenuation such as fat, air, or bone. Radiographs are however 2-D representations of 3-D anatomy and as such there is superimposition of anatomy. There is limited soft tissue contrast as all soft tissue attenuates the X-ray beam to a similar degree.

Computed Tomography (CT)

Physics

Computed tomography (CT) is derived from the Greek "tomos graphein," meaning to write a slice, and was one of the major advances in imaging in the twentieth century. CT was developed in the UK in 1972 by Sir Godfrey Hounsfield. The first scanner took several minutes both to acquire and process the image. As with all technological breakthroughs, it was not long before rapid progress was made both in resolution and time required to scan. In 1990, spiral CT was developed, and by 1998, the currently used multislice CT became available (Fig. 1.9). In CT, an X-ray beam rotates in a 360° axis around the patient. The X-ray beam is variably attenuated by the different structures as it passes through the body before it reaches the detectors on the outside of this arc. The detectors then send a digital signal to a computer, which assigns different shades of gray to the different attenuation values and reconstructs an image based on these values. These attenuation values, Hounsfield units, are set so that water has a Hounsfield value of 0 (Table 1.1). In the older single-slice machines, a single rotation, slice, produced one image. In spiral or helical mul-

Table 1.1 CT attenuation values

Tissue composition	Hounsfield units (HU)
Bone	1,000
Soft tissue	20–100
Water	0
Fat	−25 to −100
Lung	−400
Air	−1,000

tislice CT, multiple rows of detectors, 4–128, are used as the patient is moved at a set rate through the gantry. This enables a rapid acquisition. Slice thickness can be varied depending on the fine detail required.

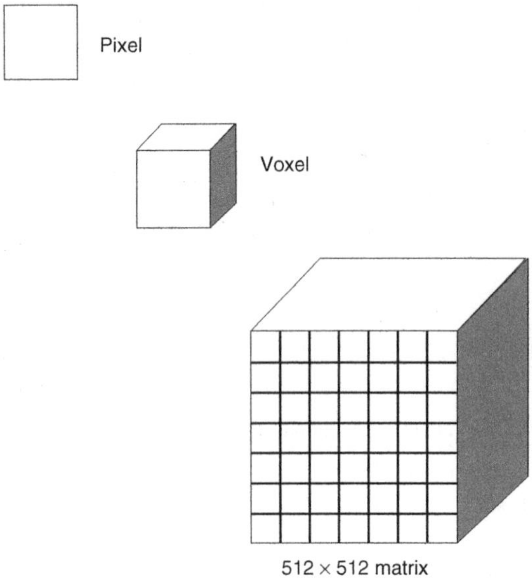

Fig. 1.10 Illustration of image components: pixel, voxel, and matrix

A CT image is composed of multiple 2-D boxes, a *pixel*, with each pixel representing the mean attenuation value of the structure within the body part that it represents (Fig. 1.10). The matrix determines the number of pixels in an image. In a 512×512 *matrix*, there are 512 pixels in both width and height of the image. Increasing the matrix increases the resolution. When slice thickness is incorporated, the pixel has a 3-D volume and is called a *voxel*. Images can be reconstructed into axial, sagittal, coronal, and oblique planes with the same resolution as the acquired imaging plane if the study was acquired as an isometric data set, i.e., the voxel has equal measurements in all directions (Fig. 1.11). If not, the reconstructions will suffer from significant artifact. CT images can also be reconstructed into 3-D images (Fig. 1.11). Surface-rendered, volume-rendered, and maximum intensity projection images can be acquired. Images in different planes can be cross-referenced to correctly identify anatomy in different planes. The image can be windowed and the gray scale can be adjusted by changing window width and level to optimize the anatomical region, e.g., lungs, bones, soft tissues, blood, etc. (Fig. 1.12).

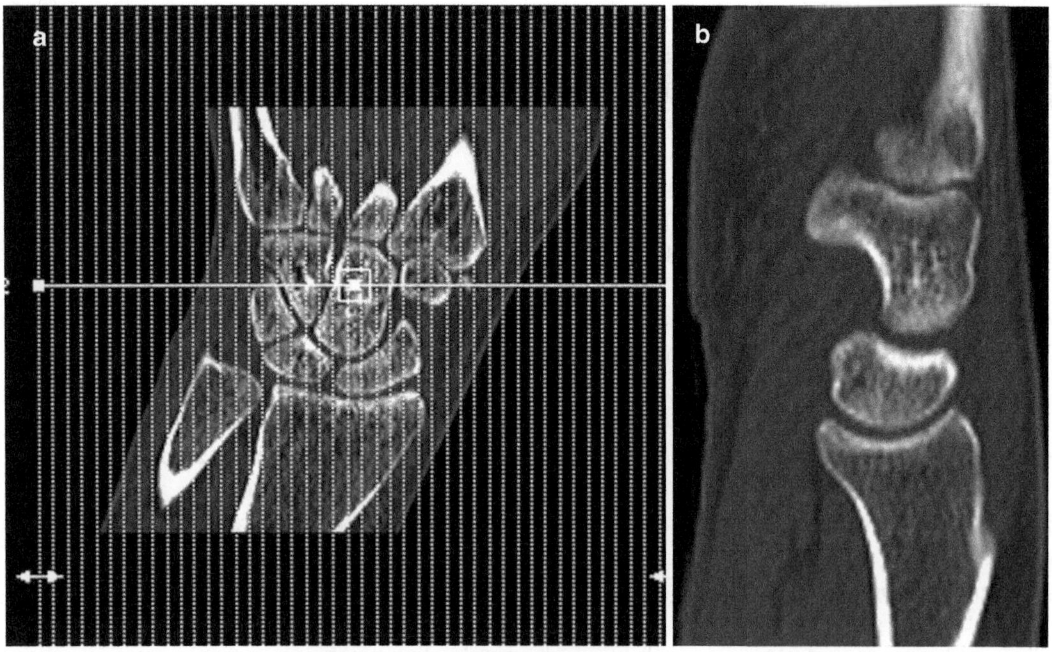

Fig. 1.11 CT wrist (**a**) low-dose localizer image in coronal plane, similar to radiograph used as template to acquire images in correct planes with respect to anatomy. (**b**) Sagittal image and (**c**) coronal image reconstructed from axial images, (**d**) 3-D image wrist

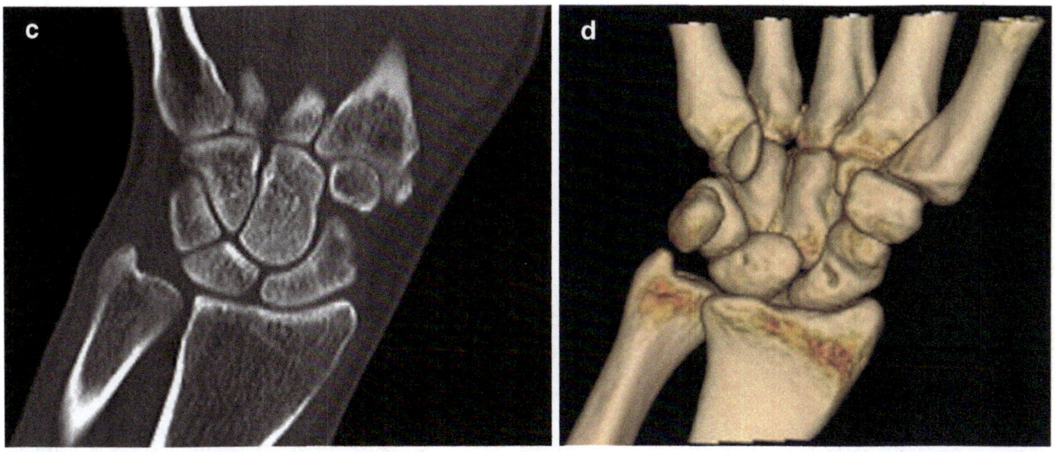

Fig. 1.11 (continued)

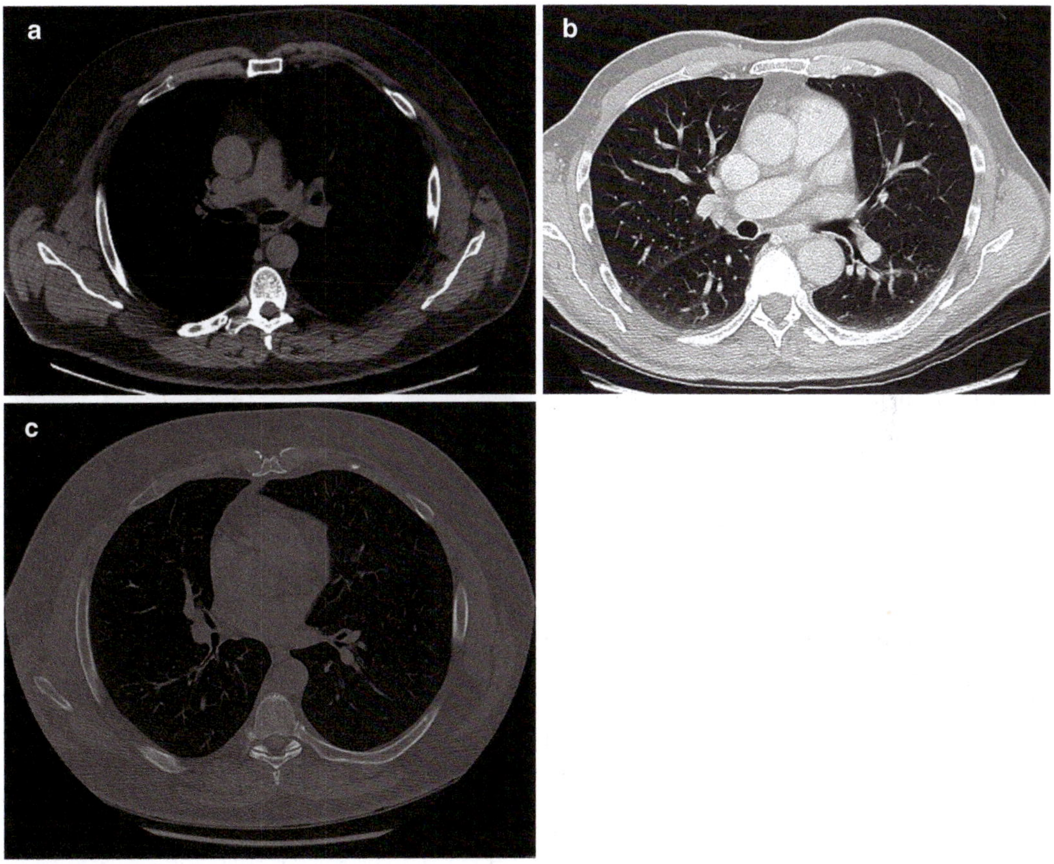

Fig. 1.12 CT windows; the same image can be manipulated by changing window width and level to optimize structure of concern, (**a**) soft tissue/mediastinal windows, (**b**) lung windows, (**c**) bone windows

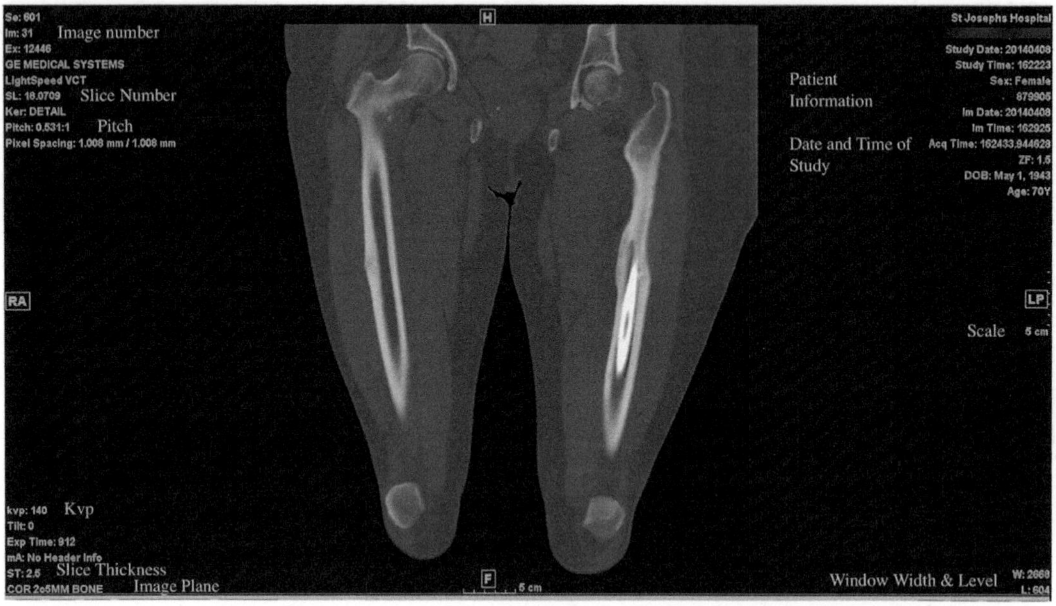

Fig. 1.13 CT image with normal information available detailing date, patient information, window level and width, etc. Patient has atypical stress fractures secondary to bisphosphonate treatment of mid-femurs with internal fixation on the left

Image Analysis and Interpretation

As detailed in the above section in radiography, the correct patient, date, and body part should be confirmed. Check the information provided on the image for matrix, slice thickness, and windowing (Fig. 1.13). The image may also indicate if contrast was used. If not, review the image for vascular structures which will be of higher attenuation than muscle if intravenous contrast has been given; if not, it is of a similar attenuation. Studies may also be acquired in different phases of contrast enhancement, e.g., arterial, venous, and delayed. Oral contrast for gastrointestinal studies may be positive and will appear white, e.g., diluted Gastrografin, or negative, dark, e.g., water. Providing detailed clinical information to the radiologist will allow a correctly protocolled study designed to answer the clinical question. Image quality may be affected by patient motion although modern scanners allow rapid acquisition, in seconds, of large body parts. In situ metal such as orthopedic hardware significantly attenuates the X-ray beam; however, modern scanners have set protocols to diminish this artifact (Fig. 1.14). Beam hardening related to bone also attenuates the beam, e.g., assessment of posterior fossa is diminished due to the thick petrous temporal bone in head CT.

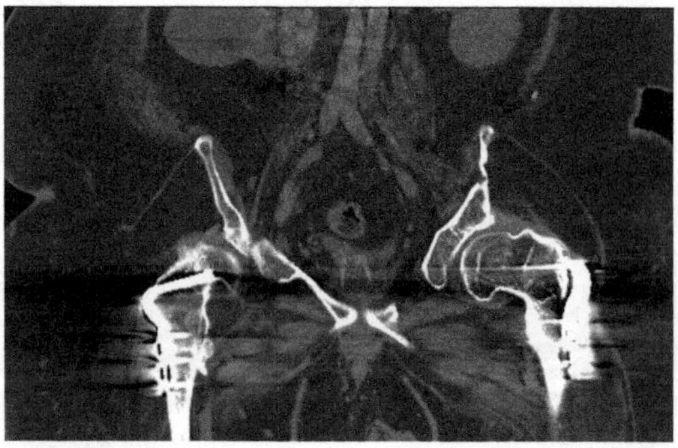
Fig. 1.14 CT artifact: beam-hardening artifact related to bilateral plates and screws of the proximal femurs with streak artifact of high attenuation superimposed over adjacent soft tissue with subsequent limitation in the assessment of pathology in this region

Terminology (Table 1.2)

Advantages/Disadvantages

CT allows the rapid noninvasive acquisition of a large data set in a short time interval. Images are digital and thus can be manipulated in multiple parameters as described above to provide high-resolution imaging, both spatial and contrast, in multiple planes. CT can compensate for

Table 1.2 CT terminology

Hounsfield units	Quantitative scale for attenuation values. Water arbitrarily set at 0 HU, air −1,000 HU, cortical bone +1,000 HU
Attenuation	Gradual loss of X-rays as they pass through the body. High attenuation regions such as the bone limit transmission of X-rays, termed high attenuating, and appear white. Low-attenuation regions appear dark, gray-black, e.g., fat and air
CT localizer radiograph	Scanned projection radiograph allows for prescription of scan including start and end points
Window level	Center point around which the window width is set
Helical or spiral scan mode	Data acquisition while the patient table is continuously moving along the Z-axis
Window center	The CT number in the center of the viewable gray scale
Automatic exposure control (AEC)	Automatic adaption of X-ray tube current to the overall patient size to limit radiation exposure while achieving good image quality
Pixel	2-D box-forming part of the image matrix represents mean attenuation values of structures within that area, has a width and height
Voxel	3-D volume, a pixel with depth, depth corresponds to slice thickness
Matrix	The CT image, matrix = total number voxels (3-D data) in the data sample, expressed as number voxels, width × height, e.g., 512×512
Window width	The range of attenuation values displayed on the gray scale, adjustable to accommodate for the limited gray scale that can be appreciated by the human eye

variable body habitus, and planes can be cross-referenced to localize anatomy in different planes. Studies along a time line can be easily compared. There is excellent bony architecture visualization but limited MSK soft tissue discrimination when compared to MRI. CT incurs a heavy radiation burden and is relatively expensive in comparison to ultrasound, but less so when compared to MRI. CT may also require the use of intravascular contrast agents, which may expose patients to adverse reactions (see contrast media section).

Ultrasound

Ultrasound is an effective and established technique in musculoskeletal imaging. Its role in diagnostic imaging is continuing to expand with the development of further clinical applications and with the advancement of ultrasound technology. It is well established as a first-line imaging modality in the investigation of musculoskeletal pathology and is rapidly gaining popularity. Ultrasound is, however, operator dependent and requires a detailed knowledge of the relevant anatomy, ultrasound artifacts, technique, and ultrasound appearance of both normal and abnormal structures for the conduction and interpretation of the study.

In 1942, ultrasound was first used as an imaging modality but took many years before clinical use. Ultrasound developed slowly until 1960, when Donald and colleagues produced the first automatic scanner. For the next decade, ultrasound was predominantly limited to evaluation of abdominal and pelvic disease. It was not until the 1970s that real-time ultrasound became available. By 1972, the first B-scan image of a joint was reported in the differentiation of a Baker's cyst and thrombophlebitis. Graf, in 1980, published his landmark paper on the use of ultrasound in the diagnosis of congenital hip-joint dislocation. In 1988, L. De Flaviis described ultrasound of the hand in rheumatoid patients including erosions 10 years after Cooperberg described features of synovial thickening and joint effusion in the rheumatoid knee. Since this time, particularly in the last decade, there has not only been a rapid development in ultrasound technology but also widespread use of ultrasound in the investigation of musculoskeletal disorders to the point where it is now firmly established as a key imaging modality. Ultrasound advances include high-resolution linear array transducers, extended field of view, tissue harmonics, compound imaging, and recently 3-D and 4-D imaging.

Physics

Ultrasound uses sound waves that are transmitted through the body. Sound waves are produced by a piezoelectric crystal that is housed in a hand-held probe, the transducer (Fig. 1.15). The crystal vibrates when an electrical current is passed through it and emits a sound wave of a certain frequency. Sound waves are reflected back at tissue interfaces and are received by the transducer to produce an image. A tissue interface is the point of change between two tissues of different acoustic impedance (AI). AI in turn is dependent on the density of the tissue and the velocity of sound through that tissue. The amount of sound reflected is proportional to the difference in AI. At soft tissue air interface, e.g., air interposed between transducer and skin, a large portion of sound is reflected; hence, a gel is used at this interface to limit reflection. When the crystal receives sound waves or echoes, it creates a current. The time interval between sending and receiving the echo back determines the depth of the tissue interface creating the echo.

Doppler ultrasound uses the Doppler effect. If we hear the siren of a moving ambulance, the frequency of the siren is higher as it approaches and decreases as it leaves. The same holds true for moving blood and an ultrasound wave. The reflected echo from the moving blood undergoes a frequency shift dependent on the direction and flow velocity of the blood, which is read by the transducer and is color-coded on the ultrasound image, hence termed *color Doppler* (Fig. 1.16). Whereas color Doppler uses the mean frequency shift, *power Doppler* uses the summation of Doppler shift frequencies and is more sensitive in detecting blood flow, depiction of flow, and edge detection. This is useful in the assessment of inflammatory changes in MSK such as joints

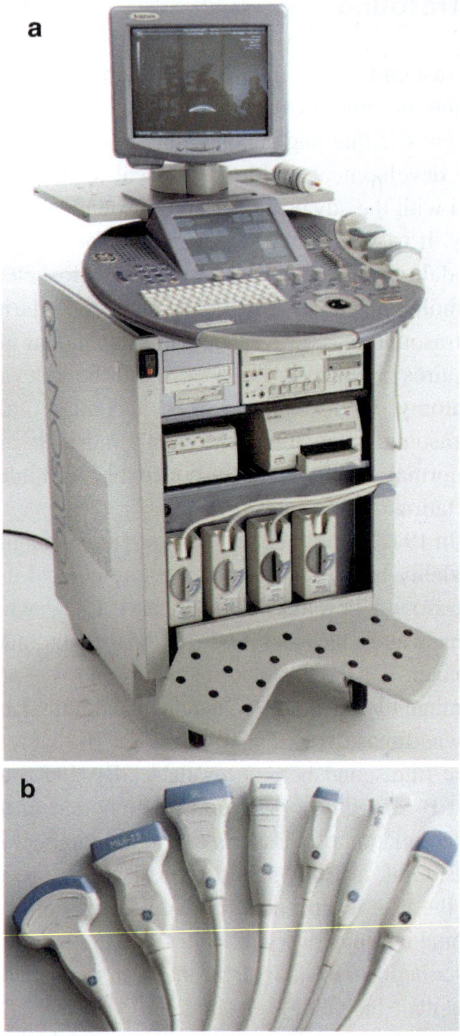

Fig. 1.15 (**a**) Image ultrasound machine, (**b**) selection of available transducers for optimization to different body parts

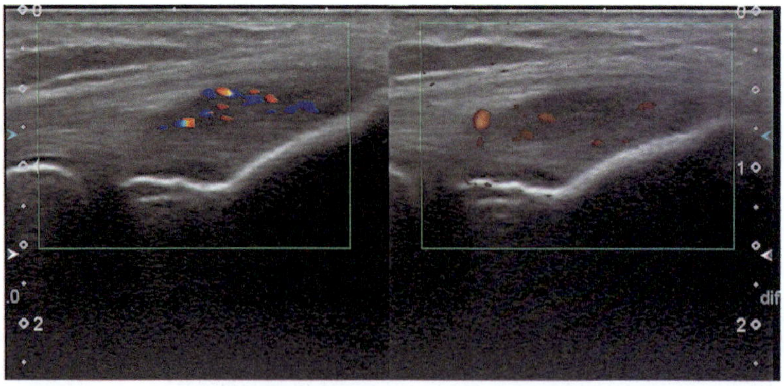

Fig. 1.16 Tendinosis: right common extensor tendon with significantly increased internal flow on Doppler; normal tendons demonstrate no internal flow on Doppler: *right* image is color Doppler, *left* power Doppler

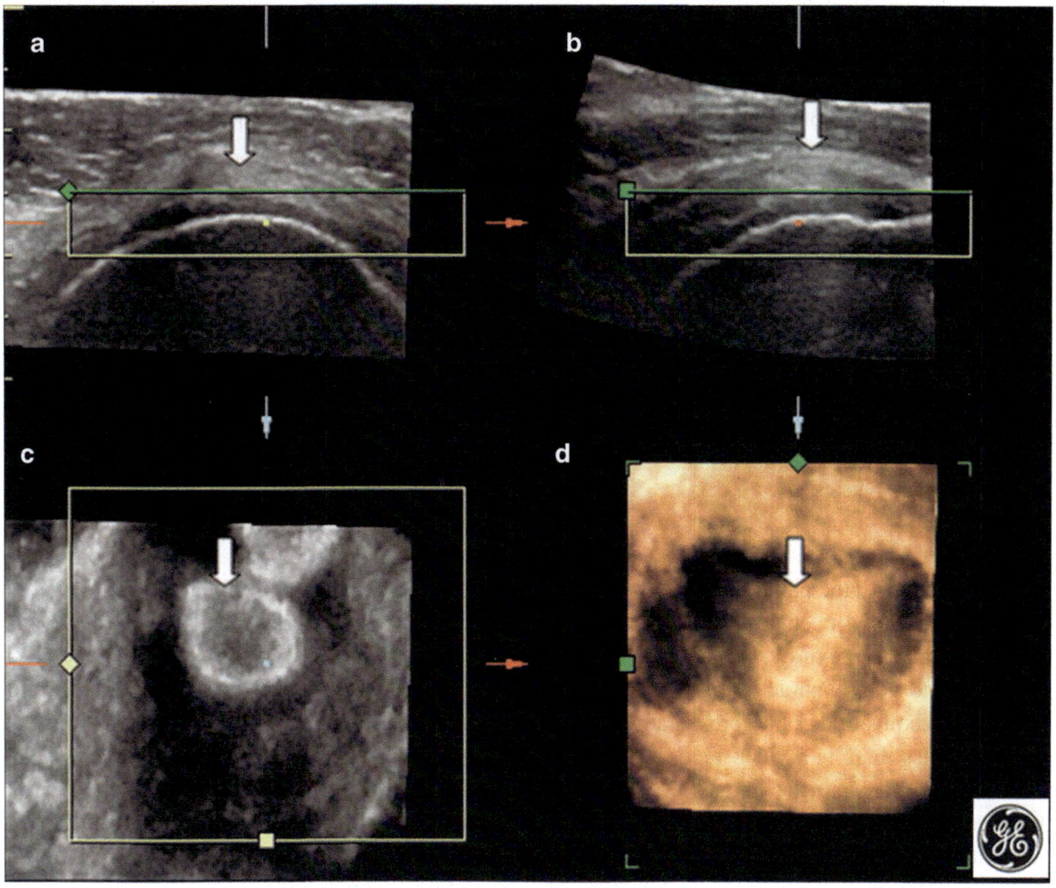

Fig. 1.17 Supraspinatus: (**a**) transverse US image demonstrating the rotator cuff interval and (**b**) corresponding transducer position. (**c**) US supraspinatus tendon using 4-D transducer, (**a**) axial, (**b**) sagittal, (**c**) coronal, and (**d**) 3-D reconstruction. *Arrows* supraspinatus tendon, *GT* greater tuberosity, *B* long head of the biceps tendon, *arrowhead* subscapularis

where blood vessels are small and increased flow may be difficult to detect with color Doppler. Intravenous contrast agents are available for ultrasound. Gas-filled microbubbles, which have high reflectivity, are injected intravenously and increase the reflected sound wave, thus increasing contrast. It is used most frequently in echocardiograms and in tumor perfusion assessment. Early studies have shown promise in the detection of slow blood flow within pannus with contrast agents versus Doppler, but further studies are required to determine indications for use. Ultrasound advances include high-resolution linear array transducers, extended field of view, tissue harmonics, compound imaging, and recently early forays into 3-D and 4-D imaging use in musculoskeletal imaging (Fig. 1.17).

Terminology (Table 1.3)

Advantages/Disadvantages

Ultrasound is a readily available, noninvasive multiplanar imaging modality that does not involve ionizing radiation and is well tolerated by patients. It allows 3-D and 4-D (dynamic 3-D) imaging. It is inexpensive in comparison to CT and MRI, is portable, and can image multiple anatomical regions in one sitting. It can assess vascularity of tissue and inflammatory response without requiring an intravenous contrast agent. Dynamic studies may reveal pathologies not visible on static imaging with CT or MRI such as intermittent tendon subluxation and muscle hernias.

Table 1.3 Ultrasound terminology

Echogenicity	Amplitude of returning/reflected echoes
Hyperechoic	High-amplitude returning echoes, appears bright, e.g., cortical bone
Hypoechoic	Limited reflected echoes, appears dark, e.g., tendon
Anechoic	No returning echoes, appears black, e.g., simple cystic fluid
Extended field of view	Position sensing technique combining a continuous ultrasound acquisition into one image
Gain (time gain compensation)	Amplification of returning echoes from deeper tissues
Focal zone	Focusing transmitted zone to a set depth, maximizes definition at level of interest

Direct contact with the patient, confirming medical history and any recent change in symptoms, allows for a directed study.

Ultrasound is a dynamic interactive examination with acquisition of representative static images, unless there is a video recording, which limits interpretation to the images acquired and the operator's experience. Ultrasound does not penetrate bone and sound is reflected from air interfaces. Therefore the internal architecture of the bone cannot be assessed. Superficial structures can be evaluated in exquisite detail; however, deeper soft tissue structures may be inadequately visualized on ultrasound. Ultrasound is operator dependent and has a long learning curve. It requires the operator to have a detailed anatomical knowledge of the structure being imaged as well as the normal and pathological ultrasound appearance.

Image Analysis and Interpretation

An ultrasound image is usually orientated cranial-caudal with the left hand side of the screen or image on the cranial side. Musculoskeletal imaging requires imaging in the anatomical planes of the structure, e.g., tendon; these images are orientated from proximal to distal. Correct study, patient, date, and body part should be confirmed (Fig. 1.18). Abnormalities that become visible only on dynamic assessment should be documented with a video clip.

Anisotropy is one of the most common and probably the most important artifact in musculoskeletal ultrasound imaging. Anisotropy is the different ultrasound echogenicity of normal tissue when the angle of insonation is not 90° to the plane of the structure being imaged. It is best identified in tendons and is less pronounced in other soft tissues including muscles, ligaments, and nerves. A common site of occurrence is within the supraspinatus tendon

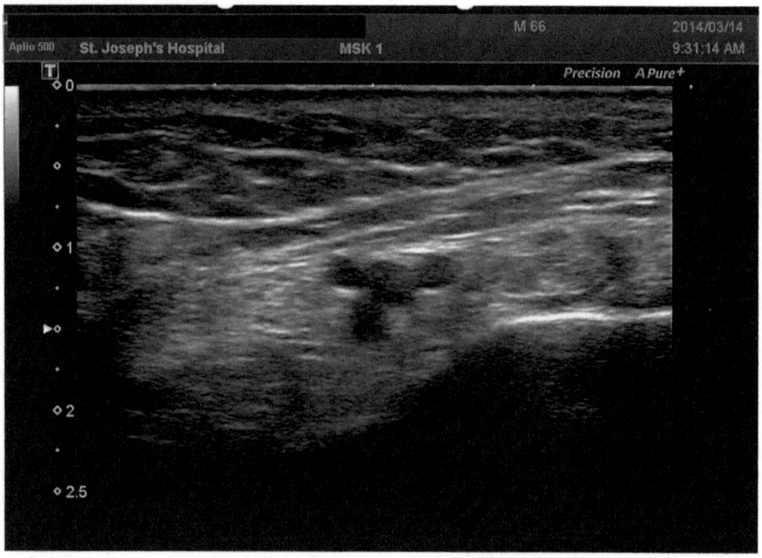

Fig. 1.18 Ultrasound image with normal information available detailing date, patient information (name has been erased), transducer setting (mid top of image, in this case "MSK1" saved setting used), depth (scale on *left side* image), and focal point (*arrowhead* projected beside scale)

because of its coronal oblique course and angulation. To separate anisotropy from pathology, the transducer is held in the same position but is angled until it is perpendicular to the tissue of interest. When imaged in the perpendicular plane, the artifactual hypoechoic appearance will resolve in normal tendons and the tissue will be of homogenous echogenicity. True pathology does not resolve with change in angulation.

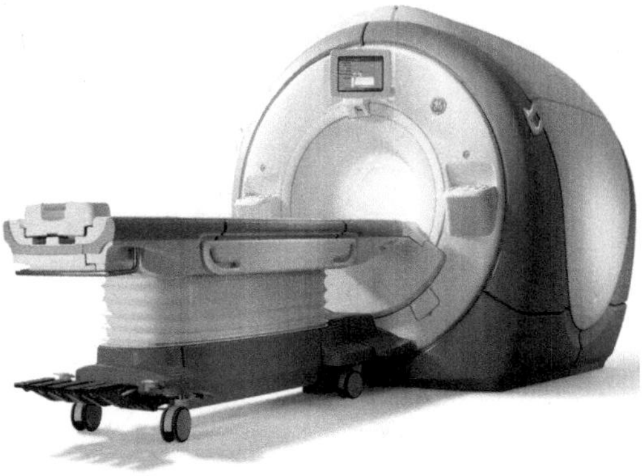

Fig. 1.19 Image MRI magnet

MRI

MRI imaging is a valuable and commonly used imaging modality in musculoskeletal imaging. There is complex physics underlying the acquisition of an MRI sequence, which are beyond the scope of this text and are not generally required by the rheumatologist. However, a basic understanding of image acquisition is required for optimal image interpretation. MRI development has provided two Nobel prizes, first for physics to Bloch and Purcell in 1962 for discovering magnetic resonance phenomenon and then for medicine in 2003 to Lauterbur and Mansfield who produced the first MRI images. Human images were produced in 1977 with a single image taking 5 min to acquire; imaging time was reduced to 5 s by 1986. Functional MRI was developed in 1992 and used initially for mapping areas of the brain. MRI has continued to develop rapidly. Clinical magnets have become more powerful with 3 T magnets in common use today with increased sensitivity and resolution.

Physics

MRI requires placing the body or body part into a strong magnetic field. Magnetic field strength is measured in tesla. Current clinical MRI scanners vary between 0.2 and 3 T (Fig. 1.19). Within the magnetic field, nuclei with odd-number nucleons, e.g., hydrogen, align themselves with the magnetic field. Hydrogen is present in both water and fat and hence is plentiful in the body and is the ideal molecule to use. The hydrogen proton is normally spinning around its own axis, much like the earth. When placed in a magnetic field, the protons behave like mini-magnets and align themselves with the magnetic field in a low energy state (Fig. 1.20). A radiofrequency pulse, with a resonant frequency specific for hydrogen, is then applied. This is absorbed as energy by the protons and they spin out of alignment. The longer the pulse is active, the more energy it imparts. As the protons return to the lower energy state, they in turn emit a radiofrequency signal (electromagnetic radiation) of a specific frequency, the Larmor frequency, which can be measured with receiver coils. T1 and T2 are the main relaxation times involved in this signal loss. T1, longitudinal relaxation, is the time to return to the original state in the *Z*-axis. T2, transverse relaxation, relates to signal loss due to dephasing (loss of synchronization) of the protons. The emitted signal decays rapidly after the radiofrequency pulse as the protons return to their low energy state.

Pulse sequences such as spin echo and gradient echo are used to emphasize tissue characteristics. Different tissues have their own relaxation times and can thus be identified separately (Fig. 1.21). Gradient coils, *Z*-, *X*-, and *Y*-axis gradients, are used to vary the strength of the magnetic field over the body to allow for spatial localization of the signal using the inverse Fourier transform. The received signal is sent to a computer, which is then plotted on a gray scale.

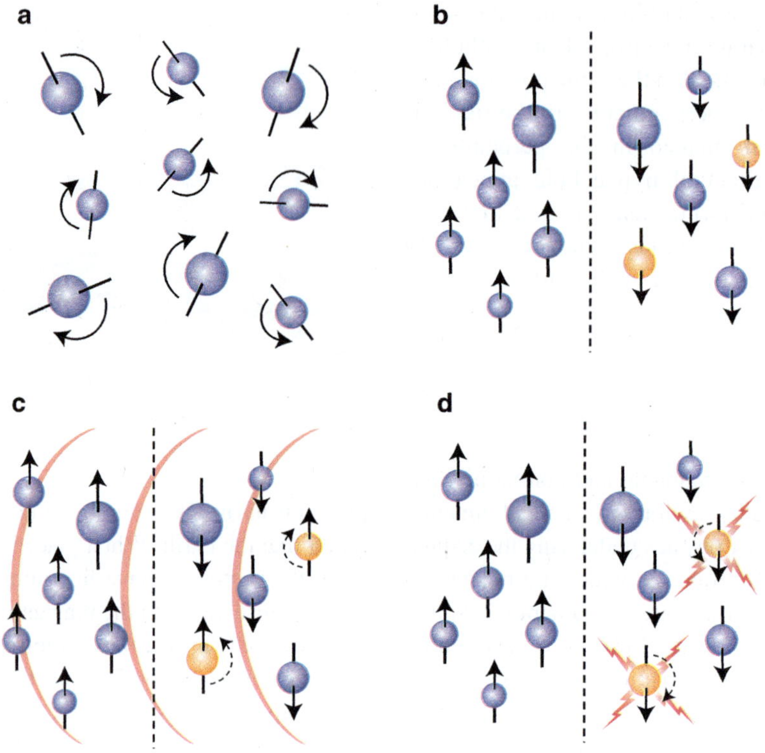

Fig. 1.20 Protons within a magnetic field: (**a**) normal atoms outside magnetic field spinning along their own magnetic fields in a random fashion; (**b**) once placed with the MRI magnet, the atoms become aligned to the magnetic field, relatively evenly distributed in the same (lower energy) and opposite (higher energy) direction to the main field; however, there are slightly more atoms aligned with the magnetic field, i.e., unmatched atoms, that are in a lower energy state (*yellow* atoms in illustration). These unmatched atoms flip their spin axis when a radiofrequency pulse (*red wave*) is applied (**c**). When the radiofrequency is turned off, they return to their lower energy state, giving off energy (**d**) which is picked up by the receiver coils and is turned into an electrical signal

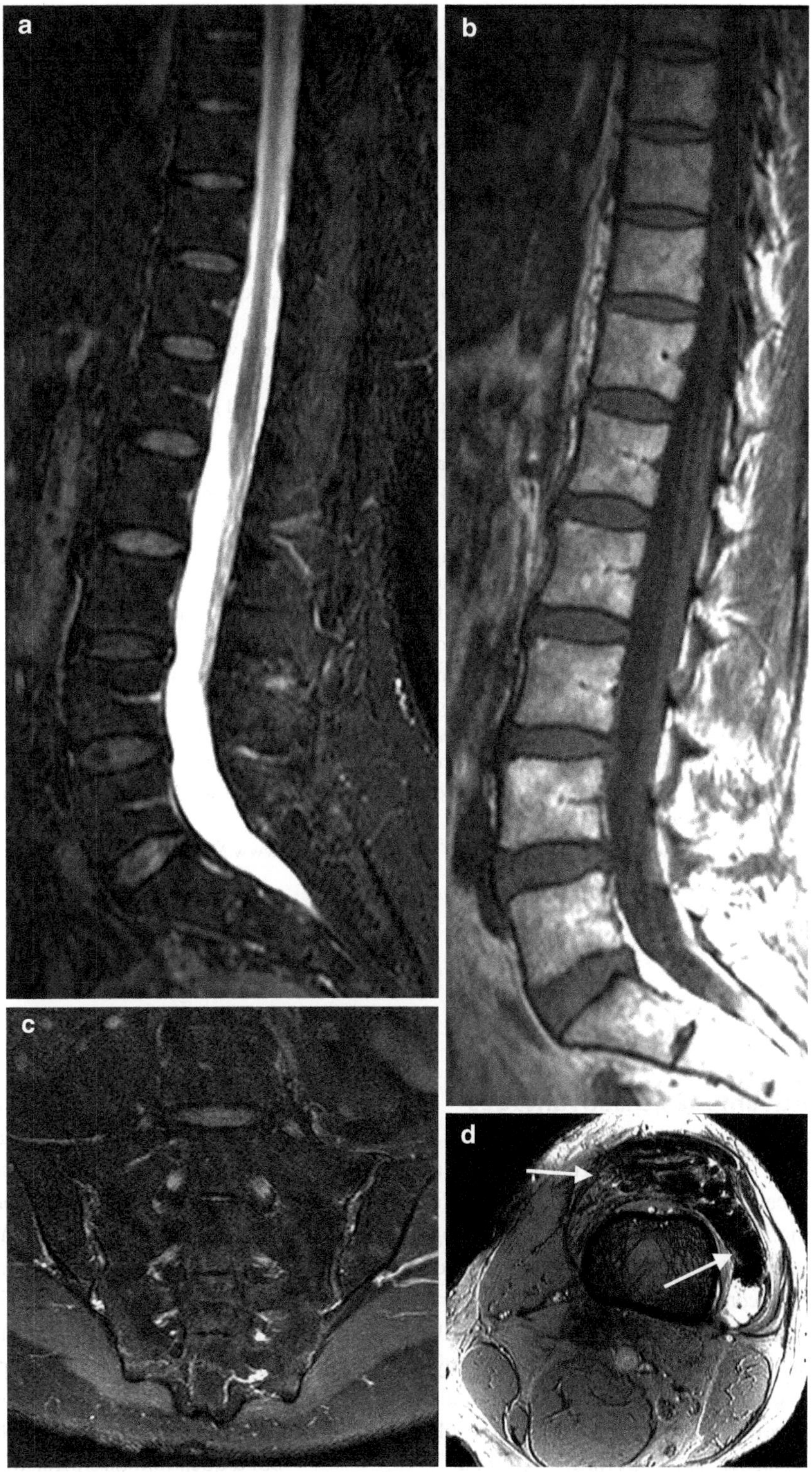

Fig. 1.21 Common sequences used in musculoskeletal MRI, (**a**) Sag T2 fat-saturated (*FS*) lumbar spine, note high signal intensity (*SI*) CSF. (**b**) Sag T1, CSF is low SI. (**c**) Cor STIR sacroiliac joints appear similar to T2FS sequence although slightly decreased resolution. (**d**) Gradient echo, axial GE, suprapatellar recess knee with blooming artifact in a patient with hemosiderin deposition secondary to PVNS (*arrows*)

Table 1.4 MRI terminology

Acquisition – process of acquiring the image data
Acquisition time – time to acquire the image data set
Coil – hardware device that can transmit or receive radiofrequency pulses during MRI study. Multiple coils available, selected so that coil is as close to the body part being imaged for optimal signal strength, e.g., spine, knee, shoulder, body, head, etc.
Fat saturation – cancellation of fat signal from area imaged. 2 methods commonly used: inversion recovery (e.g., STIR) and frequency selective (T2FS)
Field of view – area imaged
Matrix – total number of voxels (3-D data) in the data sample, expressed as number voxels, width × height, e.g., 512×512
Noise – inherent factors that negatively impact the image: patient within the magnet disturbs the magnetic field, background electrical activity, etc.
Pulse sequence – defined selection of repetitive radiofrequency and gradient pulses to produce specific tissue contrast, e.g., spin echo, turbo spin echo, gradient echo, STIR
Resolution – ability to distinguish two separate objects on an image
Signal intensity (SI) – grading of the signal from tissue into high, intermediate, and low with high SI appearing bright
Slice thickness – each image represents a 3-D volume set, the thickness of this set equates to the image slice thickness
Susceptibility artifact – local distortion magnetic field with signal loss, commonly related to ferromagnetic bodies such as metallic foreign bodies, implants, and prior hemorrhage
Tesla (T) – unit measurement of magnetic flux density (magnet strength)
T1 weighted – image where the different inherent T1 properties of tissues are maximized, uses short TE, TR
T2 weighted – image where the different inherent T2 properties of tissues are maximized, uses long TE, TR
TE – time to echo, affects the T2 weighting of an image, long TE maximizes T2 weighting
Time of flight – MR angiographic sequence, not requiring use of gadolinium, based on unsaturated blood flowing into saturated magnetized slice and thus producing high signal intensity
TR – time between each successive pulse sequence applied to same slice, controls the T1 weighting; short TR maximizes T1 weighting of tissues
For a more detailed glossary and review of MRI physics, see www.MRItutor.org

Terminology (Table 1.4)

Advantages/Disadvantages

MRI involves no ionizing radiation and provides excellent soft tissue contrast with multiplanar imaging. It can identify areas of pathology by signal intensity alone and often does not require intravenous contrast injection. In addition, intravenous contrast in MRI has a better safety profile than iodinated contrast used in CT. Vascular anatomy can also be assessed without requiring contrast, although intravenous contrast is used for high-resolution studies when detailed assessment is required.

MRI is however expensive and is not readily available in all centers. Examination time is lengthy for most examinations, usually between 20 and 40 min. Claustrophobia is a problem given the imaging time and the small bore (opening) of the MRI unit and patients may require oral sedation prior to the study. Motion is detrimental and impacts the whole sequence and not just one image and may require repeating the sequence. There are multiple contraindications to MRI, and patients/close relative must be competent to fill out a questionnaire prior to the study.

MRI Contraindications (Table 1.5)

Table 1.5 MRI contraindications

Surgical implants – type of implant and date of surgery required to ensure MRI compatibility
Intraocular metallic foreign body – may become heated or move during study. Patients at risk require orbital radiographs prior to MRI booking
Cochlear implants
Cardiac pacemaker
Electronic or magnetically controlled devices, e.g., insulin pumps
Claustrophobia – lengthy examination times and small opening of the MRI can make it difficult for predisposed patients to tolerate full examination. Discussion prior to booking, option of oral sedation, and alternative imaging modalities should be considered
Pregnancy – no documented risk to patient or fetus reported; ensure MRI is the appropriate study
For a more detailed review, see www.MRIsafety.com

Commonly Used Sequences (Table 1.6)

Table 1.6 MRI sequences

Spin echo (T1, T2, PD)	Excellent signal to noise ratio and anatomical detail, minimizes susceptibility effects, long imaging times
Fast spin echo	Shorter imaging times, blurring artifact, requires fat saturation for assessment of marrow edema
STIR – short tau inversion recovery	Excellent for identifying edema/fluid Diminished anatomical resolution when compared to T2FS
Gradient echo	Fast, susceptibility artifacts are accentuated and excellent for assessing areas with prior hemorrhage and hemosiderin deposition, good anatomical resolution cartilage, 3-D imaging, however significant loss of SI around metallic implants, limited marrow assessment and limited T2 contrast

Image Quality and Interpretation

As indicated in the above sections, confirmation of the patient's name, date, study type, and imaged body part should be confirmed (Fig. 1.22). MRI studies will usually have multiple sequences; the type of sequence will be indicated in PACS by clicking on the individual series. Alternatively looking at the image, the TE and TR times are given and one can confirm sequence as outlined in Table 1.4. Review the image for areas of simple fluid such as CSF in head and spinal imaging, bladder for pelvis, and simple joint effusion in the appendicular skeleton. This fluid will be of high signal, bright, on T2-weighted sequences and low, less than muscle, on T1 (Fig. 1.21). Then look for areas that contain macroscopic fat-like subcutaneous tissue and intermuscular and retroperitoneal spaces; if there is diffuse low signal intensity of fat, then this is a fat-saturated sequence. Motion artifact may be caused by pulsation from vascular structures, respiratory motion, or patient motion. These can cause ghostlike artifacts across the image. Technical adjustments can be made for vascular and respiratory motion to limit artifact. Chemical shift artifact is related to the different frequencies between fat and water protons at an interface and causes misregistration of fat location. Aliasing or wraparound occurs when the peripheral portion of an image is transferred to the opposite side and is related to a field of view smaller than the body part being imaged (Fig. 1.23).

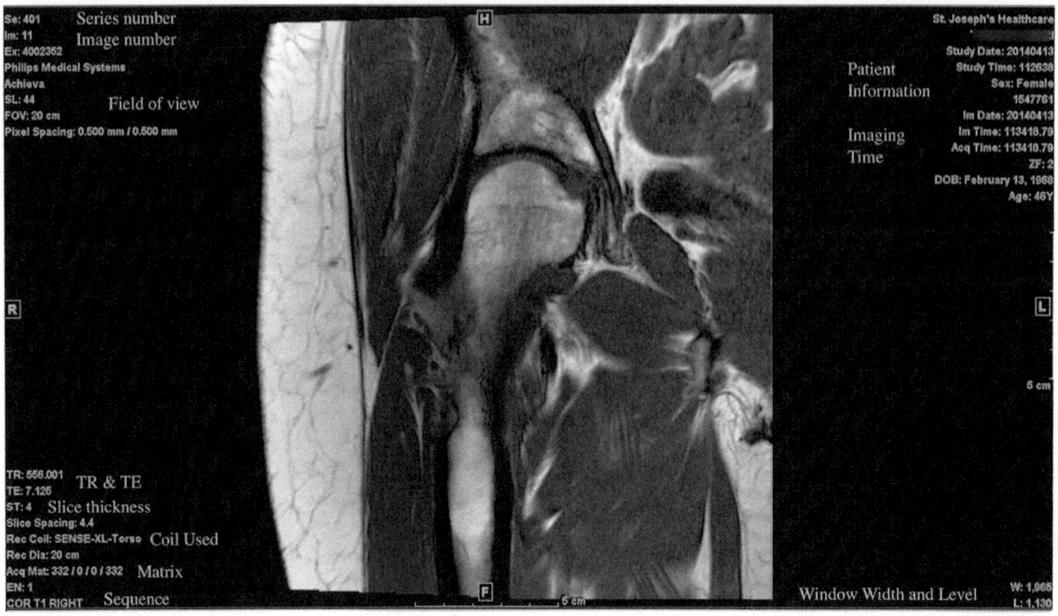

Fig. 1.22 MRI image with normal information available detailing date, patient information, MRI scanner information, sequence and parameters used, etc. (Image shown is a Cor T1 of the right hip)

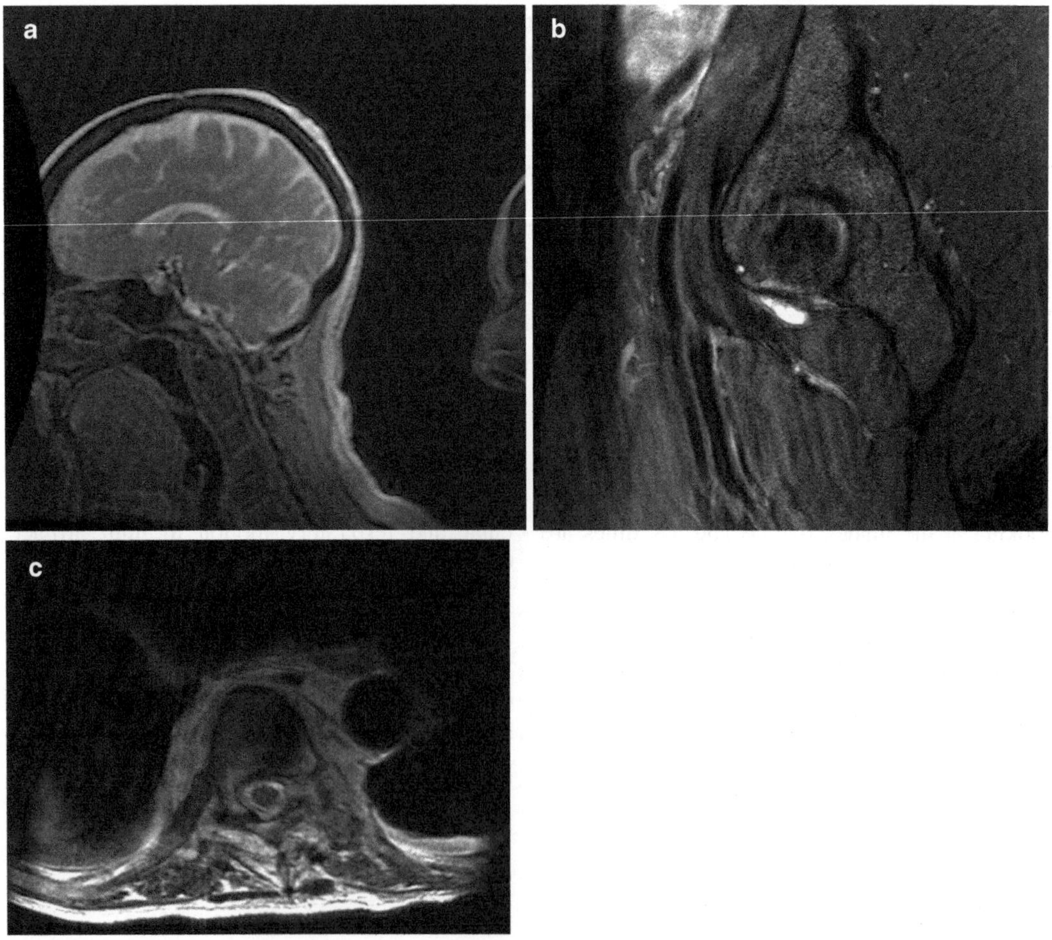

Nuclear Medicine (NM)

Nuclear medicine (NM) has two major components, therapeutic and diagnostic. We will limit this review to diagnostic and the musculoskeletal system. NM is essentially the measurement and imaging of uptake of different radionuclides taken up by different parts of the body. NM can thus provide a physiological and functional assessment of normal and pathological tissue. This unique ability however is traded off with limited image and anatomical resolution.

NM has a long and varied history. In 1896, Becquerel discovered mysterious "rays" from uranium, termed radioactivity by Marie Curie the following year. John H. Lawrence made the first clinical therapeutic application of an artificial radionuclide when he used phosphorus-32 to treat leukemia in 1936. Technetium-99m, the most commonly used radionuclide, was discovered in 1938. A major milestone in its early years was the publication of an article on the treatment of metastatic thyroid cancer with radioiodine in 1946. Nuclear medicine proliferated with the discovery of new radionuclides. In 1951, the first scintillator detector was used to detect the distribution of radioiodine in the thyroid gland. Tc-99m-labeled phosphates for bone imaging became available in 1971. There have been many advances in nuclear medicine with the development of SPECT (single-photon emission computed tomography) imaging and more recently PET (positron emission tomography). PET fusion with CT and MRI was developed to aid in anatomical localization of pathology. This has been further refined in recent years with combined PET-CT imaging and more recently PET-MRI imaging.

Physics

Radionuclide or radioisotope is a version of a chemical element that has an unstable nucleus and emits ionizing radiation during its decay to a stable form. This radiation is usually in the form of gamma rays. These differ from X-rays in that the energy usually has a shorter wavelength and is emitted from the nucleus rather than the electron. A radioisotope is usually combined with a physiologically active compound that is taken up by specific areas within the body. Diphosphonates such as methylene diphosphonate (MDP) are labeled with the radioisotope technetium-99. The MDP is taken up by bone and technetium-99 allows for localization and intensity of uptake (Fig. 1.24). The gamma rays, which are emitted in 360° from the point source, are measured by a gamma camera which has a collimator so that only gamma rays parallel to the collimator can reach the detector, hence allowing it to localize the source. The gamma ray then reaches the detector, sodium iodide crystal, which releases light, which is amplified by photomultiplier tubes to produce an electrical signal that is measured and mapped.

SPECT, single-photon emission computed tomography, involves the acquisition of multiple images from multiple angles around the patient which are then reconstructed to form 3-D imaging data sets, which can be viewed in axial, sagittal, or coronal planes (Fig. 1.25). This allows for better image contrast and localization.

PET, positron emission tomography, is used to assess the metabolic activity of cells. A positron-emitting radionuclide, produced from a cyclotron, is attached to a biologically active molecule. F-18, fluorine 18, is the commonest radionuclide used. F-18 is attached to FDG, fluorodeoxyglucose, an analogue of glucose, and can be used to assess the metabolic activity of cells. This is of primary use when assessing primary and secondary malignancies, which have a higher metabolic activity than normal cells. The PET camera has a ring of detectors attached to photomultiplier tubes. The sensitivity is significantly higher than SPECT and with higher spatial resolution. PET-CT is a combined PET and CT scanner and allows for detailed anatomical resolution as normally imaged with CT (Fig. 1.26).

Fig. 1.23 MRI artifacts: (**a**) MRI head demonstrating wraparound artifact with facial features "wrapped around" to be malpositioned on the left of the image, (**b**) flow-related artifact related to pulsations in the common femoral artery on MRI Sag T2 left hip, (**c**) image degradation with blurring secondary to patient motion on axial T2FS thoracic spine

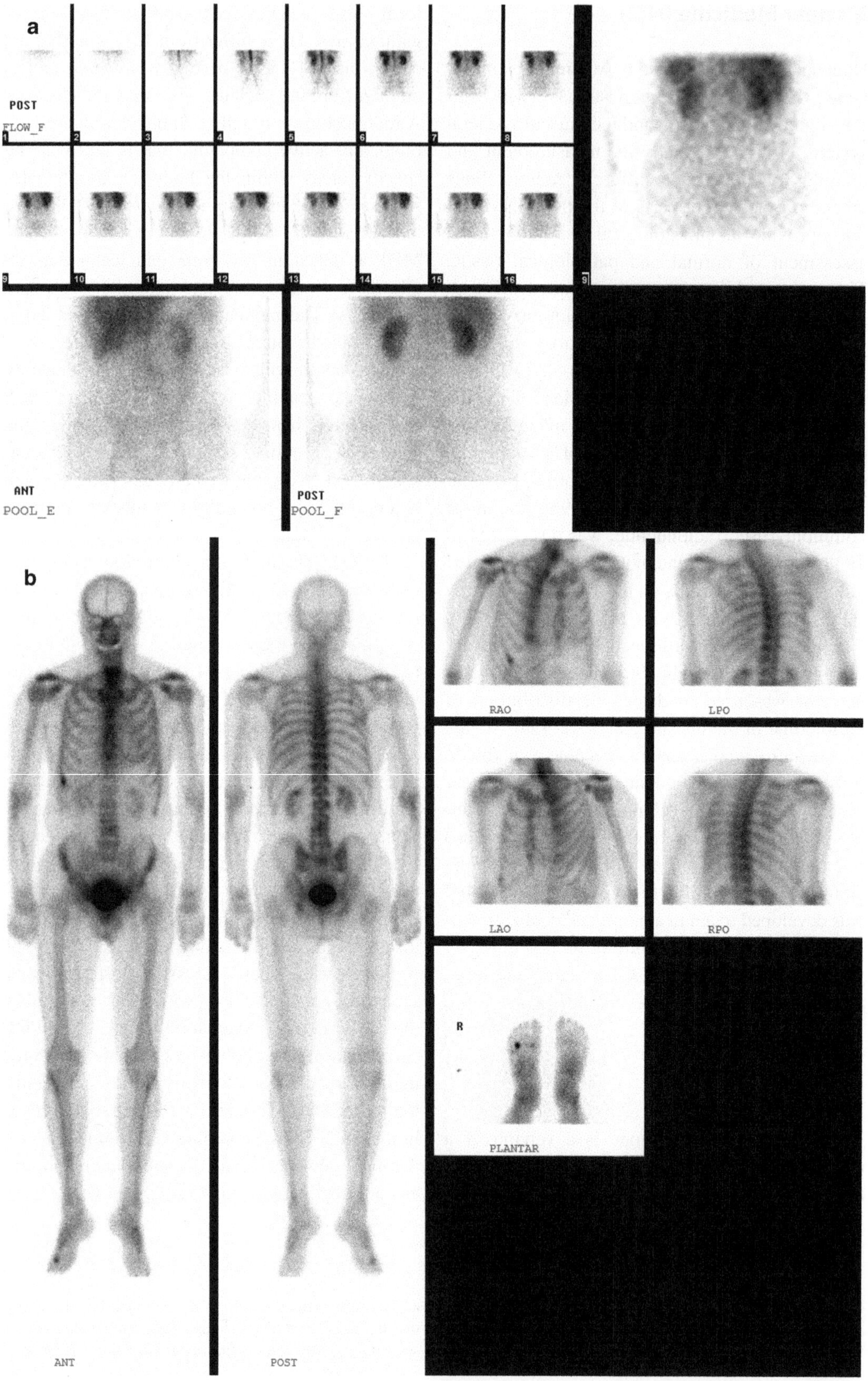
a
POST
FLOW_F
1
2
3
4
5
6
7
8
9
10
11
12
13
14
15
16
9
ANT
POOL_E
POST
POOL_F
b
RAO
LPO
LAO
RPO
R
PLANTAR
ANT
POST

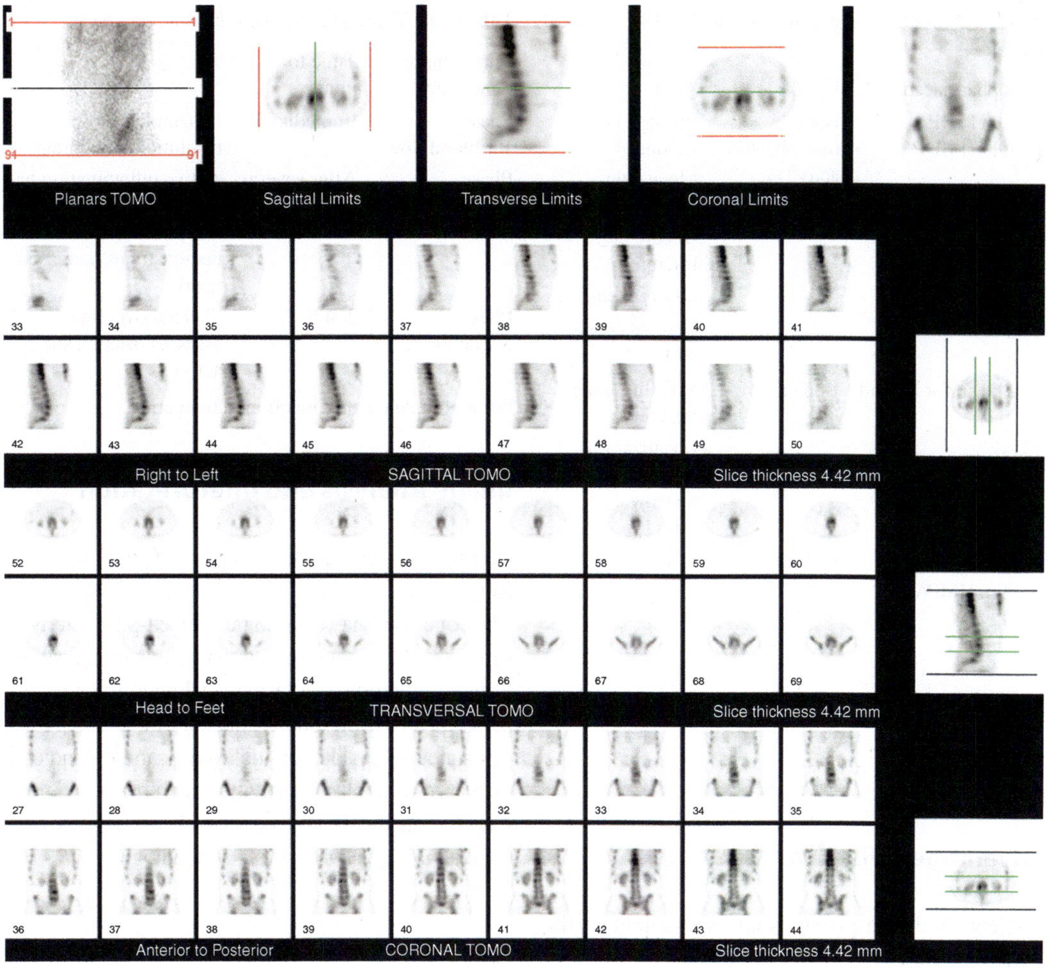

Fig. 1.25 SPECT images from same patient in Fig. 1.24

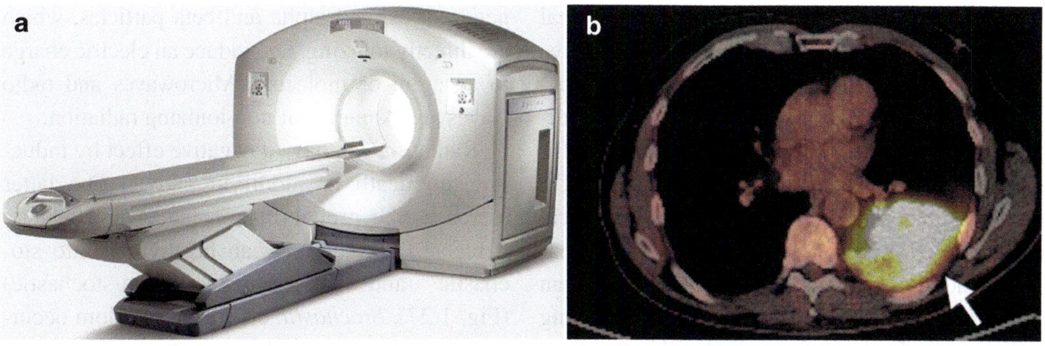

Fig. 1.26 (**a**) Image CT-PET scanner and (**b**) CT-PET fused image with increased metabolic activity and uptake in left lower lobe malignancy (*arrow*)

Fig. 1.24 Three-phase bone scan: (**a**) blood flow (immediate) and pooling (minutes) phases; (**b**) phase 3, bone phase, several hours later to assess bone metabolism and osteoblastic activity. Note increased activity in the right ninth rib secondary to fracture

Table 1.7 Radiopharmaceuticals and MSK clinical indications

Radiopharmaceuticals	Uptake	Assessment
Tc-99m MDP, Tc-99m HMDP	Bone (osteoblastic activity)	Primary bone lesions Metastatic bone disease Occult fractures Osteomyelitis Osteonecrosis RSD
Tc-99m sulfur colloid	Bone marrow	Viability bone marrow Localization prior to bone marrow aspiration
In-111	Labeled leukocyte imaging	Infection
Tc-99m HMPAO		

Advantages/Disadvantages

Nuclear medicine provides an assessment of the functional and physiological activity of different systems within the body including the skeletal (bone), cardiac, pulmonary, genitourinary, gastrointestinal, and endocrine (thyroid). It provides additional insights into normal and pathological states that may not be evident with alternative imaging techniques (Table 1.7). The limited spatial resolution is improved with SPECT and further still with PET imaging. Fusion of PET images with MRI or CT or combined PET-CT studies compensate for the limited anatomical resolution. NM however involves the use of ionizing radiation; a typical bone scan has an effective dose of 3.5 mSv. Alternate non-ionizing imaging should always be considered in the diagnostic imaging protocol, and risk-benefits of investigation should be considered. Correlation with radiographs or cross-sectional imaging is usually required.

Table 1.8 Three-phase bone scan time sequence

Three-phase bone scan	Time to image[a]	
Phase 1 – blood flow	Immediately	Resembles a low-resolution angiogram
Phase 2 – blood pool	After several minutes	Active inflammation has increased blood flow and pooling and demonstrates increased uptake
Phase 3 – delayed,	2–4 h	Skeletal overview, assesses osteoblastic activity

[a]Time to image from injection radionuclide

Image Analysis and Interpretation

Confirm correct patient, date, and type of imaging. Review prior imaging for correlation with NM study. The bone scan may be a single delayed-phase study or triple phase depending on the clinical indication. Usually inflammatory lesions including fractures are performed as triple-phase imaging (Table 1.8). Areas of increased uptake on delayed scanning indicate increased osteoblastic activity, which has a wide differential diagnosis and needs to be correlated with clinical history, examination, and radiographs.

Radiobiology

Ionizing radiation includes X-rays and gamma rays, which are indirectly ionizing via electromagnetic waves, and alpha and beta particles, which are directly ionizing, i.e., induce an electric charge to an atom or molecule. Microwaves and radio waves are examples of non-ionizing radiation.

Radiation can have a negative effect by inducing cell death or modifying DNA. The latter increases the probability of cancer and genetic defects. These effects can be divided into stochastic and deterministic (non-stochastic) (Fig. 1.27). *Stochastic* effects are random occurrences such as the induction of genetic defects and cancer, the severity but not the probability of which is independent of dose, and have no threshold below which the effect will not occur. *Deterministic* effects are directly related to

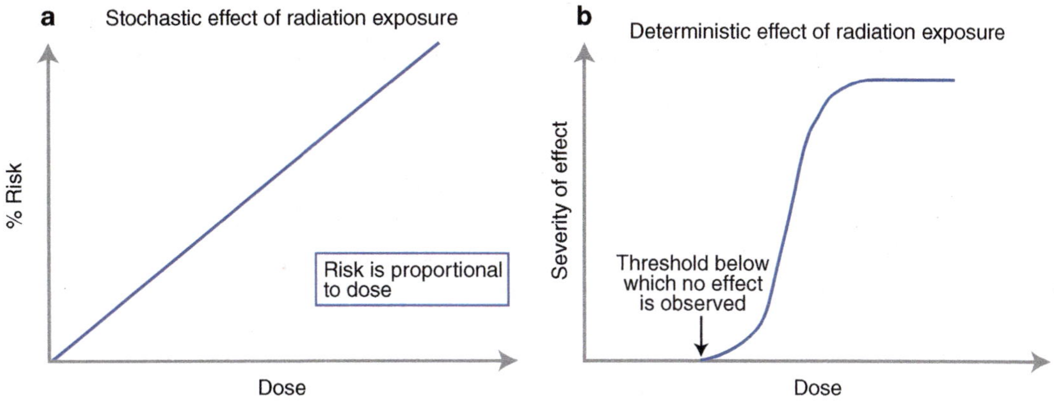

Fig. 1.27 (a) Stochastic effect of radiation exposure. (b) Deterministic effect of radiation exposure

radiation dose, the severity but not the probability of which increases with radiation dose, and have a threshold below which the effect does not occur. Examples include skin burns and cataracts. In general, children are as twice as sensitive to the negative effects of radiation compared to adults.

The *ALARA* (As Low As Reasonably Achievable) principle should always be considered when reviewing different imaging options. Essentially the study with no or lowest ionizing radiation should be used, all else being equal. If ionizing radiation is used, then the study should be optimized to achieve the optimal diagnostic images without excessive radiation dose. The risk-benefit ratio of the study is essential to consider in conjunction with the ALARA principle.

Radiation Dose

There are multiple measurements used in radiation including absorbed dose, equivalent dose, and effective dose. Effective dose will be used here for brevity and to avoid confusion. Effective dose, measured in sieverts, is a dose descriptor reflecting the radiation dose to an organ or body part and the inherent biological sensitivity of that part. It facilitates the comparison of different diagnostic imaging studies and their potential biological effect (Table 1.9). It is estimated that a study with a dose of 10 mSv will increase the possibility of fatal cancer by 1 in 2000.

Table 1.9 Radiation and imaging modalities

Imaging study	Typical effective dose (mSv)	Equivalent number of CXRs	Equivalent background natural radiation exposure (approx.)
CXR (PA)	<0.02	1	3 days
Peripheral joint radiograph	<0.01	<0.5	<1.5
Hip radiograph	0.4	20	2 months
Pelvic radiograph	0.7	35	4 months
Lumbar spine radiograph	1.0	50	5 months
Pelvic CT	4	200	20 months
Lumbar spine CT	8	400	40 months
Bone scan (Tc-99m)	4	200	20 months
MRI	0	0	0
Ultrasound	0	0	0

Radiation Exposure and Pregnancy

Women of reproductive age should be asked about the possibility of being pregnant prior to any imaging study involving ionizing radiation. The fetus is more prone to the negative effects of radiation. If the patient cannot exclude the possibility of pregnancy, then the justification and urgency of the examination should be reevaluated, and consideration for alternative imaging, with non-ionizing studies such as MRI and ultrasound, is advised. If the patient cannot exclude the possibility of pregnancy, then non-urgent ionizing studies should be restricted to the first 10 days from commencement menses, the 10-day rule. If study is urgent, then discussion should take place with the patient and the referring clinician. The study should be optimized to limit any radiation exposure to the fetus.

Contrast Agents

Discussion of contrast media will be restricted to those commonly used in musculoskeletal imaging studies. Nonionic low-osmolar iodinated contrast media are used in CT examinations and angiography and are associated with less allergic reactions (1–2 %) and nephrotoxicity than their ionic counterparts. Allergic reactions can be divided into anaphylactoid and nonidiosyncratic reactions. Anaphylactoid include urticaria, bronchospasm, and cardiovascular collapse, whereas nonidiosyncratic include vasovagal response, nausea, vomiting, and arrhythmias. Severe reactions are rare, 1/10,000, and fatalities estimated at 1/200,000. Patients at risk for renal dysfunction should have baseline creatinine clearance measured prior to the study, be well hydrated, and have nephrotoxic agents such as diuretics and NSAIDs discontinued prior to the examination.

Intra-articular iodinated contrast for confirmation of joint position for joint injection, aspiration, or arthrograms usually involves a low dose of iodinated contrast. If the patient has had a prior reaction to iodinated contrast, the patient is at risk for anaphylactoid reaction. Depending on prior reaction, the patient could be premedicated, or alternative image guidance such as ultrasound guidance or substitution of air or saline for iodinated contrast could be used. Metformin, used in the treatment of NIDDM, may rarely induce a lactic acidosis and should be indicated on the request form for any patients receiving iodinated intravascular contrast agents. There are protocols in place in departments for monitoring these patients pre- and post-contrast study, which generally include stopping metformin for 48 h after the study and recommencing only when renal function stability is confirmed.

Gadolinium is an MRI intravascular contrast that develops a magnetic moment within a magnetic field, prolonging relaxation rates of nearby protons. The effects are best appreciated on T1-weighted sequences. Reactions are uncommon with minor reaction rate of around 1 % and risk fatality of 1 in 2.5 million. Nephrogenic systemic fibrosis (NSF) is a rare disease associated with use of gadolinium agents with renal dysfunction. Fibrosis of the skin, joints, and internal organs may occur, and rarely there is a fulminant course. Patients at risk of renal dysfunction should have creatinine clearance assessed prior to administration of gadolinium-based contrast.

PACS

PACS, Picture Archiving and Communication System, is now widespread and considered standard in developed countries. PACS was a major technological advancement in imaging and has contributed significantly to patient care. It has four major components: the imaging study, a secured network, work/viewing stations, and archives. It allows for viewing of patients and prior imaging studies on high resolution a monitors at multiple sites by multiple users. Imaging studies are no longer misplaced or only accessible at one location. Multiple prior studies can be viewed side by side with the current examination.

Further Reading

1. Albert JM. Radiation risk from CT: implications for cancer screening. AJR Am J Roentgenol. 2013;201(1): W81–7.

2. Brambilla M, De Mauri A, Leva L. Cumulative radiation dose from medical imaging in chronic adult patients. Am J Med. 2013;126(6):480–6.
3. Iagnocco A, Naredo E, Bijlsma JW. Becoming a musculoskeletal ultrasonographer. Best Pract Res Clin Rheumatol. 2013;27(2):271–81.
4. Pauwels EK, Bourguignon MH. Radiation dose features and solid cancer induction in pediatric computed tomography. Med Princ Pract. 2012;21(6):508–15. doi:10.1159/000337404. Epub 2012 Mar 30.
5. Pooley RA. AAPM/RSNA physics tutorial for residents: fundamental physics of MR imaging. Radiographics. 2005;25(4):1087–99.
6. RSNA/AAPM Online Physics Modules. https://www.rsna.org/RSNA/AAPM_Online_Physics_Modules_.aspx.
7. Zhuo J, Gullapalli RP. AAPM/RSNA physics tutorial for residents: MR artifacts, safety, and quality control. Radiographics. 2006;26(1):275–97. Review.

Arthritis: A Diagnostic Approach

2

Nader A. Khalidi and John O'Neill

Arthritic disorders come in many different forms, and the key to specific diagnoses is in the meticulous taking of a history and performance of a physical exam. This will decide the type and extent of laboratory investigations and the choice of imaging techniques.

Confirming that symptoms are originating from the musculoskeletal system and are not referred, which may occur with neurologic or vascular disease, is essential. This decision making can be helped by simple questions on history such as if there is numbness or tingling, if symptoms occur at certain times, or if with certain positions (such as that of carpal tunnel syndrome which is worse at night because of the positional nature of the wrist in the flexed position), or if with pain in the buttocks or calves with ambulation (which resolves within minutes with vascular claudication upon resting or similar symptoms but take longer to resolve with neurogenic claudication).

N.A. Khalidi, MD, FRCP(C) (✉)
Program Director, Division of Rheumatology, McMaster University, Hamilton, ON L8N 1Y2, Canada
e-mail: naderkhalidi@sympatico.ca

J. O'Neill, MB, BAO, BCh, MRCPI, MSc, FRCR
Associate Professor, Musculoskeletal Imaging, Diagnostic Imaging, McMaster University/ St Joseph's Healthcare, Hamilton, ON L8N4A6, Canada
e-mail: joneill2@me.com

There are many types and subtypes of arthritides (Fig. 2.1). Some of the more common arthritides that are covered in this text and are important to keep aware of at all times include the following:

1. Osteoarthritis
2. Rheumatoid arthritis
3. Seronegative arthritis (ankylosing spondylitis, reactive arthritis, psoriatic arthritis, enteropathic arthritis)
4. Crystalline arthropathies (gout, CPPD)
5. Connective tissue disorders (SLE/scleroderma/polymyositis/dermatomyositis/Sjogren's)
6. Vasculitis
7. Infectious arthritis

Symptoms

Image interpretation should not be isolated and should be performed in conjunction with available clinical data. One must differentiate the underlying etiology of joint symptoms; the major differentials include inflammatory and mechanical etiologies. Inflammatory conditions typically are worse in the morning with stiffness lasting more than 60 min and improve with movement. Mechanical and degenerative arthritides on the other hand last less than 60 min and are worse with movement. The number and symmetry of joint involvement are helpful in determining the type of arthritis.

J. O'Neill (ed.), *Essential Imaging in Rheumatology*,
DOI 10.1007/978-1-4939-1673-3_2, © Springer Science+Business Media New York 2015

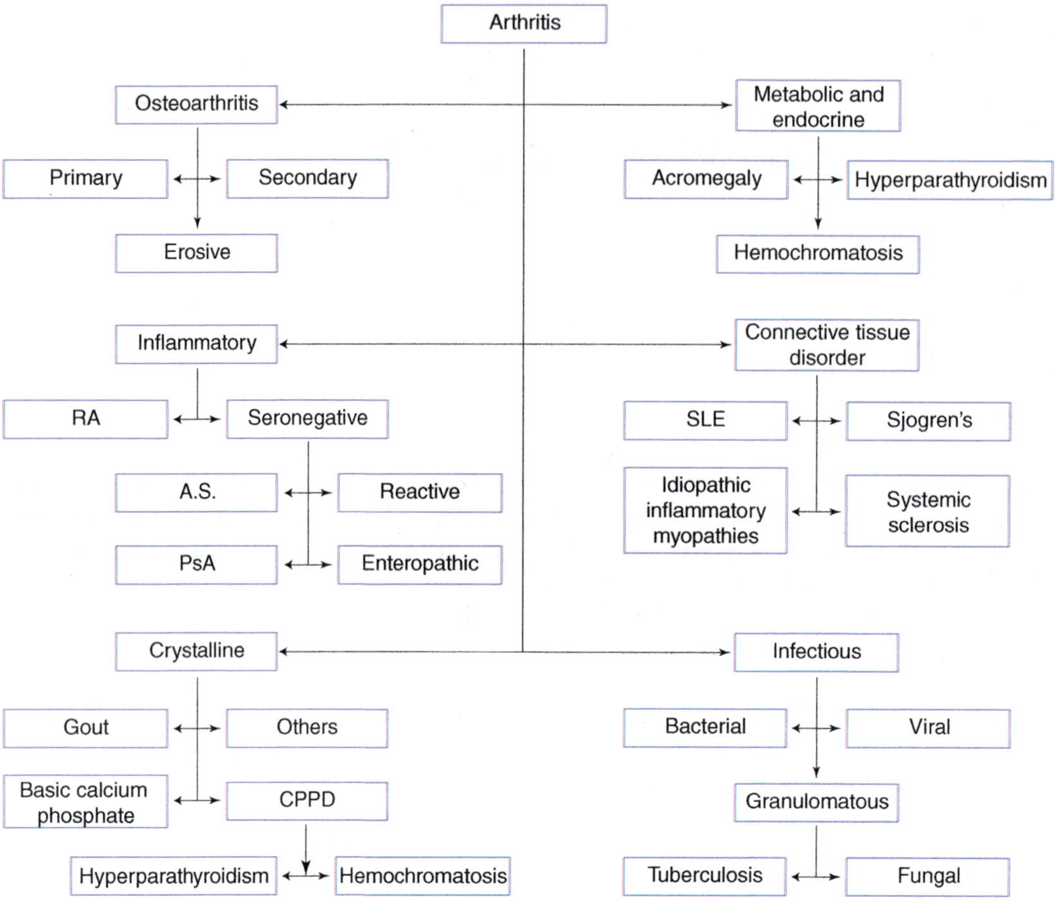

Fig. 2.1 Classification of arthritis

Table 2.1 Differential diagnosis of common causes of acute monoarthritis

Infectious (bacterial, viral)
Crystalline
Traumatic
Seronegative spondyloarthropathy (PsA, reactive)
Hemarthrosis

Table 2.2 Differential diagnosis of common causes of chronic monoarthritis

Infectious (TB, fungal, Lyme)
Seronegative arthritis (reactive, AS, PsA, enteropathic)
Noninflammatory (OA, AVN)
Pigmented villonodular synovitis
Foreign body synovitis

Typically arthritis is separated into monoarticular (one joint), oligoarticular (two to four joints), and polyarticular (more than five joints) types (Tables 2.1, 2.2, 2.3, 2.4, and 2.5). That being said, many arthritides can involve any number of joints, but typically fall into one category. Gout and CPPD are inflammatory arthritides that usually start as monoarthritis as does osteoarthritis, but as time passes, other joints can be involved. Psoriatic arthritis (PsA) can have many different presentations including monoarthritis and polyarthritis, which may or not be symmetrical.

Table 2.3 Differential diagnosis of common causes of oligoarthritis

Infectious (bacterial endocarditis, nongonococcal, disseminated GC, viral)
Postinfectious (reactive, poststreptococcal)
Seronegative arthritis (reactive, AS, PsA, enteropathic)
Oligoarticular presentation of atypical inflammatory arthritis (RA, SLE, adult onset Still's)

Rheumatoid arthritis (RA) is the classic inflammatory arthritis with a symmetric polyarthritis that almost always involves the hands. Assessment

Table 2.4 Differential diagnosis of common causes of acute polyarthritis

Infectious (viral)
Rheumatoid arthritis
Systemic lupus erythematosus
Early disseminated Lyme
HIV
Bacterial endocarditis
Psoriatic arthritis
Polyarticular gout

Table 2.5 Differential diagnosis of common causes of chronic polyarthritis

Rheumatoid arthritis
SLE
Psoriatic arthritis
Other connective tissue disorders
Polyarticular gout
CPPD (pseudo-RA)
Sarcoid arthritis
Vasculitis
Sarcoid arthropathy

of synovitis, a process whereby the synovial membrane of a joint is inflamed, is important. It is the mainstay of inflammatory conditions and occurs much more often than in osteoarthritis where it is much less intense and much less widespread.

The onset of clinical symptoms can be helpful when trying to narrow down the diagnosis to a particular disease. RA is typically subacute occurring over weeks to months rather than days. Osteoarthritis is of gradual onset, usually over many years with slow progression. Crystalline arthropathies, such as chronic CPP arthritis, can also present like osteoarthritis. Septic arthritis and acute crystalline arthritis can present acutely with rapid progression of symptoms in a matter of hours.

Weakness is another symptom that is important to further clarify. This may be subjective as in patients with polymyalgia rheumatica, where the stiffness can be so great as to cause a feeling of weakness, and when questioned, some patients state that it affected them so greatly that they had to crawl to get out of bed. However, when tested objectively, no weakness is found. This subjective stiffness and pain is symmetric and proximal. In the case of polymyositis, however, the patient has very little stiffness but is both subjectively and objectively weak when tested in the proximal musculature (shoulder and hip girdle). Weakness may alternatively be neuropathic in nature, is more often distal in nature, and is associated with other neurological symptoms.

Family history becomes particularly important when looking at the group of disorders called the seronegative spondyloarthropathies (seronegative arthritis) as they occur much more commonly in HLA-B27-positive families as well as the associated disorders of inflammatory bowel disease.

Axial Versus Peripheral Involvement

Peripheral involvement can include specific patterns like distal and proximal interphalangeal involvement (DIP/PIP) in osteoarthritis and psoriatic arthritis or proximal interphalangeal and metacarpophalangeal joint (PIP/MCP) involvement in rheumatoid arthritis, psoriatic arthritis, SLE, and pseudo-RA (crystalline arthropathy of calcium pyrophosphate dihydrate or CPPD). Acute involvement of one joint that is red, hot, and swollen should trigger one to think of a septic arthritis, gout, or pseudogout.

Axial involvement can help narrow the type of arthritis down as well. Lower back involvement is not a characteristic of rheumatoid arthritis, gout, SLE, or systemic vasculitis but is mandatory in that of ankylosing spondylitis. Peripheral involvement with axial involvement could mean osteoarthritis, ankylosing spondylitis, psoriatic arthritis, or reactive arthritis. Involvement of the cervical spine is frequent in rheumatoid arthritis as well as osteoarthritis.

Other Features

Systemic features can often point to a more definitive rheumatic etiology and these features should actively be sought after. Constitutional features of fever, anorexia, weight loss, and fatigue are more associated with an inflammatory process. Nonarticular features such as a history of bloody diarrhea or a genitourinary infection can be highly associated with an inflammatory bowel disease and enteropathic arthritis or that of a reactive arthritis respectively. Specific symptoms of dry eyes (xerophthalmia) and dry mouth (xerostomia),

Raynaud's, and specific rashes such as malar, discoid (systemic lupus erythematosus), Gottron papules, shawl sign, V-neck sign, mechanic's hands, and heliotrope rash (dermatomyositis) can help clinch the diagnosis of a connective tissue disorder. Digital ulcers, puffy fingers, and Raynaud's are all highly suggestive if not diagnostic of systemic sclerosis (scleroderma).

Laboratory Assessment

The lab is an integral part of confirming or refuting the preliminary diagnostic possibilities that have been initiated in the history and physical examination of a patient. Differential diagnoses are often narrowed to a single diagnosis after both a careful choice of laboratory investigations and radiologic undertaking.

Inflammatory markers such as an erythrocyte sedimentation rate (ESR) or C-reactive protein are almost confirmatory of an inflammatory arthritis when they are found to be elevated. One must be cautious, however, of the nonspecific nature and the need to rule out infections and malignancies as ESR and CRP are found in these conditions as well. Conversely while it is rare to see a normal ESR and CRP in rheumatoid arthritis, it is more often than not the case in the seronegative spondyloarthropathies.

More specific testing such as rheumatoid factor (RF) and anti-cyclic citrullinated peptide (anti-CCP) helps confirm the diagnosis of rheumatoid arthritis in the right clinical context. Rheumatoid factor can, however, be found in both other rheumatologic (e.g., Sjogren's and SLE) and non-rheumatologic conditions (sarcoidosis, hepatitis C, and tuberculosis). A low-titer positive RF can be seen with aging. Anti-CCP is much more specific but again can be found rarely in scleroderma and psoriatic arthritis, so the whole picture should be looked at rather than simply the results of the lab testing.

Antinuclear antibodies (ANAs) are typically found in the group of connective tissue disorders (CTD). In fact, a negative ANA should strongly suggest the search for another disease process (although rarely can be negative). ANA is positive in virtually all cases of SLE and systemic sclerosis (scleroderma), whereas in polymyositis and dermatomyositis, it is not absolutely necessary. A positive ANA in low titers can be found in the elderly. Specific antigens and patterns are related to certain subtypes of CTD but are not universally found like the presence of the ANA itself. Anti-dsDNA and anti-Sm are highly specific for SLE as that of anti-Jo-1 is of polymyositis (especially with interstitial lung disease), anti-Scl-70 for diffuse systemic sclerosis, and anti-centromere for limited systemic sclerosis. It is not unusual to see multiple antibodies in SLE (like chromatin, SSA, SSB, RNP, and Sm/dsDNA all at the same time).

Antineutrophil cytoplasmic antibodies are those that react with the cytoplasmic granules of neutrophils and are almost exclusively found in patients with ANCA-associated vasculitis (granulomatosis with polyangiitis (GPA) or microscopic polyangiitis (MPA) or less commonly in eosinophilic granulomatosis with polyangiitis (EGPA)). The patterns of the ANCA can be cytoplasmic (c-ANCA) related to the antigen serine proteinase 3 (PR3) or perinuclear (p-ANCA) related to the antigen myeloperoxidase (MPO). All other ANCAs are not really clinically relevant and so are not typically commercially available.

Arthrocentesis

Arthrocentesis remains a critical assessment tool in spite of all the advances that have been made in other laboratory assessments in rheumatology. There are very few contraindications to aspirating a joint (one of them being overlying cellulitis in order to prevent introduction of an infection into the joint). An acute, idiopathic inflammatory monoarthritis should always be aspirated to assess for a septic joint versus an acute crystalline arthropathy. Arthrocentesis is the only way to unequivocally prove an infection or the presence of gout or pseudogout. If synovial fluid analysis reveals an extreme elevation in WBC, mostly neutrophils with a positive gram stain, and no crystals, antibiotics should be initiated pending culture results. Remember though that a patient can have an infection that coexists with a crystalline arthropathy or a crystalline arthropathy can be present in any of the inflammatory polyarthritides, and careful review of the clinical history along with the synovial fluid analyses is paramount.

Imaging

Chapters 1 and 3 provide a detailed review of imaging. The following is a brief overview.

Conventional Radiography

This is the starting point for evaluation of all arthritides. Radiographs are readily available, are inexpensive, and offer excellent spatial resolution. Standard views should be obtained in at least two projections. Additional views may also be required for some joints, such as the Norgaard (ball catcher's) view, which are important in looking for erosions of the hands, e.g., radial aspects of the metacarpal heads, which may not be visible on the AP or lateral radiographs (Fig. 2.2). Occasionally asymptomatic joints should also be imaged as they may present additional helpful findings, e.g., bilateral feet radiographs may demonstrate asymptomatic erosions in suspected RA patients. Radiographs can also localize pathology that can then be assessed with other imaging modalities if clinically indicated. Radiographs can demonstrate pathology, e.g., chondrocalcinosis, and distribution patterns that may be difficult to appreciate on alternate imaging.

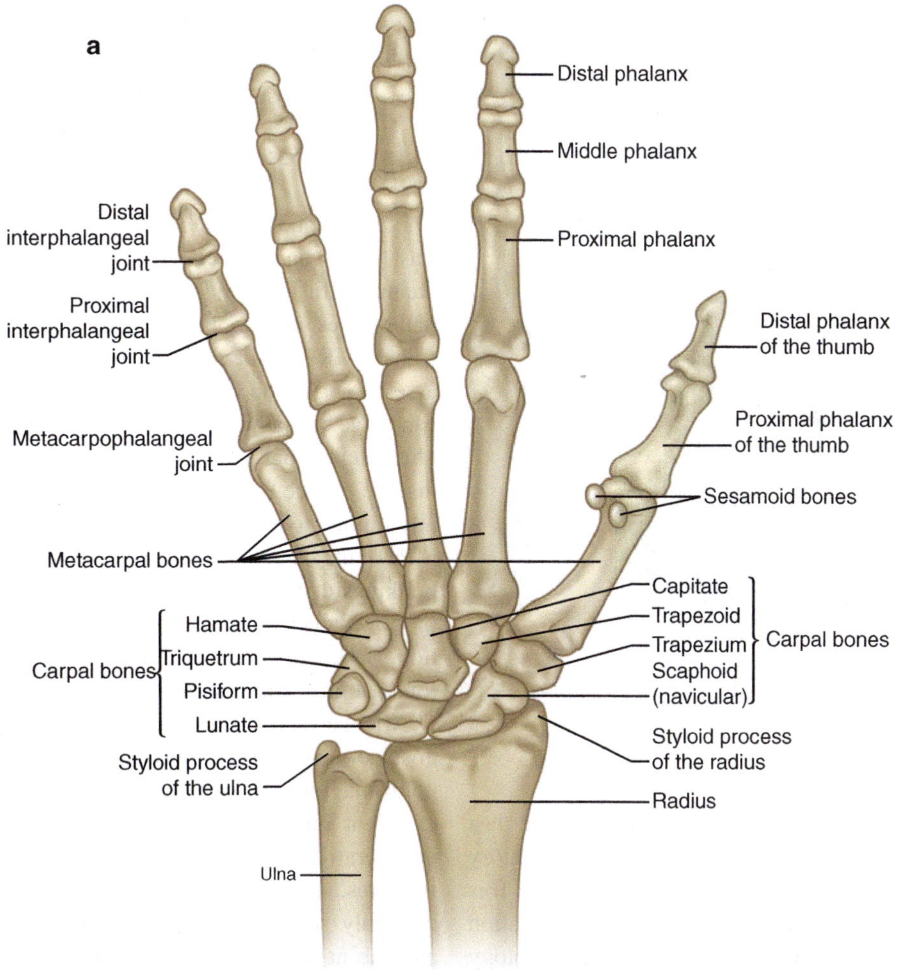

Fig. 2.2 (**a**) Normal osseous anatomy of the hand. (**b**) PA of normal bilateral hand radiographs, (**c**) Norgaard, and (**d**) lateral views

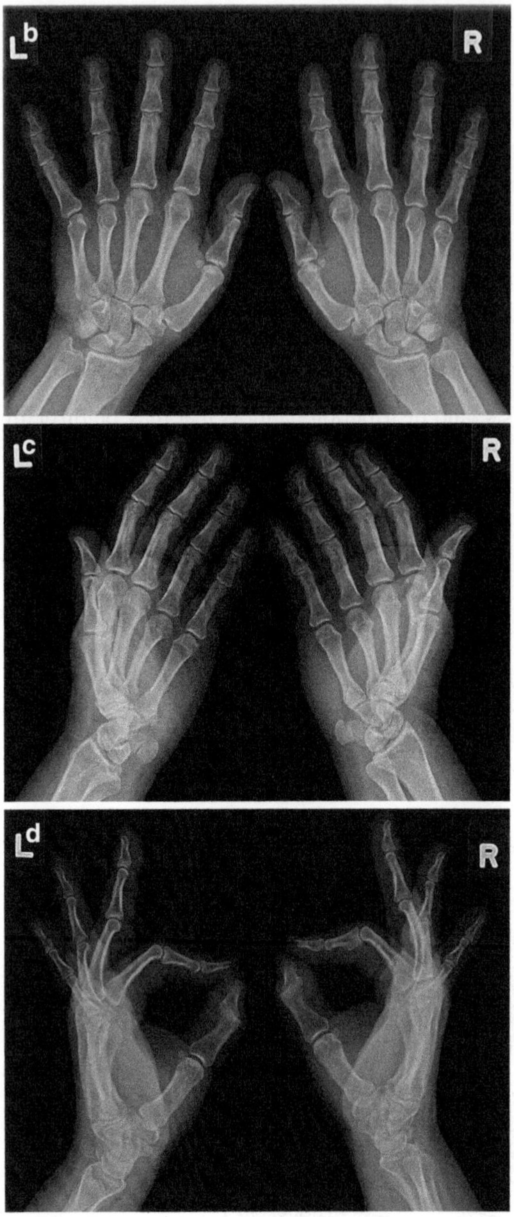

Fig. 2.2 (continued)

Ultrasound

Ultrasound has developed rapidly in the last decade in assessing patients with inflammatory arthritis, particularly in rheumatoid arthritis. It is becoming an adjunct to the clinical examination with increased direct use in the rheumatology office. The use of power Doppler has allowed for more effective analysis of synovitis and erosions in superficial joints. This allows for confirmation of active disease and allows the rheumatologist and patient to make informed decisions on treatment on the same outpatient appointment. Ultrasound can also assess for joint effusions and tendon and tendon sheath pathology and can assess multiple joints at the same setting. Ultrasound is however operator dependent and has a long learning curve. As such, many rheumatology centers are developing alongside dedicated musculoskeletal imaging centers.

Computed Tomography (CT)

CT scans offer excellent spatial resolution. It is the gold imaging standard in the assessment of erosive disease. Its general use however is limited by its significant radiation burden and the availability of ultrasound and MRI.

Magnetic Resonance Imaging (MRI)

This technique offers excellent soft tissue contrast. MRI can determine the extent of synovitis, pannus, effusions, and tendon and tendon sheath pathologies as can be demonstrated on ultrasound. MRI is not however limited to detailed assessment of superficial joints. In addition MRI can delve beneath the bone cortex, a limitation in ultrasound. Bone marrow edema and pre-erosive disease can be readily appreciated. MRI is usually limited to evaluation of a single region, e.g., MRI of the hand and elbow requires two separate bookings due to time requirements and the field of view, which is balanced against image resolution, whereas ultrasound can image multiple joints at the same examination.

MRI has had a significant impact on the diagnosis of axial spondyloarthropathy and is the gold imaging standard; see Chap. 6. MRI is an excellent imaging choice for demonstration of degenerative disk disease, AVN, insufficiency fractures, and spondylodiscitis (see Chap. 15). It is highly sensitive in diagnosing osteomyelitis and the noninfectious osteitis of the rare disorders such as SAPHO (synovitis, acne, pustulosis, hyperostosis, and osteitis) syndrome and chronic recurrent multifocal osteitis (CRMO) (see Chap. 5). Finally it has gained prominence in the evaluation of inflammatory myositis (polymyositis and dermatomyositis; see Chap. 7) and in identifying sites of biopsy for these rare muscle diseases.

Scintigraphy

Radionuclide bone scans are not as popular as they once were since the more widespread introduction of the MRI. They were used historically to evaluate the distribution of arthritis in different joints. To distinguish infections from inflammatory arthritis, indium-labeled leukocytes or gallium scans can be employed. It can be useful in determining the activity in patients with Paget's disease of the bone.

Pattern Recognition: Specific Rheumatologic Disorders

Typical distribution of affected joints and the subsequent pattern recognition are key elements in helping the clinician arrive at a diagnosis. Please see the appropriate chapters in the previous section for a more detailed review.

Osteoarthritis (Primary) (Fig. 2.3)

Hands

DIPJs, PIPJs, and the first CMCJ are classically associated with primary OA. If other joints of the hand are involved with OA, one should think of *secondary* causes to include crystal disease, RA, and trauma. The second and third MCPJs are an unusual site of primary OA and, if noted, should

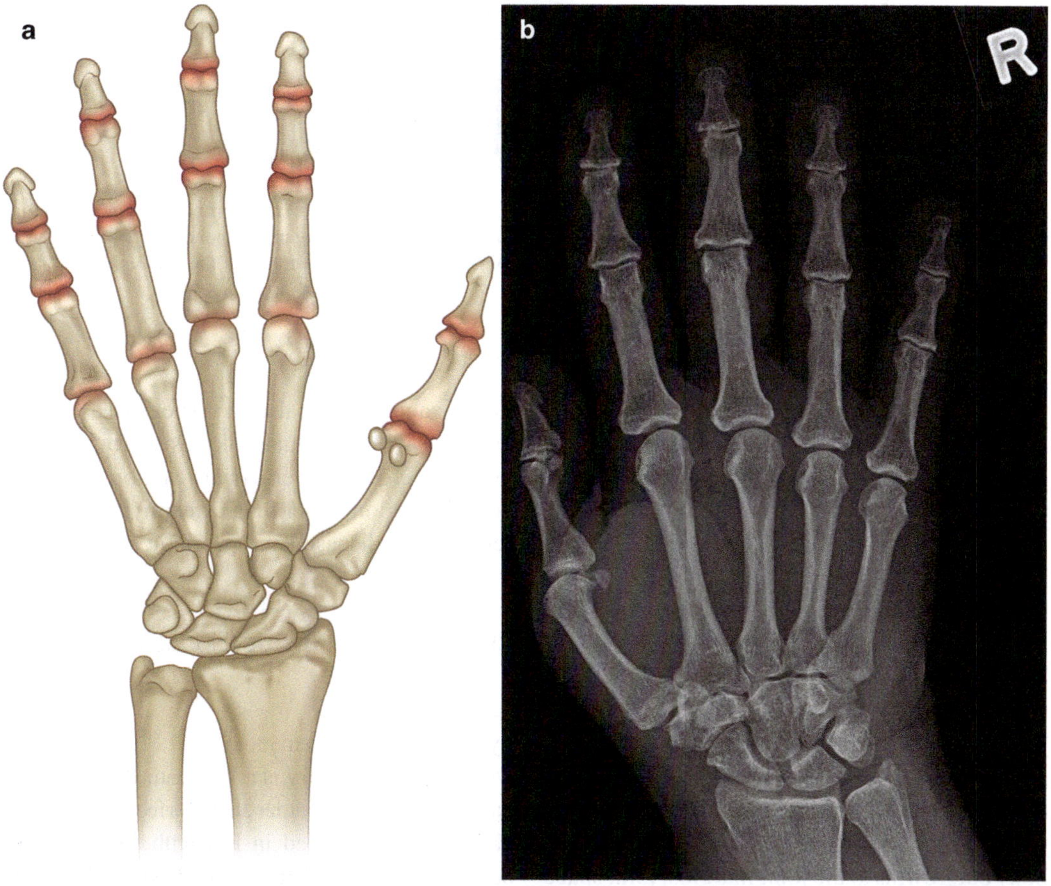

Fig. 2.3 (**a**) Common sites of involvement with osteoarthritis of the hand (*highlighted in red*). (**b**) PA radiograph of right hand with early osteoarthritis demonstrating joint space loss at the PIP and DIP joints and early subchondral cysts at the second and third DIP joints

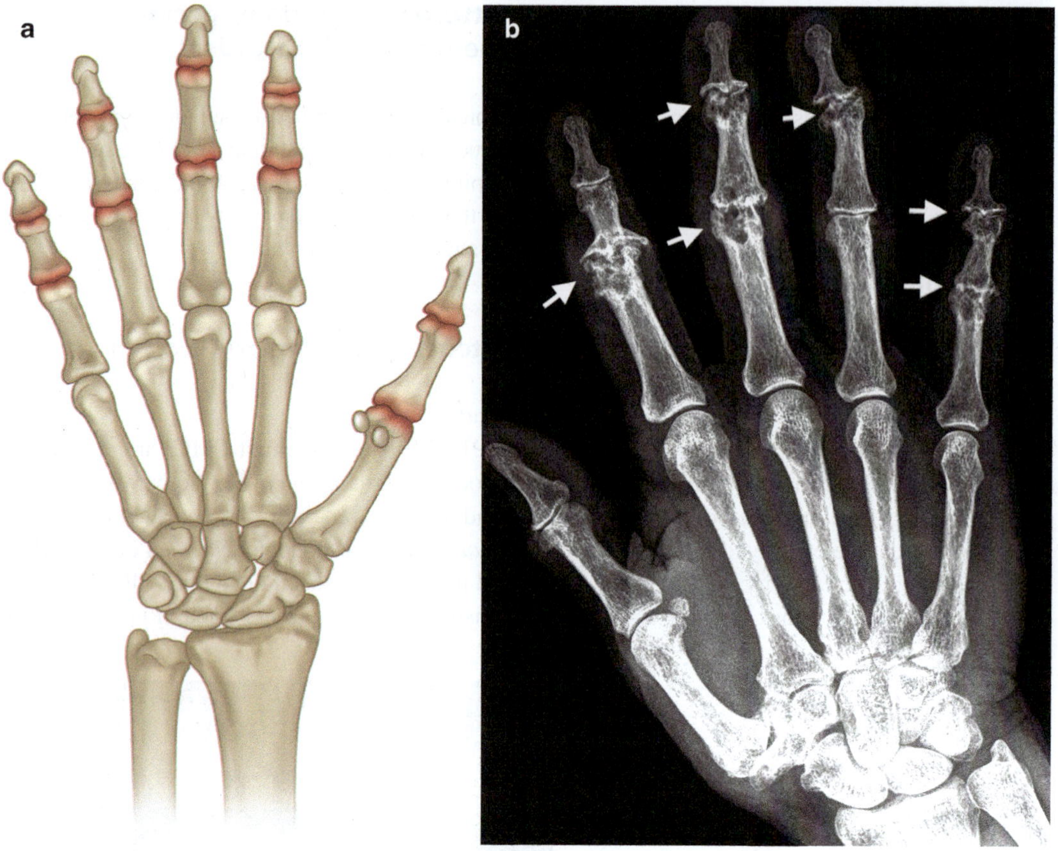

Fig. 2.4 (**a**) Common sites of involvement with erosive osteoarthritis of the hand. (**b**) PA radiograph of right hand with changes of chronic erosive osteoarthritis at the PIP and DIP joints (*arrows*) with classic central erosions and "gull wing" osteophytes (most pronounced at the second PIPJ). Note also prominent subchondral cysts at the same joints and lack of involvement of the MCPJs

prompt one to think about CPPD and more importantly its associated etiologies such as hemochromatosis (which shouldn't be missed).

Other Joints

The most classic sites involved in osteoarthritis include the acromioclavicular and sternoclavicular joints, cervical spine, lumbar spine, hips, knees, and first MTP joints.

Erosive osteoarthritis is a subset of primary OA and predominantly involves the hands (Fig. 2.4). The PIP and DIP joints are more commonly involved although any of the above joints in primary OA may be involved. There are bony outgrowths at the joint margins, joint space loss, and central erosions. The latter produces the "seagull" appearance. The disease may progress with eventual ankylosis. The lack of marginal erosions, periosteal reaction, and new bone formation, other than osteophytes, helps to separate the disease from psoriatic arthropathy.

Rheumatoid Arthritis (Fig. 2.5)

Hands

Symmetrical involvement of the PIP, MCP, and wrist joints (symmetry is a key feature in that both hands are involved rather than perfect symmetry). *Feet* are also involved in RA with similar joints being involved, i.e., PIP and MTP joints. The fifth metatarsal head is a common first site of erosion.

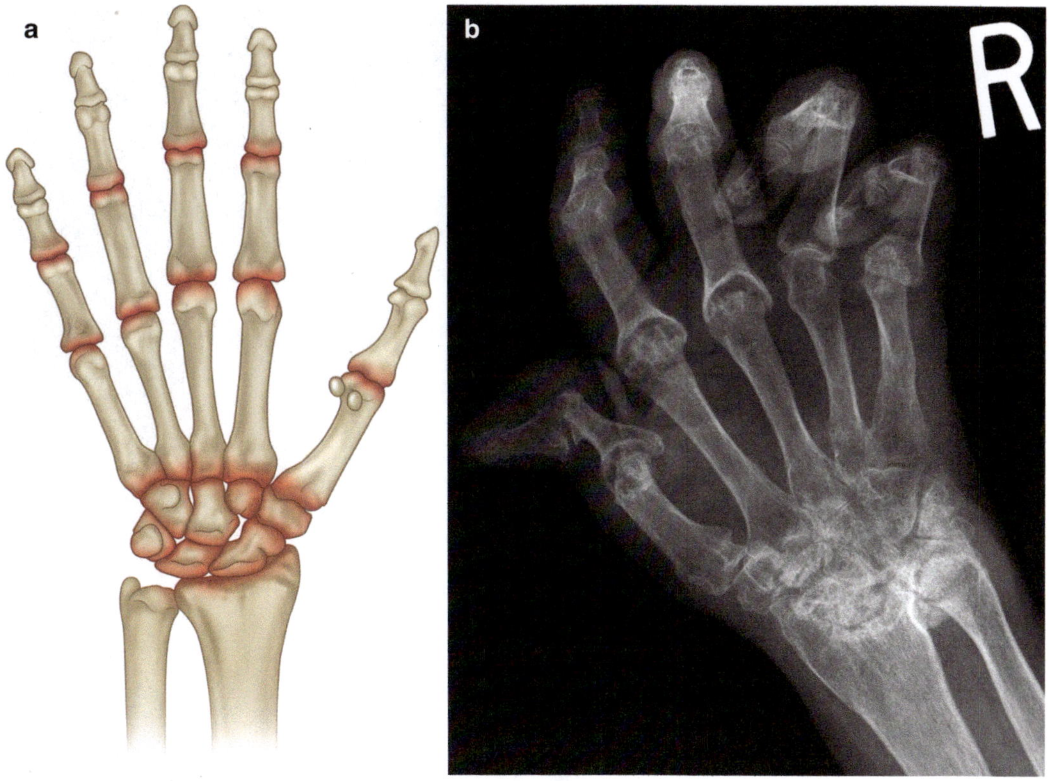

Fig. 2.5 (**a**) Common sites of involvement with rheumatoid arthritis. (**b**) PA radiograph of right hand with changes of long-standing rheumatoid arthritis (similar changes were noted in the left hand and wrist in keeping with symmetrical disease). Marked diffuse osteopenia, extensive erosions at radioulnar joint, partial collapse at proximal carpal row, erosions at the MCPJs and first IP joint, "Z" shaped deformity in the thumb, subluxation at the fifth MCPJ, and flexion deformities at the PIPJs

Other Joints

Elbows, glenohumeral, cervical spine, hips, knees, and ankles are the most common involved joints in RA. Note that lumbar spine is almost never involved. Again symmetry is typical but perfect symmetry is not absolute.

Seronegative Arthritis (Ankylosing Spondylitis, Reactive Arthritis, Psoriatic Arthritis, Enteropathic Arthritis) (Fig. 2.6)

Hands

Several patterns can be found in PsA, in particular the distal form (DIP involvement) and the symmetric polyarthritis pattern that can mimic RA (PIP, MCP, and wrist involvement). Periarticular osteopenia occurring in RA and periostitis (laying down of new bone) occurring in PsA are helpful in differentiating RA from PsA.

Other Joints

All seronegative arthritides can affect the sacroiliac joints (SI). AS by definition involves the sacroiliac joints symmetrically, whereas the other types may affect SI joints asymmetrically. Lumbar and thoracic spine are involved, but cervical spine is less commonly involved, with the exception of PsA. Lower extremity asymmetric large joint oligoarthritis is classic and is found in the hip, knee, and ankle joints.

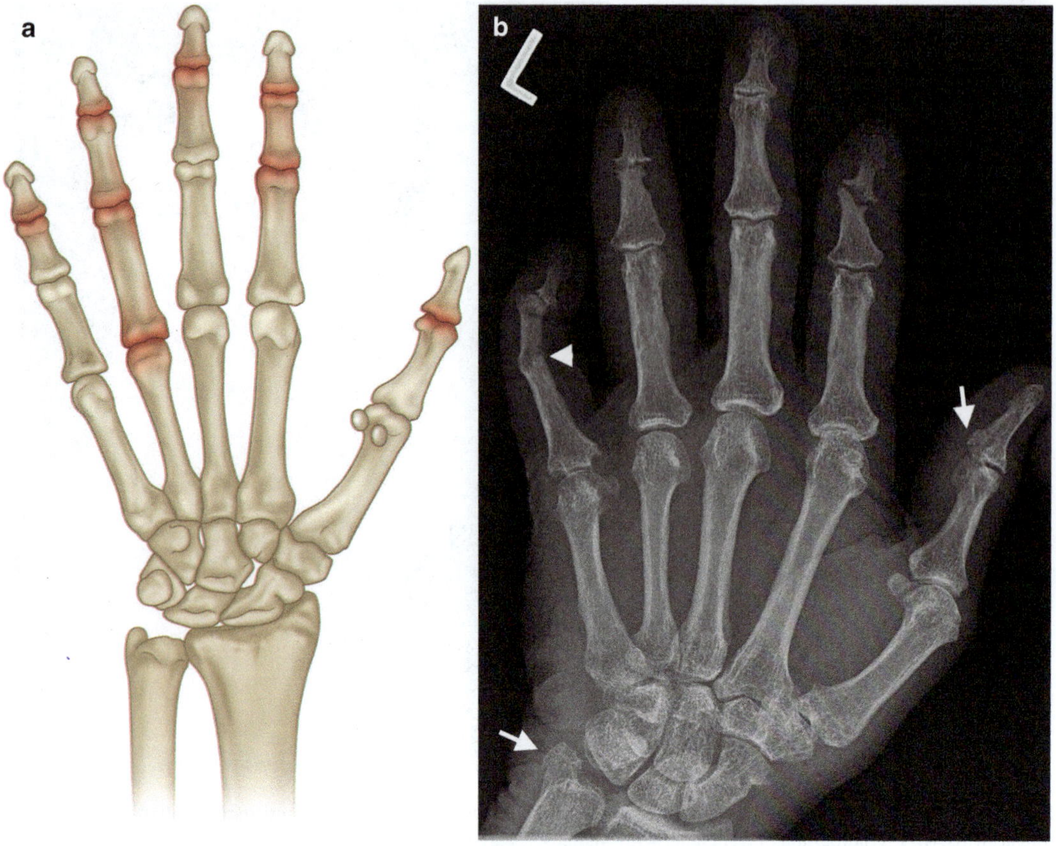

Fig. 2.6 (**a**) Common sites of involvement with seronegative arthritis. (**b**) PA radiograph of the left hand in a patient with long-standing psoriatic arthritis (asymmetrical changes were present on the right hand). Normal bone density, new bone formation at ulnar styloid and base of the first distal phalynx (*arrows*), marginal erosions at the distal scaphoid and the fifth MCPJ and DIPJ, central and marginal erosions at the second and fourth DIPJs, and joint fusion at the fifth PIPJ (*arrowhead*)

Crystalline Arthropathies (Gout, CPPD) (Fig. 2.7)

Hands

Any joints of the hands can be affected in gout or CPPD arthropathy. When these diseases become chronic and recurrent, they often mimic rheumatoid arthritis. In the case of CPPD, this clinical presentation is termed pseudo-rheumatoid arthritis. Plain radiographs would be of great help especially if it shows OA of the second and third MCPs as well as calcification in the cartilage of the triangular fibrocartilage complex (TFCC) of the wrist.

Other Joints

Almost any other joints can be involved in crystalline arthropathies, but involvement of the spine, except for atlantoaxial joint, is unusual. The first MTP is classically the first joint to be involved in gout (podagra).

Connective Tissue Disorders (SLE/Scleroderma/Polymyositis/Dermatomyositis/Sjogren's) (Fig. 2.8)

Hands

SLE often involves the hands in the typical RA distribution (PIPs, MCPs, and wrists) and can

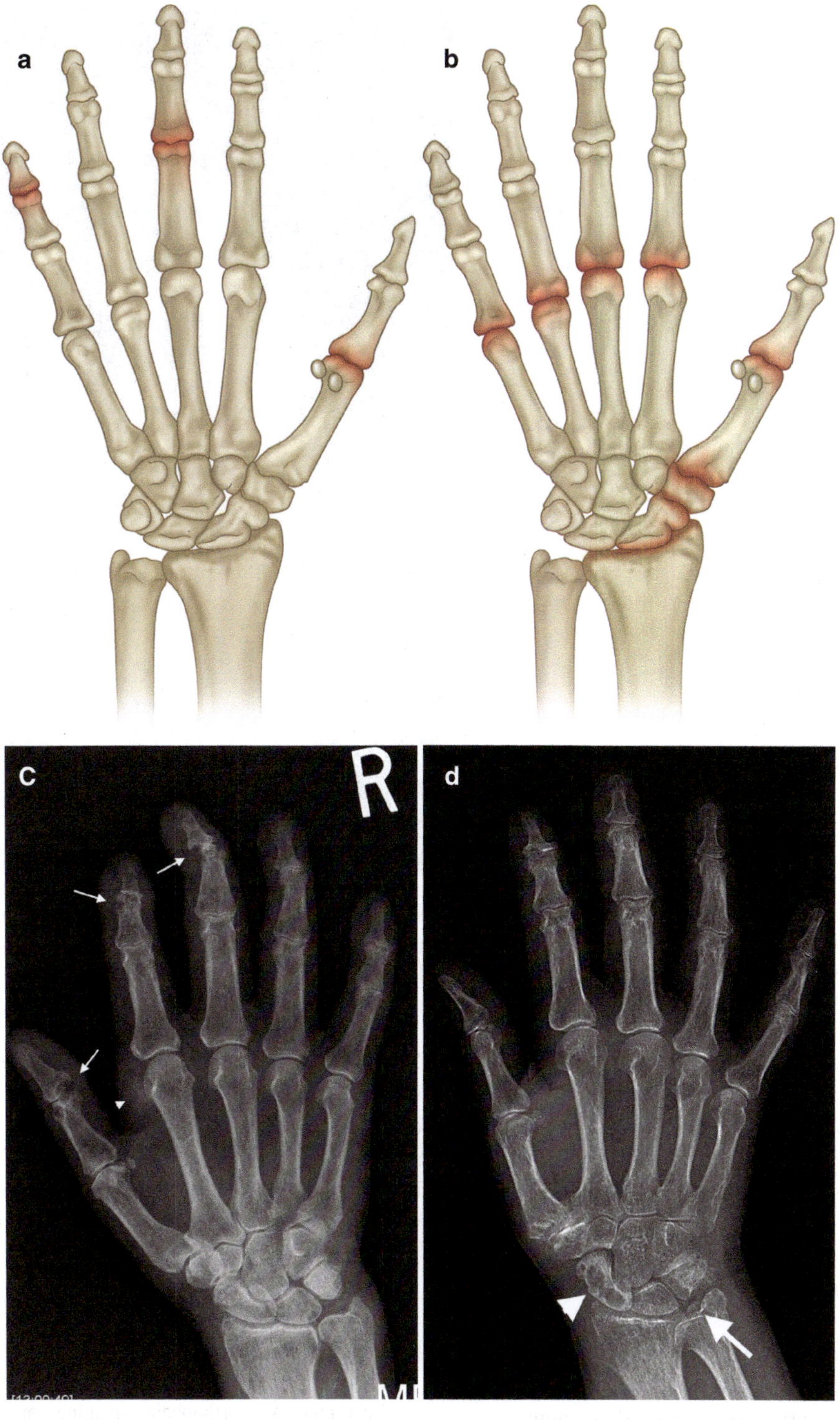

Fig. 2.7 Common sites of involvement with (**a**) gout and (**b**) CPPD arthropathy. (**c**) PA radiograph of the right hand in a patient with a 15-year history of gout and chronic renal failure with marginal erosions (*arrows*), some with overhanging edges (first IPJ), and gouty tophus (*arrowhead*). Note absence of periarticular osteopenia. There was asymmetrical left hand involvement (not shown). (**d**) PA radiograph of the right hand with chondrocalcinosis triangular fibrocartilage (*arrow*), normal bone density, mild joint space loss at the MCPJs, moderate degenerative changes at the first CMC, and crystal-related prominent subchondral cysts of the scaphoid. Incidental mild osteoarthritis, age-related, at the PIP and DIP joints in (**c**, **d**)

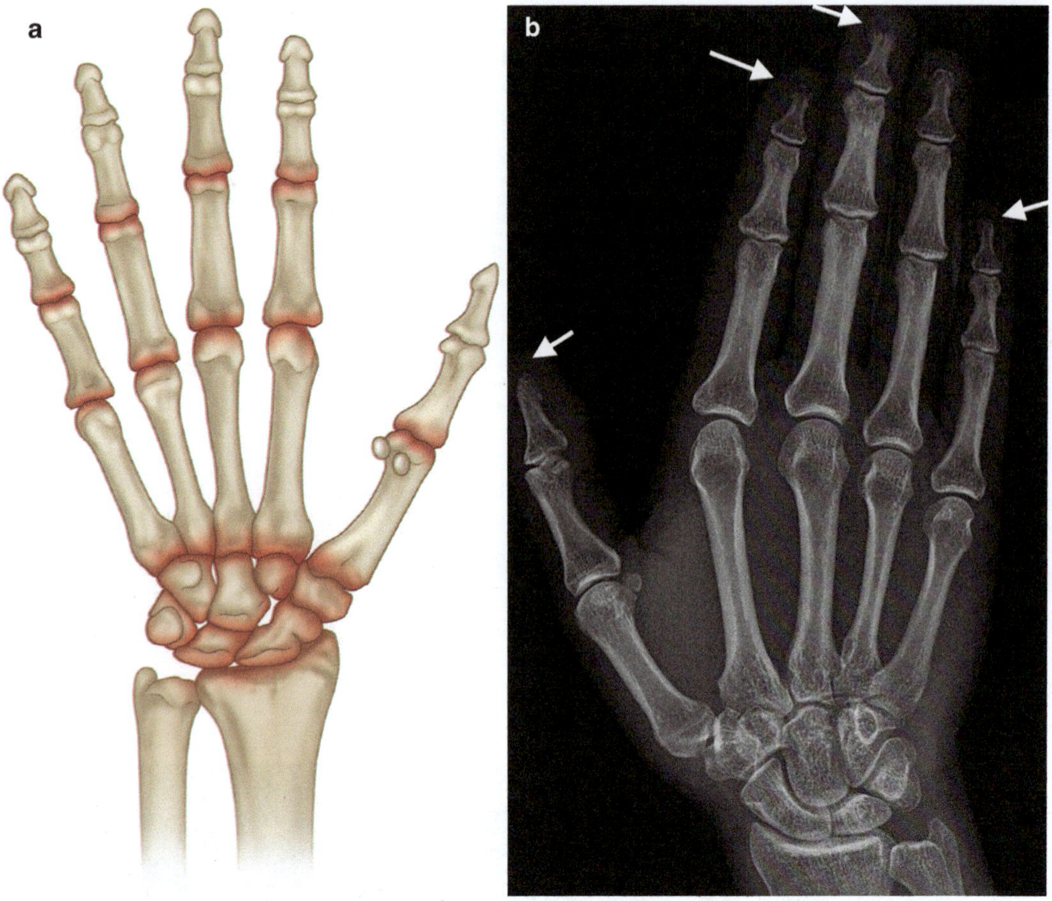

Fig. 2.8 (**a**) Common sites of involvement with connective tissue disease. (**b**) PA radiograph of the right hand with scleroderma demonstrating resorption at phalangeal tufts (*arrows*), acro-osteolysis. No significant overlying soft tissue atrophy or soft tissue calcification noted in this patient but are commonly encountered in scleroderma (see Chap. 7)

have the same deformities as RA (swan neck and boutonnière), but the lack of erosions on plain radiographs is a key differentiating factor in long-standing disease. The pattern of reversible joint deformity is termed Jaccoud arthropathy.

Vasculitis

There is no particular pattern seen in vasculitis. Joint involvement is almost exclusively peripheral and it is rare to see axial involvement.

Infectious Arthritis

There is no particular pattern seen in infectious arthritis and any joint can be involved. Sternoclavicular joints are more commonly seen in patients who abuse intravenous illicit drugs and should alert the clinician to this possibility if noted on physical exam. Chronic infections such as TB can affect any joint and when it affects the spine, it is referred to historically as Pott disease.

Further Reading

1. Greenspan A. Orthopedic imaging: a practical approach. 5th ed. Philadelphia: Lippincott Williams and Wilkins; 2011.
2. Hochberg MC, Silman AJ, Smolen JS, Weinblatt ME, Weisman MH, editors. Rheumatology. 5th ed. St. Louis: Mosby; 2011.
3. Klippel JH, Stone JH, Crofford LJ, White PH, editors. Primer on rheumatic disease. 13th ed. Atlanta: Springer, USA: Arthritis Foundation; 2008.

3 Image Analysis

John O'Neill

In order to understand the imaging appearance of normal tissues, it is essential to know the normal internal anatomy of those tissues and what gives rise to the imaging appearance. The following is a brief description of normal MSK anatomy and pathology and its multimodality imaging appearance. With the rapid growth of musculoskeletal ultrasound, we have expanded the description on ultrasound technique.

Muscle

Anatomy

There are three different varieties of muscle found in the human body: skeletal, smooth, and cardiac. This description will focus on the structure and imaging appearance of the skeletal muscle.

Muscle is composed of individual fibers, cylindrical or prismatic in shape. Each fiber in general measures up to 1.5 in. in length and 0.02 in. in breadth. The length of individual fibers is, however, highly variable. A sheath, the sarcolemma, surrounds individual fibers. A bundle of fibers is called a fasciculus. The fasciculi are prismatic in shape and align parallel to one another, oblique or parallel to the longitudinal axis of the muscle. The endomysium, composed of connective tissue, separates individual muscle fibers. It is derived from the perimysium, which envelops the fasciculus, whereas the epimysium invests the entire muscle (Fig. 3.1). Nerves and blood vessels are supported within this connective tissue framework.

Muscles have an origin, a belly, and an insertion. The origin and insertion attachment sites can be multiple including bones, cartilage, ligaments, and skin. By definition, the insertion is the attachment that has the greatest movement on muscle contraction. There are multiple different arrangements of fiber orientation with respect to the tendon including quadrilateral, fusiform, triangular, and pennate, which in turn can be unipennate, bipennate, or multipennate (Fig. 3.2).

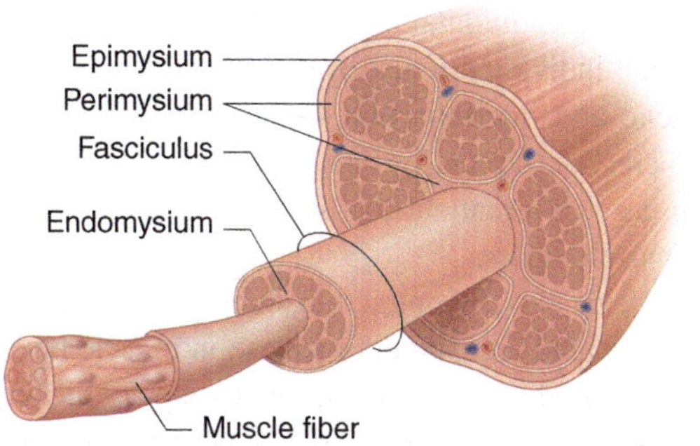

Fig. 3.1 Muscle fiber anatomy: cross-sectional illustration

J. O'Neill, MB, BAO, BCh, MRCPI, MSc, FRCR
Associate Professor, Musculoskeletal Imaging,
Diagnostic Imaging, McMaster University/
St Joseph's Healthcare,
Hamilton, ON L8N4A6, Canada
e-mail: joneill2@me.com

J. O'Neill (ed.), *Essential Imaging in Rheumatology*,
DOI 10.1007/978-1-4939-1673-3_3, © Springer Science+Business Media New York 2015

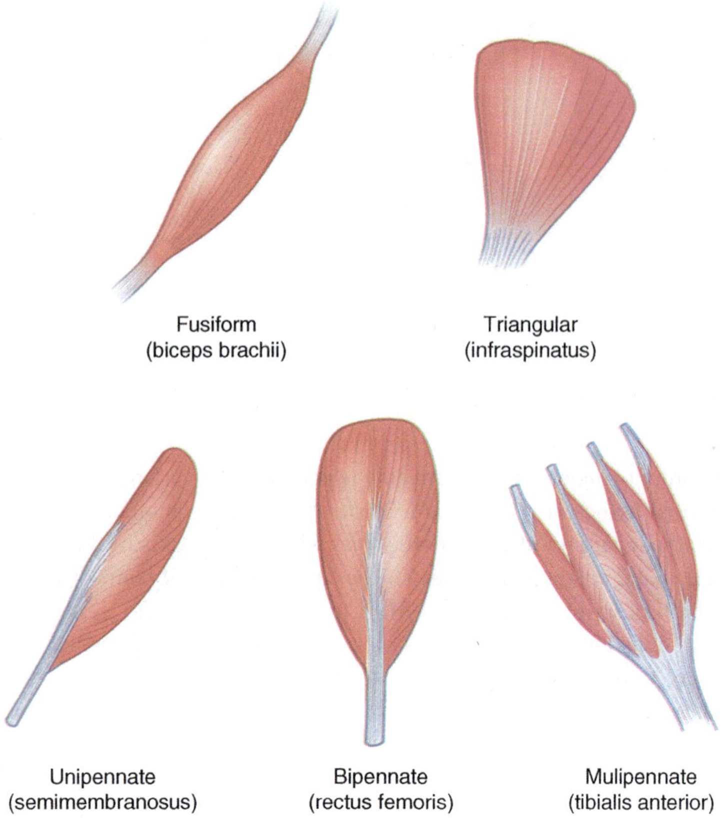

Fig. 3.2 Muscle structure: illustration demonstrating some of the different arrangements of fiber orientation

Ultrasound of Muscle

The fasciculi can be identified as separate structures on ultrasound. They are best identified in the longitudinal plane as hypoechoic cylindrical structures, separated by the hyperechoic intervening connective tissue, the perimysium (Fig. 3.3). Individual fibers and the endomysium are not individually discernible. The epimysium, fascia, and intermuscular fat are all thin linear hyperechoic structures on ultrasound. Ultrasound can also differentiate the different arrangements of muscle fibers.

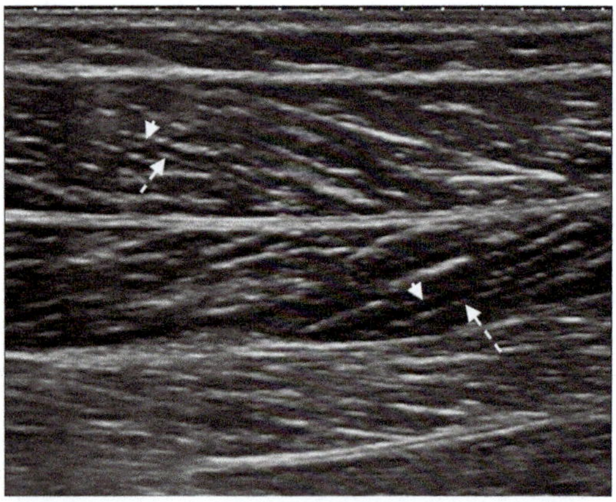

Fig. 3.3 Longitudinal US image of the medial gastrocnemius muscle demonstrating multiple linear hypoechoic cylindrical structures, the fasciculi. A muscle fasciculus (*arrowhead*) is shown separated by the thin hyperechoic intervening connective tissue, the perimysium (*dashed arrow*). Note the bipennate structure of the muscle

During muscle contraction, there is a shortening of fibers and an apparent increase in muscle bulk (Fig. 3.4). The hypoechoic fascicles appear thicker and give a more hypoechoic appearance to the muscle in the contracted state. When comparing the echotexture of the contralateral muscle, it is

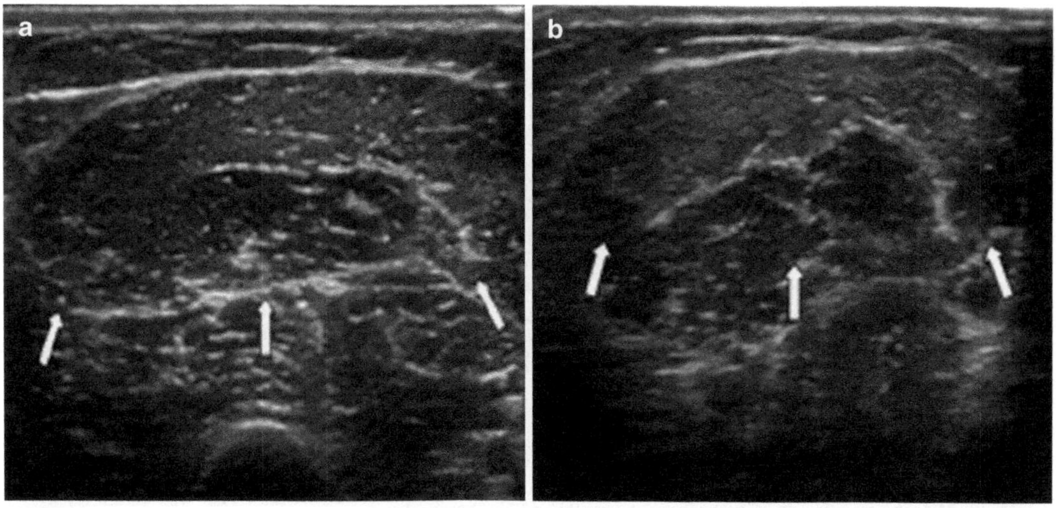

Fig. 3.4 Muscle contraction: transverse US image of the anterior mid-arm biceps muscle, short and long heads (*arrows*), (**a**) pre- and (**b**) post-muscle contraction. In (**b**), there is an apparent increase in muscle bulk and the hypoechoic fascicles appear thicker and slightly more hypoechoic

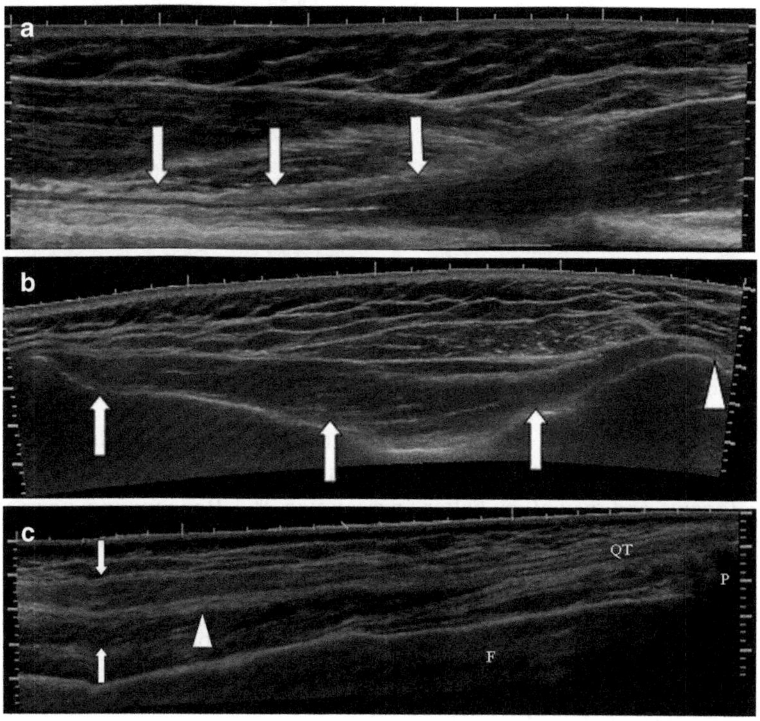

Fig. 3.5 Extended field of view imaging of the (**a**) long head biceps (*arrows*) at the musculotendinous junction, (**b**) Infraspinatus muscle arising from the infraspinous fossa (*arrows*) and inserting onto the greater tuberosity humerus (*arrowhead*) and (**c**) extended field of view rectus femoris at musculotendinous junction, tendon is central (*arrowhead*) surrounded by muscle (*arrows*)

important that they are in the same state of relaxation or contraction. Abnormal contraction patterns may explain different functional capabilities in patients with similar pathology.

In general, linear array transducers are preferred with higher frequencies for superficial muscles. Deeper muscles may require the use of a curvilinear probe with a frequency of 5 MHz to allow for deeper penetration. Extended field of view can allow for the full length of the muscle to be captured on one image (Fig. 3.5). 3-D and 4-D are new applications that are in

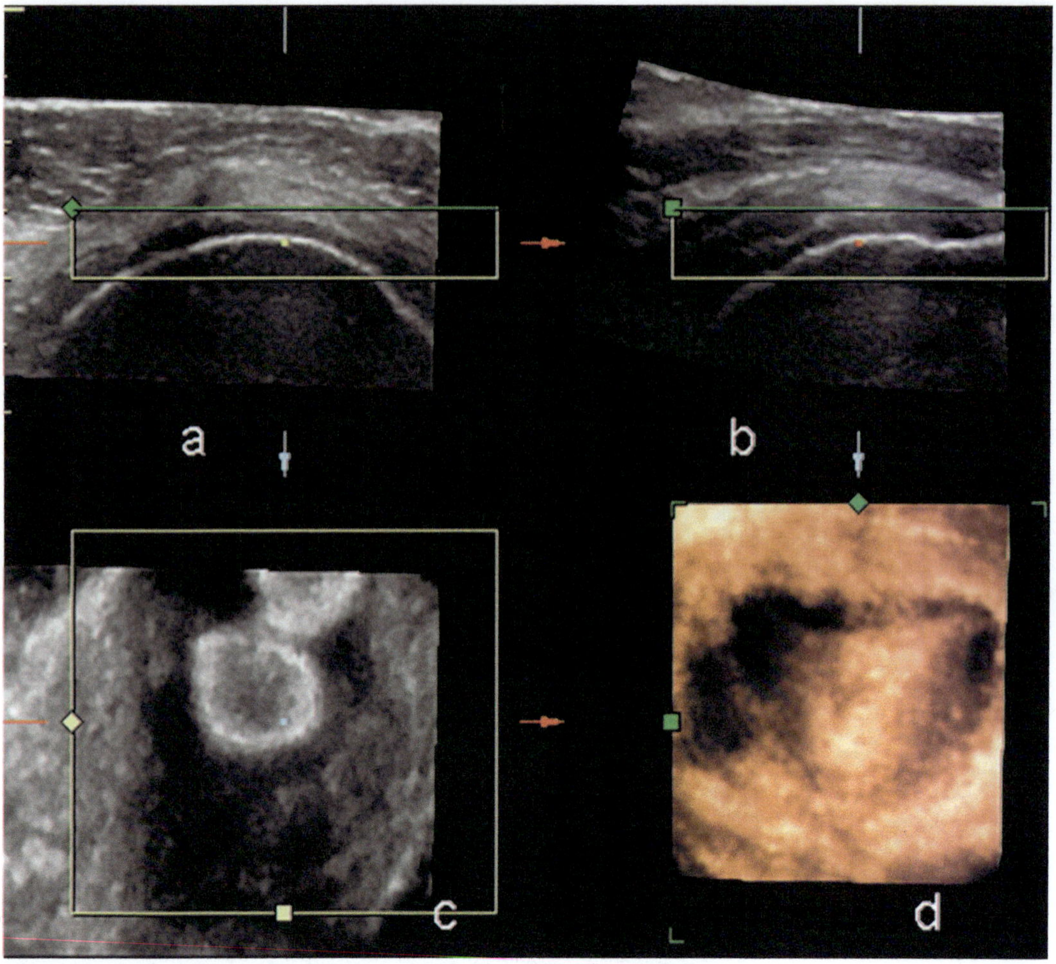

Fig. 3.6 Supraspinatus tendon using 4-D transducer: (**a**) axial, (**b**) sagittal, (**c**) coronal, and (**d**) 3-D reconstruction

their early stages of development in musculoskeletal ultrasound. 3-D will allow multiplanar reformats and may allow better appreciation of the extent of pathology and surrounding anatomical relationships (Fig. 3.6). This may be of particular benefit to clinicians not used to viewing ultrasound images.

Ultrasound Technique

The probe is held perpendicular to the axis of the muscle and scanned in the longitudinal and transverse plane. If the patient has significant point tenderness, we normally scan the area surrounding this point first until we identify a normal ultrasound appearance and then move slowly over the symptomatic region. Recognizing normal anatomy and landmarks will allow for an easier assessment of adjacent pathology. Applying gel liberally and floating the probe over the area of interest to avoid compression are useful techniques in these circumstances. This allows the patient to relax and to tolerate a full study. Comparison to the contralateral side is helpful in delineating subtle abnormalities. Doppler may reveal the presence of normal transversing blood vessels and areas of increased/decreased internal flow in pathology.

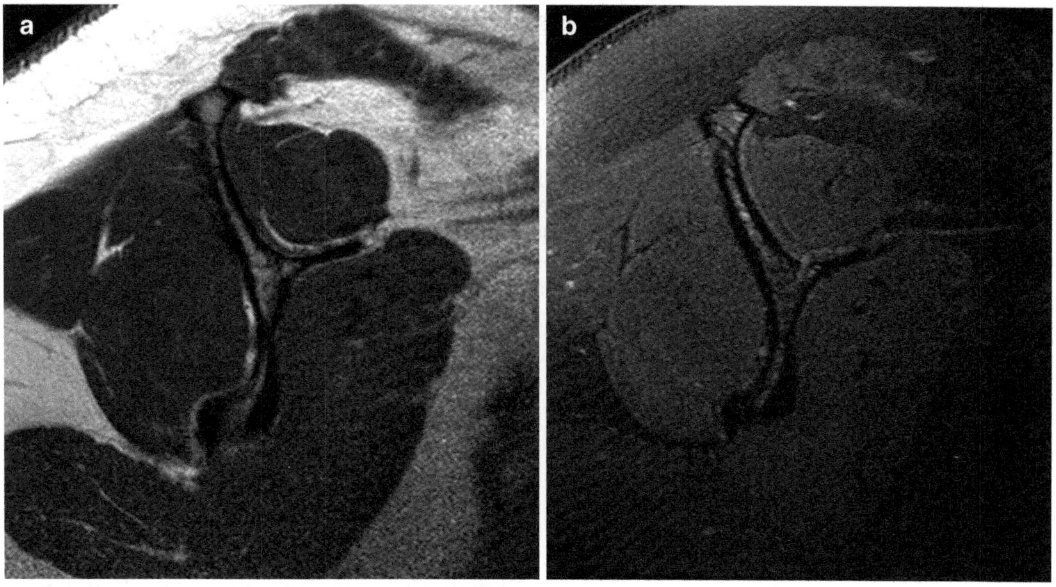

Fig. 3.7 MRI of a normal muscle: (**a**) rotator cuff muscles on T1 and (**b**) T2FS

MRI of the Muscle

The muscle is of intermediate SI on all imaging sequences. Individual fascicles can be appreciated on MRI. Advanced imaging techniques such as diffusion tensor MRI allow for identification of individual fibers and fiber disruption in trauma via tractography, but are not commonly used in daily practice. On T1-weighted sequence, fat is of high SI and is interposed between fascicles, intramuscular, and between different muscles, intermuscular. This imparts a marbled appearance to the muscle (Fig. 3.7). T2 has a similar appearance. With fat saturation there is a decrease in SI due to loss of signal from fat (Fig. 3.7b). It is therefore more difficult to separate different muscle groups with fat saturation. Tendons, depending on muscle type, can be seen as low SI structures, ovoid in cross section and linear in longitudinal plane in relation to the muscle.

Muscle Pathology

Muscle injuries are most common at or just proximal to the myotendinous junction. They can be classified as internal and external. Internal injuries are usually related to contraction, whereas external injuries are related to compression and penetration. In cases where the injury mechanism is not compatible with imaging findings, a predisposing condition such as a benign/malignant lesion or prior injury at the same site should be sought. Injuries can be classified into three grades (Table 3.1, Fig. 3.8). The initial injury site is occupied by hematoma which appears as a complex fluid collection, initially ill-defined interspersed between disrupted muscle fibers and later becoming defined as a localized collection of fluid displacing adjacent muscle fibers.

MRI demonstrates a complex collection; internal signal intensity is variable depending on the age of hematoma. There is no internal enhancement but the capsule may enhance, although contrast is rarely required unless a predisposing intramuscular lesion is suspected. Ultrasound demonstrates a complex collection of heterogeneous echotexture. *Ultrasound* allows for a dynamic evaluation, with the patient actively contracting or the examiner passively moving

Table 3.1 Grading muscular injuries and imaging findings

Grade	Type	Ultrasound findings	MRI
Grade 1	Microscopic tear	Normal or may demonstrate minimal fluid, thickened hypoechoic myotendinous junction	Edema with T2 high SI with feathery appearance, +/– hemorrhage
Grade 2	Partial tear	Partial disruption fibers; defect may be occupied by fluid, hypoechoic or heterogeneous in appearance; fluid may track proximally or distally, exaggerating the true size of injury	Fiber disruption of up to 50 % with focal defect filled with high T2 SI fluid/hemorrhage, surrounding edema
Grade 3	Complete tear	Complete disruption fibers, proximal muscle retraction, defect occupied initially by fluid (hematoma)	High SI T2 fluid-filled defect, +/– retraction

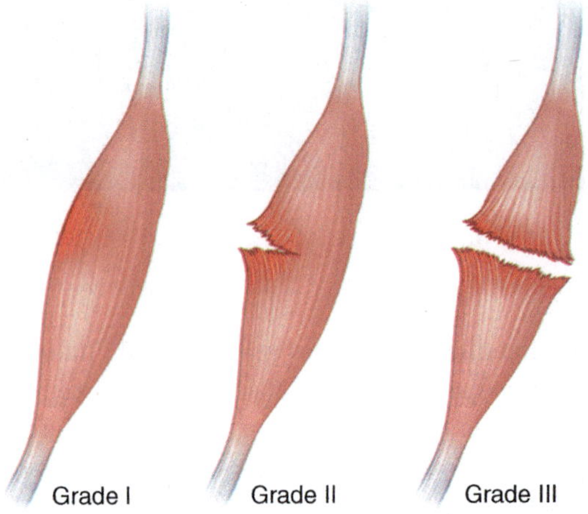

Fig. 3.8 Grading muscular injuries

and stretching the muscle of interest, which can allow for assessment of contraction patterns and aid in identifying the full extent of a muscle tear. Both imaging studies demonstrate related fiber disruption; however, this may be best appreciated on ultrasound in superficial injuries. *CT* is of limited value given limited soft tissue differentiation compared to MRI and ultrasound, and in addition it incurs a significant radiation dose. A low attenuating fluid collection and muscle defect can be identified albeit at a lower resolution and sensitivity than above imaging studies. *Radiography* may demonstrate localized ill-defined soft tissue thickening if involving the appendicular skeleton with loss of fat planes. Nuclear medicine studies are not indicated.

The hematoma eventually reabsorbs and depending on the severity of the injury and subsequent treatment will either heal or undergo fibrosis and scarring. Fibrosis on ultrasound appears as irregular hyperechoic foci with volume loss and areas of low signal intensity on MRI. In severe partial or complete tears, the muscle may become atrophied and undergo fatty degeneration. Comparison with the contralateral side, presuming that this is normal, allows for accurate assessment atrophy where there is visible loss of volume on ultrasound. A cross-sectional measurement comparison can be made for estimation. Fatty degeneration demonstrates increased echotexture compared to the normal hypoechoic muscle on ultrasound. Fatty atrophy is best assessed on T1-weighted MRI in orthogonal plane to the muscle (Fig. 3.9). This can be divided into four grades (Table 3.2).

Pyomyositis, a suppurative bacterial infection of the muscle, most often occurs in the immunocompromised patient. This is reviewed in detail in Chap. 13. *Staphylococcus aureus* is the most commonly isolated organism. *Ultrasound* findings depend on the stage of presentation and whether an abscess has formed. Initially the muscle is tender on probe placement and is swollen with a hyperechoic echotexture (Fig. 3.10). Later, as areas of necrosis and abscesses develop, hypoechoic foci become evident. An *abscess* has developed when these foci have a defined wall. They demonstrate increased through transmission, i.e., tissues directly posterior to the abscess demonstrate increased echotexture in comparison to adjacent similar tissue at the same depth (Fig. 3.11). The abscess is usually of heterogeneous echotexture. Doppler will demonstrate increased flow within the adjacent muscle and within the wall of the abscess. *MRI* demonstrates

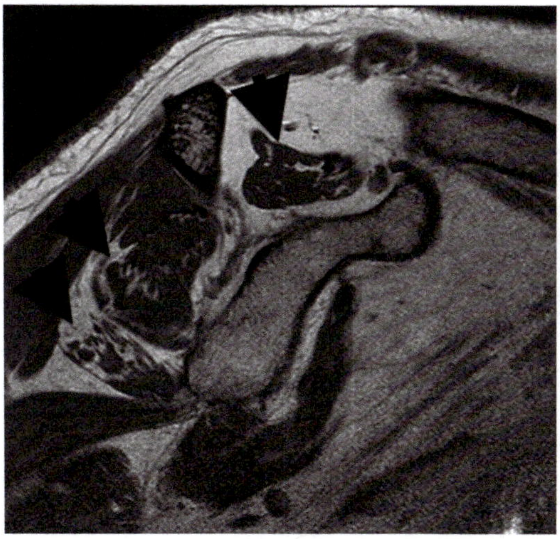

Fig. 3.9 Sag T1 rotator cuff muscles demonstrating atrophy and fatty infiltration (*black arrowheads*) of the supraspinatus, lower infraspinatus, and teres minor and atrophy without fatty infiltration of the subscapularis. See Fig. 3.7 for normal appearance

Table 3.2 Grading muscle fat infiltration

Grade 0	Normal
Grade 1	Volume fatty tissue less than residual normal muscle
Grade 2	Volume fatty tissue equal to residual normal muscle
Grade 3	Volume fatty tissue greater than residual normal muscle

ill-defined edema as high SI on T2-weighted sequences, best appreciated with fat saturation or STIR. This is of low SI on T1. The muscle may be enlarged and fluid appears as linear high SI on T2 along fascial planes. Abscess formation appears as a heterogeneous encapsulated lesion of low SI on T1 and high SI on T2 with rim enhancement with contrast (Fig. 3.11). It may demonstrate restricted diffusion on diffusion-weighted imaging (DWI). *CT* is limited in assessment and may demonstrate an enlarged muscle with low-attenuation cystic lesion with rim enhancement.

Plain radiography demonstrates no specific findings and may be normal. Soft tissue swelling may be present with loss of fat planes. Radiographs are useful for assessment of superficial or deep soft tissue air. *Nuclear medicine* with use of indium-labeled white cells can localize sites of infection but incurs a significant radiation dose and is not commonly used if nonionizing modalities are available. Differential diagnosis in diabetic patients includes *muscle infarction*, usually in poorly controlled diabetes. This most commonly involves the thigh musculature and presents with severe pain and muscle enlargement. MRI demonstrates diffuse edema with possible hemorrhage. If contrast is given, non-enhancing areas may be seen with surrounding rim enhancement in keeping with an area of infarction.

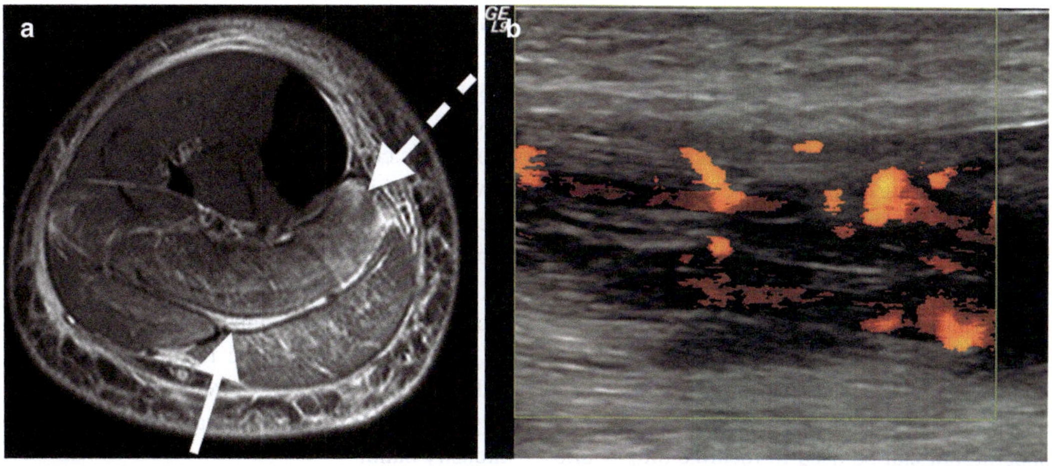

Fig. 3.10 Pyomyositis: (**a**) axial T2FS MRI in patient with pyomyositis with diffuse increased muscular edema (*dashed arrow*) and fascial fluid (*arrow*) and (**b**) longitudinal ultrasound image with power Doppler demonstrating hypoechoic muscle with marked increase flow

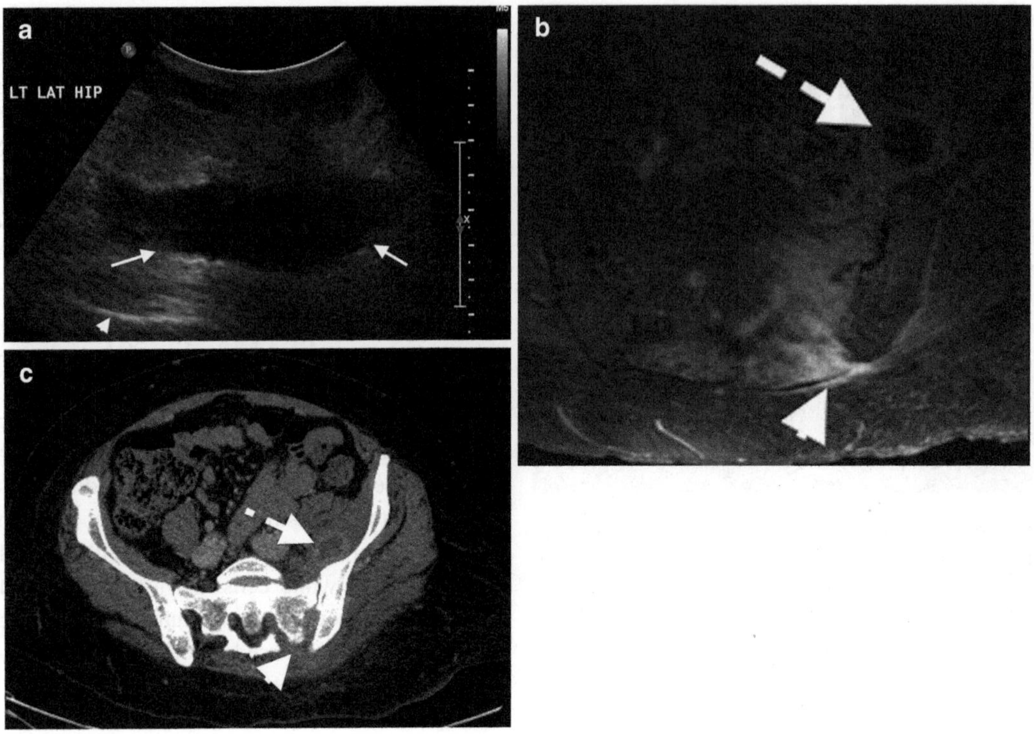

Fig. 3.11 Abscess: (**a**) soft tissue abscess over the left hip on ultrasound demonstrating a hypoechoic walled-off collection (*arrows*), (**b**) axial T1FS post-contrast MRI of septic arthritis on the left sacroiliac joint (*arrowhead*) with anterior abscess with central low signal intensity (*dashed arrow*) and surrounding enhancing muscle, pyomyositis, and corresponding CT on the same patient, and (**c**) with rim enhancement iliacus abscess

Idiopathic Inflammatory Myopathies

This group includes dermatomyositis, polymyositis, and sporadic inclusion body myositis. *MRI* is the imaging gold standard. Sporadic areas of increased ill-defined edema, depicted best on T2 fat-saturated sequences, are noted, usually affecting several muscle groups and most often involving the shoulder or pelvic girdle. MRI is useful for directing biopsy sites. Chronic disease demonstrates areas of atrophy and fatty infiltration. This is reviewed in detail in Chap. 7. *Ultrasound* may demonstrate muscle edema as areas of increased echotexture with increased flow on Doppler. Ultrasound findings are nonspecific but can be used to localize biopsy sites when correlated with MRI. CT and plain radiography have no role in the primary imaging of myopathies.

Fascia

Anatomy

Fasciae are divided into superficial and deep fasciae. The superficial fascia lies deep to the skin and is composed of fibroareolar tissue. It is of variable thickness and connects the skin to the deep fascia. The superficial fascia may contain superficial muscles or serve as attachment, e.g., platysma myoides. On *ultrasound*, the appearance of superficial fascia is determined by the content of adipose tissue, hypoechoic, and separated by thin hyperechoic linear bands (Fig. 3.12). MRI demonstrates a low signal intensity band.

The deep fascia is a dense fibrous membrane that invests muscles and deeper structures. It is of variable thickness, becoming thicker on more

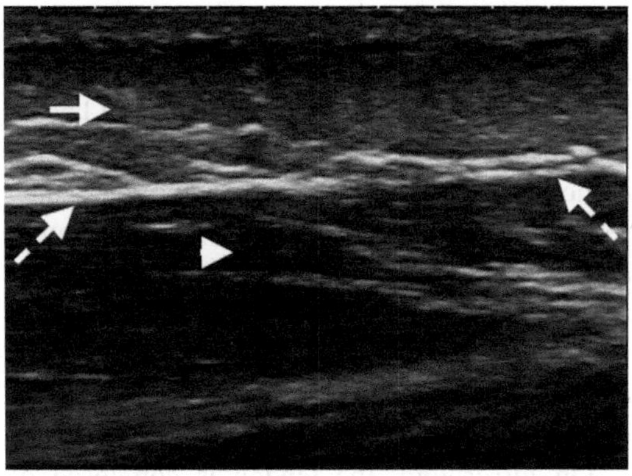

Fig. 3.12 Fascia: longitudinal US image of the proximal thigh demonstrating the superficial fascia containing adipose tissue (*arrow*) separated by thin hyperechoic linear bands. The deep fascia (*dashed arrows*) is thin and hyperechoic, enclosing the deeper hypoechoic muscle (*arrowhead*)

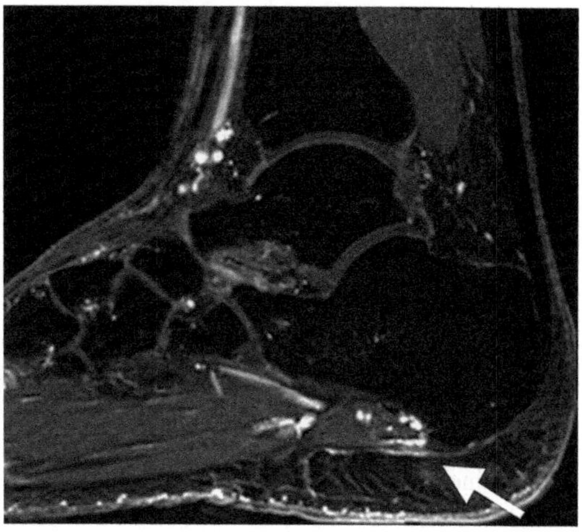

Fig. 3.13 Plantar fasciitis on Sag T2FS MRI of the right ankle with thickened plantar fascia of high signal intensity (*arrow*) at calcaneal attachment

exposed regions; e.g., it is thicker on the lateral aspect of the leg versus the medial aspect. It forms a sheath for muscles and occasionally as a site of attachment. It gives off the intermuscular septa, which separate various muscles and compartments and attach to the periosteum. In the regions of joints, the deep fascia can become thickened to form the retinacula, as part of fibro-osseous tunnels, maintaining the underlying tendons and nerves in place. On *ultrasound*, the deep fascia is hyperechoic with an identifiable fibrillar pattern of variable thickness. The hyperechoic intermuscular septa can be seen arising from the fascia. *MRI* demonstrates the deep fascia as low signal intensity on all imaging sequences. CT can identify fascia, fascial thickening, and perifascial fluid but is less sensitive than MRI; however, CT is excellent at detecting air. NM has no role in imaging fascia.

Fascial Pathology

Plantar fasciitis is a common condition with inflammation of the plantar fascia at its calcaneal origin. It can be diagnosed with ultrasound or MRI (Fig. 3.13). *Necrotizing fasciitis* is a bacterial infection of the soft tissues that causes rapid tissue necrosis and rapidly spreads via fascial planes. It can be mono- or polymicrobial and may result from minor injuries. If it is clinically diagnosed, surgical debridement should not be delayed. MRI is the gold imaging standard and demonstrates fluid signal intensity along thickened fascial planes with adjacent edema of the musculature. Cellulitis on the other hand demonstrates edema confined to the subcutaneous tissues. CT may demonstrate thickening along fascial planes but is less sensitive than MRI but may demonstrate soft tissue air bubbles, which may not be appreciated on MRI. Radiographs may identify air within the soft tissues. Ultrasound and NM have no primary role in imaging necrotizing fasciitis. Necrotizing fasciitis is reviewed in detail in Chap. 13.

Eosinophilic fasciitis, Shulman's syndrome, is a rare disorder. It is a localized scleroderma-like disease with bilateral peripheral symmetrical skin induration associated with peripheral eosinophilia. MRI is again the gold imaging standard and demonstrates fascial thickening on T1, high SI on T2FS or STIR sequences, and marked enhancement post contrast. MRI findings correlate with disease activity. Ultrasound can be cross-referenced with MRI using bony landmarks and is useful for localizing a biopsy site. Eosinophilic fasciitis is reviewed in detail in Chap. 7.

Tendon

Anatomy

Tendons are composed of tightly packed type I collagen fibers with intervening fibroblasts. Bundles of parallel fibers form primary (subfascicle), secondary (fascicle), and tertiary bundles. They are loosely bound in a loose connective tissue sheath, the endotendineum, and the peritendinal connective tissue. The latter encloses several subfascicles to form a fascicle. The peritendineum also contains the supplying blood vessels and nerves. The epitendineum is a thicker fibroelastic sheath surrounding the whole tendon. At the musculotendinous junction, the sarcolemma intervenes, i.e., there is no direct continuity of muscle and tendon fibers. At the attachment site to bone, the tendon fibers attach to the periosteum, to the fibrocartilage, or directly to the bone. Tendons can also insert onto fascia. Tendons can be round (e.g., biceps), oval (e.g., Achilles), or flattened (e.g., patellar tendon) in cross section. They are surrounded by a synovial sheath in regions that are exposed to friction on motion. The synovial sheath is composed of two layers, one of which is reflected along the surface of the tendon. The sheath contains synovium, which secretes a thick viscid fluid to reduce friction and encourages smooth gliding of the tendon. In areas where a synovial sheath is not required, the tendon is surrounded by the paratenon, a layer of loose connective tissue encasing the epitendineum (e.g., Achilles tendon).

On *ultrasound*, the tendon is composed of dense linear hyperechoic bands forming a fibrillar pattern, when evaluated in the tendon's longitudinal axis (Fig. 3.14). On transverse images, the tendon is hyperechoic with multiple hyperechoic foci or dots. The hyperechoic appearance is due to the specular reflections at the interface between the fascicles and the peritendineum. Normal tendons are not compressible. The paratenon is identified as a thin hyperechoic line surrounding the tendon (Fig. 3.14b). The synovial sheath is best visualized when fluid is present between

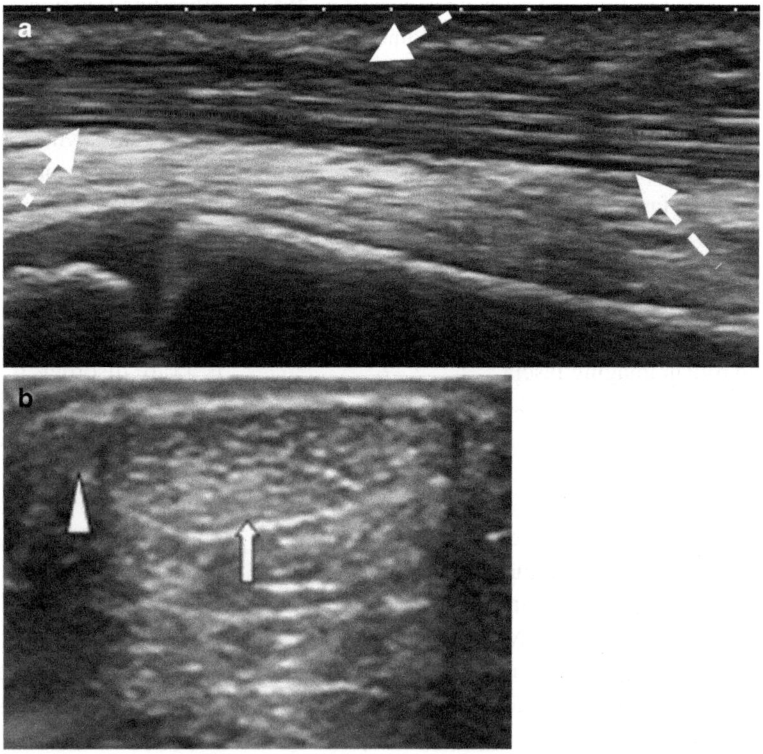

Fig. 3.14 Ultrasound of the tendon: (**a**) longitudinal ultrasound of the tibialis anterior with normal fibrillar pattern and (**b**) transverse US image of the oval Achilles tendon (A) (*arrow*) and adjacent plantaris tendon (*arrowhead*) medially; the paratenon is identified as the thin hyperechoic rim surrounding the AT

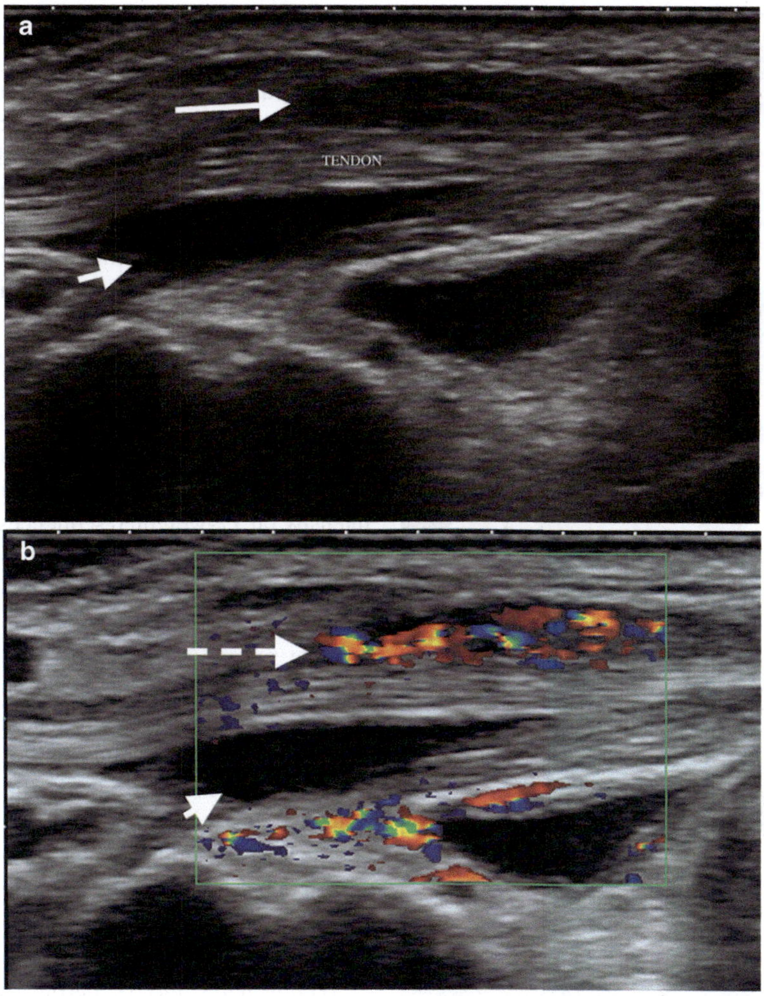

Fig. 3.15 Fourth extensor compartment tenosynovitis of the wrist on ultrasound: (**a**) tendons surrounded by fluid (anechoic, *short arrow*) and soft tissue thickening/synovial proliferation (*long arrow*) which demonstrates increased flow on Doppler (*dashed arrow*) (**b**)

its layers (Fig. 3.15). A small amount of fluid may normally be present. In some tendons, the fibers have to change course slightly prior and at insertion and often appear hypoechoic due to anisotropy. Realigning the transducer so it is perpendicular to the change in orientation will resolve most of the hypoechoic appearance in normal tendons; the remaining hypoechoic appearance is related to the interdigitating fibrocartilage.

On MRI, tendons are of low SI on all imaging sequences (Fig. 3.16). Magic angle is a common MRI imaging artifact and occurs when a structure, commonly tendons and ligaments, lies at 55° to the main magnetic field. This creates apparent increased SI within the tissue, simulating pathology. Common sites are the critical zone of the supraspinatus tendon proximal to its insertion onto the greater tuberosity, the proximal patellar tendon, and the peroneal tendons as they course under the lateral malleolus (Fig. 3.17). Magic angle is present only on sequences with a short TE such as T1, PD, and GE. Magic angle is not evident on long TE sequences such as T2 and STIR, and this allows differentiation from true pathology.

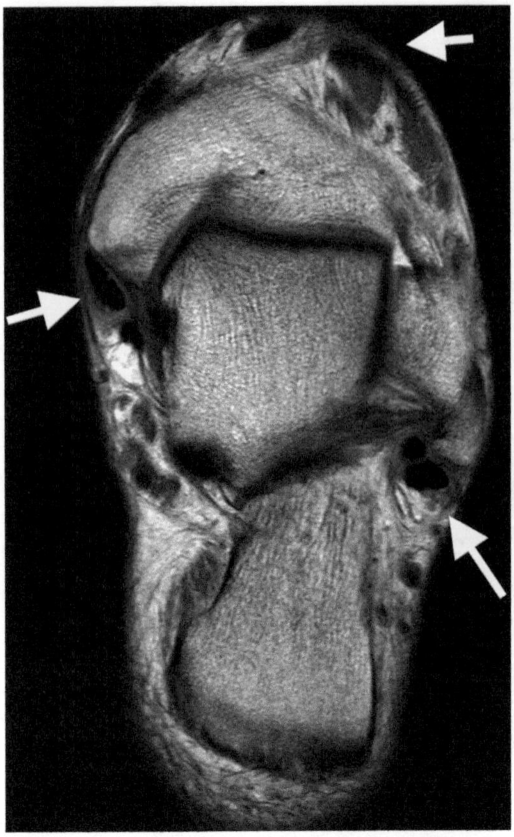

Fig. 3.16 Axial oblique T2 MRI image of the ankle demonstrating multiple round and oval low signal intensity normal tendons (*arrows*)

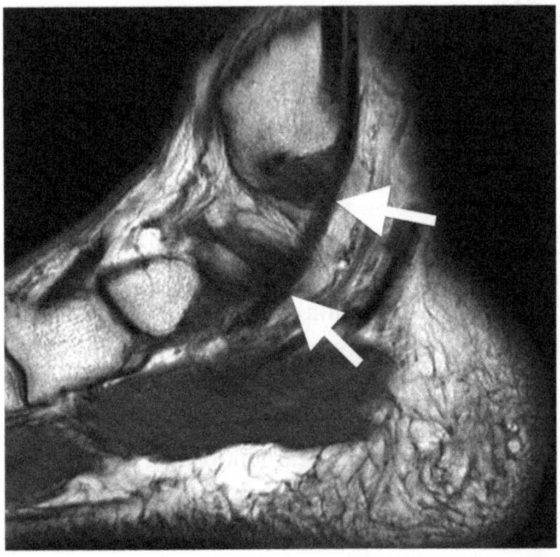

Fig. 3.17 Magic angle effect on Sag T1 ankle: tendon (*arrows*) appears of increased signal, intermediate signal intensity, but remains of normal signal on Sag T2 (not shown). See text for full explanation of magic angle

Tendon Pathology

Tendinopathy or tendinosis refers to tendon degeneration and is usually hypoxic or myxoid in origin. The term tendinitis is usually avoided, as there is usually no acute inflammatory component. On *ultrasound*, the tendon may be enlarged, be attenuated, or be of normal caliber. The normal fibrillar pattern is usually lost and is replaced by hypoechogenicity (Fig. 3.18). The tendon may demonstrate increased internal flow on Doppler interrogation. Comparison with the contralateral tendon can be helpful to identify subtle findings. On *MRI*, the tendon may be enlarged, be attenuated, or be of normal caliber. Increased internal signal intensity on T2-weighted sequences is in keeping with increased water content (Fig. 3.19). Post-gadolinium imaging demonstrates abnormal enhancement within the tendon and may also demonstrate enhancement of the tendon sheath or paratenon. Note that enhanced studies are not required for the diagnosis of tendinopathy. *CT* is not as sensitive or specific as ultrasound or MRI in assessing morphological change. It may demonstrate tendon enlargement, attenuation, split tendons, or complete tears. Current imaging description will therefore concentrate on ultrasound and MRI imaging appearances of tendon pathology.

Tendon tears may be partial, full thickness, or complete (Fig. 3.20). Partial tears may be contained within the tendon, interstitial tears. Interstitial tears on *ultrasound* are identified as a

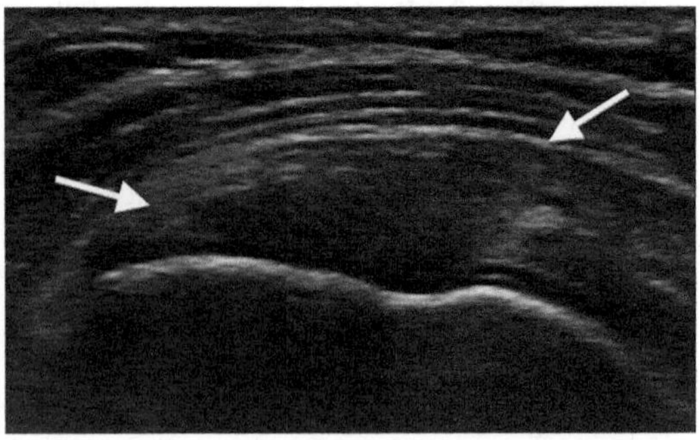

Fig. 3.18 Tendinosis on ultrasound: there is loss of the normal fibrillar pattern in this supraspinatus tendon (*arrows*) with generalized hypoechogenicity

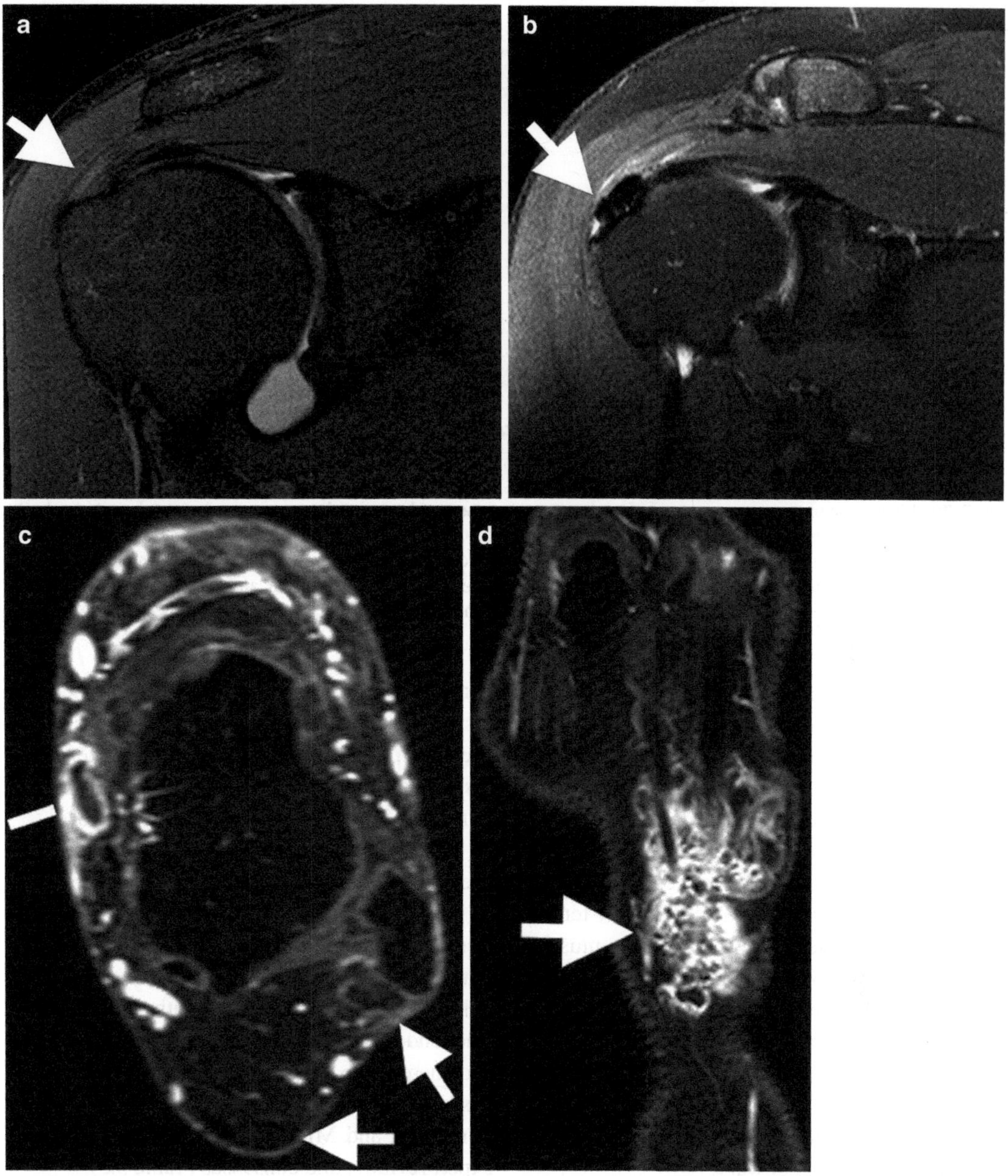

Fig. 3.19 Tendinosis on MRI; (**a**) mild tendinosis of the supraspinatus tendon with mild increased signal on Cor T2FS (*arrow*), (**b**) calcific tendinosis of the supraspinatus with calcium deposit of low signal (*arrow*) on Cor T2FS, and (**c**) axial T1FS post contrast tendinosis (*arrows*) demonstrated by heterogenous tendons of increased signal and tenosynovitis (*line*). (**d**) Cor T1FS post contrast of the wrist in a patient with rheumatoid arthritis demonstrating enhancing, active, tenosynovitis on the fourth extensor compartment with internal low signal intensity bodies, "rice bodies" (*arrow*)

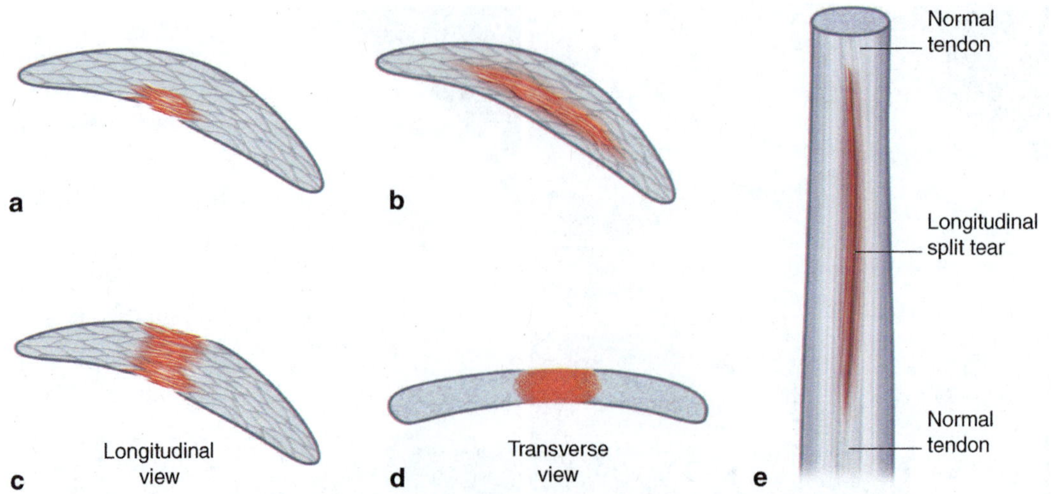

Fig. 3.20 Illustration of the common types of tendon tears: (**a**) partial-thickness tear, may be from superficial or deep surface. (**b**) Interstitial tear, does not extend to surface tendon. (**c**) Full-thickness tear in longitudinal axis: tear extends from superficial to deep margin; some tendon fibers remain intact as shown in (**d**) transverse axis. (**e**) A longitudinal split tendon where there are two or more tendon bundles. Other tendon tears include a complete tear with no residual intact fibers, an attenuated tendon, and tendon avulsion from bony attachment with or without avulsed bony component

hypoechoic or anechoic cleft within the tendon. On *MRI*, linear internal clefts of fluid signal intensity are identified (Fig. 3.21). Tears may progress and develop a longitudinal split of the tendon. Ultrasound and MRI will then demonstrate more than one tendon bundle. The number of tendon bundles, percentage of involved tendinous fibers, and positional relationship to the parent tendon should be noted. Be aware of accessory muscles and tendons which can simulate a split tear, e.g., peroneus quadratus is an accessory tendon adjacent to the peroneus longus and brevis at the level of the lateral malleolus and usually inserts upon the calcaneus and has its own muscle belly. It may simulate a tear of the peroneus brevis or longus tendons to the unwary.

Alternatively the tear may extend and involve the superficial fibers, a surfacing partial tear. Ultrasound and MRI both demonstrate fiber discontinuity. The defect may be occupied by granulation tissue or fluid. The defect appears hypoechoic/anechoic on ultrasound and demonstrates a fluid signal intensity defect on MRI. A full thickness tear requires extension to the opposite tendon surfaces, e.g., superficial to deep surface. It implies however that some tendinous fibers remain intact. Tendon tear area should be measured in orthogonal planes and include the percentage of fibers involved. When all fibers are disrupted, it is termed a complete tear. Measurement retraction between the tendon ends, residual distal tendon fibers remaining attached to bone, and bony avulsions should be assessed.

Tenosynovitis is active distension of the tendon sheath with fluid or synovium. Fluid may normally be present in tendon sheaths but is usually minimal. Some tendon sheaths communicate with joints and may have significant fluid within, e.g., flexor hallucis longus communicates with the ankle joint. The tendon sheath in these cases is not thickened and there is no synovial thickening. OMERACT has developed definitions for tenosynovitis on ultrasound and MRI based on literature reviews, expert reviews, and consensus (Table 3.3).

In tendons without a tendon sheath, a *paratenon* is present and may demonstrate similar changes in peritendinitis as seen in tenosynovitis. On ultrasound, fluid may partially or completely surround the tendon with or without increased peritendinous flow on Doppler (Fig. 3.23). OMERACT defines peritendinitis on MRI as signal characteristics consistent with increased water content or abnormal post-gadolinium enhancement adjacent to a tendon, in an area without a tendon sheath. The *entheseal complex*, the site of union of the tendon or ligament to the bone, can be patho-

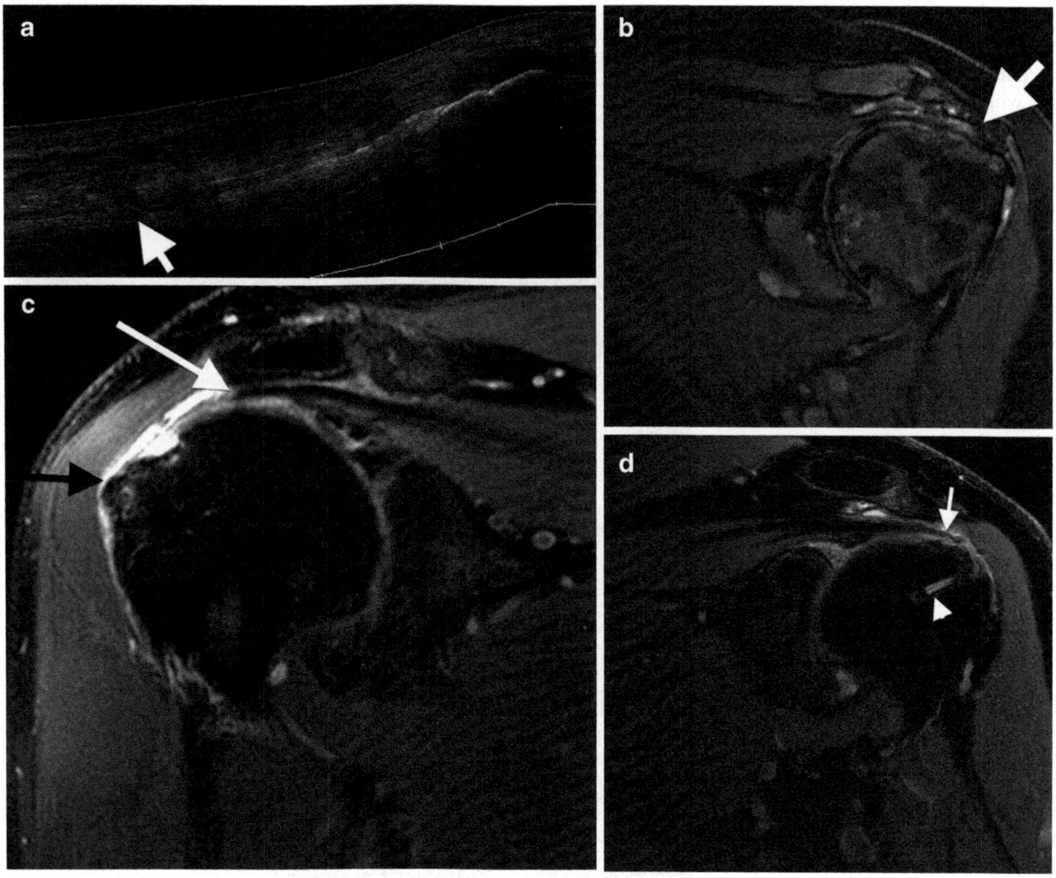

Fig. 3.21 Tendon tears: (**a**) extended field-of-view longitudinal ultrasound image of a tendinotic Achilles tendon with proximal partial thickness tear (*arrow*). Cor T2FS MRI images of (**b**) the left shoulder in a patient with long-standing rheumatoid arthritis with secondary degenerative changes demonstrating attenuation, and tendinosis of the supraspinatus tendon. (**c**) Full-thickness tear of the supraspinatus with tendon retraction (*white arrow*) and bursal distension (*black arrow*). (**d**) Recurrent full-thickness tear of the supraspinatus (*arrow*); note the suture (*arrowhead*)

logically involved in many conditions and is commonly involved in seronegative arthropathies. Radiographs may demonstrate bone erosions or new bone formations (enthesophytes) extending from the enthesis into the distal tendon. There may be loss of definition of the tendon and fat planes and adjacent increased soft tissue attenuation at sites of known bursae. MRI features include thickening distal tendon at bone attachment and increased internal signal intensity on T2, which may enhance post gadolinium. The bone may demonstrate erosion and adjacent bone marrow edema close to the attachment site, which may enhance post gadolinium with/without adjacent bursal distension. This is reviewed in greater detail in Chap. 5.

Table 3.3 OMERACT ultrasound and MRI definitions

Hypoechoic or anechoic thickened tissue with or without fluid within the tendon sheath, which is seen in two perpendicular planes and which may exhibit Doppler signal (Fig. 3.22). *OMERACT ultrasound definition of tenosynovitis*
Signal characteristics consistent with increased water content, high SI on T2FS/STIR and low SI on T1, or abnormal post-Gd enhancement of a thickness greater than the width of the normal synovium. *OMERACT MRI definition of tenosynovitis*
Abnormally hypoechoic and/or thickened tendon or ligament at its bony attachment seen in two perpendicular planes that may exhibit Doppler signal and/or bony changes including enthesophytes, erosions, or irregularity. Tendon may occasionally contain hyperechoic foci consistent with calcification. *OMERACT ultrasound definition of enthesitis*

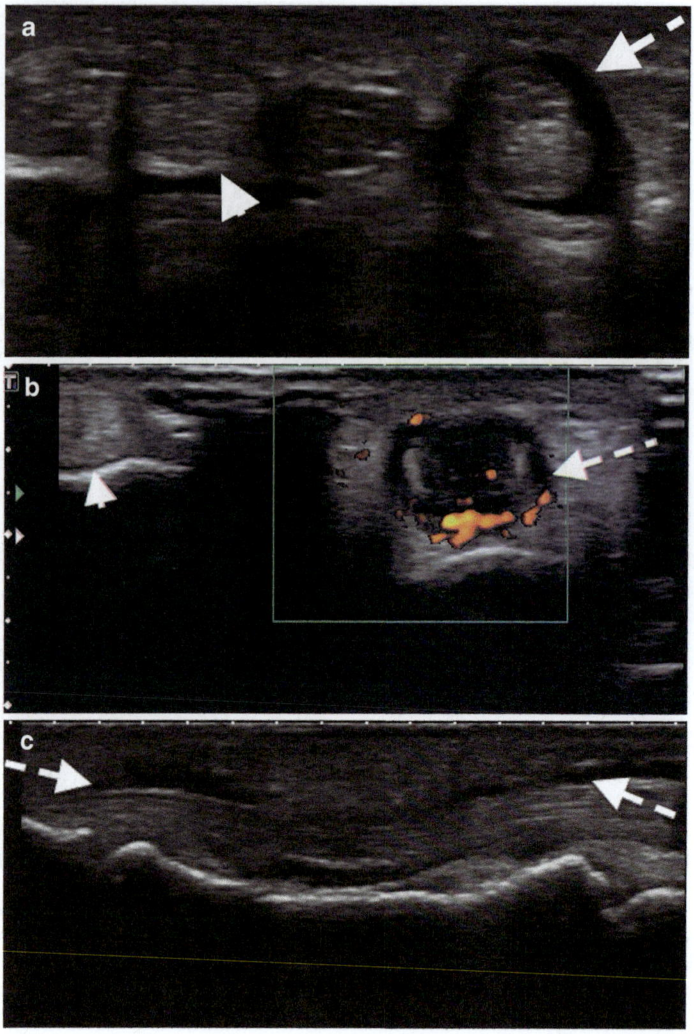

Fig. 3.22 Ultrasound of the third common flexor tendons – (**a**) transverse, (**b**) with power Doppler, and (**c**) longitudinal – demonstrating fluid distension tendon sheath (*dashed arrow*) surrounding the tendon with increased peritendinous flow on Doppler. Note normal second common flexor tendon and sheath (*arrowhead*)

Calcific tendinosis commonly occurs in hydroxyapatite crystal deposition disease (HADD) and calcium pyrophosphate deposition disease (CPPD). The imaging findings are described in detail in Chap. 8. Tendon calcification usually commences as periarticular amorphous cloud-like calcification and gradually becomes more defined and denser. Calcification may change in size and shape over time, may be reabsorbed, and may occasionally reappear. There are four recognized stages: formative, calcific, resorptive, and reparative. Patients may or may not be symptomatic during these phases. The periarticular soft tissues of the shoulder are commonly involved, particularly the supraspinatus. This can be identified on *radiograph* as focal calcification overlying the greater tuberosity on external rotation. *Ultrasound* demonstrates hyperechoic foci within a tendon, usually close to insertion (Fig. 3.24). Depending on the formative stage, the calcification may be cloud-like without posterior shadowing, well-defined hyperechoic foci with posterior shadowing, or hyperechoic foci without shadowing. Documenting whether the patient is symptomatic directly over the area of calcification during the ultrasound examination may be helpful in determining whether the calcific tendinosis is the cause of symptoms. Ultrasound can also identify the underlying cortical changes and any related bursitis.

CT is rarely required in the diagnosis of calcific tendinosis and is more often identified as an incidental finding. Depending on the phase of development, calcification is identified within tendons but may also be seen within ligaments and intra-articularly as amorphous and heterogeneous or well-defined solid calcification. *MRI* is somewhat limited in the evaluation of tendinous calcification as tendon and calcific deposits will both be of low signal intensity on T1- and T2-weighted sequences and are best visualized on sequences that demonstrate the susceptibility artifact of calcification such as gradient echo sequence whereby the calcification will demonstrate significant decreased SI and will appear black (Fig. 3.19b).

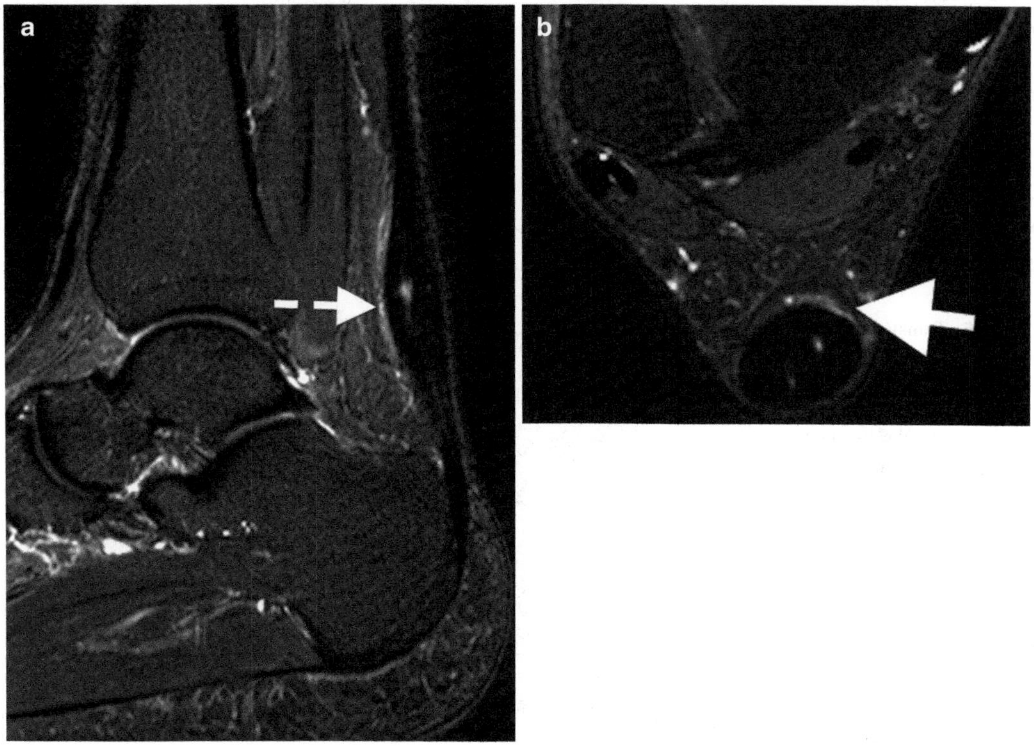

Fig. 3.23 MRI of a tendinotic Achilles tendon: (**a**) Sag and (**b**) axial T2FS of a thickened mid-tendon with interstitial tear and anterior margin rim of high signal intensity (*dashed arrow*) of the paratenon in keeping with peritendinitis

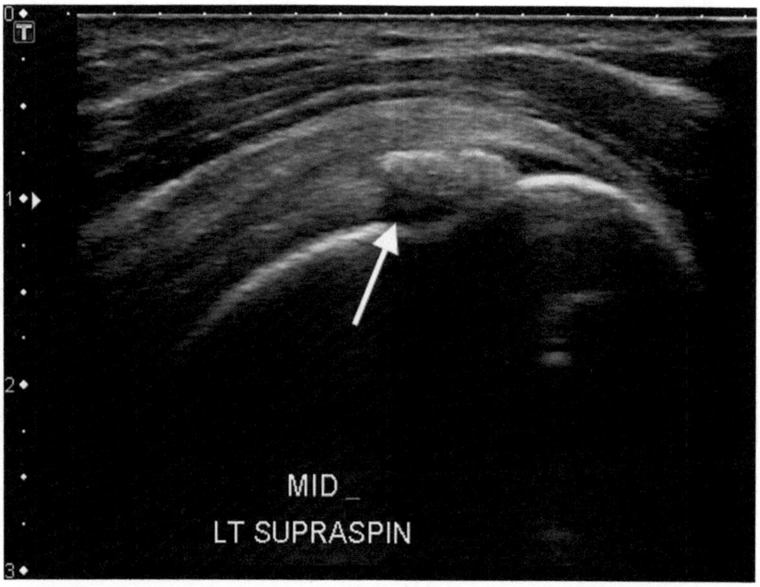

Fig. 3.24 Ultrasound of a calcific tendinosis of the supraspinatus tendon demonstrating internal echogenic focus with posterior shadowing (*arrow*)

Ligament

Anatomy

Ligaments are fibrous structures with histology similar to tendons. They are usually, but not exclusively, situated around joints and attach bone to bone, helping to maintain correct joint position, stability, and alignment. Their attachment to the bone, like tendons, is an enthesis. Ligaments can be well-defined structures easily visualized on ultrasound, e.g., medial collateral ligament of the knee, or represent focal thickening of the joint capsule and may not be discernible as separate structures on ultrasound.

On *ultrasound*, ligaments have a hyperechoic linear appearance. They are often better visualized when they are stretched; e.g., the anterior talofibular ligament is stretched by mild plantar flexion foot and medial orientation forefoot (Fig. 3.25). Linear array transducers with high frequency are optimal. Smaller footpads allow for better manipulation of the transducer along the path of the ligament. Ligaments on *MRI* have a similar imaging appearance to tendons and are of low SI on all imaging sequences and have uniform thickness. As indicated above they are also prone to magic angle artifact. The anterior cruciate ligament of the knee is an exception to the standard low SI and has a striated appearance (Fig. 3.26).

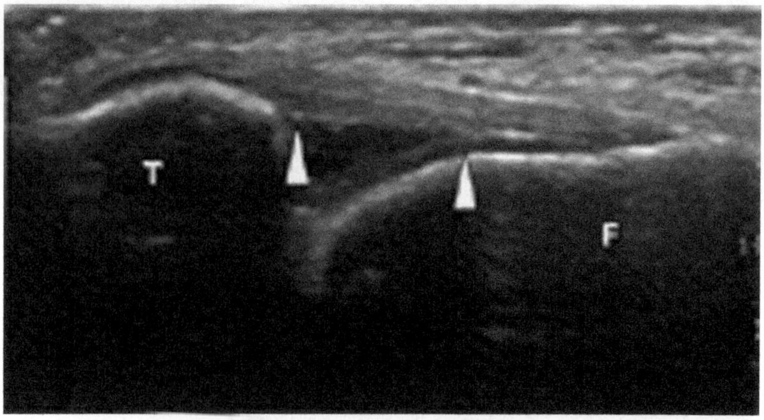

Fig. 3.25 Transverse oblique US of the distal tibiofibular joint in the longitudinal axis of the anterior talofibular ligament (*arrowheads*). *T* talus, *F* fibula

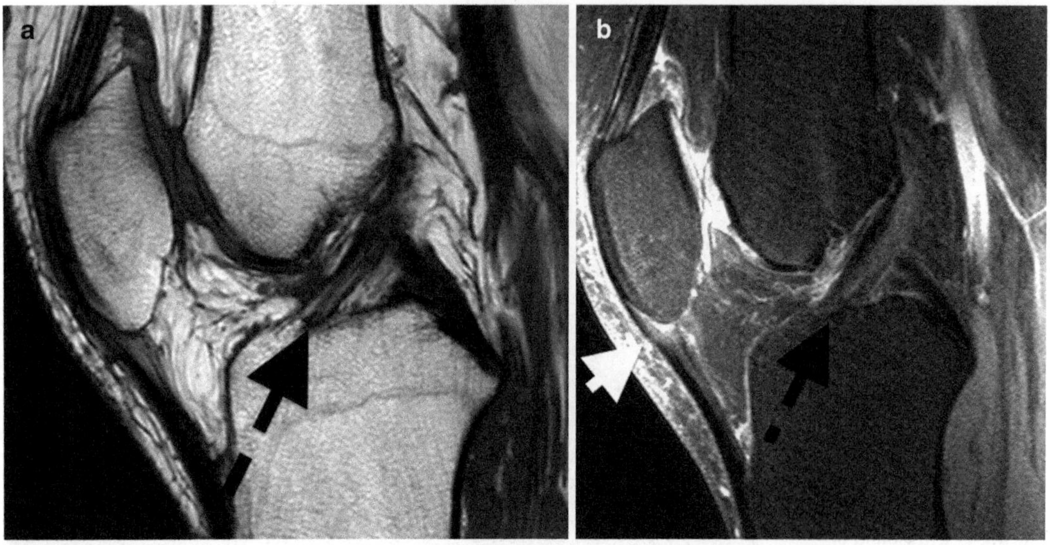

Fig. 3.26 ACL striated appearance (*dashed arrows*) on Sag (**a**) T1 and (**b**) T2FS MRI. Note also tendinosis and partial deep surface tear of the proximal patellar tendon (*white arrow*)

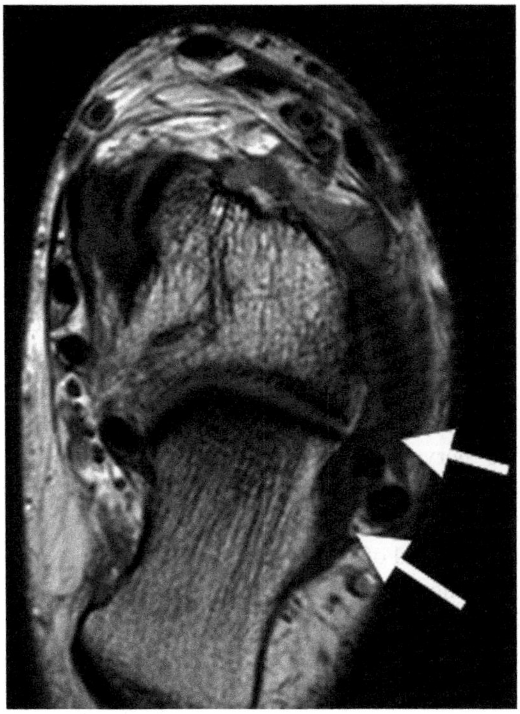

Fig. 3.27 MRI, axial oblique T2, of the calcaneofibular ligament (*arrows*) which is thickened and of intermediate signal intensity as it passes deep to the peroneal tendons, type 2 strain injury

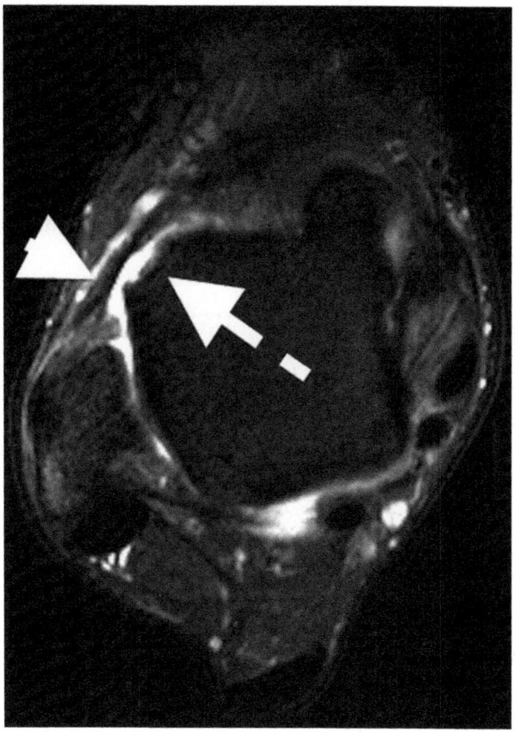

Fig. 3.28 Axial T2FS MRI of the ankle with osseous avulsion (*dashed arrow*), anterior talofibular ligament at fibular attachment, ligament is thickened, intermediate signal (*arrowhead*) with surrounding edema and small joint effusion

Ligament Pathology

Ligament pathology occurring at the entheseal complex has a similar imaging appearance as detailed in the tendon section above. Ligaments are also prone to *traumatic injury* and can be graded 1–3. Grade 1 sprains are minimal injuries with microscopic tears. The ligament is intact and of normal appearance on ultrasound and MRI. There may be surrounding edema and hemorrhage that parallels the ligament on its superficial or deep surface. A grade 2 sprain indicates a partial thickness tear with disruption fibers. This can be further subdivided to account for the percentage fibers involved. Ultrasound and MRI in the acute stage demonstrate fiber discontinuity with surrounding edema and hemorrhage. MRI may also show related bone contusion at ligament attachment as high SI on T2-weighted sequences. In chronic cases, the ligament may heal by fibrosis in which case the ligament is thickened with heterogeneous hypoechogenicity on ultrasound and low signal thickening on MRI (Figs. 3.27 and 3.28). Grade 3 is a complete tear with no residual intact fibers.

Nerve

Anatomy

A peripheral nerve is a cordlike structure containing a large number of individual nerve fibers. The nerve fibers are grouped together into bundles known as fascicles (Fig. 3.29). The fascicles are enclosed in a connective tissue sheath or membrane known as the epineurium. Each fascicle is in turn covered by a sheath of connective tissue, the perineurium. The individual nerve fibers within the fascicle are also enclosed by a sheath of connective tissue, the endoneurium. Extending inward from the epineurium is the interfascicular epineurium, which is a thin septum, adding further support to the nerve bundles and their vascular supply. Similar septa extend inward from the perineurium. The individual nerve fibers are continuous and do not branch or coalesce. The nerve may branch giving off one or more fasciculi and unite with other fasciculi.

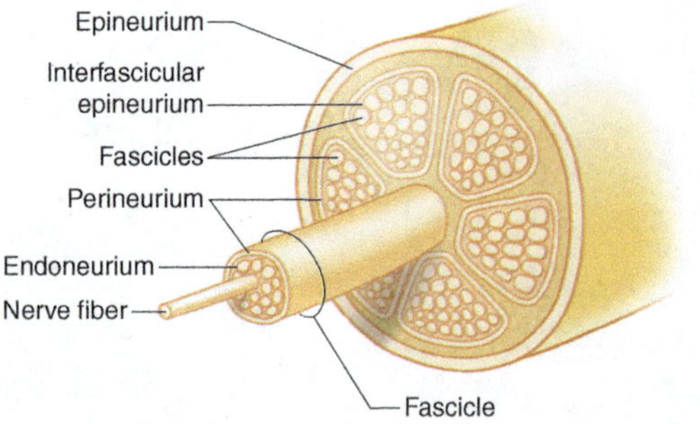

Fig. 3.29 Illustration of the peripheral nerve: cross-sectional anatomy

Ultrasound

The longitudinal axis of the nerve demonstrates a fascicular pattern of uninterrupted hypoechoic bands with intervening linear interrupted hyperechoic bands (Fig. 3.30). The hypoechoic bands represent the fasciculi and the hyperechoic bands the supporting interfascicular epineurium. The epineurium is hyperechoic and has similar appearance with perineural fat and may not be separable on ultrasound. On axial study, the nerve is composed of fasciculi seen as multiple hypoechoic dots, which may be of varying size, intermingled in a hyperechoic background of the supporting connective tissue. Identification of individual fascicles will depend on a number of factors, including the depth of the nerve and the frequency of the transducer.

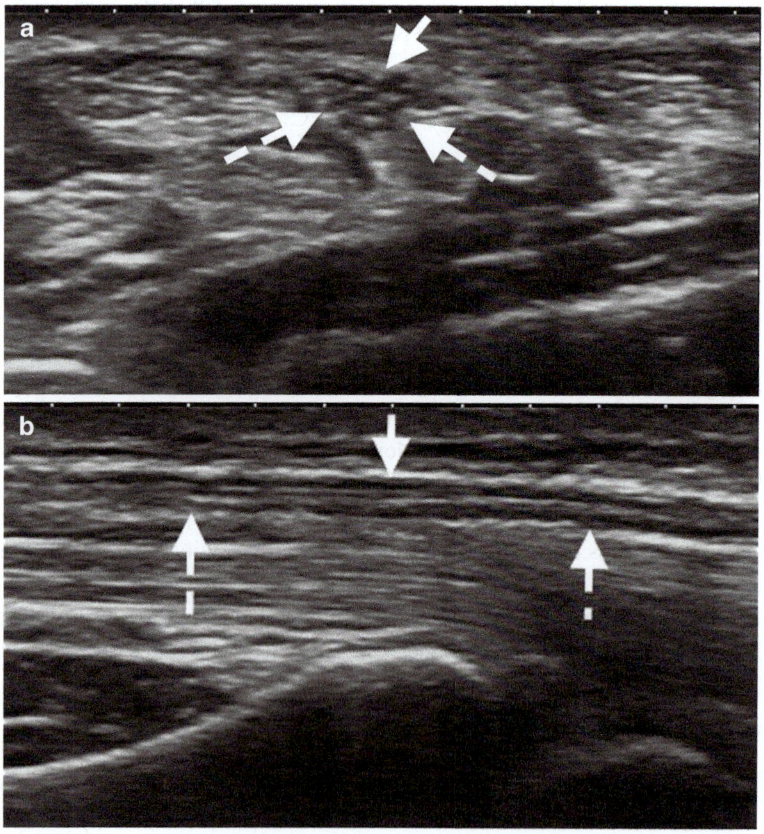

Fig. 3.30 Median nerve (*arrows*) proximal to carpal tunnel: (**a**) transverse and (**b**) longitudinal ultrasound images; note the uninterrupted hypoechoic linear bands with intervening linear interrupted hyperechoic bands

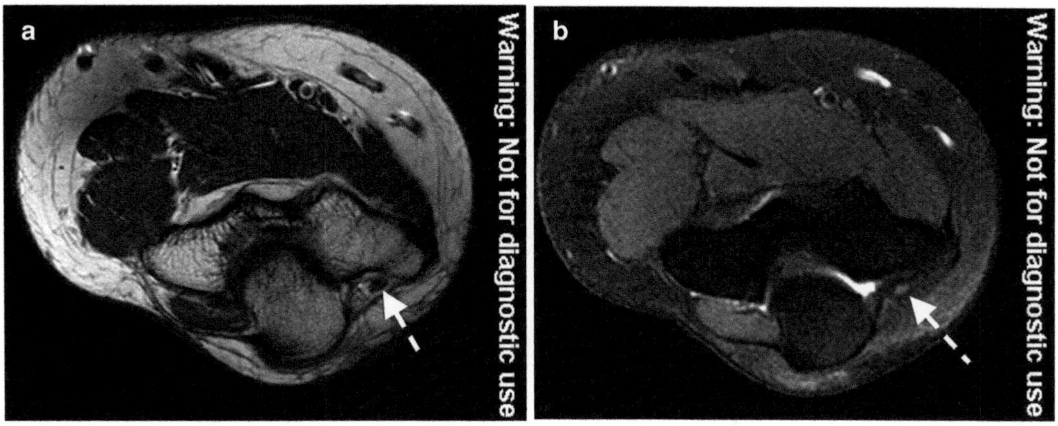

Fig. 3.31 MRI of the ulnar nerve (*dashed arrow*) within the cubital tunnel at the elbow on axial (**a**) T1 and (**b**) T2FS

In general, the greater the depth and the lower the frequency of the transducer, the lower the resolution. Nerves may become more uniformly hypoechoic when they pass through narrow passages, such as fibro-osseous tunnels, with the fascicles becoming tightly packed and less intervening hyperechoic connective tissue.

Tendons and nerves can have a similar appearance and size. Tendons have a fibrillar pattern versus the fascicular pattern of nerves; tendons are more prone to the artifact of anisotropy, are not normally compressible, and demonstrate more motion on active movement of the adjacent muscles. Small, hypoechoic perineural vessels can be distinguished from the adjacent nerve with color or power Doppler. When nerves pass through fibro-osseous tunnels, they are held in place by retinacula. Dynamic assessment is important to exclude subluxation or dislocation of the nerve.

MRI

On MRI, nerves are oval or round in cross section with similar/mildly increased signal intensity to muscle on T2- and T1-weighted sequences. Signal intensity may increase on T2 as the nerve passes through a fibro-osseous tunnel (Fig. 3.31). In cross section, the fascicles appear like dots in a honeycomb-like pattern. Due to the oblique course of many nerves, it is usually easier to follow the course of the nerve in the axial plane. In long axis, larger peripheral nerves demonstrate interposed fat between individual fascicles. More recently neurography with diffusion-weighted imaging has become available in some centers.

CT is not as sensitive as MRI or US in the assessment of peripheral nerves. On *CT*, nerves can be identified separate from adjacent soft tissues when they are surrounded by fat. They have similar attenuation to muscle. Perineural vessels are best identified separate from the nerve in contrast-enhanced studies.

Nerve Pathology

Compression or entrapment neuropathy is the commonest presenting pathology that the rheumatologist encounters. Nerves are particularly prone to compression neuropathy at anatomical sites of constriction such as fibrous and fibro-osseous tunnels (Table 3.4). The nerve may become enlarged because of repeated episodes of short-lived compressions, which may interfere with vascular supply and eventually induce fibrotic changes of the nerve sheaths, resulting in axonal degeneration. The enlarged nerve becomes too large for the anatomical tunnel in which it exists. This causes further microtrauma as the nerve, which normally slides unimpeded, becomes constrained by the confines of the tunnel.

The nerve may become compressed by normal variants such as anomalous muscles and tendons and adjacent pathologies including tendinopathy,

Table 3.4 Common nerve compression/entrapment sites

Nerve	Location	Syndrome
Suprascapular nerve	Suprascapular or spinoglenoid notch	Suprascapular nerve syndrome
Axillary nerve	Quadrilateral space	Quadrilateral space syndrome
Median nerve	Distal humerus	Supracondylar process syndrome
	Cubital fossa	Pronator syndrome
	Proximal forearm	Anterior interosseous nerve syndrome
	Wrist carpal tunnel	Carpal tunnel syndrome
Ulnar nerve	Elbow – cubital tunnel	Cubital tunnel syndrome
	Wrist – Guyon's canal	Guyon's canal syndrome
Radial nerve	Humeral spiral groove	Saturday night syndrome
	Elbow	Radial tunnel syndrome
	Proximal forearm	Posterior interosseous nerve syndrome
Sciatic nerve	Greater sciatic foramen/intrapiriformis	Piriformis syndrome
Lateral femoral cutaneous nerve	Deep to inguinal ligament	Meralgia paresthetica
Common peroneal nerve	Fibular neck	Peroneal tunnel syndrome
Tibial nerve	Popliteal fossa	Popliteal entrapment syndrome
Posterior tibial nerve	Tarsal tunnel at and below medial malleolus	Tarsal tunnel syndrome
Interdigital nerve of the foot	Beneath the intermetatarsal ligament at the level of the metatarsal heads	Morton's neuroma

distended joint capsule, fibrous bands, ganglion cysts, bony growths including exostosis and osteophytes, and benign and malignant tumors.

Ultrasound demonstrates an enlarged nerve centered to the area of compression with the nerve gradually returning to normal size and imaging appearance proximally and distally. At the site of compression, there may be an abrupt change in the contour of the nerve. Individual fascicles are thickened and there is loss of interposed connective tissue and fat. The cross-sectional area of the nerve is measured and can be compared with the more proximal normal appearing nerve (Fig. 3.32). Dynamic evaluation with ultrasound allows for assessment of subluxation or dislocation that may be intermittent. Dynamic ultrasound can also identify adjacent tissues, which may only compress the nerve in certain positions, e.g., enlarged medial head triceps compressing the ulnar nerve within the carpal tunnel in elbow flexion. Denervation edema may be evident as increased echotexture but may be subtle; correlation with adjacent normal muscle or the contralateral side is advised. Chronic denervation atrophy and fatty infiltration are demonstrated as loss of muscle bulk and increased internal echotexture which decreases through transmission, respectively.

MRI demonstrates changes in size and signal intensity of the nerve. The size changes are as described in the ultrasound appearance above. Signal intensity increases on T2-weighted sequences and is most pronounced at the site of compression (Fig. 3.33). MRI is a static study and intermittent subluxation/dislocation may not be identified. Related findings of denervation are best appreciated on MRI. The adjacent musculature innervated by the involved nerve is of increased signal intensity on T2 in the acute phase. In chronic denervation, edema subsides and the muscle undergoes atrophy and fatty infiltration. *CT* is limited in the assessment of nerve pathology and is not a primary imaging modality in the evaluation of peripheral nerves. It may demonstrate changes to nerve size and contour and underlying bony changes such as osteophytes. It has however poor discrimination of adjacent soft tissue pathology. Radiographs are limited but are occasionally used to exclude bone pathology in the area of concern.

Vasculitis-related neuropathy can occur in multiple rheumatologic conditions such as rheumatoid arthritis, Sjogren's syndrome, Wegener's granulomatosis, and polyarteritis nodosa (PAN). Patients can develop multiple mononeuropathies. The nerve maintains a nor-

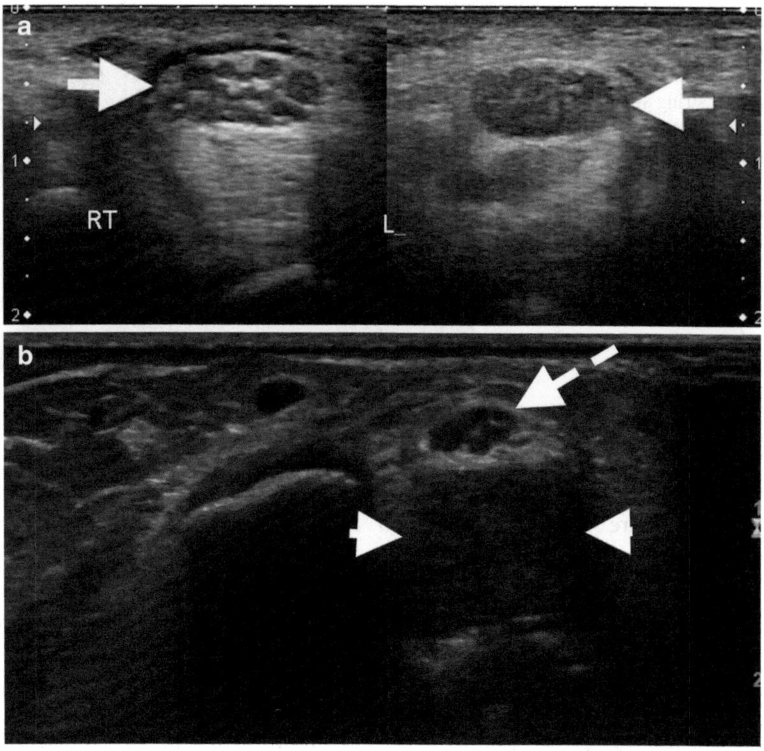

Fig. 3.32 (**a**) Ultrasound of bilaterally enlarged (25 mm squared cross-sectional area) median nerves (*arrows*) demonstrating marked thickening of the fascicles (*hypoechoic dots*) and loss of interfascicular connective tissue. (**b**) Enlarged ulnar nerve (*dashed arrow*) at cubital tunnel; nerve is subluxed due to displacement by significant synovial tissue (*arrowheads*) in this patient with rheumatoid arthritis

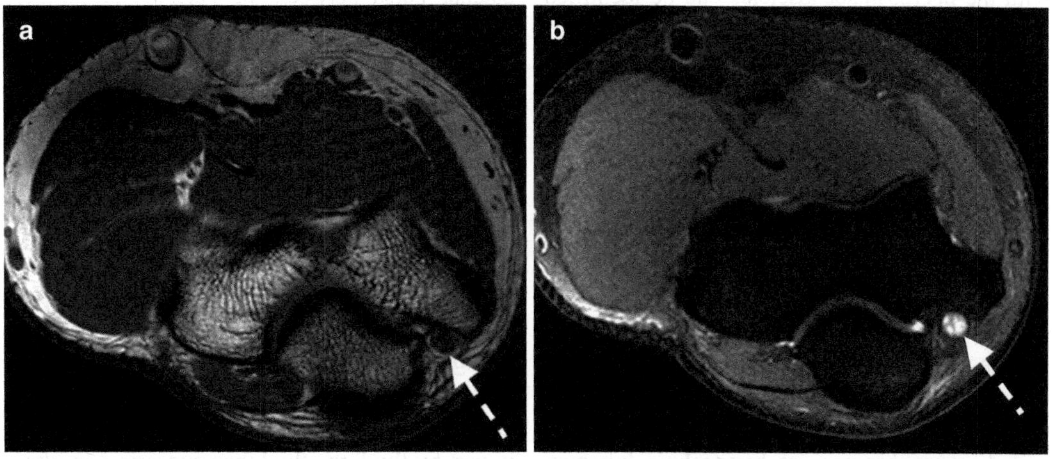

Fig. 3.33 MRI of ulnar neuropathy within the cubital tunnel: (**a**) axial T1 and (**b**) axial T2FS demonstrating enlarged ulnar nerve (*dashed arrow*) with increased signal intensity on T2. Compare to Fig. 3.31 for normal appearance

mal imaging appearance, which helps exclude other etiologies such as entrapment neuropathy.

Nerve injury can manifest in increasing grades of severity as neurapraxia, axonotmesis, and neurotmesis. Neuropraxia involves localized damage to the nerve sheath with the axon remaining intact. Depending on the extent of injury, recovery can be from several hours to 3 months, e.g., Saturday night syndrome with compression of the radial nerve classically by having the arm draped over the back of a chair, compressing and causing ischemia of the radial nerve. Imaging is usually normal. In axonotmesis, the axon is disrupted while the sheath remains intact; recovery, if it occurs, takes weeks to months. In the most severe form, neurotmesis, the axon and the sheath are tran-

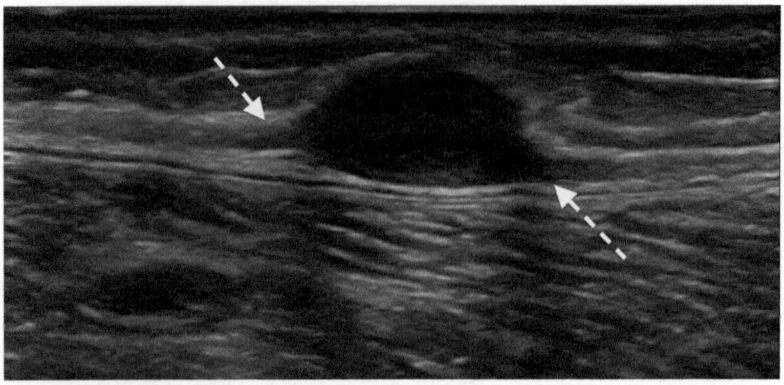

Fig. 3.34 Schwannoma of the sural nerve on longitudinal ultrasound. Note "string sign" (*dashed arrows*) of the eccentric peripheral nerve entering and leaving the hypoechoic lesion

sected and require surgical repair. Retracted nerve fibers with surrounding edema and soft tissue thickening are seen on *ultrasound* and *MRI*. Denervation edema can be seen in acute cases and muscle atrophy with fatty infiltration in chronic cases. Post-traumatic neuromas usually occur within one year of injury. They are the result of nerve partial or complete transection and form due to disorganized attempt at repair. Ultrasound demonstrates a hypoechoic mass in continuity with the nerve; intact fascicles can be identified adjacent to the neuroma in cases of previous partial transection. MRI demonstrates a normal nerve entering a fusiform heterogeneous mass of intermediate SI on T1 and intermediate to high SI on T2. The neuroma enhances post gadolinium.

Peripheral nerve and nerve sheath *tumors* include the benign neurofibroma and schwannoma, respectively. Neurofibromas on imaging are demonstrated as focal fusiform enlargement of the nerve. The nerve can be identified centrally entering and exiting the lesion, the string sign. The perineural fat is displaced peripherally around the mass, the split-fat sign. On *ultrasound*, neurofibromas are hypoechoic but may have a central fibrotic hyperechoic focus producing a target-like appearance. Doppler may demonstrate internal flow but usually less than schwannomas. *MRI* may have a similar target appearance with low signal intensity on T2 centrally and peripherally higher signal intensity. Schwannomas are eccentric to the nerve (Fig. 3.34). On ultrasound, the tumors are hypoechoic and produce increased through transmission and can simulate a cyst. Doppler demonstrates increased flow within.

Bursa

Anatomy

Within the body there are three subdivisions of synovial membranes: articular, synovial sheath, and bursal. The bursal synovial membrane is further subdivided into mucosae and synovia. The former is present within the subcutaneous tissue, between the skin and underlying bony prominence (e.g., prepatellar bursa between the patella and skin). It becomes distended, for example, when there is increased friction between the bone and overlying soft tissue. Bursae synoviae are located deeper and lie between the muscle or tendon and the bone and again serve to reduce friction. Occasionally, these deeper bursae will communicate with the joint, e.g., subscapularis bursa with the shoulder joint and iliopsoas bursa with the hip joint.

Imaging and Pathology

Bursae are not usually discernible unless distended in part by fluid, the fluid then appearing on *ultrasound* as anechoic between the hyperechoic tissue layers representing adjacent fat planes and capsule (Fig. 3.35). Internal synovial tissues may be heterogeneous in echotexture. Separating fluid from the synovium can sometimes be difficult. Active synovitis will demonstrate internal flow on Doppler interrogation, whereas fluid will not. Chronic fibrotic synovial thickening may demonstrate no flow. In this case compression of the bursa with the probe will cause fluid to move away, whereas synovium does not, although may demonstrate some loss of volume. The same holds true in joint synovial assessment. *MRI* will demonstrate a fluid signal intensity lesion, low on T1 and high on T2 (Fig. 3.36). Signal intensity however

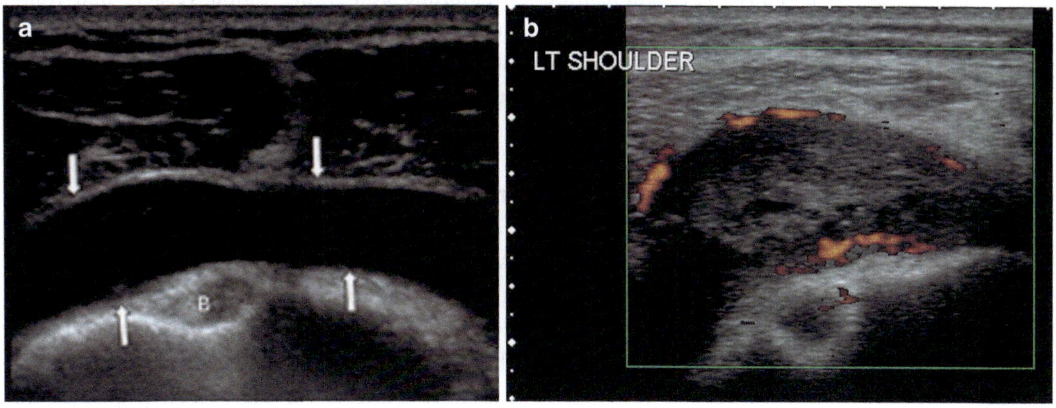

Fig. 3.35 Ultrasound of the subacromial-subdeltoid bursa: (**a**) anechoic fluid distension bursa (*arrows*) in a patient with bursal distension secondary to rotator cuff tear and (**b**) distension bursa with heterogenous soft tissue and increased peripheral flow on power Doppler in a different patient with septic arthritis and bursitis

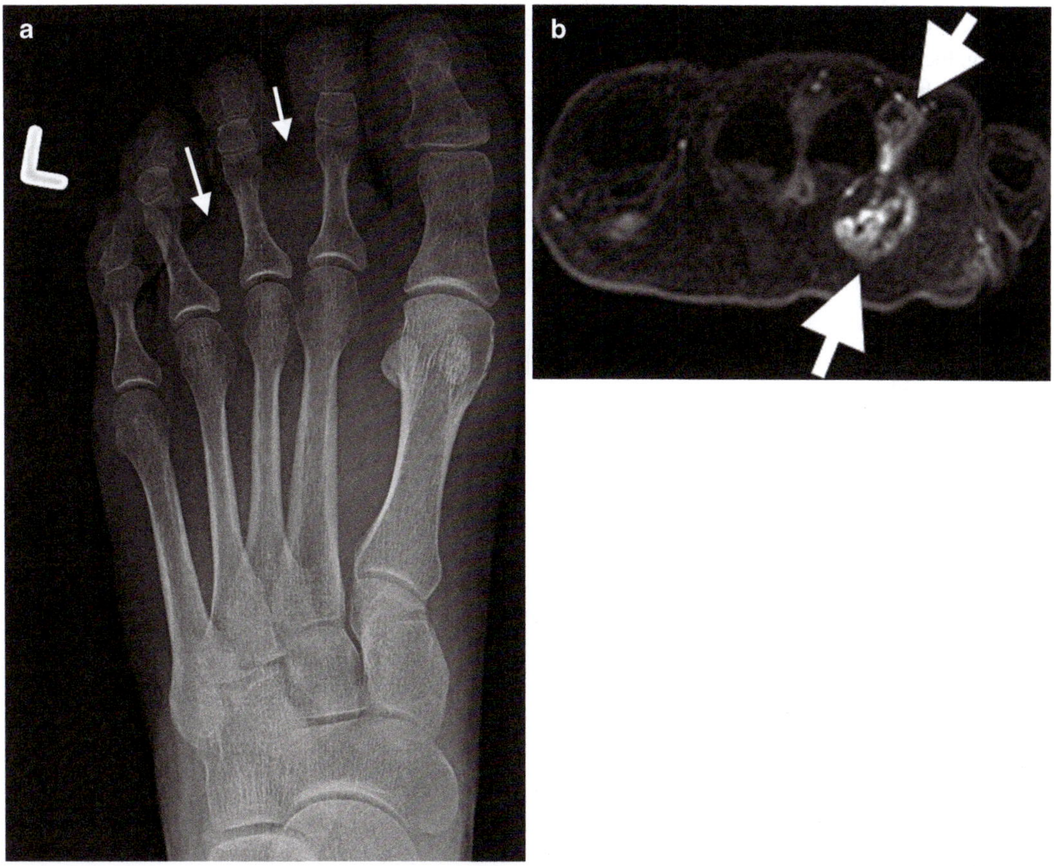

Fig. 3.36 (**a**) AP left foot radiograph in a patient with rheumatoid arthritis and soft tissue prominence on the second and third interspaces (*arrows*) and (**b**) axial T1FS post contrast demonstrating enhancing, predominantly peripheral, intermetatarsal bursa (*arrows*)

may be heterogeneous particularly if there is synovial thickening within which can be similar to fluid signal intensity but often has a slightly lower signal. A post-gadolinium study will demonstrate bursal wall enhancement as well as enhancement of any internal synovium. *CT* may not identify bursa unless significantly distended. They are noted as low-attenuating fluid-filled sacs occurring in expected locations. *Radiographs* may suggest the presence of bursa in expected locations where there is loss of normal soft tissue-fat interfaces (Fig. 3.36a). Examples include the olecranon bursa, prepatellar bursa, and retrocalcaneal bursa.

Bone

Anatomy

There are two main ingredients to bone, compact and cancellous. Compact bone forms the outer covering, the cortex, encasing the inner cancellous or spongy bone. The latter has a honeycomb distribution of trabeculae, which support the marrow cavity (Fig. 3.37). Trabeculae become more pronounced at sites of normal physiological stress, e.g., the femoral head and neck. The compact bone is, in turn, encased by a periosteal membrane containing blood vessels that transverse the cortex. A detailed description of the hematopoietic marrow is provided in the MRI section below on normal marrow imaging.

Imaging

Although *ultrasound* has limitations when imaging bone, it does offer excellent anatomical detail of the cortical surface of superficial bone (Fig. 3.38). The high resolution provided by ultrasound allows for the detection and assessment of subtle cortical changes. Occult fractures not seen on radiographs can sometimes be identified as focal cortical defects on ultrasound when involving superficial bones. This is most commonly seen in our department in non-displaced occult humeral fractures. Erosions of superficial bones, e.g., metacarpal heads, that are sometimes not visible on plain radiographs can be demonstrated on ultrasound (Fig. 3.39). The

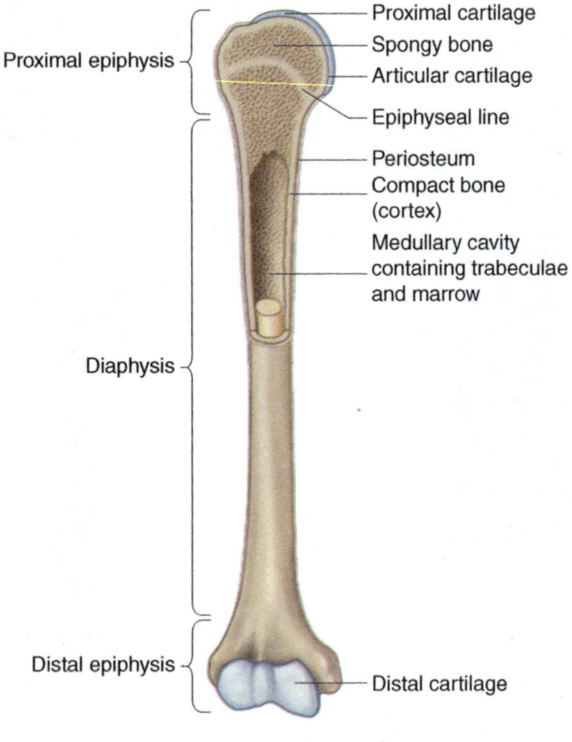

Fig. 3.37 Normal bone anatomy

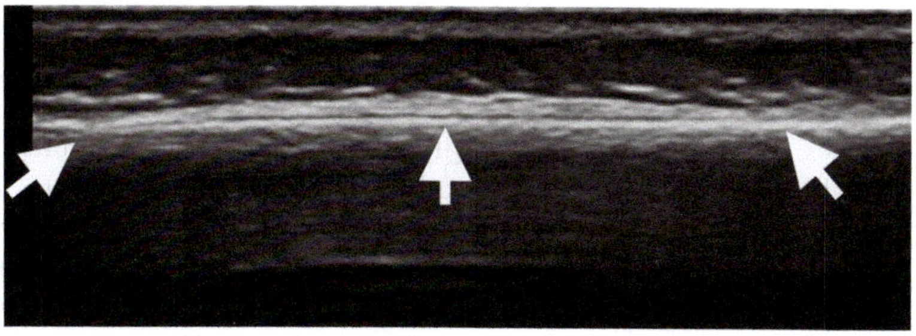

Fig. 3.38 Ultrasound of the cortex bone demonstrated as a smooth echogenic line (*arrows*). There is no anatomical detail deep to this line as sound waves are reflected from the cortex

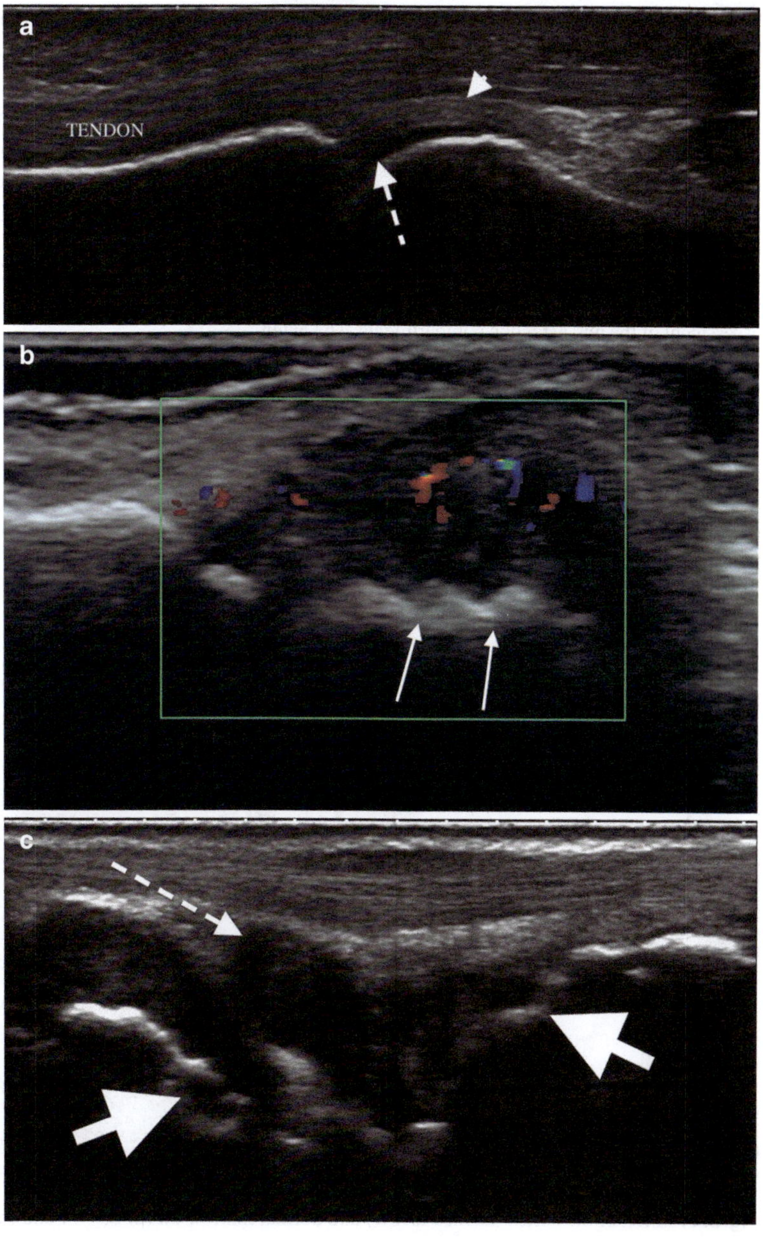

Fig. 3.39 Ultrasound longitudinal images of (**a**) normal MCPJ that demonstrates overlying flexor tendons, hypoechoic articular cartilage (*dashed arrow*), and echogenic triangular complex (*small arrow*). (**b**) Active synovitis of the MCPJ with early erosions (*arrows*) that were not visible on x-ray and (**c**) dorsal wrist with synovitis (*dashed arrow*) and multiple erosions of the carpal bones (*arrows*)

cortical surface, however, is highly reflective on ultrasound. This causes the cortex to be visualized as a well-defined hyperechoic continuous line but obscures the deeper medullary cavity. Deeper cortical surfaces usually require a lower frequency transducer. The overlying normal periosteum is not normally identifiable separate from the bone and the adjacent soft tissues. Knowledge of the bony anatomy is essential in the full ultrasound evaluation of the musculoskeletal system. Bony landmarks will often form an easily identifiable location to assess the overlying soft tissues, e.g., Lister's tubercle at the dorsal wrist and the third extensor compartment (Fig. 3.40).

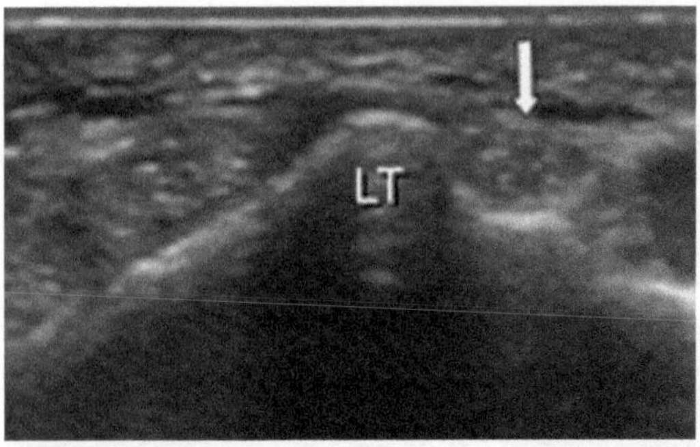

Fig. 3.40 Lister's tubercle (*LT*) on the dorsal aspect of the distal radius is an important bone landmark in the assessment of the dorsal tendon compartments. The extensor pollicis longus tendon (*arrow*) lies on its ulnar aspect and is separated from the second compartment by LT

Cortical and medullary bones have different signal intensities on *MRI* (Fig. 3.41). Cortical bone is of low signal intensity on all imaging sequences due to lack of resonation of tightly packed protons, which therefore produces no signal. Cortex should be smooth and continuous without interruption. Fat and hematopoietic cells resonate and produce a signal and occupy the medullary cavity; the supporting thin trabecular bone does not resonate.

Hematopoietic tissue produces red and white blood cells, platelets with a supporting reticulum of macrophages, and undifferentiated non-phagocytic cells. There is a significant portion of fat cells within this hematopoietic tissue. The amount of hematopoietic tissue, red marrow, present is age dependent. At birth, red marrow is

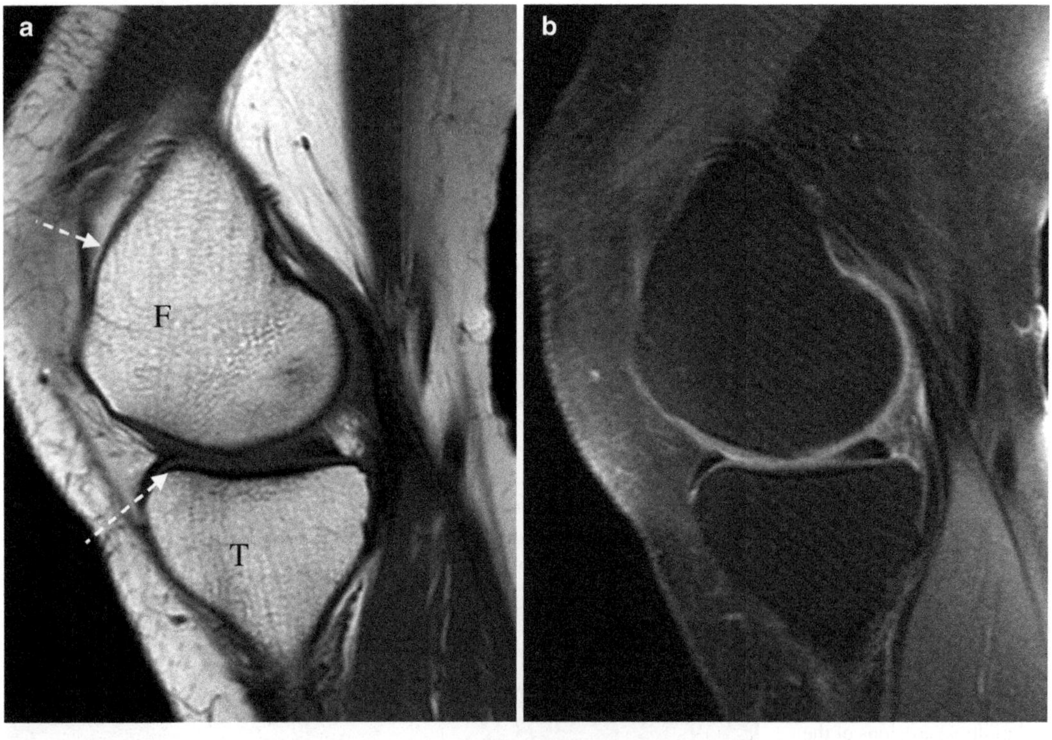

Fig. 3.41 MRI of the cortex (*dashed arrow*) and normal marrow on (**a**) Sag T1 and (**b**) Sag T2FS. *F* femur, *T* tibia

present throughout with sparing of ossified epiphyses and apophyses. Red marrow regresses with age in a fixed pattern until early adulthood where red marrow occupies the axial skeleton and proximal metaphyses of the long bones. In the elderly, red marrow regresses further in the axial skeleton. Yellow marrow due the high fat content is of high signal intensity on T1 and intermediate on T2 and follows signal intensity of subcutaneous fat (Fig. 3.41). With fat saturation, it loses signal and hence is of low signal on T1FS, T2FS, and STIR sequences. Red marrow is of intermediate signal intensity on T1, slightly higher than adjacent muscle or intervertebral disk (Fig. 3.42). On T2, red marrow is of lower signal intensity than yellow marrow, but distinction between the two types of marrow is limited on T2. With fat suppression red marrow is of intermediate signal and can be distinguished from yellow marrow, which loses signal intensity.

CT allows for excellent resolution of bone cortex and trabecular pattern but is less sensitive than MRI in assessing marrow pattern (Fig. 3.43). Yellow marrow has low attenuation due to fat content; attenuation however on CT also varies due to the number and thickness of trabeculae in the region of interest. Hematopoietic marrow has a higher attenuation than yellow marrow but is still relatively low due to its high fat content. *Radiography* has excellent resolution of bony architecture and is the first-line imaging investigation for bone pathology. There are well-recognized pathological processes that are easily discriminated on radiographs, e.g., bone tumors, but may be difficult to accurately diagnose on more advanced imaging such as MRI.

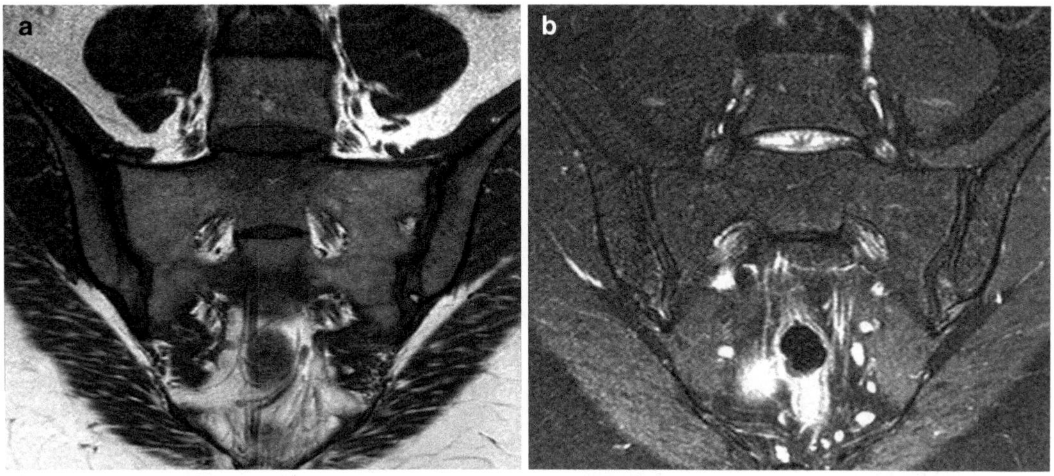

Fig. 3.42 MRI of the sacroiliac joints. (**a**) Cor T1; note marrow signal intensity is heterogenous and lower than Fig. 3.41a due to hematopoietic tissue. (**b**) Cor T2FS provides fat suppression and loss of signal intensity of the marrow

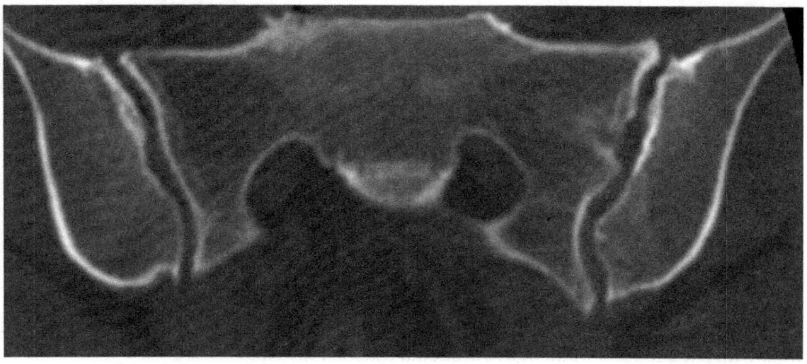

Fig. 3.43 Coronal reformatted CT, on bone windows, of the sacroiliac joints

Pathology

Bone marrow edema on *MRI* is of high SI on T2 but is poorly differentiated from adjacent marrow that is also of high SI without the addition of fat saturation (FS). The edematous marrow is therefore best depicted on STIR or T2FS sequences where it is of high SI, and the normal adjacent marrow is suppressed due to lack of signal from fat and is of low SI (Fig. 3.44). A more uniform suppression of fat is present on STIR sequence than on T2FS at a cost of decreased resolution on STIR. On T1, marrow edema is of low SI. CT, ultrasound, and radiography are unable to identify bone marrow edema.

Periosteal reaction is the formation of new bone in response to injury or other stimuli of the periosteum. There are many types of periosteal reaction which suggest the aggression of the underlying etiology (see Fig. 17.2). Underlying etiologies include trauma, infection, inflammation (arthritis), metabolic disease (hypertrophic osteoarthropathy), vascular disease (venous stasis), and neoplasm. Periosteal reaction may have a single layer or multiple layers or onion skin appearance, be spiculated, have a hair-on-end and sunburst appearance, or demonstrate the Codman's triangle. *Radiographs* are excellent in identifying and assessing the full extent of reaction and identifying inciting pathology (Fig. 3.45a). On *MRI*, periosteal reaction may be identified as a rim of high SI on T2 sequences and low on T1 (Fig. 3.45). There may be surrounding soft tissue injury with edema and hemorrhage. *CT* is very sensitive for detecting periosteal reaction. In the early phase, it appears as a subtle, usually thin, and linear increased attenuation along the cortical surface of the bone, eventually forming mature bone, depending on the underlying etiology, upon the cortex. *Ultrasound* is sensitive in identifying periosteal reaction in superficial bone as a hyperechoic linear region directly applied to the underlying cortex but will require further evaluation with radiographs to assess the underlying bone in greater detail.

A *fracture* is identified as a break in the cortex and can be complete, involving both cortices, or incomplete with disruption of only one cortex. The imaging appearance will depend on the etiology, age of the fracture, and healing response. Types include traumatic fracture, stress fracture, insufficiency fracture, and pathological fracture (Fig. 3.46). A stress or fatigue fracture is caused by repetitive stress on normal bone, whereas an insufficiency fracture occurs in the bone with abnormal mineralization that is unable to bear normal stress. A pathological fracture indicates underlying bone pathology, such as tumor or

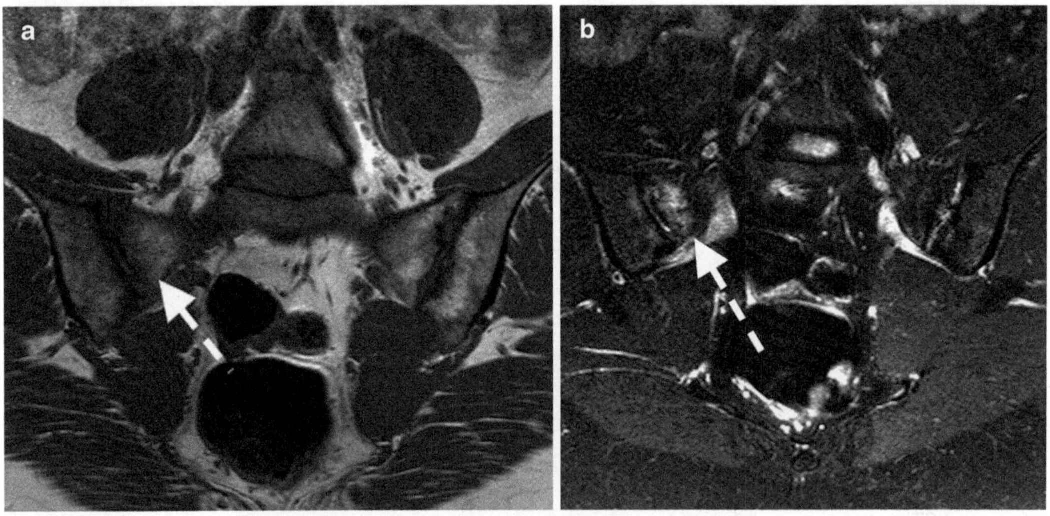

Fig. 3.44 MRI of a marrow edema: (**a**) Cor T1 and (**b**) T2FS sacroiliac joint in a patient with acute or chronic sacroiliitis with subchondral bone marrow edema (*dashed arrow*)

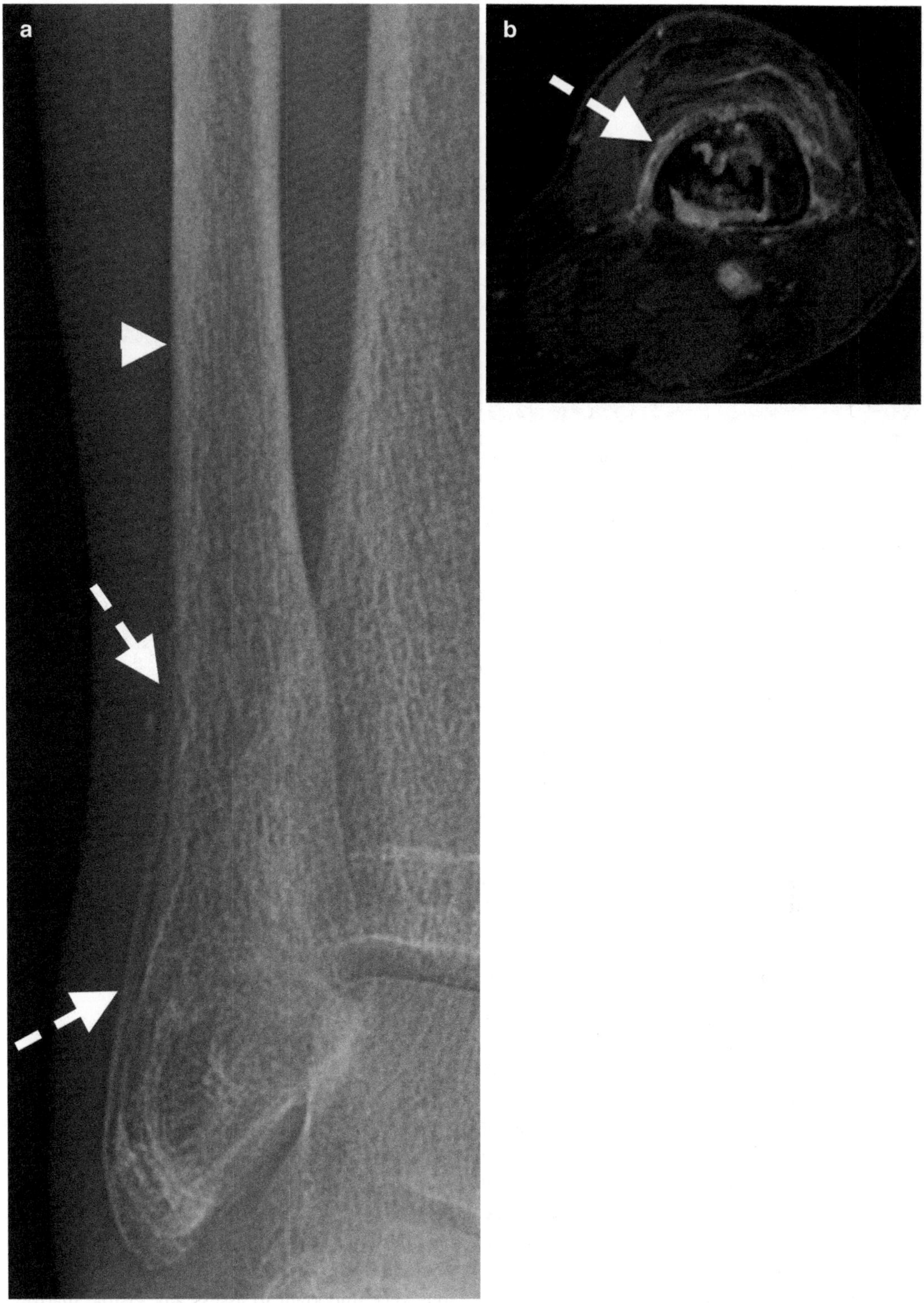

Fig. 3.45 Periosteal reaction: (**a**) AP distal fibula with lateral periosteal reaction (*dashed arrows*) and underlying cortical loss secondary to overlying soft tissue infection and early osteomyelitis; note normal cortex (*arrowhead*). (**b**) Different patient: axial T2FS of the distal femur with aggressive periosteal reaction (*dashed arrow*) secondary to underlying malignant bone tumor

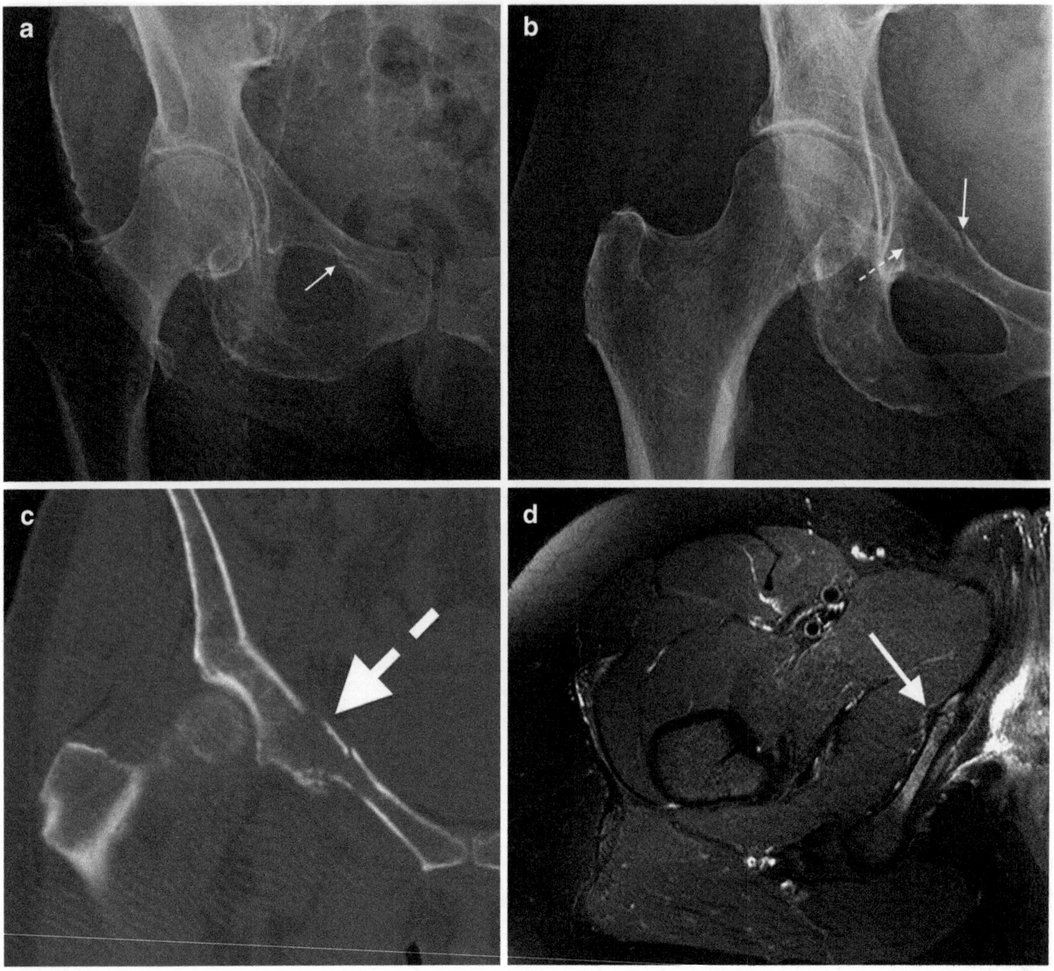

Fig. 3.46 Fractures: (**a**) insufficiency fracture of the right superior pubic ramus after minor trauma in an elderly patient with osteoporosis. (**b**) Fracture (*arrow*) of the right superior pubic ramus through an ill-defined osteolytic lesion (*dashed arrow*); renal cell carcinoma metastatic deposit, i.e., a pathological fracture, also demonstrated on (**c**) coronal reformatted CT. (**d**) Stress fracture (*arrow*) in a 27-year-old female marathon runner of the right inferior pubic ramus on axial T2FS MRI with callus formation and bone marrow edema

infection, which weakens the structural integrity of the bone. Radiographs are the first line of investigation. The parent bone should be assessed for density and underlying marrow for predisposing bone pathology, periosteal reaction and type, and location. In addition, the level of trauma should be sufficient to cause the subsequent bone injury. Patient history and clinical condition in conjunction with the above factors will determine whether further investigation is required. Discussion with your radiologist with respect to the optimal imaging algorithm is always appreciated.

Marrow disorders are best assessed on MRI. CT and radiographs may identify marrow abnormality but are significantly less sensitive. *MRI* identifies marrow disorders as a change in the expected marrow SI pattern for the patient's age. Marrow disorders include proliferative and replacement disorders, marrow depletion, vascular abnormalities, and miscellaneous conditions (Fig. 3.47). It is thus very important to assess any visible marrow on any examination to confirm a normal appearance and not to miss incidental pathology. A full detailed description is beyond the scope of this text.

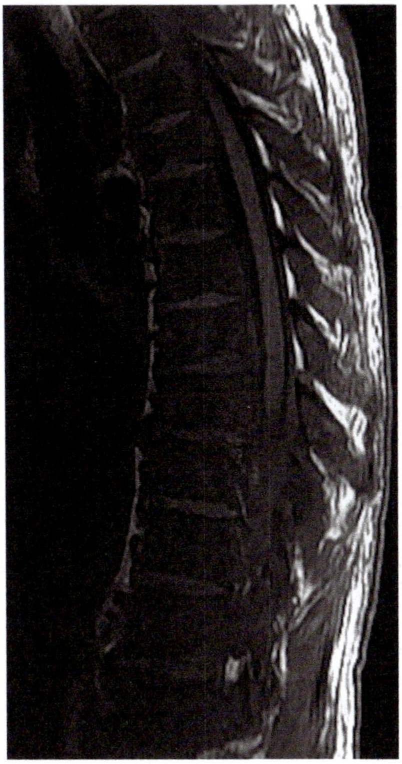

Fig. 3.47 Sag T1 thoracic spine with diffuse loss of normal high signal intensity marrow due to replacement with diffuse prostatic metastatic disease

Joints

Anatomy

A joint is the juncture of two or more bones. Motion may or may not be present at a joint. There are multiple types of joints including synovial, cartilaginous, and fibrous. Synovial, the commonest type, has synovium lining the joint capsule which extends across the articular surfaces, attaching to the joint margin. The area between the capsule insertion and the margin of the articular cartilage is known as the bare area (Fig. 3.48). This is a common site for early erosive disease as there is no cartilage present. Erosion rate of cartilage by pannus is lower when compared to cortical erosion. Bone erosion, synovitis, cartilage, and subchondral sclerosis and cysts are described in detail below.

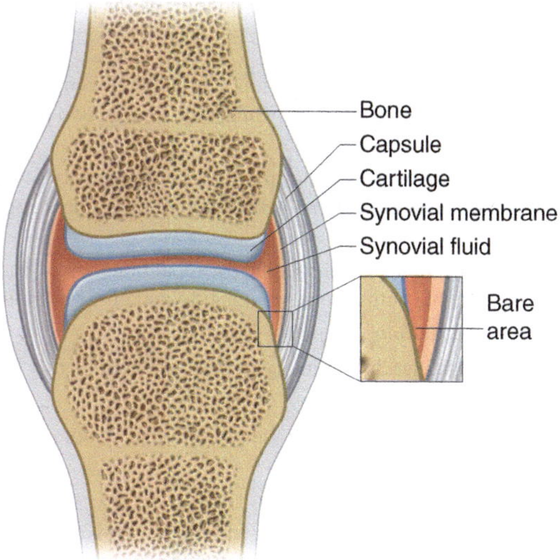

Fig. 3.48 The bare area, that part of bone within a joint covered by synovial membrane but without a protective cartilage surface

Pathology

We will adopt the OMERACT definition of erosion and synovitis for ultrasound and MRI (Table 3.5). The ultrasound definition for erosion is also appropriate for CT. Radiographs do not require visualization of an erosion in two planes, remembering that radiographs are 2-D representation of 3-D anatomy and can be defined as a focal nontraumatic intra- or extra-articular cortical defect secondary to local pathology.

Osteoarthritis: Subchondral Sclerosis, Cysts, and Osteophytosis

The subchondral region or endplate is located deep to the articular surface, separated only by a thin layer of calcified articular cartilage (Fig. 10.2). When there is loss of the overlying cartilage, as in osteoarthritis, the subchondral bone is directly exposed to the stresses across the joint. The subchondral bone reacts to this stress with trabecular collapse and flattening and appears ivory-like with polished surface, *eburnation*. The subchondral regions in areas of lower stress become increasingly vascularized. This stimulates endo-

Table 3.5 OMERACT imaging definitions for joint-related pathology

MRI erosion
A sharply marginated bone lesion, with typical signal characteristics*, with correct juxta-articular localization and typical signal characteristics, which is visible in two planes with a cortical break seen in at least one plane (Fig. 3.49)**
*On T1w images: loss of normal low signal intensity of cortical bone and loss of normal high signal intensity of trabecular bone. Quick post-gadolinium enhancement suggests presence of active, hypervascular pannus tissue in the erosion
**This appearance is nonspecific for focal bone loss. Other lesions may mimic erosions but are generally distinguishable with associated imaging and clinical findings
Ultrasound erosion
An intra-articular discontinuity of the bone surface that is visible in two perpendicular planes (Fig. 3.50)
Bone proliferation
Abnormal bone formation in the periarticular region, such as at the enthesis (enthesophytes) and across the joint (ankylosis) (Fig. 3.51)
MRI periarticular inflammation
Signal characteristics consistent with increased water content*or abnormal post-Gd enhancement** at extra-articular sites including the periosteum ("periostitis") and the entheses ("enthesitis"), but not the tendon sheaths (Fig. 3.52)***
*High signal intensity on T2w FS and STIR images.**Enhancement is judged by comparison between T1w images obtained before and after IV Gd contrast.***Defined as tenosynovitis
MRI synovitis
An area in the synovial compartment that shows increased post-gadolinium (post-Gd) enhancement* of a thickness greater than the width of the normal synovium (Fig. 3.53)
*Enhancement (signal intensity increase) is judged by comparison between T1-weighted (T1w) images obtained before and after intravenous (IV) gadolinium (Gd) contrast
Ultrasound synovial hypertrophy
Abnormal hypoechoic (relative to subdermal fat, but sometimes may be isoechoic or hyperechoic) intra-articular tissue that is non-displaceable and poorly compressible and which may exhibit Doppler signal (Figs. 3.39 and 3.54)
Ultrasound synovial fluid
Abnormal hypoechoic or anechoic (relative to subdermal fat, but sometimes may be isoechoic or hyperechoic) intra-articular material that is displaceable and compressible, but does not exhibit Doppler signal (Fig. 3.55)
Joint space narrowing
Reduced joint space width when compared to normal joint. On MRI assessed in a slice perpendicular to the joint surface

chondral ossification with new bone formation, *osteophytes*. They are usually marginal, growing as an extension of the joint margin. New bone formation may also occur centrally in areas of full cartilage loss and appear as new bone formation at the cortical surface, often with an irregular margin. *Subchondral cysts* develop between the deformed trabeculae in areas of eburnation. They are of variable size. The overlying cortex may be intact or may have a focal defect, allowing communication of the cyst with the joint space.

The imaging findings of osteoarthritis are summarized here but are reviewed in detail in Chap. 10. On *radiographs*, eburnation is noted as subchondral sclerosis and may demonstrate flattening and collapse of its surface. Osteophytes are noted as new bone forming at the periphery of the joint space. Subchondral cysts are variable in size, have a thin sclerotic margin, and may demonstrate communication with the joint space, e.g., intra-articular gas may extend into cyst. The overlying cortex is usually intact or demonstrates a focal defect. Occasionally it may be difficult to differentiate a subchondral cyst from an erosion if there is collapse of the articular margin of the cyst. Subchondral cysts are however associated

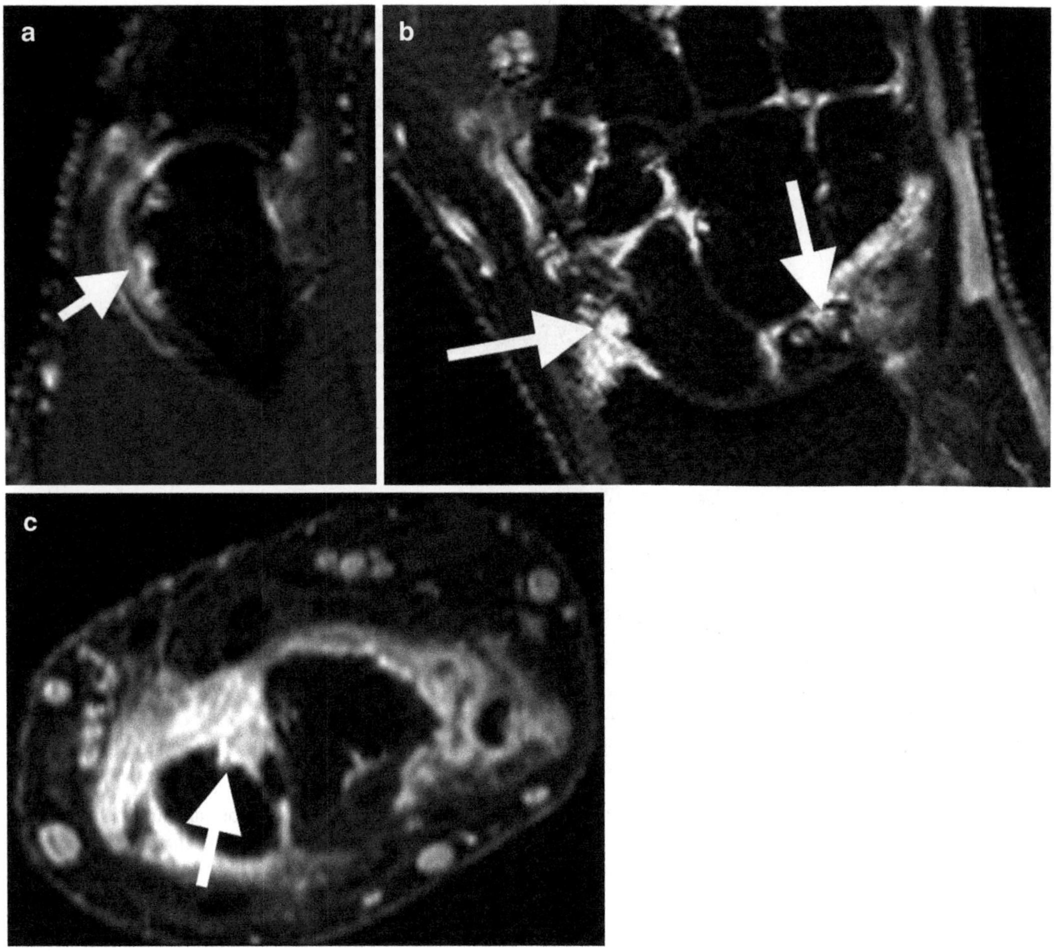

Fig. 3.49 MRI of an erosion. (**a**) Cor T1FS PG of the 2nd MCPJ with active synovitis and erosion with defined cortical breach metacarpal head (*arrow*). (**b**) Cor T1FS PG of the wrist of the same patient with active synovitis and erosions of the scaphoid and lunate (*arrows*), with lunate erosion also demonstrated on (**c**) axial T1FS PG

with joint space loss, subchondral sclerosis, and osteophytosis. Additional studies other than radiographs are rarely required; however, the above changes can be detailed on other imaging modalities when performed for alternative indications. *CT* demonstrates exquisite detail of subchondral changes as described in the radiographic section. CT is occasionally used for assessment of residual bone mass, e.g., glenoid, prior to joint replacement. Subchondral sclerosis on *MRI* is of low SI on both T1- and T2-weighted sequences. Subchondral cysts may contain proteinaceous material or joint fluid if they communicate with the joint and are of high SI on T2 and usually low SI on T1. Ultrasound is not recommended as it cannot assess the subchondral region. Ultrasound when used for assessment of joint fluid or synovitis will demonstrate associated changes such as joint space loss, cartilage thinning and loss in the periphery of superficial joints, cortical irregularity, and osteophytosis. Nuclear medicine imaging is not indicated.

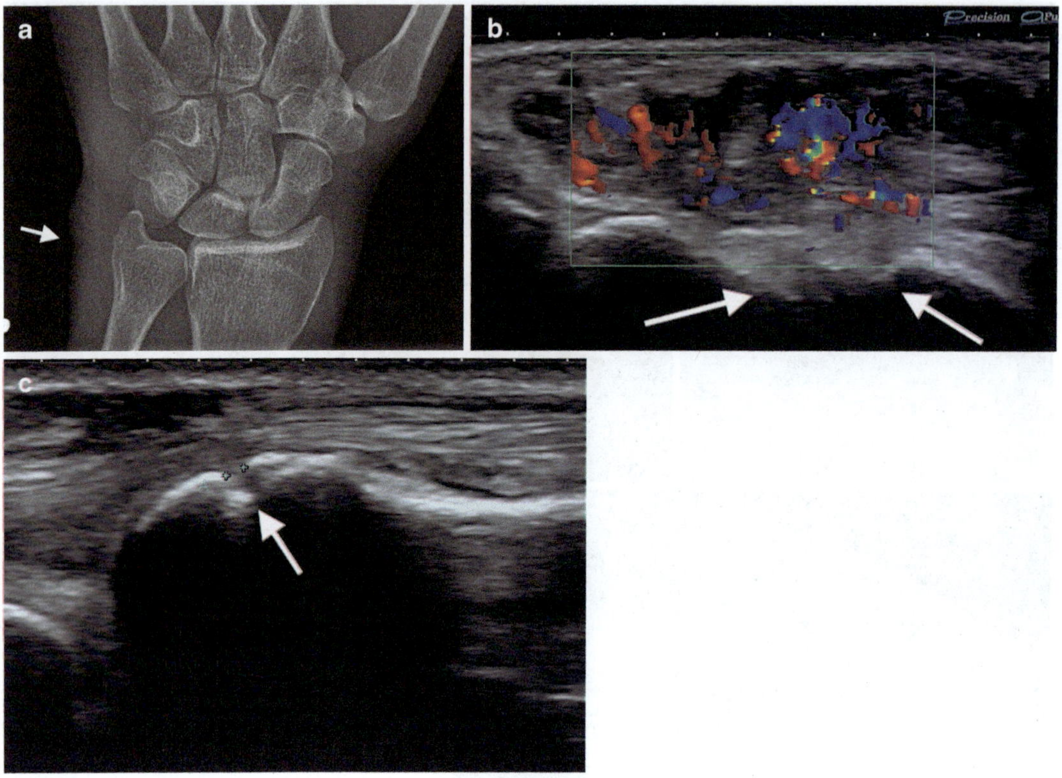

Fig. 3.50 Patient with rheumatoid arthritis. (**a**) AP radiograph of the wrist with soft tissue swelling over ulnar styloid process with subtle cortical changes. (**b**, **c**) Longitudinal ultrasound demonstrates extensor carpi ulnaris tendinosis and tenosynovitis with focal erosion (*arrows*) of the ulnar styloid

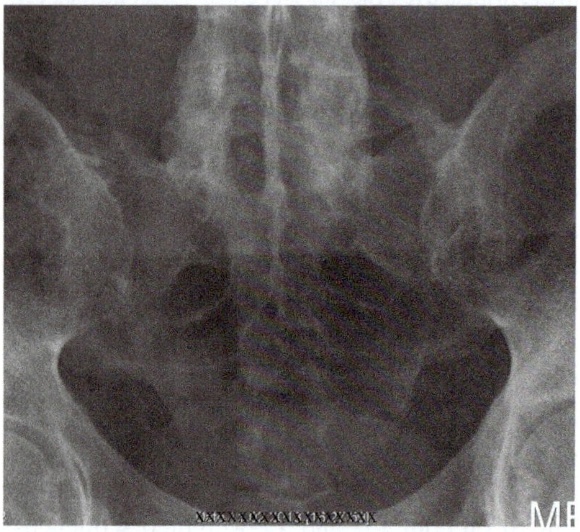

Fig. 3.51 AP radiograph of the sacroiliac joint with bilateral ankylosis in a patient with long-standing ankylosing spondylitis

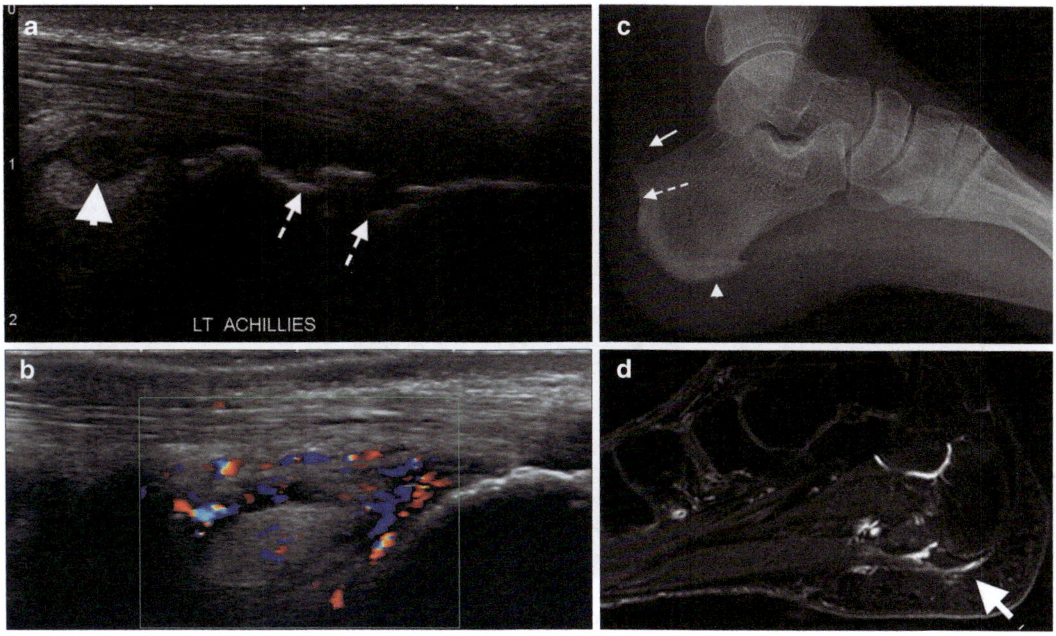

Fig. 3.52 An 18-year-old male with a 2-year clinical history of unresponsive distal Achilles tendinosis. (**a**) Longitudinal ultrasound with erosions of the calcaneus (*dashed arrows*) and distended retrocalcaneal bursa which demonstrates marked flow on color Doppler (**b**), also noted within distal tendon. (**c**) Lateral ankle radiograph demonstrating erosions of the calcaneus (*dashed arrow*), soft tissue thickening in the region of retrocalcaneal bursa (*arrow*), and new bone formation on the deep margin of the calcaneal spur (*arrowhead*). On discussion with the patient, he also complained of right sacroiliac inflammatory pain. Patient was referred to a rheumatologist for evaluation of spondyloarthropathy. (**d**) Sag T1FS post contrast in a different patient with enthesitis at plantar fascia insertion on the calcaneus with thickened enhancing fascia (*arrow*) and underlying bone marrow edema

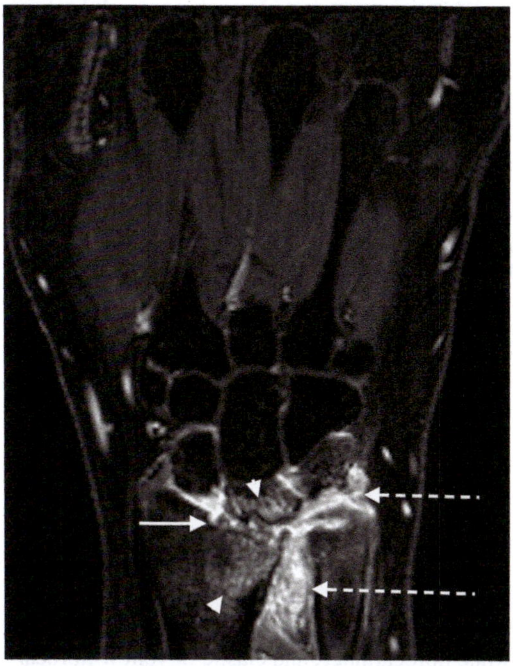

Fig. 3.53 Cor T1FS MRI post contrast in a patient with rheumatoid arthritis demonstrating active enhancing synovitis (*dashed arrows*) of the radiocarpal and distal radioulnar joints with enhancing bone marrow edema (*arrowhead*), erosions (*arrow*), and synovitis

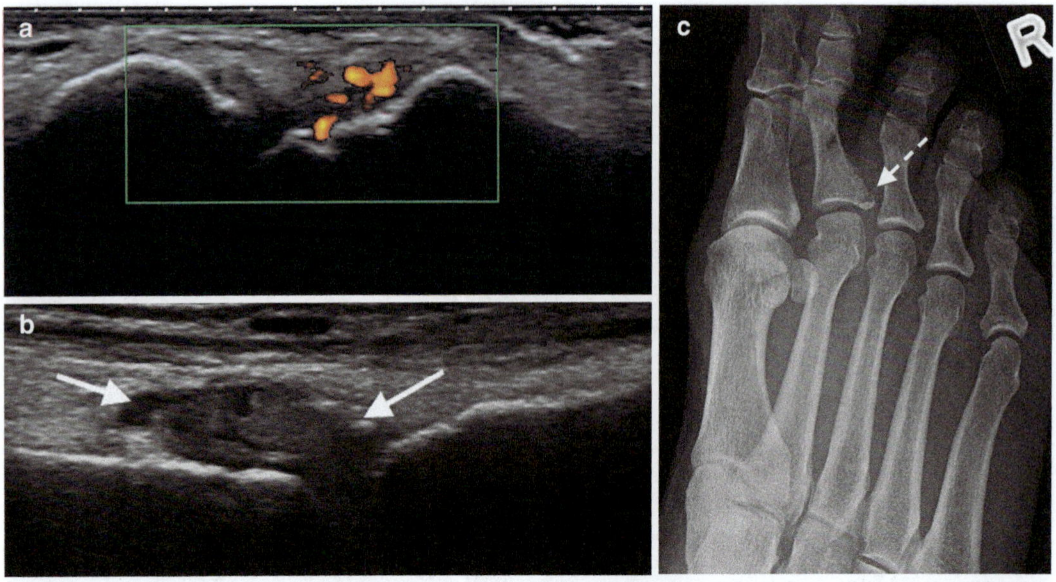

Fig. 3.54 Ultrasound synovitis. (**a**) Active synovitis of the MCPJ with moderate increased internal flow on power Doppler. (**b**) Longitudinal ultrasound in a different patient with clinical suspicion of gout demonstrates synovial thickening of the right second MTPJ; focal cortical defect noted during study. (**c**) Oblique radiograph demonstrates chronic bony avulsion. This highlights that synovitis may be related to many pathologies and not just an inflammatory arthropathy

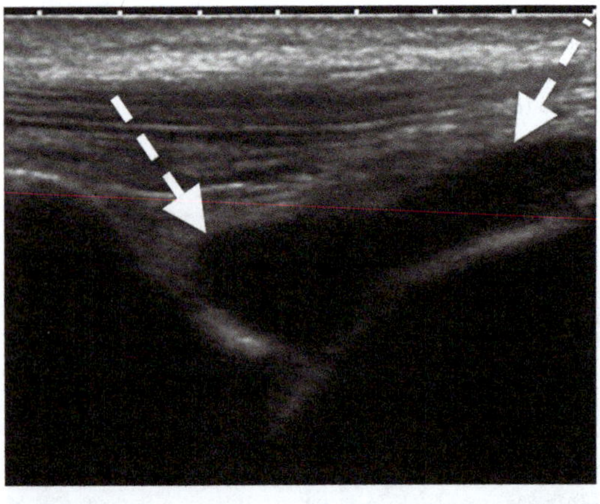

Fig. 3.55 Ultrasound joint effusion at the ankle demonstrating intra-articular anechoic fluid (*arrows*). This was displaceable on compression and demonstrated no internal flow on Doppler (not shown)

Cartilage

Anatomy

Cartilage can be divided into hyaline cartilage, white fibrocartilage, and elastic or yellow fibrocartilage. The latter is present in only select regions, e.g., the auricle of the external ear. Articular cartilage, costal cartilage, and temporary cartilage are composed of hyaline cartilage. With the exception of articular cartilage, cartilage is covered by perichondrium. Articular cartilage is of varying thickness, being thicker in points of greater stress and on convex rather than concave surfaces. It provides a degree of elasticity and shock absorption and helps to dissipate stress across a joint.

On *ultrasound*, articular cartilage has a smooth, well-defined surface and border and is uniformly hypoechoic (Fig. 3.56). In children, cartilaginous centers prior to ossification are not visible on plain radiographs but are clearly visible on ultrasound as hypoechoic structures with early ossification beginning centrally as a zone of hyperechogenicity (Fig. 3.57).

MRI is the gold imaging standard in assessing cartilage. Appearance is dependent on imaging sequence. There has been a rapid proliferation of research into different imaging sequences for articular cartilage including 3-D imaging. These sequences are most often used in research and clinical trials and are slowly making their way into clinical practice. Their integration is limited

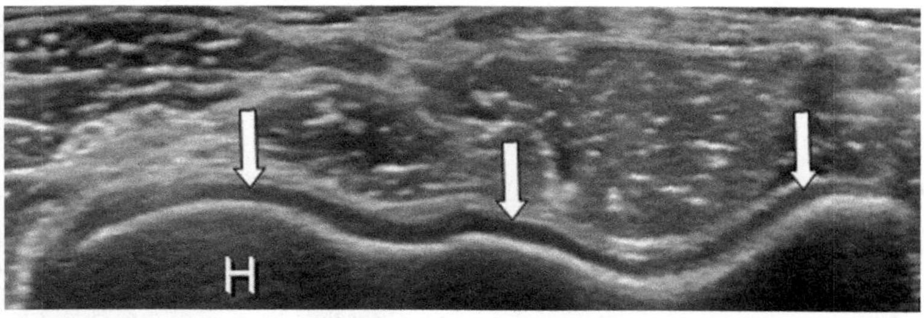

Fig. 3.56 Articular cartilage: transverse US demonstrating the uniformly well-defined hypoechoic normal articular cartilage (*arrows*) of the articulating surface distal humerus (*H*)

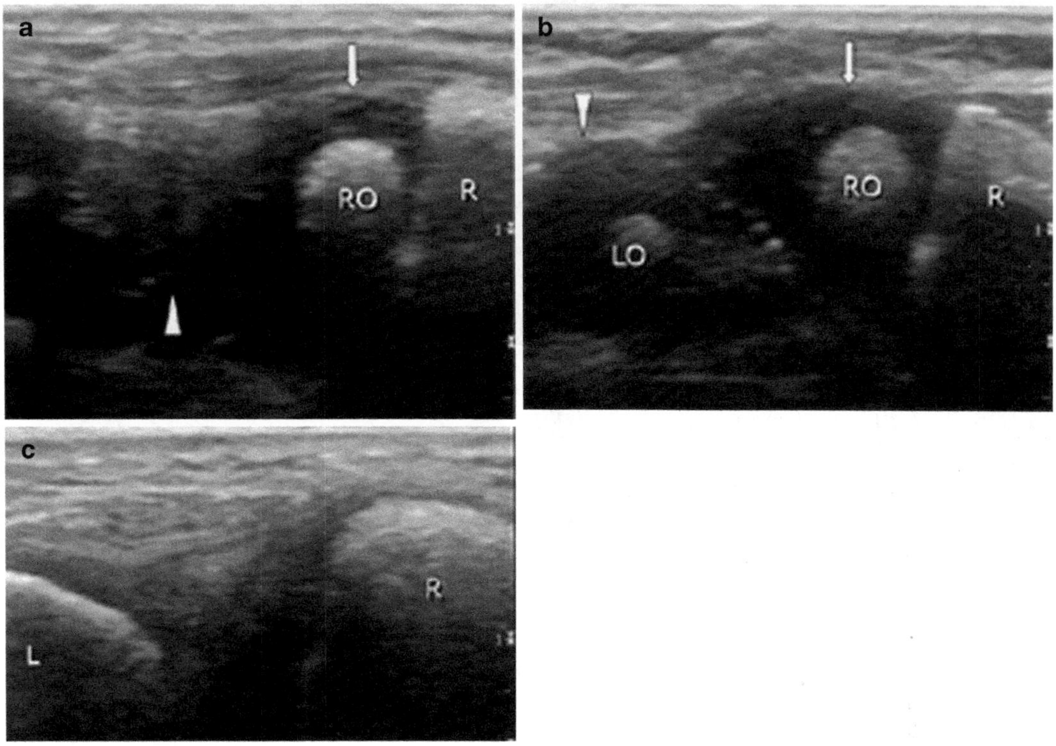

Fig. 3.57 Cartilaginous centers prior to ossification are clearly visible on ultrasound as hypoechoic structures with early ossification beginning centrally as a zone of hyperechogenicity. (**a**) Longitudinal US of a 2-year-old girl demonstrating early ossification center of the distal radius (*RO*) surrounded by the hypoechoic cartilaginous center; no ossification has commenced within the lunate (*arrowhead*) which remains uniformly hypoechoic. (**b**) Early ossification center is now visible in the lunate (*LO*) in this 4-year-old boy and (**c**) normal adult appearance

by access to software or magnet upgrades and the length of time required to acquire the study. We will concentrate on the commonly used sequences used in everyday clinical practice including T1, T2, and gradient echo (GE) (Fig. 3.58). Articular cartilage on T1 is of intermediate signal intensity and is easily distinguished from the underlying low signal intensity cortex. There is less clear definition however of the articular surface from joint fluid. T1 is therefore limited in assessment of cartilage. On T2 sequence fat saturation is preferred to help distinguish joint fluid from cartilage. Fluid is of high signal intensity and will extend into cartilage defects increasing their conspicuity. The cartilage is of intermediate signal intensity on T2. GE can be acquired as 3-D T1w sequence with the cartilage being of high signal intensity. The Outerbridge arthroscopic grading system for chondromalacia is adapted for MRI (Table 3.6, Fig. 3.59).

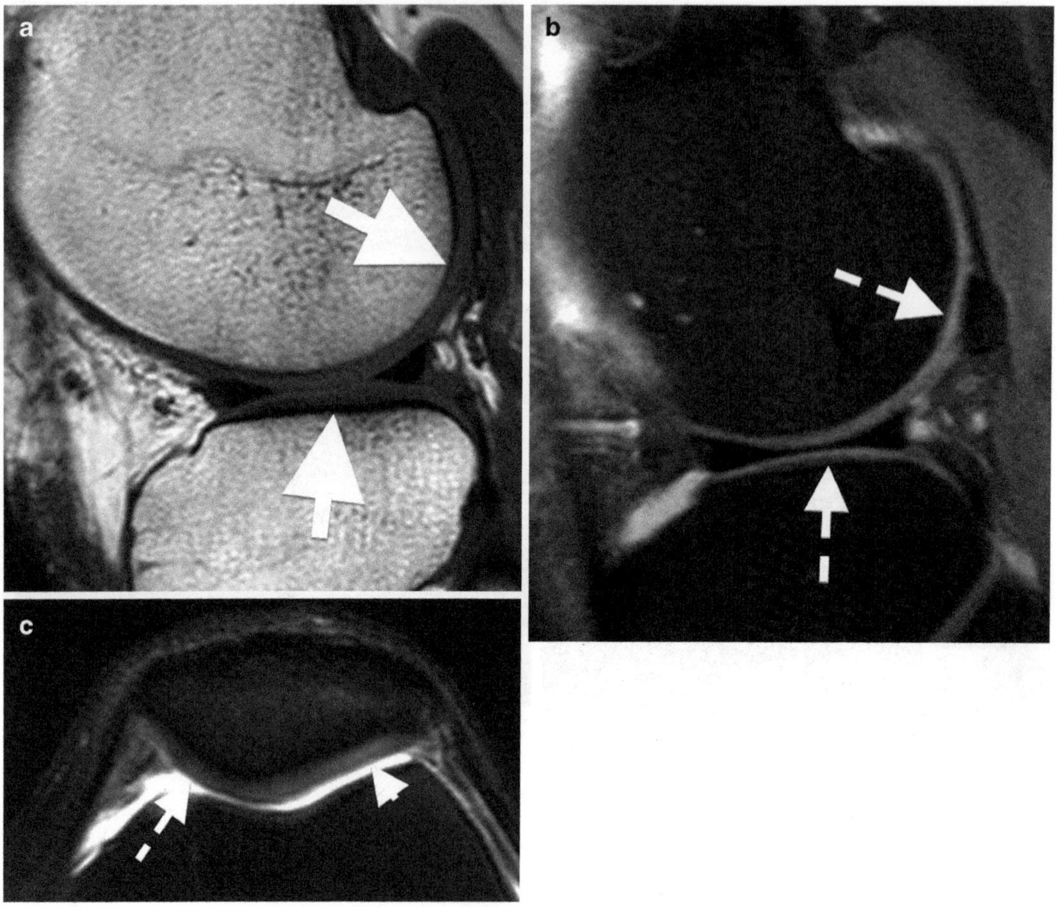

Fig. 3.58 MRI of the normal cartilage (*arrows*) of the knee on (**a**) Sag T1, (**b**) Sag T2FS, and (**c**) axial T2FS (*dashed arrow*) with grade 1 chondromalacia of the lateral patellar facet (*arrowhead*)

Table 3.6 Outerbridge arthroscopic grading chondromalacia

Grade	Arthroscopy	MRI
Grade 0	Normal	Normal
Grade 1	Softening, swelling, fibrillation surface	Signal intensity change, fibrillation
Grade 2	Fibrillation, fissuring extending to a depth of 1–2 mm	Fissuring extending up to 50 % cartilage depth
Grade 3	Fissuring extending greater than 50 % cartilage depth, no involvement of the subchondral bone	Fissuring extending greater than 50 % cartilage depth but not full thickness
Grade 4	Complete loss of cartilage with exposed bone	Full thickness cartilage loss, may be associated with subchondral sclerosis, edema, or cyst formation

Fibrocartilage is a variable mixture of white fibrous tissue and cartilaginous tissue with a large component of collagen fibrils. It provides elasticity and flexibility. The menisci of the knee, temporomandibular and sternoclavicular joints, the glenoid and hip labra, and the triangular fibrocartilage of the wrist are composed of fibrocartilage. On ultrasound, fibrocartilage is hyperechoic with well-delineated borders (Fig. 3.60). Because of its position within the joints, it is not always fully accessible on a full ultrasound examination.

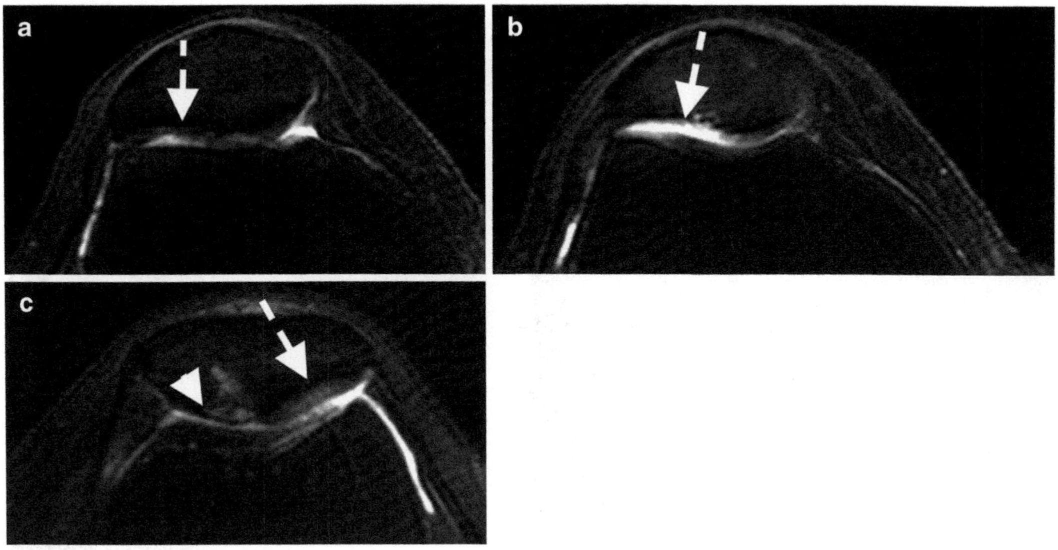

Fig. 3.59 MRI axial T2 of the patellofemoral articulation. (**a**) Lateral facet cartilage loss with areas greater than and less than 50 % loss (*dashed arrow*), (**b**) full-thickness cartilage loss of the lateral facet, (**c**) full-thickness cartilage loss with subchondral bone marrow edema and cyst formation of the lateral facet (*arrowhead*) and cartilage edema of the medial facet (*dashed arrow*)

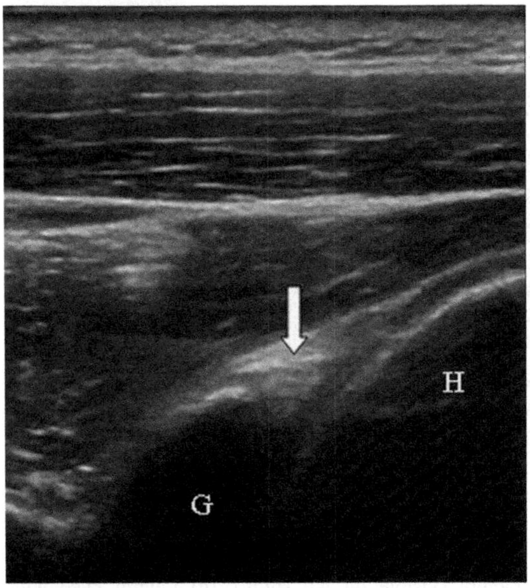

Fig. 3.60 Fibrocartilage: the posterior glenoid labrum (*arrow*) is demonstrated here as a well-defined hyperechoic triangular structure between the articulating surfaces of the glenoid (*G*) and the humerus (*H*)

Joint Effusion

All joints contain a small amount of fluid for normal lubrication. A joint effusion is an abnormal increase in the normal fluid volume and may be related to many etiologies including trauma, degenerative disease, inflammatory arthropathies, and infection. Effusions cause displacement of intra-articular fat pads, if present (e.g. elbow and ankle), and periarticular soft tissue swelling as the capsule expands. Knowledge of anatomical insertion sites of the joint capsule and careful review of periarticular fat planes for displacement are helpful in the radiographic assessment of effusions. Many effusions can be assessed on radiographs (Fig. 3.61). Ultrasound is helpful in assessing joints with smaller effusions or less readily assessed on radiographs, such as the hip joint. Fluid may be anechoic or heterogenous and appearance does not guide underlying diagnosis. Doppler interrogation should always be performed to assess for synovial hypertrophy. CT will demonstrate joint distension, however CT is not used for the primary evaluation of an effusion. Effusion may be low attenuating but may be higher in complex effusion or hemarthrosis. MRI is usually reserved for deeper joints that may be more difficult to assess with ultrasound (Fig. 3.62). Simple effusions will be of low signal intensity on T1 and high on T2.

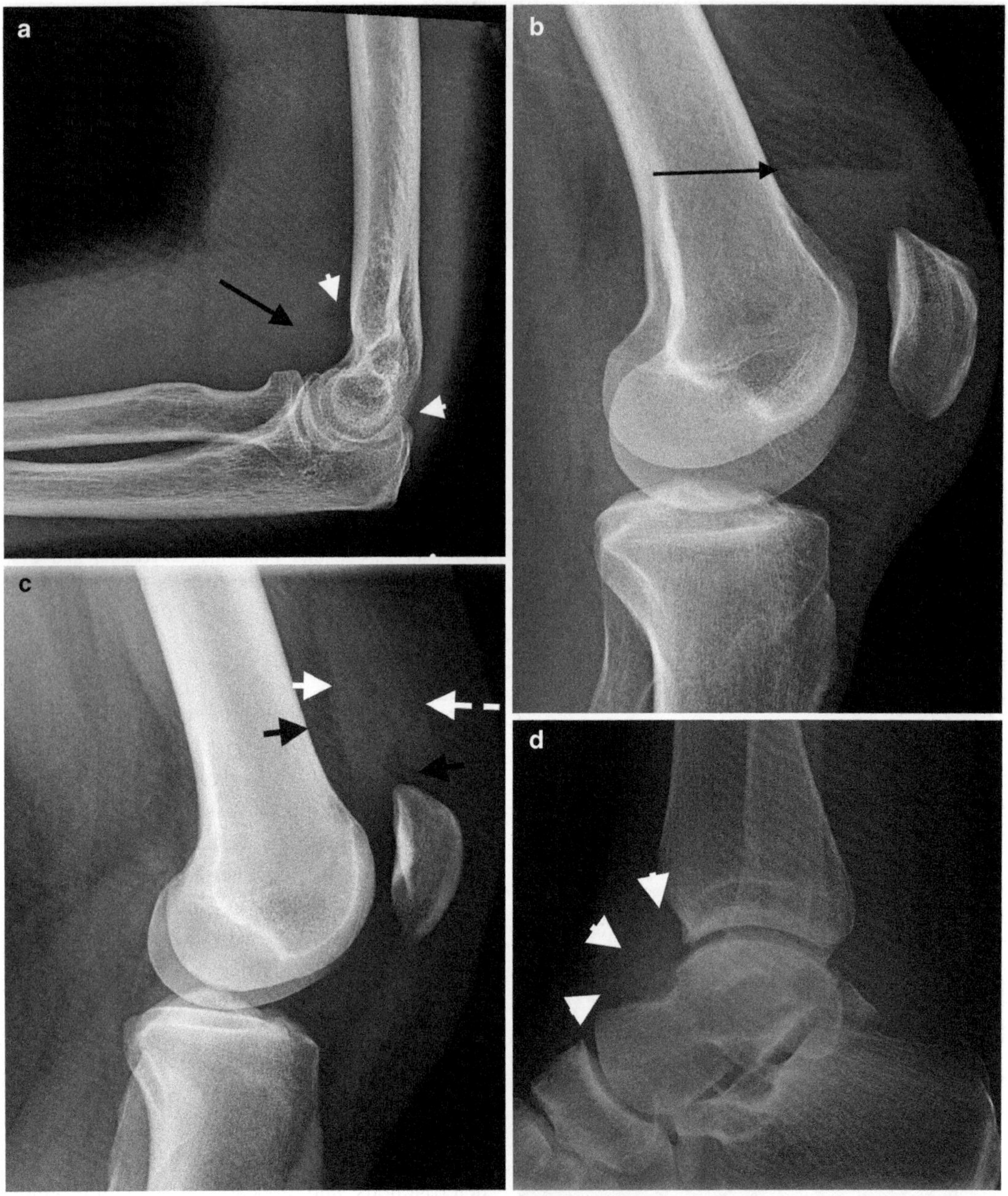

Fig. 3.61 Joint effusions: (**a**) lateral elbow radiograph with moderate effusion (*black arrow*) and sail sign, displacing the anterior fat pad superiorly, and the posterior fat fad becomes visible (*arrowheads*). (**b**) Lateral standing knee radiograph with fat fluid level (*arrow*) in keeping with lipohemarthrosis in patient with lateral tibial plateau fracture (visible on AP study). (**c**) Lateral knee with suprapatellar effusion (*white arrow*). Note the anterior and posterior fat pads (*black arrows*), post quadriceps and pre-femoral, respectively. (**d**) Lateral ankle radiograph with moderate effusion (*white arrowheads*). This demonstrates points of anterior capsular attachments

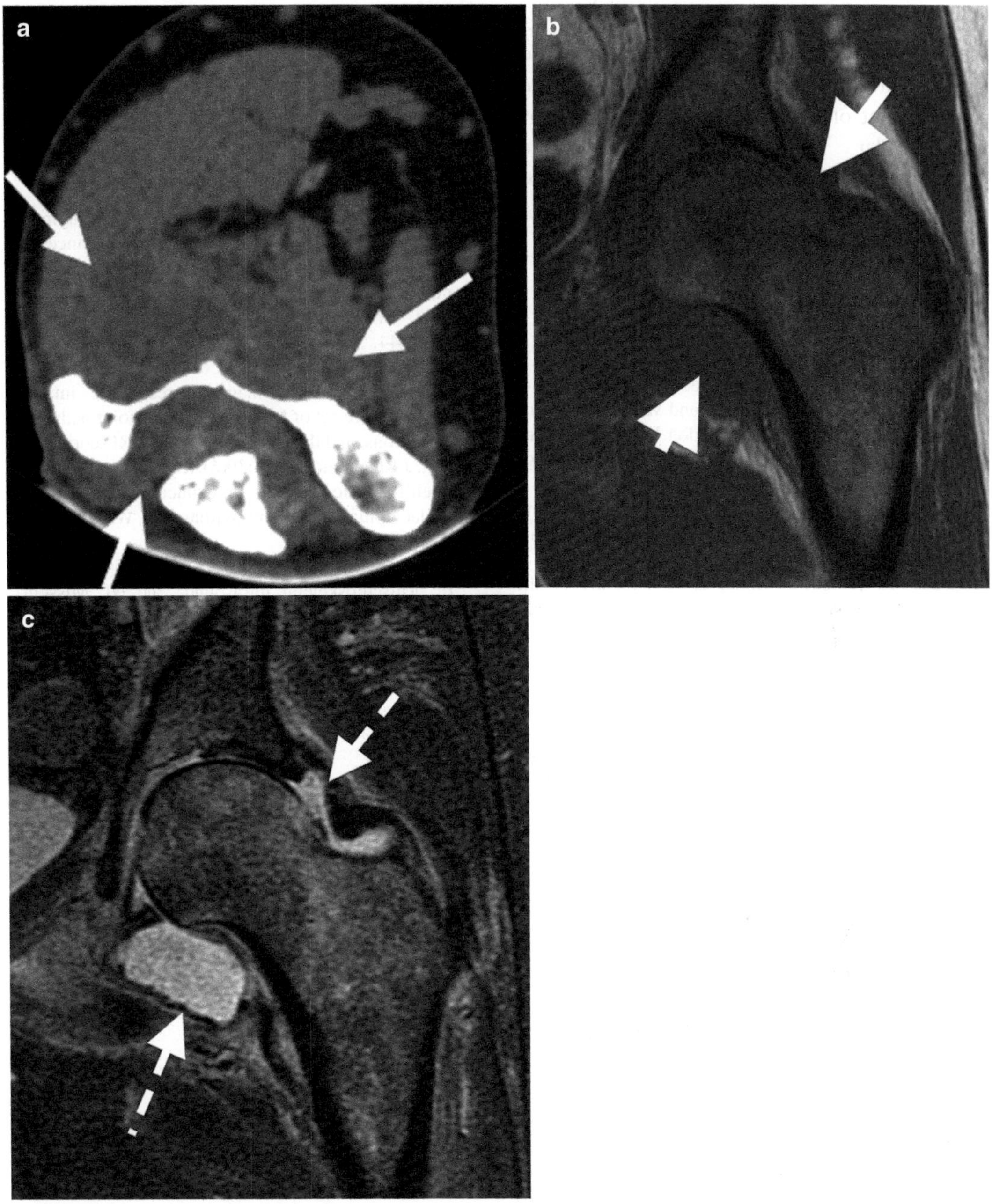

Fig. 3.62 (**a**) Axial CT elbow with complex effusion in patient with chronic hemophilia. (**b**) MRI Cor T1 and (**c**) T2 of complex effusion (*arrows*), as SI is intermediate on T1, suggesting effusion is complex (would be of low SI in simple effusion) in a patient with septic arthritis of the left hip

Joint fluid will not enhance if study is performed immediately post injection contrast. After approximately 10 min, there may be apparent enhancement of an effusion secondary to slow intra-articular permeation of gadolinium. Immediate enhancement is in keeping with active synovitis.

Further Reading

1. Alcalde M, D'Agostino MA, Bruyn GA, OMERACT Ultrasound Task Force. A systematic literature review of US definitions, scoring systems and validity according to the OMERACT filter for tendon lesion in RA and other inflammatory joint diseases. Rheumatology (Oxford). 2012;51(7):1246–60.
2. Gray H. General anatomy or histology. In: The complete Gray's anatomy. 16th ed. London: Longman, Green, and Co.; 1905. p. 1–72.
3. Gruber H, Kovacs P. Sonographic anatomy of the peripheral nervous system. In: Peer S, Bodner G, editors. High resolution sonography of the peripheral nervous system. 1st ed. Berlin: Springer; 2003. p. 28–32.
4. Hammer HB, Haavardsholm EA. Advances in imaging. Curr Opin Rheumatol. 2012;24(3):299–305.
5. Martinoli C, Bianchi S, Dahmane M. Ultrasound of tendons and nerves. Eur Radiol. 2002;12:44–55.
6. O'Neill J. Musculoskeletal ultrasound: anatomy and technique. New York: Springer; 2008.
7. Østergaard M, Pedersen SJ, Døhn UM. Imaging in rheumatoid arthritis–status and recent advances for magnetic resonance imaging, ultrasonography, computed tomography and conventional radiography. Best Pract Res Clin Rheumatol. 2008;22(6):1019–44.
8. Østergaard M, Peterfy C, Conaghan P. OMERACT rheumatoid arthritis magnetic resonance imaging studies. Core set of MRI acquisitions, joint pathology definitions, and the OMERACT RA-MRI scoring system. J Rheumatol. 2003;30(6):1385–6.
9. Snell R. Basic anatomy. In: Clinical anatomy. 7th ed. Philadelphia: Lippincott Williams & Wilkins; 2004. p. 1–48.
10. van Holsbeeck M, Introcaso J. Sonography of tendons. In: Musculoskeletal ultrasound. 2nd ed. Missouri: Mosby; 2001. p. 77–81.

Image-Guided Interventional Diagnosis and Treatment

4

John O'Neill

Overview

Image-guided diagnosis and treatment have grown significantly in the last decade. A major component in this growth is the use of ultrasound as an imaging guide in the treatment of musculoskeletal pathology (Table 4.1). Fluoroscopic arthrography and joint injections, however, remain the most commonly requested procedures and are reviewed in detail.

Imaging Modalities

Ultrasound is an ideal imaging technique for image-guided therapy (Figs. 4.1 and 4.2). Ultrasound is readily available and inexpensive and involves no ionizing radiation. It provides direct communication with the patient throughout the procedure. Assessment of the soft tissue mass, localization of solid components suitable for biopsy, and assessing lesional and adjacent soft tissue vascularity with Doppler are all possible with ultrasound. The dynamic real-time imaging allows for continuous imaging of needle tract and localization of injectate throughout the procedure. In addition, alternate sources of pathology can be identified and assessed, e.g., identification of a periarticular bursa in a patient with suspected septic arthritis. If a joint effusion is present, aspiration of the joint and bursa may be required but as separate procedures.

CT is usually reserved for musculoskeletal procedures not suitable for ultrasound guidance (Fig. 4.3). Deep soft tissue masses, where ultrasound may have difficulty visualizing the mass, are suitable for CT guidance. All masses where there is any possibility of malignancy require review by an oncology surgeon prior to procedure, so the correct access path is employed as this will be resected at the time of surgery. Bone biopsies can be performed under *fluoroscopy* or CT, the latter allowing for greater precision.

Fluoroscopy is most commonly employed for joint injections and aspirations. Fluoroscopy is also used for image-guided biopsy of bone lesions, vertebroplasty, and kyphoplasty. *MRI* is currently not used for MSK-guided procedures due to cost, time restraints, the requirement of non-ferromagnetic instruments, and the ready availability of ultrasound and CT.

Procedures

Tenotomy or dry needling is performed in selected cases for tendinopathy or partial tears. The involved tendons should not be involved by

J. O'Neill, MB, BAO, BCh, MRCPI, MSc, FRCR
Associate Professor, Musculoskeletal Imaging, Diagnostic Imaging, McMaster University/ St Joseph's Healthcare, Hamilton, ON L8N4A6, Canada
e-mail: joneill2@me.com

J. O'Neill (ed.), *Essential Imaging in Rheumatology*,
DOI 10.1007/978-1-4939-1673-3_4,

Table 4.1 Common ultrasound-guided procedures

Pathology	Procedure
Tenosynovitis	Ultrasound-guided aspiration/injection
Tendinopathy	Ultrasound-guided tenotomy, blood injection, steroid injection, PRP injection
Tendon tears (partial)	Ultrasound-guided tenotomy, blood injection, PRP injection
Ganglion	Ultrasound-guided aspiration, wall disruption, and steroid injection
Joint	Ultrasound-guided aspiration +/– injection, synovial biopsy (CT or fluoroscopy for deeper joints)
Bursa	Ultrasound-guided aspiration +/– injection
Calcific tendinosis	Ultrasound-guided barbotage
Soft tissue lesion	Biopsy (usually in consultation with soft tissue tumor surgeon), ultrasound-guided for superficial lesions (CT guidance for deeper lesions)
Miscellaneous	Muscle biopsy for diagnosis myositis, Morton's neuroma injection, trigger finger, perineural diagnostic and therapeutic injections, e.g., carpal tunnel syndrome

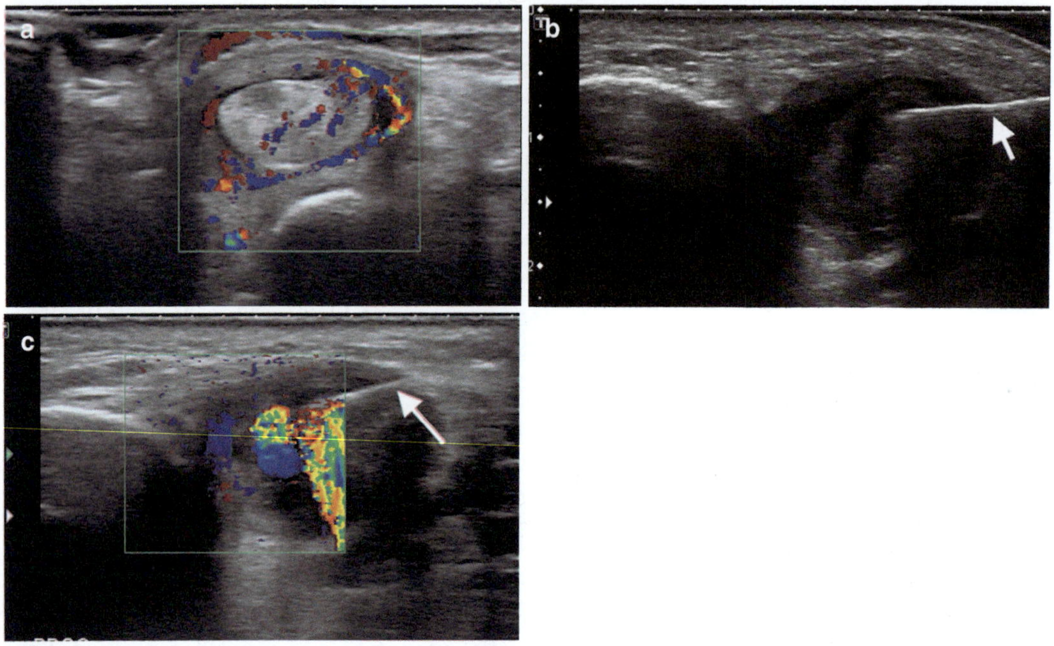

Fig. 4.1 A 59-year-old female patient with marked posterior tibialis (PT), tendinosis, and tenosynovitis. (**a**) Transverse ultrasound level of the medial malleolus demonstrating thickened heterogenous tendon and distended tendon sheath with increased flow within on color Doppler. (**b**) Needle (*arrow*) within PT tendon sheath. (**c**) Color Doppler demonstrating motion injectate during injection

a systemic process as can be seen in seronegative arthropathies, which usually require treatment of the underlying systemic disease. A 22G needle repeatedly transverses the local pathology under ultrasound guidance, disrupting areas of fibrosis and chronic inflammation and inducing an acute injury. Localized intratendinous hemorrhage occurs with an influx of platelets, containing multiple growth factors, which in turn stimulate healing. Activity related to the treated tendon is limited for 2 weeks, and then a graduated return to normal activity is employed. Education with respect to the initiating pathology is required to prevent recurrent tendinopathy.

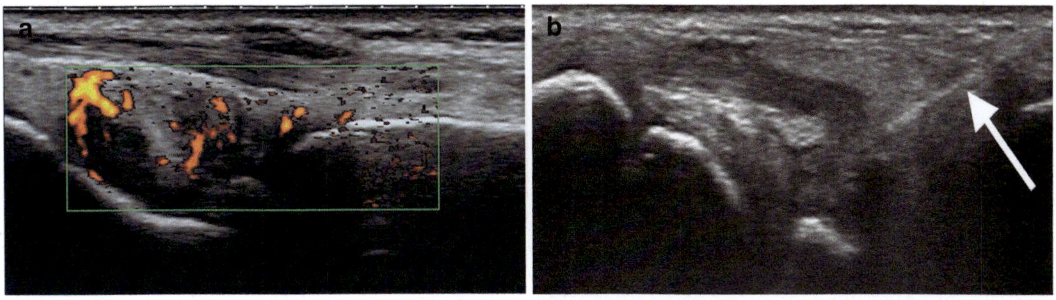

Fig. 4.2 A 29-year-old female with subacute right wrist synovitis of unknown etiology for ultrasound-guided synovial biopsy. (**a**) Active synovitis of the dorsal radiocarpal joint with moderate flow on power Doppler and (**b**) synovial biopsy needle (*arrow*)

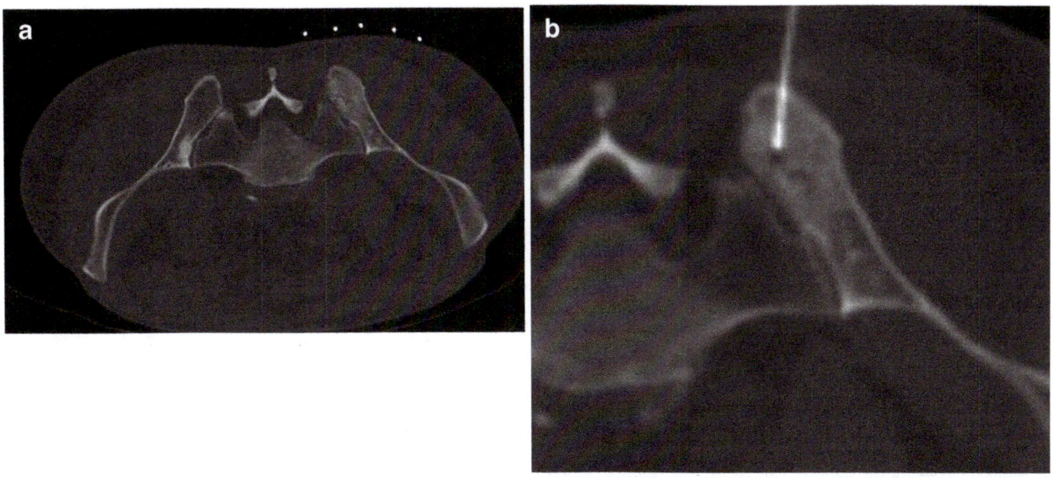

Fig. 4.3 A 68-year-old male with right pelvic pain. (**a**) Axial CT with patient prone demonstrates ill-defined sclerotic lesion of the right posterior ilium and (**b**) CT-guided bone biopsy with in situ needle. Lesion confirmed to be metastatic deposit from prostate carcinoma

Physiotherapy is often used in conjunction with tenotomy after a period of 2–4 weeks. An extension of tenotomy is whole blood injection and plasma-rich platelet (*PRP*) injections (Figs. 4.4 and 4.5). Tenotomy is performed as described above. After tenotomy, 3–5 ml of the patient's whole blood or PRP is directly injected into the tendon at the tenotomy site. PRP requires centrifuging 10–20 ml of the patient's whole blood. This allows separation of plasma and RBCs. Platelets are concentrated in the plasma, ideally at least five times the blood concentration, and hence contain a greater proportion of growth factors, which should have a greater impact on healing. Further research is required directly comparing tenotomy, blood injection, and PRP injection. The most common tendons treated in our center include the common extensor tendon at the elbow, the Achilles tendon, the common flexor tendon, and the patellar tendon.

Barbotage, calcific tendinosis disruption and aspiration, is used in selected cases for treatment of symptomatic calcific tendinosis. Identification of calcific tendinosis on imaging should be correlated with the patient's symptoms. It is most commonly identified within the rotator cuff. Symptoms directly over the area of calcification and lack of adjacent pathology should be assessed

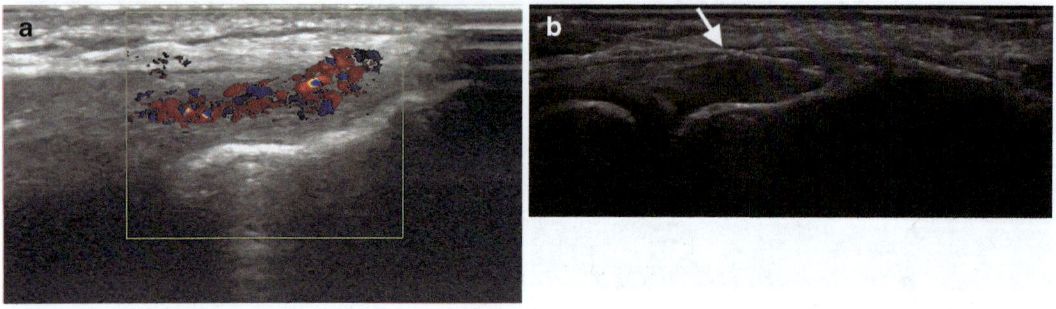

Fig. 4.4 A 44-year-old male with chronic extensor tendinosis at the elbow unresponsive to conservative treatment. (**a**) Pre-procedural ultrasound demonstrates tendon heterogeneity and significant internal flow on power Doppler; patient had also severe tenderness with mild probe compression over this region. (**b**) Needle (*arrow*) transversing the tendon as part of tenotomy immediately pre-PRP injection

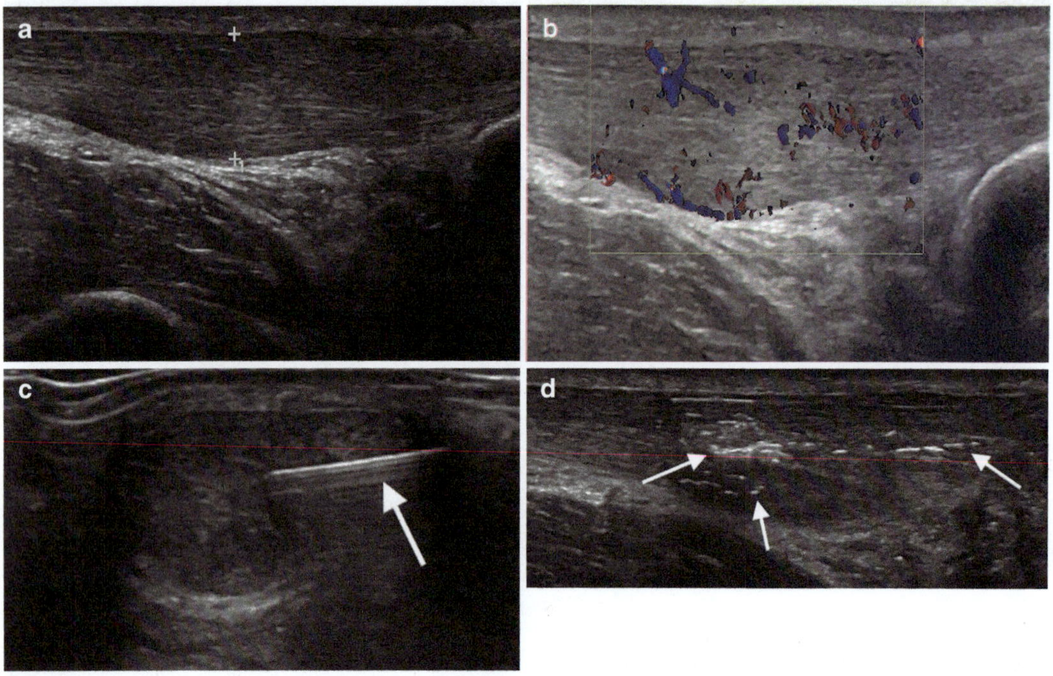

Fig. 4.5 A 52-year-old male with Achilles tendinosis with limitation activity and pain on compression of the mid-Achilles. (**a**) Longitudinal ultrasound demonstrates mid AT tendinosis with (**b**) increased internal flow on color Doppler. (**c**) Tenotomy needle (*arrow*) on transverse image and (**d**) longitudinal ultrasound image post PRP injection demonstrating the expected proximal and distal propagation of the injectate (*arrows*)

prior to barbotage. If there is a generalized tendinopathy without exaggeration of symptoms over the area of calcific tendinosis, we will often advise a conservative treatment for tendinopathy in the first instance. In those cases selected for barbotage, the calcification is identified under ultrasound, and a 20–22G needle is repeatedly passed through the calcification while flushing and aspirating with local anesthetic (Fig. 4.6). Some centers use a two-needle approach, one for injection of local anesthetic and the second to aspirate. Steroid should be injected into any overlying bursa, e.g., subacromial-subdeltoid bursa when performed for the supraspinatus tendon, to limit

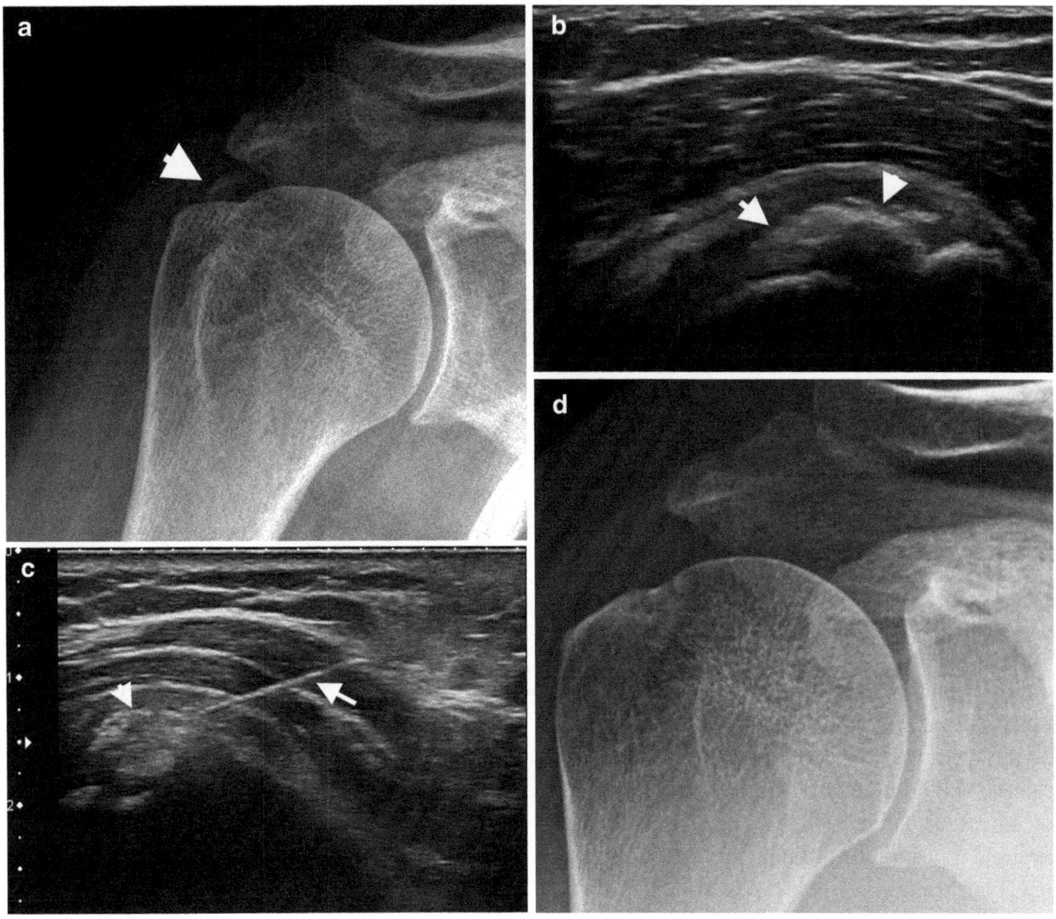

Fig. 4.6 A 28-year-old female with calcific tendinopathy of the supraspinatus tendon with persistent pain and limited range of motion for 1 year. (**a**) AP radiograph demonstrates calcification of the supraspinatus tendon (*arrowhead*). (**b**) Longitudinal ultrasound with hyperechoic calcific deposit corresponding to radiograph (*arrowheads*), patient had tenderness on probe compression directly over the calcification. (**c**) Needle (*arrow*) transversing the calcification (*arrowhead*) which is already partially disrupted after previous passes by the needle. (**d**) Follow-up radiograph 3 months post-procedure with no residual calcification. Patient reported complete relief of symptoms

secondary bursitis due to potential leakage of crystals into the bursa. Radiographs are taken pre- and post-procedure and at 3 months. There is often residual calcification immediately post barbotage that is gradually reabsorbed on follow-up.

Arthrography

Arthrography, injection of a contrast into a joint space, may be performed for diagnostic or therapeutic purposes (Table 4.2). A conventional arthrogram is usually performed as a fluoroscopically guided injection of a joint but may be performed under ultrasound or CT guidance in selected cases. Intra-articular position is confirmed by injection of a small amount of iodinated contrast

Table 4.2 Indications for joint-related procedures

Aspiration for infection, crystals
Assessment loosening joint prosthesis
Diagnostic arthrogram
Pre-MRI or CT arthrograms
Therapeutic steroid, anesthetic, and viscosupplementation injectates

into the joint space. Depending on the procedure, the joint is further distended with contrast for MRI or CT arthrogram, gadoliniums versus iodinated-based contrast respectively, or alternate injectate for therapeutic or diagnostic injection. The latter may include an anesthetic agent, viscosupplementation, or steroids. Anesthetic may be short or long acting and may help identify the origin of pain. This is commonly used for diagnostic hip injections where the symptoms may be related to intra-articular pathology of the hip, which will be relieved with anesthetic, whereas referred pain from degenerative lumbar spine disc disease or periarticular pathology will not be relieved. Use of a visual analogue score sheet for the patient pre- and post-procedure can be useful in grading any relief from anesthetic. We also advise patients to maintain a pain diary to document any long-term relief from therapeutic injections.

In patients who are allergic to iodinated contrast, several options are available including use of air or saline instead of iodinated contrast. Therve should be no resistance or induced pain on injection saline, and one should be able to aspirate a portion of the injectate. Alternatively, if CT arthrogram is being performed, then air can be substituted for iodinated contrast. The procedure can be also performed under ultrasound guidance.

MRI and CT arthrography have replaced arthrography alone as the gold standard in the assessment of internal joint derangement. Cases are usually decided on a per patient basis depending on clinical symptoms, prior imaging, and management options.

There are usually different options with respect to points of injection for any particular joint. Choice depends on the location of the suspected pathology with every effort made not to inject into the area of pathology, e.g., if torn ligament is suspected, then one should not transverse that ligament on gaining access to joint as this may obscure or complicate the imaging appearance of pathology. Also patients should be kept in the most comfortable position possible to limit any unintentional movement during the procedure. All procedures are performed under strict aseptic

Table 4.3 Pre-procedure checklist

Confirm clinical indication
Review prior imaging/intervention
If proceeding to MRI arthrogram, exclude any contraindications to MRI
Obtain brief history from the patient and note any changes in clinical symptoms since referral
Exclude any skin conditions at the site of injection, e.g., cellulitis
Exclude bleeding diathesis/anticoagulant therapy
Obtain written informed consent
Perform visual analogue score if giving therapeutic or diagnostic intra-articular anesthetic after joint manipulation pre- and post-procedure

Table 4.4 Arthrogram-related complications

Infection	Symptoms usually develop after 24 h, 1:10,000–20,000
Chemical synovitis	Steroid-induced synovitis commencing usually several hours after injection and lasting less than 48 hrs
Pain	e.g., extra-articular injection
Hemorrhage	Intra-/extra-articular
Vasovagal reactions	
Allergic reactions	Uncommon
Avascular necosis (AVN)	Steroid injection, uncommon, risk increases with repeated injections into same joint

conditions. Pre-procedure checklist is detailed in Table 4.3. Complications of arthrograms are uncommon (Table 4.4). Helpful tips for joint-related procedures are outlined in Table 4.5. Joint injections are a common procedure in the outpatient clinic. As such, a more detailed description of image-guided joint injections and arthrograms is provided below.

Technique

Patient preparation and pre-procedure workup are performed as outlined above and in Table 4.3. All procedures are carried out under strict aseptic technique and use of local anesthetic. The procedures described below are those for MRI or CT arthrograms and can be modified appropriately for aspiration, injection, or conventional arthrogram.

Shoulder Arthrography

Joint aspiration, steroid injections, and treatment of adhesive capsulitis are common indications. MRI shoulder arthrograms are reserved in our center for patients with instability for the assessment of labrum/capsule/ligamentous injuries and rarely complex or postoperative rotator cuff tears requiring further evaluation after standard MRI or ultrasound. CT arthrograms can be performed in those with contraindication to MRI or where MRI is not available. It is also very useful in the detailed assessment of associated bone injuries. There are three common access points for shoulder arthrogram. Choice depends on suspected location pathology, patient comfort, overlying skin pathology, and operator experience. An anterior or posterior approach can be performed.

Anteriorly one may inject into the rotator interval (Fig. 4.7a) or transverse the mid subscapularis (Fig. 4.7b). The patient lies supine, extended upper limb held in external rotation and palm facing up and held in this position with the use of a sandbag. External rotation increases the accessible joint surface: however, if one over-rotates, then the injection becomes more difficult as the capsule is stretched over the humeral head. The rotator interval injection point lies over the medial and superior third humeral head, level with the superior margin of the base coracoid process. This is the most shallow of the three injections and a 3.5 cm 22G needle can usually be used. The trans-subscapularis approach is directed over the junction of the mid and inferior thirds of the humeral head, approximately 5 mm lateral to the subchondral humeral

Table 4.5 Helpful tips for joint procedures

Performing an ultrasound prior to joint aspiration for infection can be very helpful in confirming joint distension and excluding periarticular collections/bursae
All joints should be aspirated prior to therapeutic or diagnostic injection to diminish dilution effect
Knowing the site of capsular attachments of a joint will facilitate a more confident injection technique
Never inject into resistance
Pre-procedure radiographs may be required for arthrograms. For the wrist, a standard PA and lateral and fist-clenched PA are required. A standing centered AP bilateral hip and ipsilateral Dunn view are performed pre-hip arthrogram
Discussion with your radiologist is always welcomed particularly with respect to the optimal study for a patient

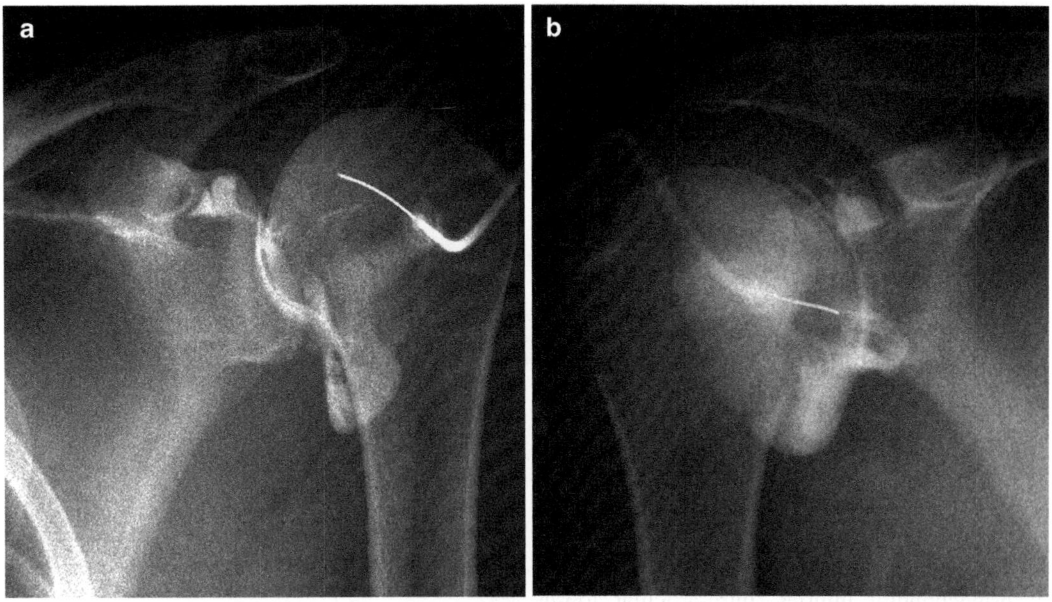

Fig. 4.7 Shoulder arthrogram: fluoroscopic images acquired demonstrating needle position for (**a**) rotator interval and (**b**) trans-subscapularis approaches

cortical margin. This avoids any contact with the labrum. This approach requires a 22G spinal needle, as do all major joints unless otherwise specified (Fig. 4.3). The posterior approach is performed with the patient prone and a 45° sponge under the affected shoulder. The arm is held in external rotation with the palm facing down. The posterolateral margin of the acromion is palpated; a site 3–4 cm inferior and 2 cm medial to this is selected. The needle is advanced in the direction of the anteriorly positioned coracoid process, to the humeral articular cartilage, keeping above the physeal line.

Under strict aseptic conditions, with the use of local anesthetic and fluoroscopic guidance, the needle is slowly advanced, perpendicular to the point of access for anterior injection and obliquely for posterior approach as described above, until the needle abuts the humeral head. Position is confirmed with 1–2 ml of iodinated contrast. If contrast does not flow immediately away from the needle tip, stop the injection and reevaluate. Confirm that the arm is in external rotation when performing the anterior approach. If needle is in correct position, rotate the needle bevel so it points toward the joint and reattempt injection. If unsuccessful a second time, then the needle should be repositioned. Once intra-articular position is confirmed, the appropriate contrast, 10–12 ml, for CT or MRI arthrogram is then injected. We use dilute iodinated contrast with our gadolinium injectate, so we can perform alternative imaging with CT in those who cannot complete their MRI arthrogram study, e.g., due to claustrophobia. Limiting motion of the injected joint will decrease any post-procedural extravasation contrast into the surrounding soft tissues. Ideally the patient should be imaged as soon after injection as possible to maximize the amount of joint distension; we aim to have less than 30 min between the procedure and study.

Elbow Arthrography

MR arthrogram indications include assessment of osteochondral injuries, intra-articular loose bodies, and ligamentous disruption. There are two main approaches, lateral and posterolateral. The former is the most common site of access. The ulnar nerve and its close approximation to the joint limit a medial approach. I will often prefer to use ultrasound guidance if there are multiple sites of suspected pathology or if I cannot palpate the ulnar nerve within the cubital tunnel. For the lateral approach, the patient lies prone with the elbow flexed at 90° above the head. Injection point is the mid-radiocapitellar joint space (Fig. 4.8). As stated above, if this is the site of clinical concern, an alternate injection site should be chosen. In the posteromedial approach, the patient lies supine with the arm pronated and semiflexed raised above the head. The ulnar nerve lies within the cubital tunnel, which can be palpated. The site of injection is between the cubital tunnel and olecranon, targeting the olecranon fossa. A 3.5 cm 22G needle is used with the patient prepped and draped in a standard fashion. Confirmation of intra-articular position is confirmed with 1–2 ml iodinated contrast, and then 8–10 s of the required contrast is injected. Any joint fluid is aspirated prior to injection.

Wrist Arthrography

Wrist arthrograms are commonly performed for the assessment of the TFCC (triangular

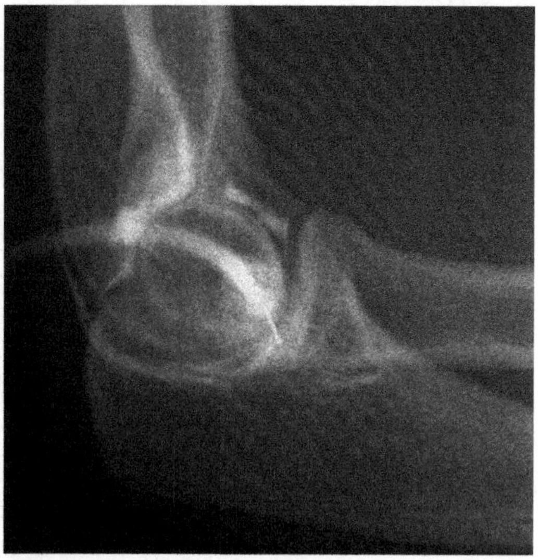

Fig. 4.8 Elbow arthrogram: fluoroscopic image acquired demonstrating needle position for a lateral radiocapitellar joint space approach

fibrocartilage complex) and the integrity of the intrinsic ligaments, the scapholunate and lunotriquetral ligaments. Careful patient selection is required.

Pre-procedure radiographs are required for wrist MRI/CT arthrograms. A standard PA and lateral and fist-clenched PA are performed to confirm alignment and to assess ulnar variance. A sagittal MRI will often demonstrate lunate rotation, which is often positional and will be normally aligned on radiograph in the absence of related pathology (Fig. 4.5). Ulnar variance may change and be progressively more positive with a clenched fist, i.e., ulnar neutral variance may become ulnar positive variance. The majority of wrist injections are single radiocarpal injections at our institution however an occasional triple wrist arthrogram may be performed, commencing with the midcarpal, then distal radioulnar, and finally the radioscapoid joint (Fig. 4.9). MR arthrogram theory is to distinguish the joint compartments and integrity of the ligaments and TFC by having gadolinium-based contrast only in the middle joint space, i.e., radiocarpal. On T1-weighted images, this contrast will be of high signal intensity, whereas the remaining joints will be of low signal intensity thus confirming integrity. If a tear is identified during the fluoroscopic injection, then the type of contrast is modified accordingly, e.g., if contrast leaks from midcarpal to radiocarpal joint, then iodinated contrast injection is stopped and tubing flushed with gadolinium-based contrast which is then injected into the midcarpal space. Gadolinium will then diffuse into the radiocarpal space and allow differentiation from the distal radioulnar joint (DRUJ), which will have no Gd within, presuming an intact TFCC.

The dorsal triquetrolunohamate space is the optimal site for the midcarpal injection, which is the first injection. Once intra-articular position is confirmed, 2–3 ml of iodinated contrast is injected under cinefluoroscopic guidance at 2 frames/s. Contrast may extend to the proximal carpal row but will not pass into radiocarpal space unless a tear is present. The wrist is gently moved in ulnar and radial deviation. If an SL or LT tear is identified, the injection is stopped and injectate is exchanged for gadolinium-based contrast and a further 2 ml is injected. The DRUJ is the second injection, again from a dorsal approach with needle position over the proximal ulnar-articulating surface. 1–2 mls is injected under fluoroscopic guidance. If a full thickness tear is noted upon DRUJ injection, then 2 ml gadolinium-based contrast is injected into the DRUJ; contrast will then transverse into the radiocarpal space. If the first or second injections reveal no tears, then the radiocarpal space is approached on the radial and dorsal aspect, lateral to the S-L ligament and just distal to the distal margin of the radius, remembering that the radius has a cupped distal margin. 2 mls of gadolinium-based contrast is then injected into the radiocarpal space.

Hip Arthrography

MRI or CT arthrography of the hip is most often performed for the assessment of the acetabular labrum. Many centers particularly with 3T MRI availability will restrict MRA as often the non-arthrographic 3T MRI will demonstrate excellent anatomy and delineate underlying labral and cartilage pathology. As indicated above, intra-articular anesthetic injection with pre-/post-pain assessment will help confirm intra-articular pathology as the potential cause of symptoms. A standing centered AP bilateral hip and unilateral Dunn view are performed pre-procedure to assess acetabular coverage and femoral head/neck dysplasia. The patient is then prepped in a standard fashion in a supine position. The hip is maintained in neutral or slight internal rotation with the knees semiflexed with the use of a support pad. The capsule attaches to the lower femoral neck anteriorly. The optimal site is at the lateral margin of the mid femoral neck. Lateral approach avoids the femoral neurovascular bundle. After intra-articular position is confirmed with 1–2 ml of iodinated contrast, the joint is distended with 10–12 ml appropriate contrast as outlined above (Fig. 4.10).

Knee Arthrography

Knee joint injection is the most common therapeutic joint injection performed at our institution. It has increased in use particularly with the development of viscosupplementation. MRI or CT

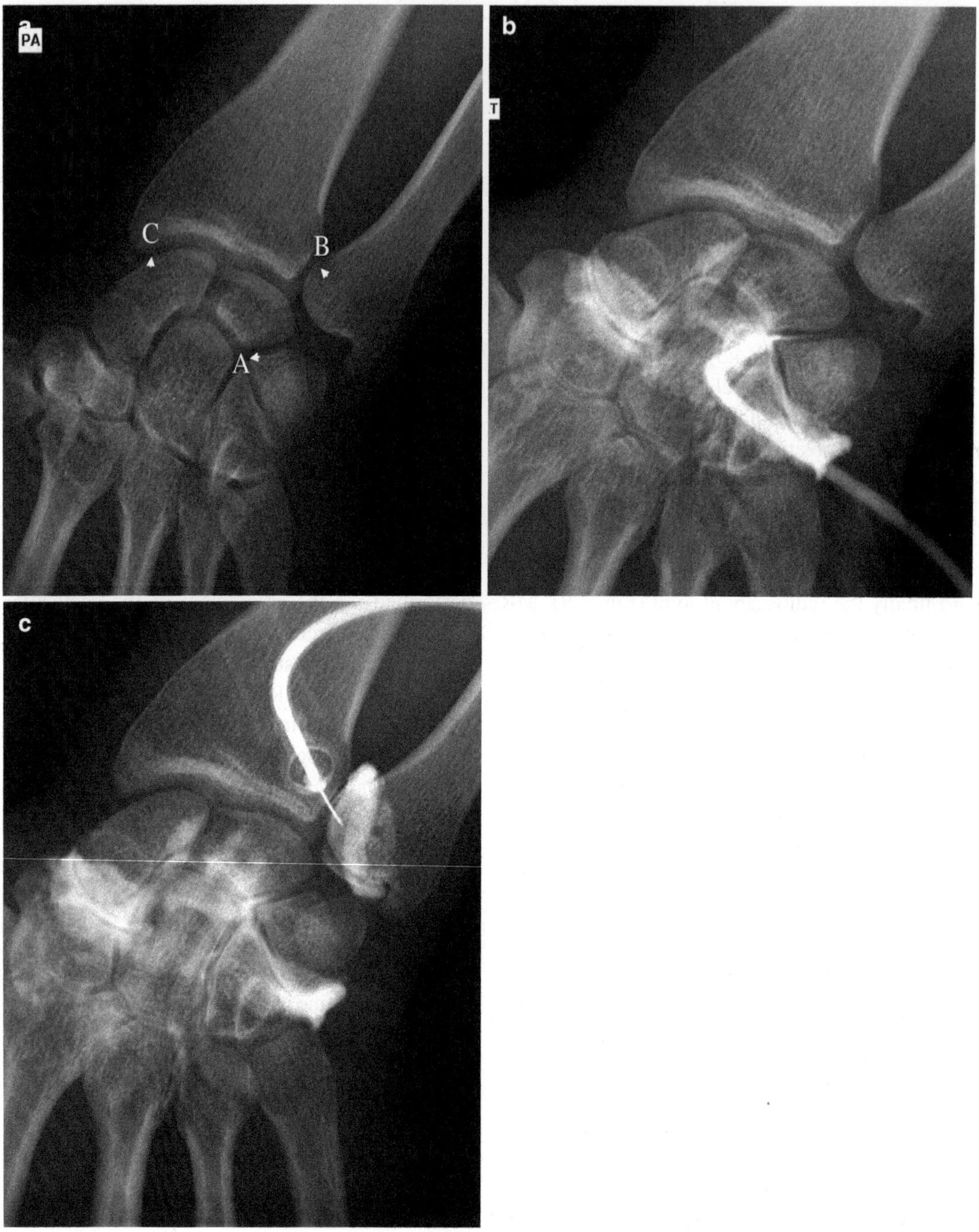

Fig. 4.9 Wrist arthrogram (**a**) demonstrates points of access (*arrowheads*) for midcarpal (*A*), distal radioulnar (*B*), and (*C*) radiocarpal joint approaches. (**b**) Fluoroscopic images acquired during midcarpal and (**c**) distal radioulnar joint access

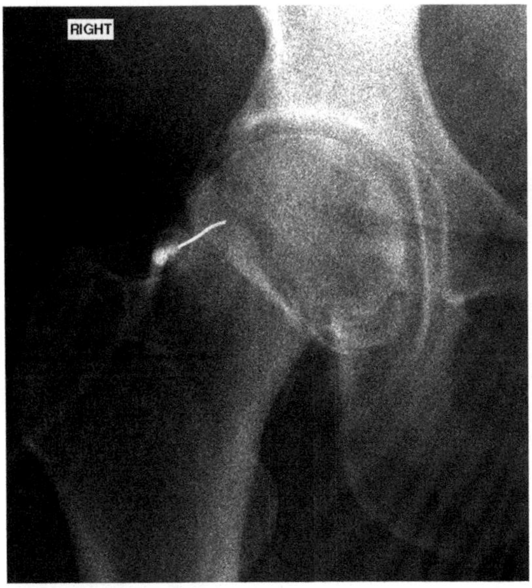

Fig. 4.10 Hip arthrogram: fluoroscopic images acquired demonstrating needle position for a hip joint space approach

arthrograms are less common procedures. These are usually reserved for patients with a prior history of partial meniscectomy, of at least 25 % meniscal resection, and assessment of prior cartilage repair or osteochondral injuries. Usually these patients have a standard MRI performed initially in our center and only proceed to arthrogram if standard imaging is insufficient in delineating and diagnosing pathology. There can be variability between institutions depending on equipment and specialist availability, and discussion with the radiologist is always welcomed.

The patient lies supine with the knee semiflexed to 45° and supported by a pad placed under the knee. There are several approaches to the knee joint. A medial or lateral patellofemoral are the commonest approaches. The deep articular margin of the patella, at junction of the mid and superior one third, is palpated. This joint space usually lies deeper than one expects and is a common reason for failure at initial attempt. This is the site of needle position which is then angled at 25–45° to the superior margin of the patellofemoral joint. The procedure is then performed in a standard fashion as outlined above (Fig. 4.11a).

An anterior medial or lateral oblique approach can also be employed. The point of access lies at the lower patellar margin, medial or lateral to the patellar tendon, orientated to the ipsilateral femoral condyle (Fig. 4.11b). After aspiration of joint fluid, 20–40 ml of the appropriate contrast is injected once intra-articular injection is confirmed with 1–2 ml iodinated contrast.

Ankle Arthrography

Indications for ankle arthrogram have overlapped with standard MRI ankle. The choice of optimal study depends on symptoms, prior imaging studies, and treatment options. Indications include assessment of osteochondral injuries, intra-articular loose bodies, lateral ligamentous complex, and syndesmotic injury and ankle impingement. The patient lies supine with mild plantar flexion ankle. The dorsalis pedis artery is palpated. Injection point lies medial to the artery. Note that the capsule joint extends to the talar neck, and the distal body talus is the optimum site for injection, avoiding damage to any articular cartilage more proximally. The patient is prepped in the standard fashion as described above, and a 3.5 cm 22G needle is used to access the joint. 7–10 mls of the appropriate contrast is injected once intra-articular injection is confirmed with 1–2 ml iodinated contrast (Fig. 4.12). Note that the ankle joint may communicate with the posterior subtalar joint in 10 % of normal patients. Post-procedure ambulation is limited to prevent capsule rupture, and the patient is then transferred to MRI or CT via wheelchair.

Subtalar Arthrography

The subtalar joint is usually accessed for therapeutic steroid injection or diagnostic anesthetic injection to confirm origin of hindfoot pain. The patient lies in a lateral position, and the ankle raised on a support pad in neutral position. A 25G 3.5 cm needle can be used. The inferior and lateral margin of the lateral malleolus is used as the palpable bony landmark; needle placement is just posterior to the peroneal tendons. Intra-articular injection is confirmed with 1 ml iodinated contrast (Fig. 4.13).

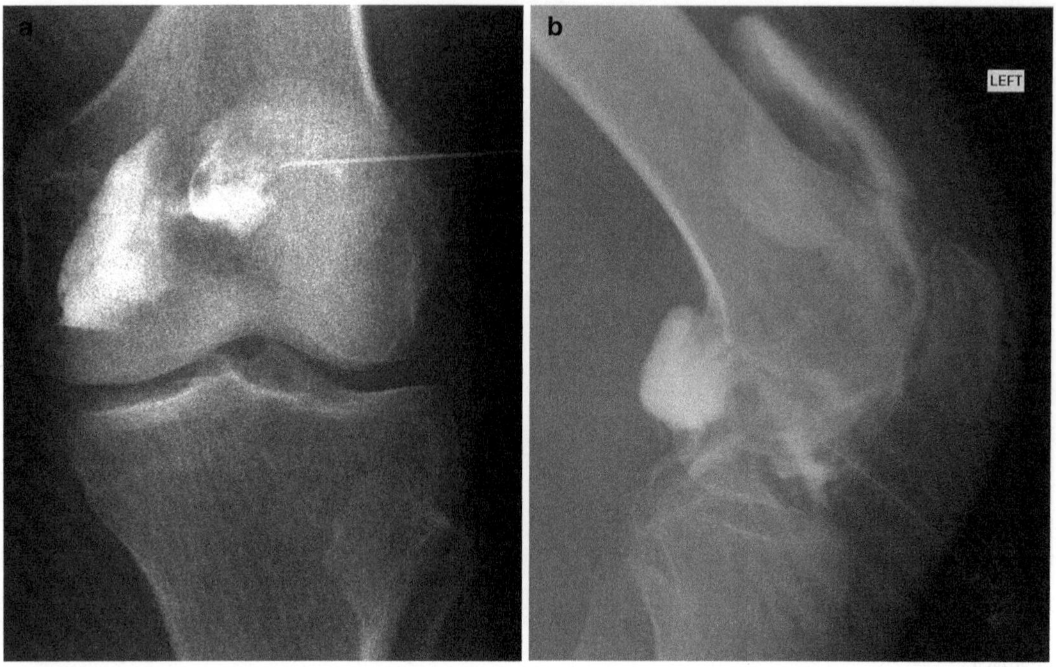

Fig. 4.11 Knee arthrogram: fluoroscopic images acquired during (**a**) a lateral patellofemoral approach and (**b**) a lateral oblique approach

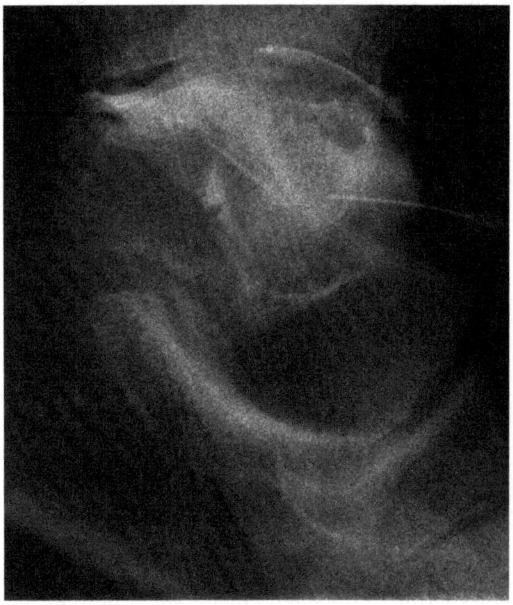

Fig. 4.12 Ankle arthrogram: fluoroscopic images acquired during anterior joint approach

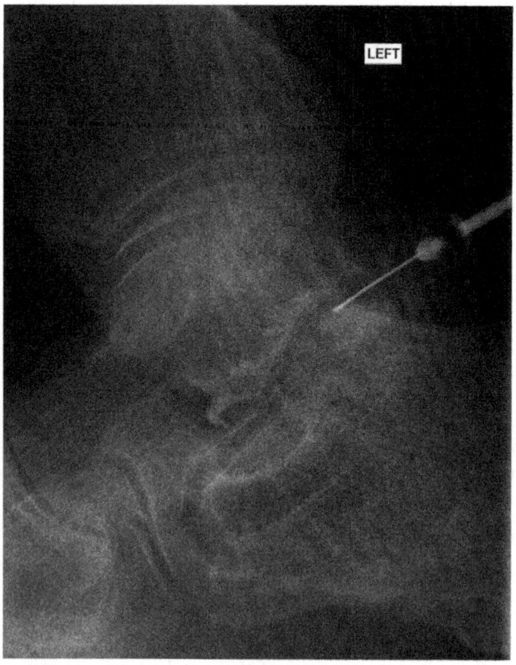

Fig. 4.13 Subtalar arthrogram: fluoroscopic images acquired during lateral subtalar joint approach

Small Joint Arthrography

The small joints of the hand and foot and acromioclavicular and sternoclavicular joints are usually accessed under ultrasound guidance. Ultrasound can confirm the presence of joint effusion, synovitis, and erosive or degenerative changes and assess the overlying tissues for bursal distension or tenosynovitis. The needle can be identified throughout its course to the joint avoiding neurovascular bundles and tendons. The needle appears as a linear hyperechoic line with posterior reverberation at 90° to transducer (Fig. 4.2b). Occasionally because of the size of the joint and transducer position, only a portion of the needle can be identified at any one time. It is essential that the needle tip be visualized as the needle is advanced. Intra-articular position is confirmed by identifying the needle tip within the joint and by injecting 1 ml anesthetic or saline injection, visualized as a dynamic hypoechoic fluid distension of the joint. The joint is aspirated prior to injection to prevent dilution of injectate.

Further Reading

1. Joines MM, Motamedi K, Seeger LL. Musculoskeletal interventional ultrasound. Semin Musculoskelet Radiol. 2007;11(2):192–8.
2. Koski JM, Hammer HB. Ultrasound-guided procedures: techniques and usefulness in controlling inflammation and disease progression. Rheumatology. 2012;51 Suppl 7:vii31–5.
3. Nguyen RT, Borg-Stein J, McInnis K. Applications of platelet-rich plasma in musculoskeletal and sports medicine: an evidence-based approach. PM R. 2011; 3(3):226–50.
4. Resnick D. In: Resnick D, editor. Diagnosis of bone and joint disorders. 4th ed. Philadelphia: WB Saunders Co. Ltd; 2002.
5. Stephens MB, Beutler AI, O'Connor FG. Musculoskeletal injections: a review of the evidence. Am Fam Physician. 2008;78(8):971–6.

Part II

Imaging in Rheumatology

5 Inflammatory Arthritides

Maggie J. Larche

Rheumatoid Arthritis

Overview

Rheumatoid arthritis (RA) is an autoimmune erosive inflammatory arthritis of unknown aetiology. The triggering event is unclear but blood markers suggesting autoimmune activation include high inflammatory markers and positive antibodies such as rheumatoid factor (RF). RF is positive in around 50–80 % of patients with RA depending on the stage of the disease, but the disease may also be "seronegative", i.e. negative RF, particularly in early disease. More specific autoantibodies have been described and the anti-citrullinated peptide antibodies (Anti-CCP or ACPA) are in routine clinical use currently.

Rheumatoid factor is an IgM autoantibody directed against the Fc portion of the IgG molecule. It is generally measured by one of two immunological techniques: latex fixation or nephelometry. While up to 80 % of patients with RA have a positive RF, RF is not specific for RA and can be positive in patients with a variety of autoimmune diseases including SLE, Sjogren's syndrome, scleroderma and other connective tissue diseases (CTDs). It can also be positive in some infectious diseases including bacterial endocarditis, TB and syphilis. Around 2 % of healthy individuals may test positive for RF (usually at a low titre). The group of patients with RA but with a negative RF are termed "seronegative RA" and tend to have less erosive diseases.

Anti-citrullinated peptide antibodies (ACPA) including anti-cyclic citrullinated peptide (anti-CCP) are more specific (around 97 %) and have the same sensitivity for RA as RF. They are found in around 50 % of patients with RA. Citrullination is a posttranslational modification of the amino acid arginine, and autoantibodies directed against citrulline are specific for RA. A positive ACPA test is predictive of the development of erosions.

Like many autoimmune diseases, RA affects women more commonly than men with a peak incidence around 40 years of age. The prevalence is around 1 % of the adult population.

RA is characterised by synovial proliferation and inflammation (Fig. 5.1). This results in soft tissue swelling due to synovitis or tenosynovitis, new vessel formation in the synovium (neovascularisation), bony erosions, bone marrow oedema, cartilage destruction and periarticular osteopenia, which are the pathological hallmarks of RA. Erosions occur in up to 80 % of patients with RA within 20 years, and within 3 years of symptom onset, 19 % of patients have erosions. Erosions are clearly linked with functional disability.

The advent of new treatments for RA (termed "biologics") in the late 1990s along with a more

M.J. Larche, MBChB, MRCP(UK), PhD
Associate Professor, Division of Rheumatology, Department of Medicine, McMaster University, Hamilton, ON L8N 1Y2, Canada
e-mail: mlarche@mcmaster.ca

J. O'Neill (ed.), *Essential Imaging in Rheumatology*,
DOI 10.1007/978-1-4939-1673-3_5, © Springer Science+Business Media New York 2015

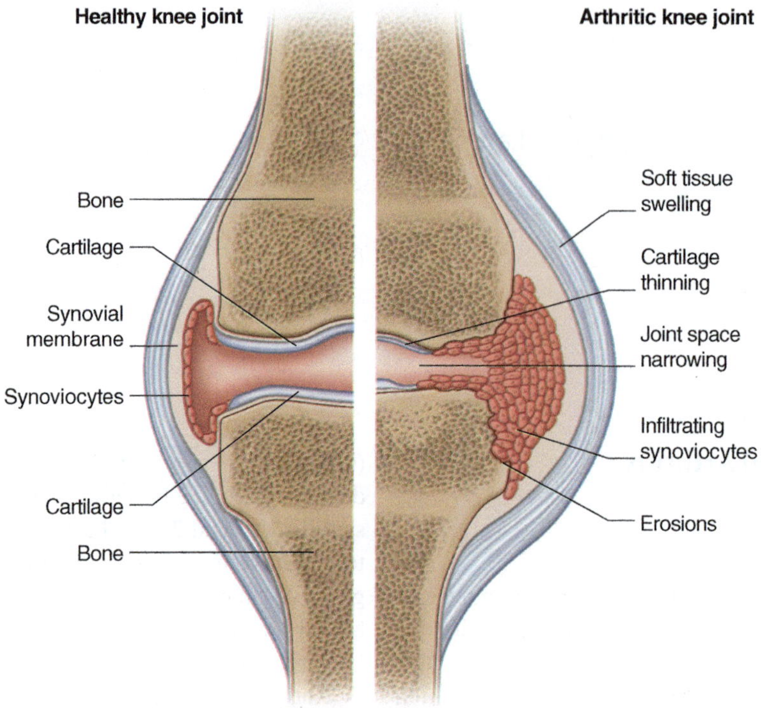

Fig. 5.1 The development of erosive disease and synovitis in rheumatoid arthritis

intensive approach to control of inflammation – the so-called treat-to-target approach – has revolutionised the management of RA, and outcomes continue to improve with fewer erosions, less deformity and improved functional ability.

The 2010 American College of Rheumatology/European League Against Rheumatism (ACR/EULAR) classification criteria describe the diagnosis of definite RA based on joint involvement, including pattern and duration of swollen or tender joints (which may be confirmed by imaging evidence of synovitis), inflammatory markers, and RF and ACPA serological tests (Table 5.1).

Presentation

RA has a propensity for women with a female–male ratio of 3:1, with women particularly affected in their 40–60s. There is a genetic component with a modest familial predisposition to the disease – for example, in monozygotic twins, there is a concordance of around 7 %. Up to 70 % of Caucasian patients with RA have the gene encoding for HLA-DR4 or DR1 (the so-called shared epitope). In addition, environmental factors associated with the development of RA include cigarette smoking, obesity and exposure to silica dust and air pollution increasing the risk, while alcohol and the use of the oral contraceptive pill seem to reduce the risk. The small joints of the hands and feet are particularly commonly affected, but any synovial joint can become involved.

Symptoms at onset include the following:

- Pain and swelling in the synovial joints
- Morning stiffness lasting more than 1 hour
- Fatigue

Diagnosis depends on a combination of factors including more than 6 weeks of tender or swollen joints (a homunculus is a convenient method of documenting tender and swollen joint counts; Fig. 5.2), a raised inflammatory response and a positive rheumatoid factor or anti-CCP (or ACPA) antibody test (Table 5.1).

Table 5.1 ACR/EULAR 2010 classification criteria

Target population: Patients who have at least 1 joint with definite clinical synovitis; with synovitis not better explained by another disease	
Classification criteria	Score
Joint involvement (any swollen or tender)	
1 large joint	0
2–10 large joints	1
1–3 small joints	2
4–10 small joints	3
>10 joints (at least one small)	5
Serology	
Negative RF and negative ACPA	0
Low-positive RF or low-positive ACPA	2
High-positive RF or high-positive ACPA	3
Acute phase reactants	
Normal ESR and normal CRP	0
Abnormal ESR or abnormal CRP	1
Duration of symptoms	
<6 weeks	0
>6 weeks	1
Score ≥6 = definite RA	

Adapted from Aletaha D, Neogi T, Silman AJ, Funovits J, Felson DT, Bingham 3rd CO, Birnbaum NS, Burmester GR, Bykerk VP, Cohen MD, Combe B, Costenbader KH, Dougados M, Emery P, Ferraccioli G, Hazes JM, Hobbs K, Huizinga TW, Kavanaugh A, Kay J, Kvien TK, Laing T, Mease P, Ménard HA, Moreland LW, Naden RL, Pincus T, Smolen JS, Stanislawska-Biernat E, Symmons D, Tak PP, Upchurch KS, Vencovský J, Wolfe F, Hawker G. Rheumatoid arthritis classification criteria: an American College of Rheumatology/European League against rheumatism collaborative initiative. *Arthritis Rheum.* 2010;62(9):2569–81 with permission from BMJ Publishing Group Ltd

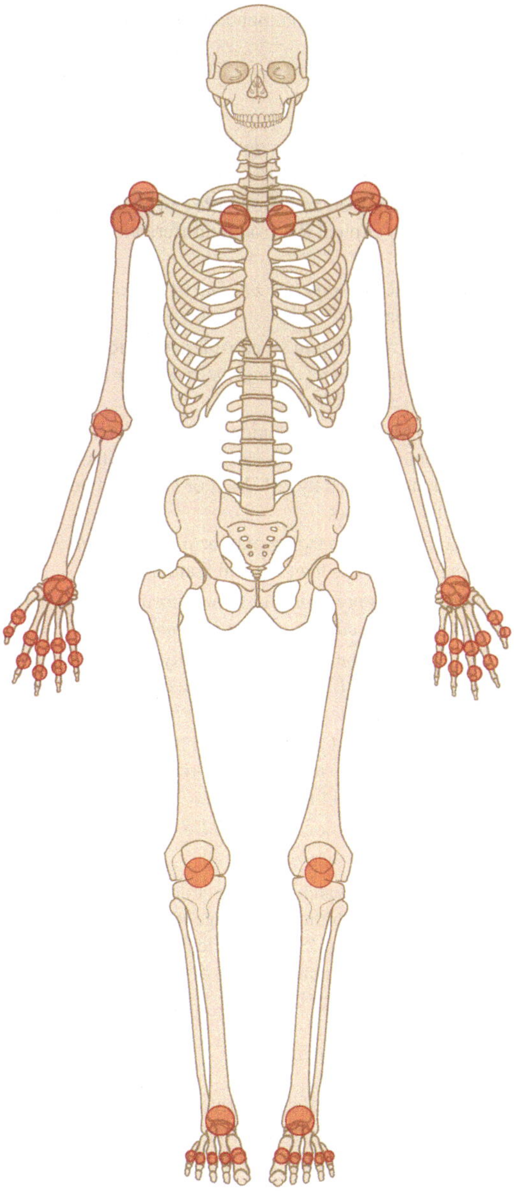

Fig. 5.2 Homunculus used to depict location of swollen and/or tender joints. The affected joints are marked off – usually two are used, one for swollen joints and one for tender joints

Imaging changes are not part of these initial classification criteria, although plain radiographs are usually performed at baseline to aid with diagnosis, assess radiographic severity of the disease and serve as a useful baseline for comparison with follow-up studies. Furthermore, both MRI and US are often used to delineate synovitis, effusion and erosions in a patient with questionable swollen joints on clinical examination at presentation.

A plain chest radiograph is essential prior to commencing pulmonary toxic drugs like methotrexate and prior to commencing biologic drugs as these have a propensity to reactivate covert mycobacterial infections.

In addition to baseline assessments, plain radiographs of the affected joints, US and/or MRI, can be used to monitor the progression of disease and response to treatment.

Table 5.2 EULAR recommendations for the use of imaging in rheumatoid arthritis

Recommendation	Strength of recommendation (0–10 scale –0 = not recommended; 10 = highly recommended)	Level of evidence
1. When there is *diagnostic doubt*, CR, US or MRI can be used to improve certainty of diagnosis	9.1	III
2. Inflammation seen on US or MRI can be used to *predict progression* to clinical RA from undifferentiated inflammatory arthritis	7.9	III
3. US and MRI are *superior to clinical examination* in detecting joint inflammation	8.7	III
4. *US and or MRI* should be considered if CR does not show damage and may *detect damage at an earlier time point* – especially in early RA	9.0	IV
5. BME on MRI is a strong independent *predictor of subsequent radiographic progression* in early RA. Synovitis on MRI or US, and erosions detected by CR, MRI or US could be used as prognostic indicators	8.4	III
6. Inflammation on imaging may be *more predictive of a therapeutic response* than clinical features	7.8	III–IV
7. US and MRI may be useful in monitoring disease activity, as they allow *improved detection of inflammation*	8.3	III
8. CR should be considered periodically to evaluate joint damage. *MRI (and possibly US)* is more responsive to change in joint damage and can *monitor disease progression*	7.8	III
9. CR (in flexion and neutral) should be used to *monitor instability of the C-spine*. MRI should be performed if CR positive or if specific neurological findings	9.4	III
10. In clinical remission, *MRI and US can detect persistent inflammation*	8.8	III

Adapted from Colebatch AN, Edwards CJ, Østergaard M, Van Der Heijde D, Balint PV, D'Agostino MA, Forslind K, Grassi W, Haavardsholm EA, Haugeberg G, Jurik AG, Landewé RB, Naredo E, O'Connor PJ, Ostendorf B, Potocki K, Schmidt WA, Smolen JS, Sokolovic S, Watt I, Conaghan PG. EULAR recommendations for the use of imaging of the joints in the clinical management of rheumatoid arthritis. *Ann Rheum Dis*. 2013;72(6):804–14 with permission from BMJ Publishing Group Ltd

Key:

CR conventional radiography

Categories of evidence:

III – nonexperimental descriptive studies such as comparative studies, correlation studies and case-control studies

IV – expert committee reports or opinions or clinical experience of respected authorities, or both

A recent position statement has been published from EULAR with recommendations for imaging in RA. The recommendations include evidence for imaging in diagnosis, comparison with clinical examination alone, detection of damage, prediction of therapeutic responses and monitoring disease activity and progression and remission. These recommendations are summarised in Table 5.2. They particularly address the additional utility of MRI and US:

- In the detection of subclinical inflammation
- As a more accurate assessment of inflamed joints than clinical examination alone
- In monitoring disease activity
- In determination of remission
- In prognosis

RA is a systemic disease with several possible extra-articular features including pulmonary nodules and interstitial lung disease, systemic vasculitis, renal failure, pyoderma gangrenosum, scleritis, arrhythmias and coronary artery disease.

Table 5.3 Imaging and clinical features of the different stages of rheumatoid arthritis with radiographs, ultrasound and MRI

	Different stages of RA in hands		
	Early	Intermediate	Late
Imaging modality	Ultrasound or MRI best for imaging synovitis, effusions and tenosynovitis. MRI can also identify pre-erosive disease. Plain radiographs for periarticular osteopenia		Plain radiographs visualise destructive changes. MRI and US can additionally visualise active inflammatory changes
Imaging features	Soft tissue swelling	Soft tissue swelling including tenosynovitis	Soft tissue damage resulting in ulnar deviation and finger drop
	Periarticular osteopenia	Osteopenia	Osteopenia
	Possible marginal erosions	Marginal erosions progressing to larger erosions	Progression of destructive erosive disease, subluxations and deformities
	Joint space widening secondary to effusion and synovitis	Joint space narrowing	Joint space narrowing, ankylosis
Characteristic *clinical* features	Soft tissue swelling – particularly MCPJs, PIPJs and wrists	Possible finger drop due to tendon rupture ulnar deviation	MCP subluxation, swan neck and boutonniere's deformities. Ulnar deviation

Several imaging modalities could be employed to assess these features. The MSK features, rather than the extra-articular features, of RA will be the focus of this text.

Imaging Features

Radiographs

Radiographs are an essential component of any imaging algorithm in the assessment of structural damage in RA. They have several advantages over other imaging modalities: multiple joints can be assessed at the same time (most frequently hands, wrists and feet are requested); radiographs are accessible to most practitioners; well validated methods of interpreting radiographs are established and several pathological features can be identified such as:

- Soft tissue swelling
- Effusions
- Erosions
- Osteopenia
- Cartilage loss

Furthermore, radiographs are affordable and can detect early osteopenia which neither MRI nor US can visualise. However, plain radiographs are a two-dimensional representation of a three-dimensional structure. This is resolved in part by the addition of tomosynthesis that may represent a more sensitive tool for detecting structural changes (see Chap. 1). In addition, radiographs have low sensitivity particularly early in the course of the disease prior to the development of erosions. This is particularly relevant currently, as there is a clinical drive to detect and treat the disease early in its course to prevent irreversible structural damage and to maintain function, hence the increasing use of ultrasound and MRI in early disease (Table 5.3). Initial radiographic assessment should include posterior-anterior, oblique and lateral projections of the hands and feet. Radiographs are advised even if asymptomatic due to high yield of erosions.

Soft tissue swelling is often the first sign of synovitis and may be secondary to synovial proliferation, effusion or tenosynovitis. This can be visualised as loss of the fat planes and as

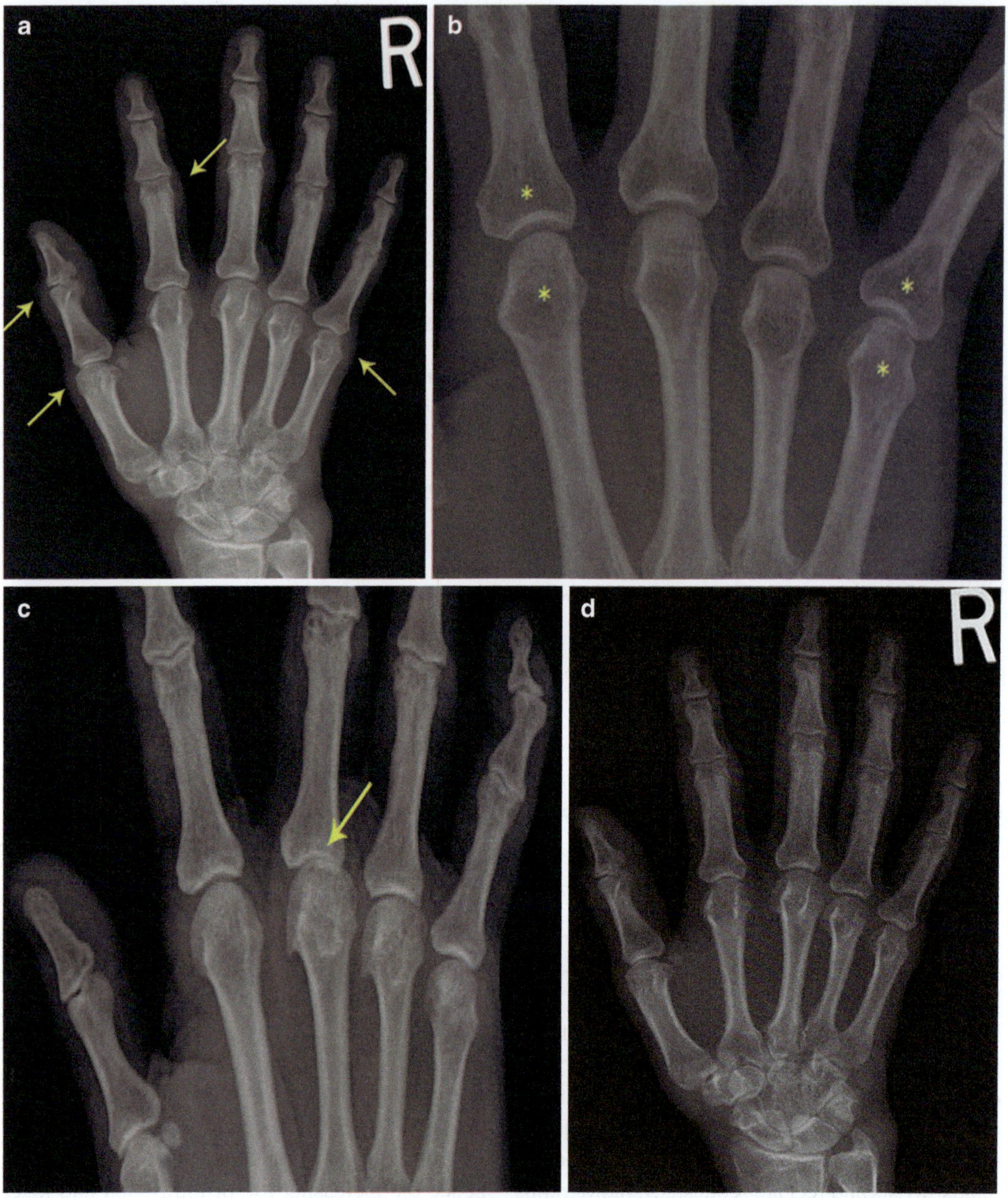

Fig 5.3 (**a**) Soft tissue swelling of the MCPJs and PIPJs (*arrows*). (**b**) Periarticular osteopenia (*asterisks*). (**c**) Joint space narrowing at 3rd MCP joint (*arrow*). (**d**) Normal R hand radiograph for comparison

fusiform swelling around the joints (Fig. 5.3). Soft tissue swelling can be subtle and careful review of the periarticular soft tissues of the same joints is required to identify early changes, i.e. assess and compare the periarticular soft tissues at the MCPJs separately from the PIPJs.

Osteopenia is an early radiographic change of active disease (Fig. 5.3b). Osteopenia is thought to be related to high levels of inflammatory cytokines, particularly tumour necrosis factor (TNF)-alpha and interleukin (IL)-6 and IL-17. It is one of the first features of RA and usually predates erosions.

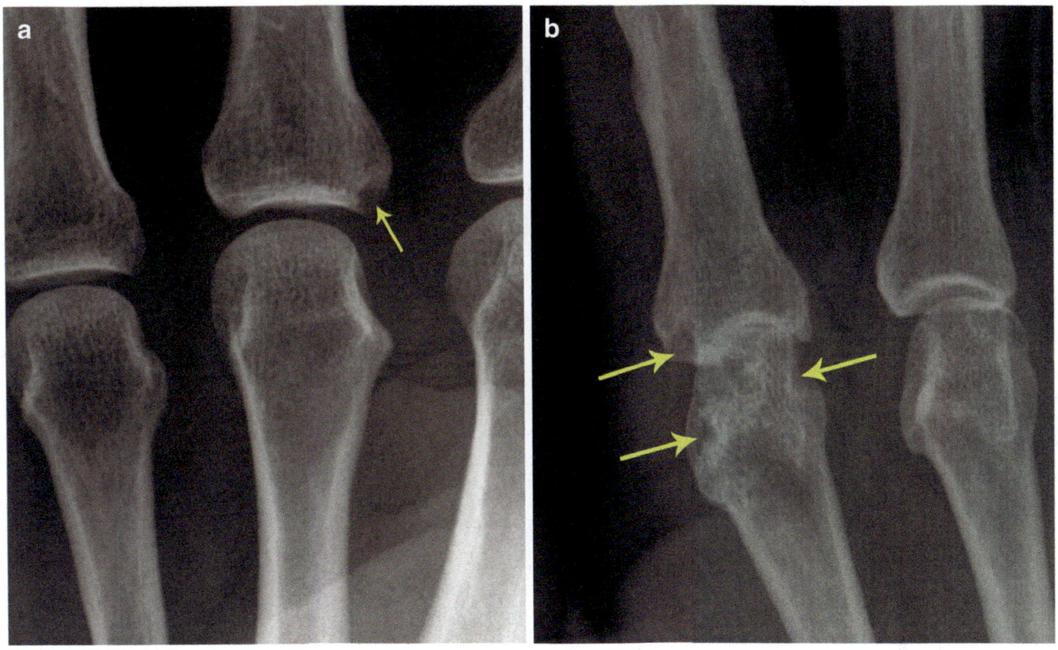

Fig. 5.4 Marginal erosions in (**a**) a 43-year-old woman with a 2-year history of arthralgia and arthritis symptoms. Small MCP marginal erosion (*arrow*); (**b**) 58-year-old man with 10-year history of moderately active RA despite DMARD treatment. Multiple larger erosions affecting metacarpal and proximal phalanx bones (*arrows*)

Joint space narrowing (*JSN*) occurs due to cartilage thinning resulting from the presence of inflammatory cytokines and invasion of synovitis. On plain radiographs, joint space loss is assessed by measuring the distance between the joints, comparing with the other joints in that limb, e.g. MCPJs, and comparing with the other side (Fig. 5.3c). In RA, cartilage loss is usually uniform across the whole joint compared to OA where the cartilage loss is often focal and with subsequent asymmetrical joint space loss.

Erosions and ankylosis are hallmark features of RA. As the disease progresses, erosions develop at the intracapsular articular margins (known as "marginal erosions") (Fig. 5.4). This region is an area of exposed bone without articular cartilage where the joint capsule inserts, referred to as the "bare area". A combination of synovial proliferation and invasion ("pannus") along with high levels of inflammatory cytokines is thought to contribute to the development of marginal erosions. Other pathological changes include tenosynovitis with underlying erosions, for example, at the ulnar styloid (see Fig. 5.9), and cartilage destruction and osteopenia inducing compression erosions. Marginal erosions begin as small cortical breaks. These progress to larger defects in the bony cortex, associated with osteopenia. There is a lack of periosteal sclerosis or new bone formation, which would be typical in psoriatic arthritis or gout (see Fig. 5.32). Progression of erosions occurs without adequate treatment (Fig. 5.5a–d). With progression, there can be bony collapse followed by destruction and ankylosis most commonly seen in the carpal bones (Fig. 5.6).

Joint Involvement

Characteristic Hand Deformities

The characteristic joint involvement in RA is depicted in Fig. 5.2 using the homunculus. The hand and wrist are most commonly involved in RA.

The second and third MCPJs are the most common and earliest joints involved, with frequent involvement of the second and third PIPJs.

Synovitis with joint destruction, tenosynovitis, ligamentous instability and tendon rupture

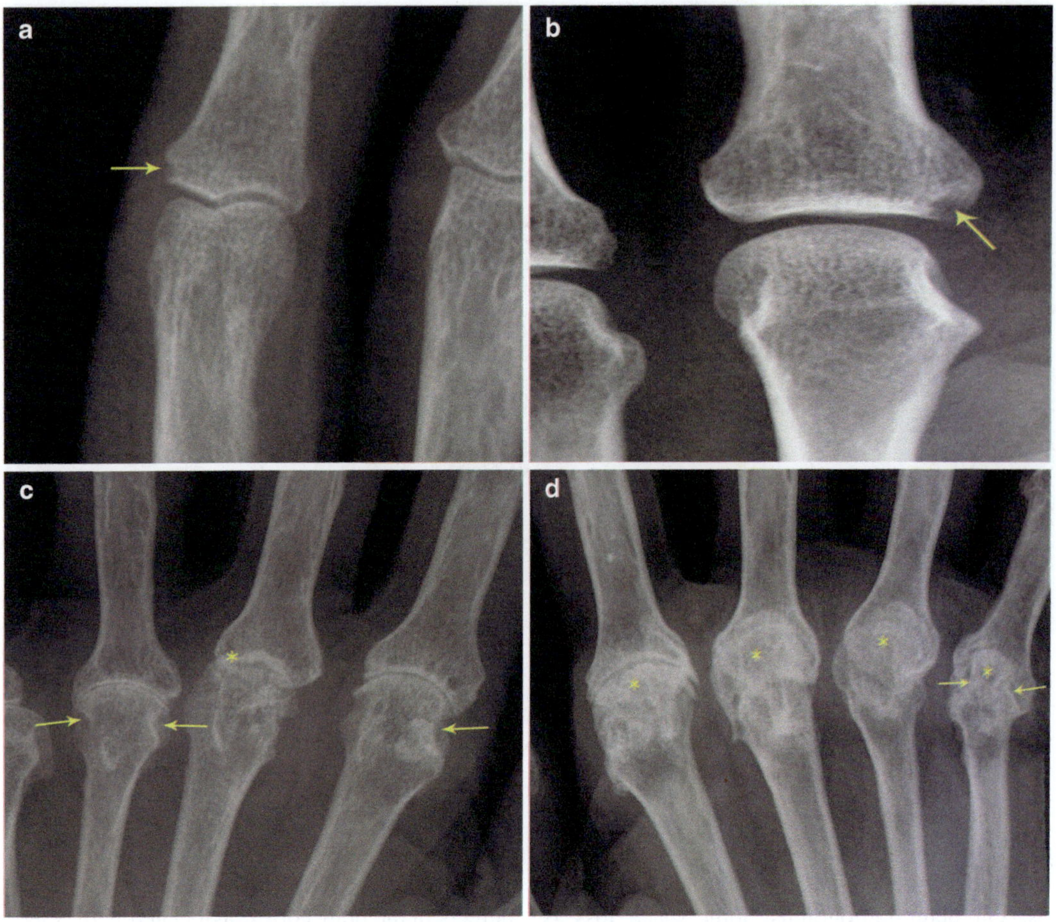

Fig. 5.5 Progression of erosions in four different patients. (**a**) Marginal erosion at PIP (*arrow*); (**b**) larger marginal erosion (*arrow*); (**c**) large erosions (*arrows*) with marked joint space narrowing at MCP (*asterisk*); (**d**) erosions (*arrow*) with joint space narrowing and subluxation at MCP (*asterisk*)

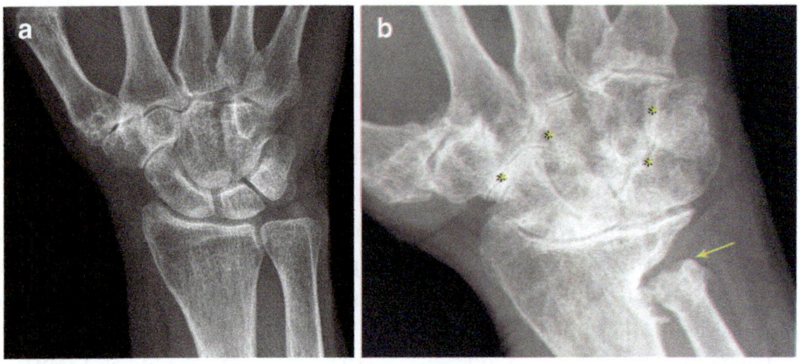

Fig. 5.6 Carpal ankylosis in two different patients: (**a**) early carpal ankylosis at capitate and hamate and capitate and trapezoid and crowding of the carpal bones in a 58-year-old woman with RA for 15 years and (**b**) severe carpal ankylosis (*asterisk*) in a 74-year-old woman with long-standing disease. Note ulnar translocation of the proximal row of carpal bones. Note also large ulnar erosion (*arrow*)

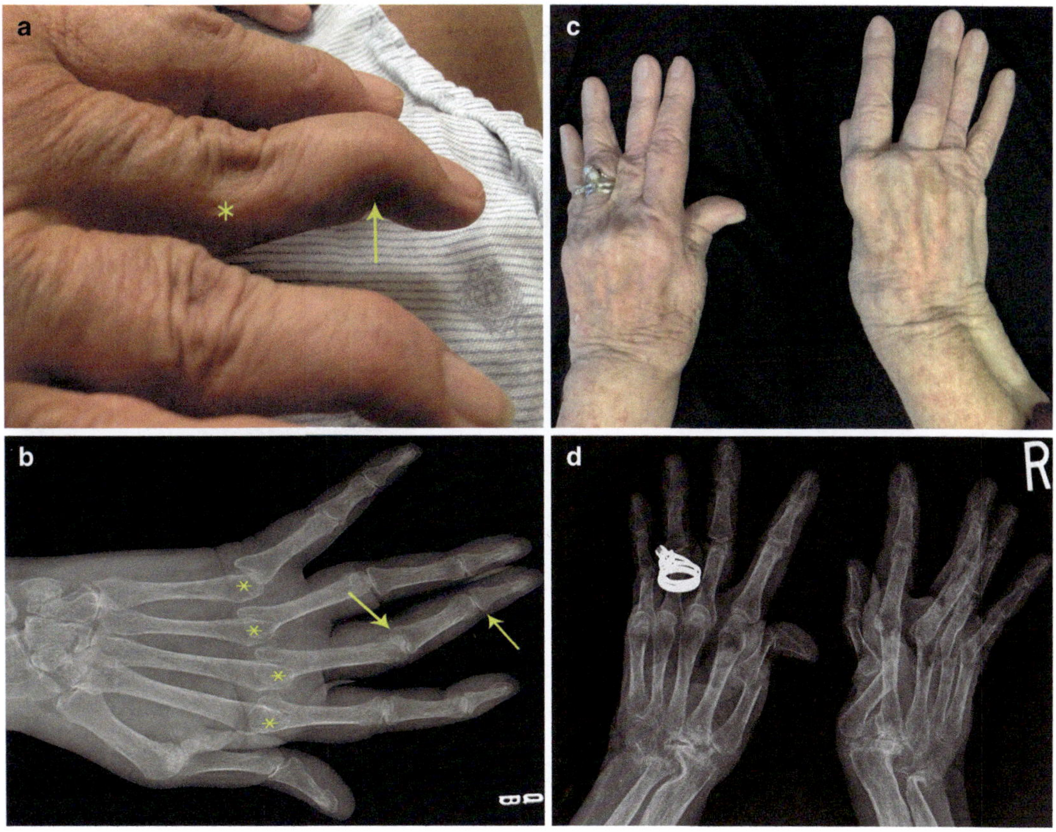

Fig. 5.7 (**a**) Swan neck deformity with flexion of the DIP (*arrow*) and hyperextension at PIP with (**b**) corresponding radiographic features in a 64-year-old woman with long-standing RA; (**c**) 77-year-old woman with a 50-year history of RA and multiple deformities including subluxation, ulnar deviation, boutonniere's deformity of right third finger and Z thumb; (**d**) corresponding radiograph

lead to the characteristic deformities of RA – swan neck (Fig. 5.7a) and boutonnière deformities, ulnar deviation (Fig. 5.7c), subluxation at the MCPJs (Fig. 5.7c) and finger drop. In anatomical terms, swan neck deformities relate to hyperextension at the PIP and flexion at the DIP, while boutonniere's is caused by flexion at the PIP and hyperextension at the DIP (Fig. 5.8).

Wrists

In the wrist, there are multiple sites of involvement, including the radiocarpal, intercarpal and distal radioulnar joint, with their own specific radiographic findings. Malalignment generally occurs because of the complex biomechanical forces from tendons and ligaments resulting in subluxations of the carpal bones on the radius or ulna.

Deformities at the wrist include the following:

- Erosions at the ulnar styloid (Fig. 5.9)
- Radial deviation of wrist which may accompany ulnar deviation of fingers
- Ulnar translocation of the proximal row of carpals (See Fig. 5.6b)
- Dorsal or volar slip of the scaphoid in relation to the lunate
- Distal ulnar subluxation with interruption of the distal radioulnar ligaments which may result in the "piano key sign" where pressure on the distal ulna results in impingement on the carpals

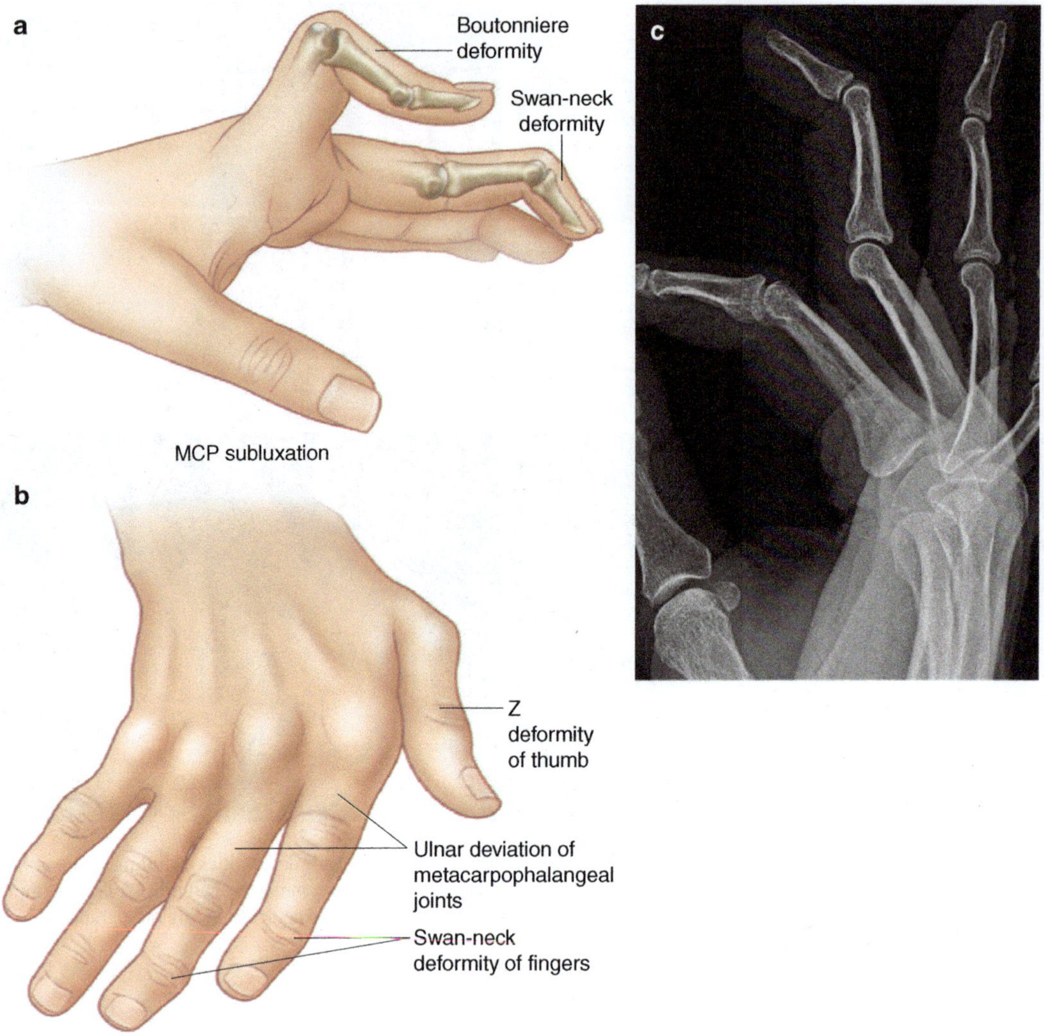

Fig. 5.8 (**a**) Swan neck and boutonniere's deformities, (**b**) chronic deformities in rheumatoid arthritis, (**c**) magnified lateral hand radiograph demonstrating swan neck deformity

Feet and Ankles

In up to 20 % of patients with newly diagnosed RA, the MTP joints are the presenting joints. Deformities and erosions in the MTPJs mimic those in the MCPJs with marginal erosions, soft tissue swelling, joint space narrowing, misalignment and eventual ankylosis. Erosions are particularly commonly seen on the lateral aspect of the fifth MTPJ (Fig. 5.10).

The tibiotalar joint demonstrates cartilage loss with bony erosions around the distal tibiofibular articulation. The intertarsal joints are affected in a similar manner to the intercarpal joints in the hands.

Large Joints

In the knee, hip, elbow and shoulder joints, articular cartilage loss is the predominant finding on plain radiography. Soft tissue swelling (either synovitis or effusion) is also a common feature, particularly in the knee with an increased soft tissue density in the suprapatellar pouch or anterior displacement of the patella visible on lateral knee x-ray. Erosions are the hallmark radiological feature of RA and can be found in any large joints including the knee and elbow (Fig. 5.11a, b). Hip joint effusions can be determined on AP radiographs as a widened distance between the lateral aspect of the acetabulum and the medial femoral head. Often

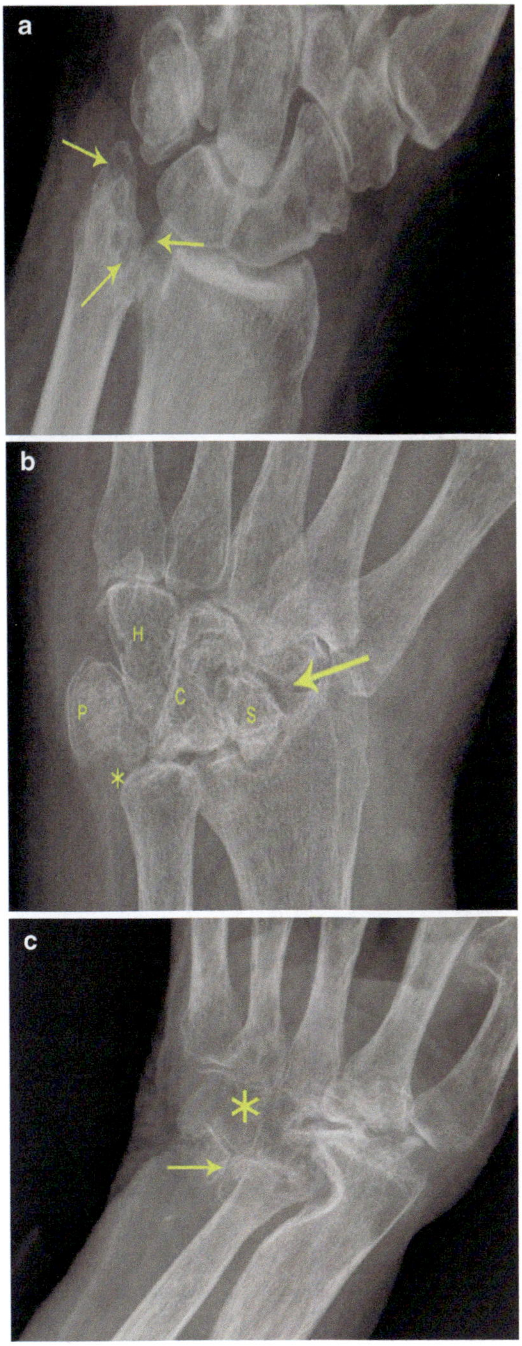

Fig. 5.9 (**a**) Erosions at ulnar styloid (*arrows*) in a 53-year-old man with newly diagnosed RA but symptoms for around 5 years; (**b**) osteolysis of the ulnar styloid (*asterisk*) with ulnar migration (*arrow*) of many of the carpal bones (*S* scaphoid, *C* capitate, *P* pisiform, *H* hamate); (**c**) complete destruction of the carpus (*asterisk*) and the ulnar styloid (*arrow*)

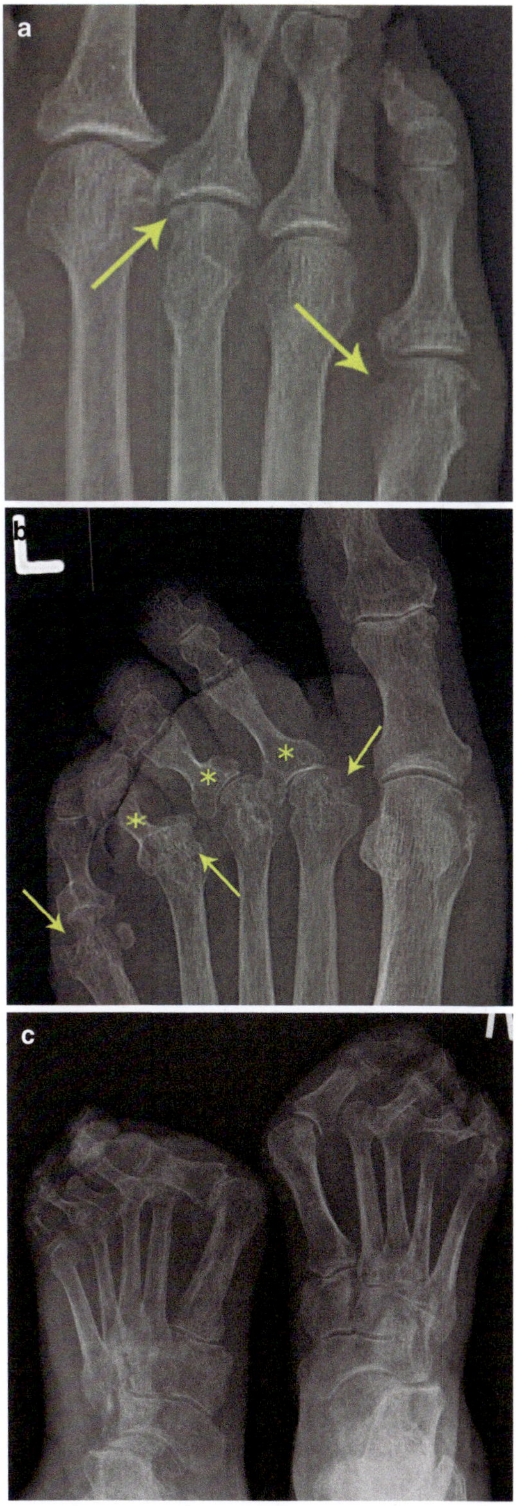

Fig. 5.10 (**a**) Erosions at MTPJ (*arrows*) in a 74-year-old woman with 20-year history of RA. (**b**) Erosions (*arrows*) and subluxation and lateral deviation (*asterisks*) of phalanges in a 58-year-old man with inadequately treated RA. (**c**) Severe destructive arthropathy of the feet

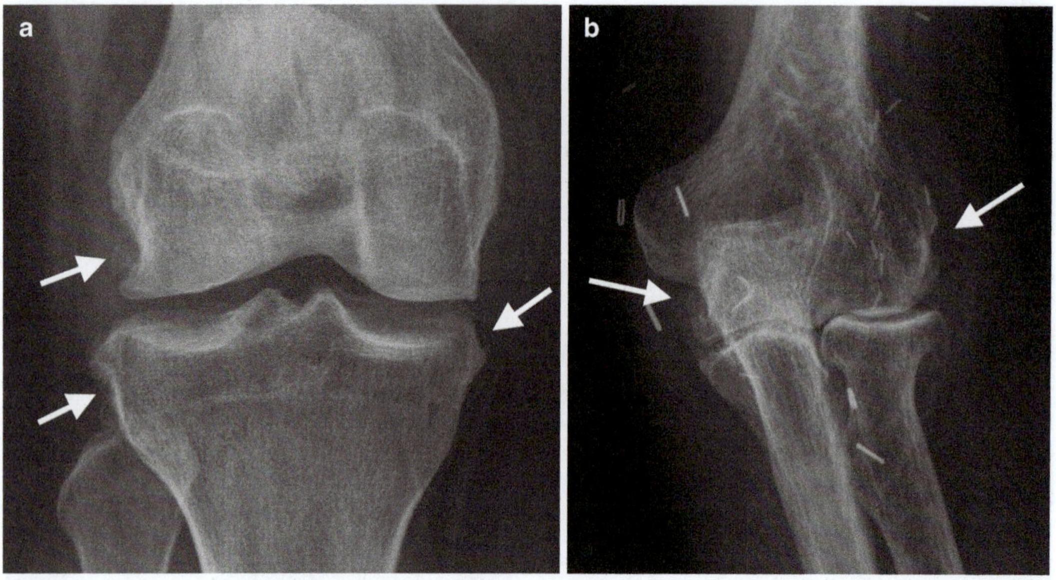

Fig. 5.11 (**a**) AP radiograph of the knee in a 24-year-old female patient with long-standing RA with multifocal erosions (*arrows*) with sclerotic margins suggesting erosions are inactive. (**b**) Marginal erosions elbow different patient with RA. Incidental note of the multiple surgical clips (*arrows*)

this is asymmetrical, and comparison can be made with the unaffected side. Cartilage loss in the hip in patients with RA is usually uniform throughout the joint and results in migration of the femoral head superiorly and medially in the direction of the femoral neck angulation. This can result in the femoral head protruding in to the pelvis: a condition known as acetabular protrusion.

In the elbow, effusions and synovitis can be recognised on plain radiography as first disappearance of the anterior fat pad followed by distension of the posterior fat pad (Fig. 5.12). Cartilage loss and erosion are visible at any of the articulations in the elbow.

Similarly in the shoulder, diffuse uniform cartilage loss and disruption of the rotator cuff tendons result in superior and medial migration of the humerus. Narrowing of the acromiohumeral distance to <6 mm suggests a chronic complete rotator cuff tear involving at least the supraspinatus and often the infraspinatus tendons (this would be best imaged by US or MRI). There can be progression with involvement of the subscapularis and long head biceps and development of a rotator cuff arthropathy.

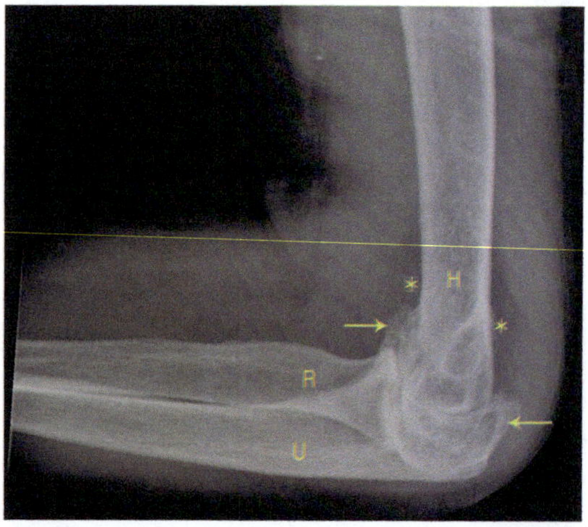

Fig. 5.12 Left elbow of a 71-year-old man with long-standing seropositive RA showing large effusion (*asterisks*) and secondary osteophytosis (*arrows*). *H* humerus, *R* radius, *U* ulna

Spine

The cervical spine is the most commonly affected part of the spine in RA, with up to 70 % of patients demonstrating involvement. Patients may have asymptomatic disease. The atlantoaxial joint is most commonly involved. This is the articulation between the C1 vertebral body, known as the atlas, and the C2, the axis. The axis has a large superior process, the odontoid peg, which articulates with the anterior arch of the atlas. Synovium can be found between the odontoid

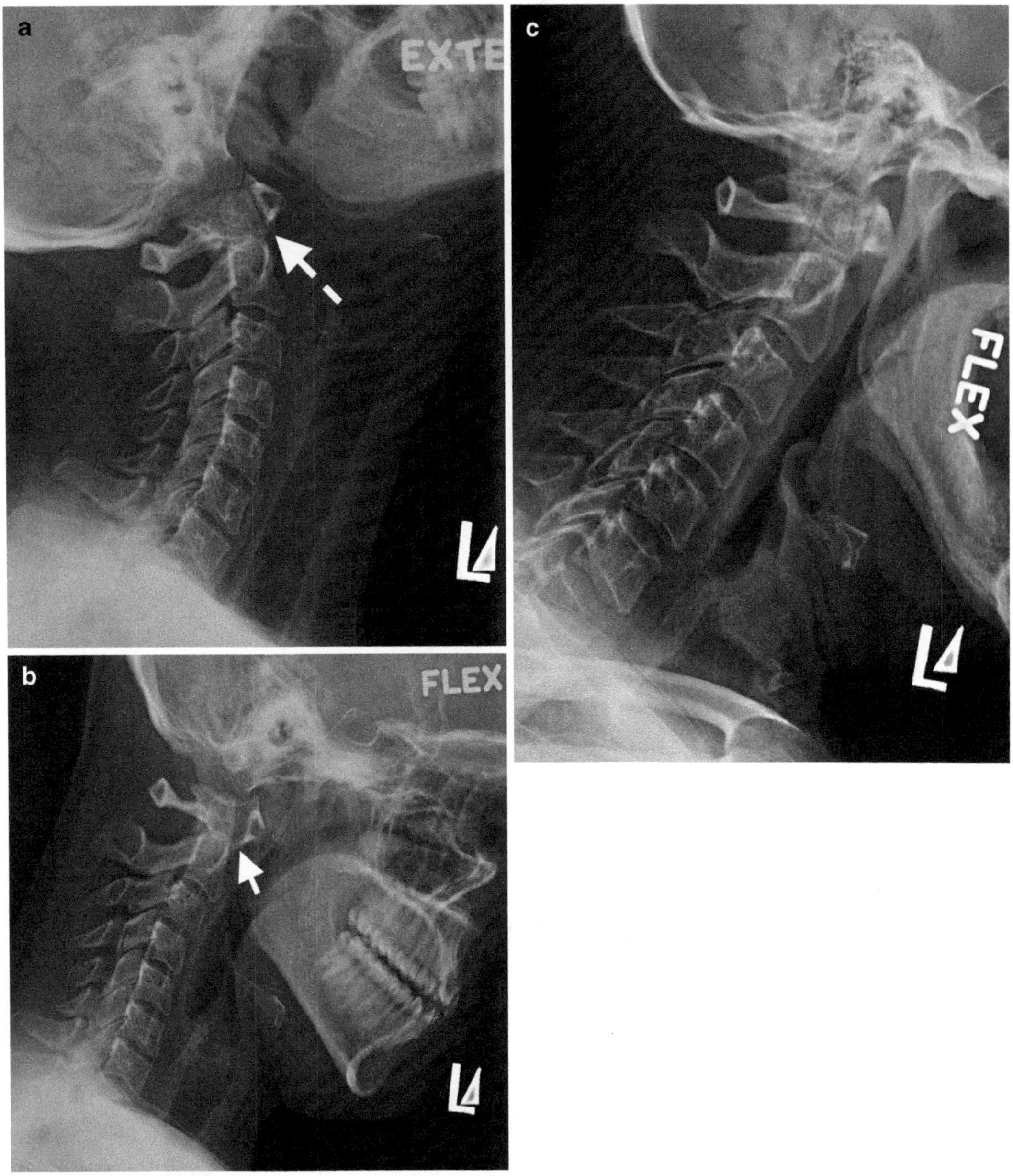

Fig. 5.13 Lateral cervical spine radiographs showing atlantoaxial instability in a 75-year-old woman with long-standing RA in a routine pre-op assessment, (**a**) in extension with normal atlantoaxial interval (*dashed arrow*) which increases significantly in flexion, (**b**) in keeping with instability. Alignment remainder cervical spine is maintained, (**c**) normal flexed cervical spine for comparison

process (also referred to as the dens) and the atlas and between the odontoid process and the transverse ligament (Fig. 5.13a–c, X-rays, and Fig. 5.14a, b illustration of bones in C spine c CT scan of C-spine involvement). The transverse ligament runs posterior to the odontoid process and maintains stability of the atlantoaxial joint. In rheumatoid synovitis, the integrity of the transverse ligament is compromised, allowing for anterior subluxation of C1 on C2. Furthermore, the odontoid process can be eroded resulting in further instability of the cervical spine and potential

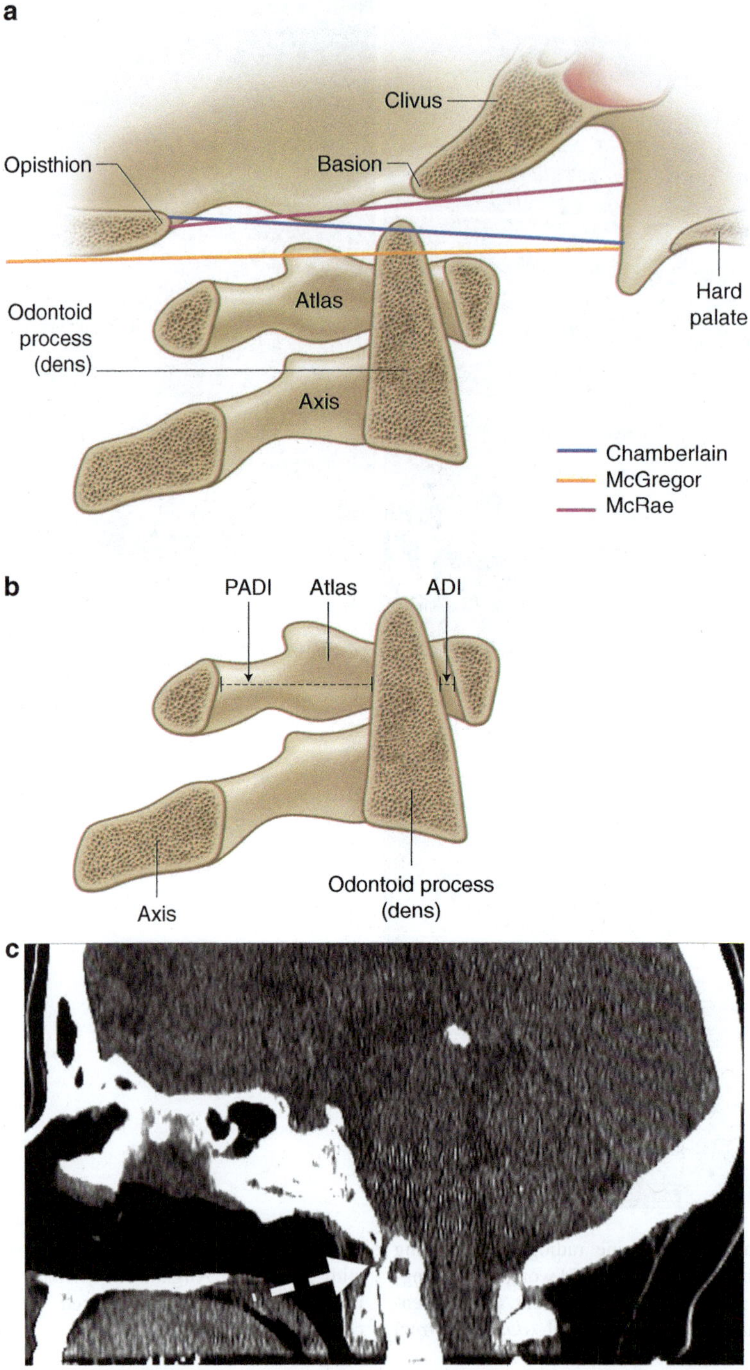

Fig. 5.14 (**a**, **b**) Illustration of the bones in the C-spine with measurements of anterior and posterior atlantodental interval (AADI, PADI). (**c**) A 63-year-old female RA: basilar invagination (*dashed arrow*) noted as an incidental finding for CT of the paranasal sinuses

spinal cord compression. Flexion views of the cervical spine allow for more accurate assessment of instability with measurement of the posterior atlantodental interval (PADI). This is the distance between the posterior aspect of the odontoid and the anterior surface of the posterior arch of the atlas and should be >14 mm. Axial CT imaging of the neck better delineates erosions of the dens and spinal cord compression. The most extreme neck pathology in RA involves atlantoaxial impaction where the odontoid peg migrates superiorly into the cranium and compromises the spinal cord. With the advent of more intensive therapies for RA, these complications are becoming much less frequent.

Extra-articular Manifestations

The extra-articular manifestations of RA can be imaged by plain radiographs, CT, MRI, US, radioisotope bone scanning, angiography or bone densitometry where appropriate. Other radiographic features include rheumatoid pulmonary nodules or pulmonary fibrosis (either idiopathic or secondary to methotrexate) on plain chest radiograph (Figs. 5.15 and 5.16), avascular necrosis (Fig. 5.17) or osteopenia/osteoporosis secondary to long-term corticosteroid use. Other imaging modalities are better suited to outlining the extra-articular manifestations such as:

- Entrapment neuropathies, popliteal cysts or bursal or tendon involvement best imaged by US or MRI
- Vasculitis best imaged by conventional angiography or MRA or CTA
- Septic arthritis or osteomyelitis by bone scintigraphy or MRI
- Chest pathologies by HRCT
- Felty's syndrome by CT or US
- Spinal cord compression by MRI
- Osteoporosis by bone densitometry

Secondary osteoarthritic changes and surgical correction are common with long-standing severe RA (Fig. 5.18).

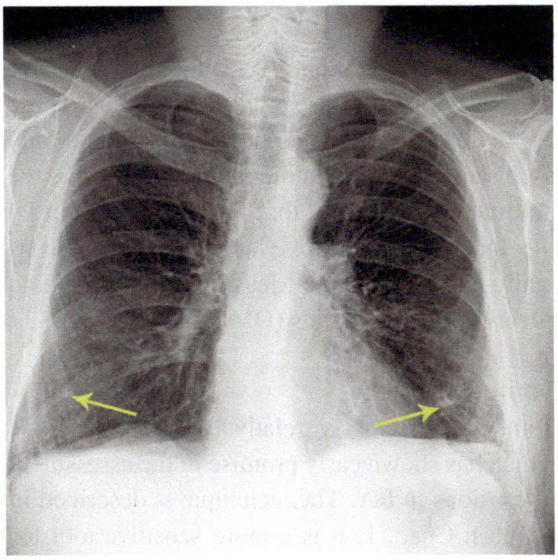

Fig. 5.15 Chest radiographs showing multiple pulmonary nodules (*arrows*)

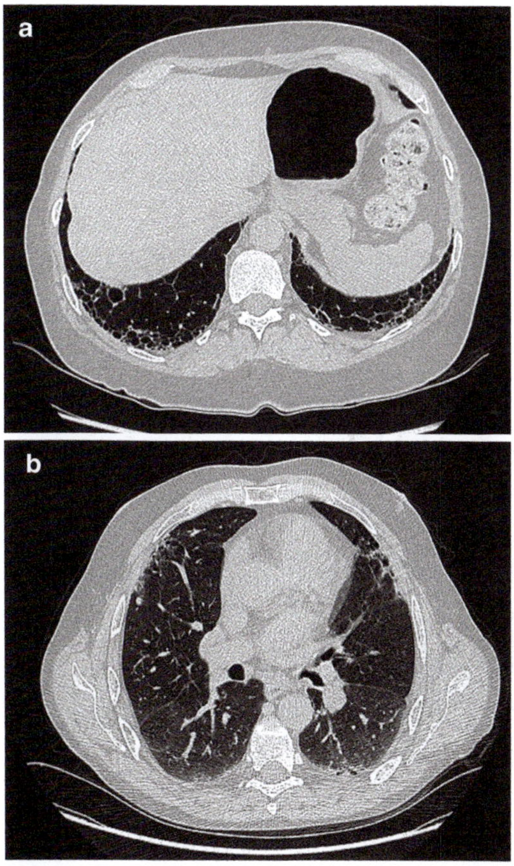

Fig. 5.16 CT chest showing (**a**) basal pulmonary fibrosis with honeycombing and (**b**) ground glass opacification on the dorsal side

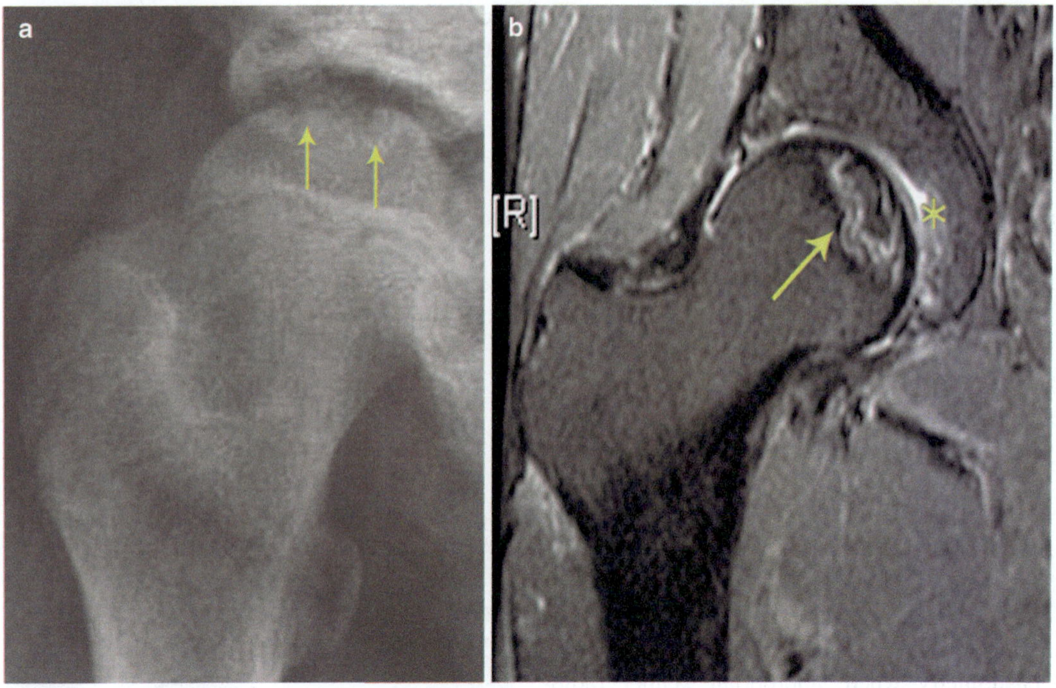

Fig. 5.17 Avascular necrosis (AVN) in a 56-year-old man treated for 30 years with 15 mg prednisone for RA. (**a**) Plain radiograph with collapsed femoral head (*arrows*) and (**b**) corresponding T2-weighted MRI showing BME and collapsed femoral head (*arrow*), and small effusion (*asterisk*)

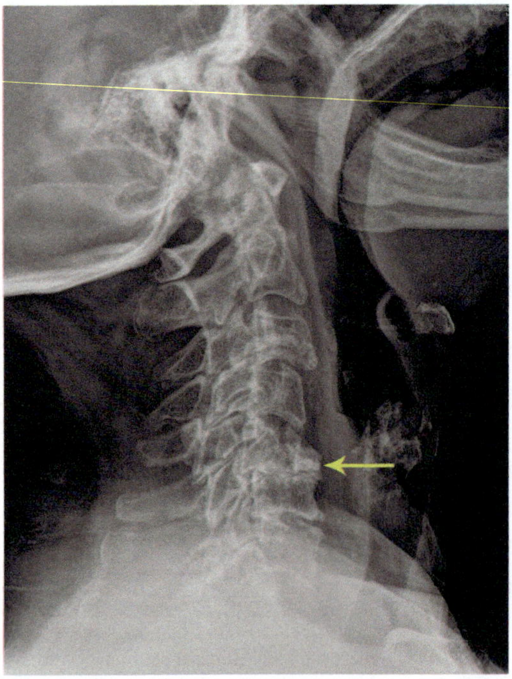

Fig. 5.18 Secondary OA in the C-spine of a woman with long-standing RA with large anterior osteophyte (*arrow*)

Rheumatoid nodules are typically seen on the extensor surface of MCPJs and PIPJs. Figures 5.15 and 5.19 depict some of the extra-articular features of RA.

Several radiographic scoring methods have been developed for use in clinical studies. These are reviewed in Appendix. The most commonly used scoring system in rheumatoid arthritis is the modified Sharp score that has been adopted by the Outcome Measures in Rheumatology formally called Outcome Measures in Rheumatoid Arthritis Clinical Trials (OMERACT) group.

Tomosynthesis

Tomosynthesis is a relatively new technique which has shown early promise in the assessment of erosions in RA. The technique is described in detail in Chap. 1. It is a more sensitive tool for detecting erosions. An example of a clearly defined erosion visualised by tomosynthesis is shown in Fig. 5.20. This technique requires further research but is likely to be a useful tool for assessing erosions in the future.

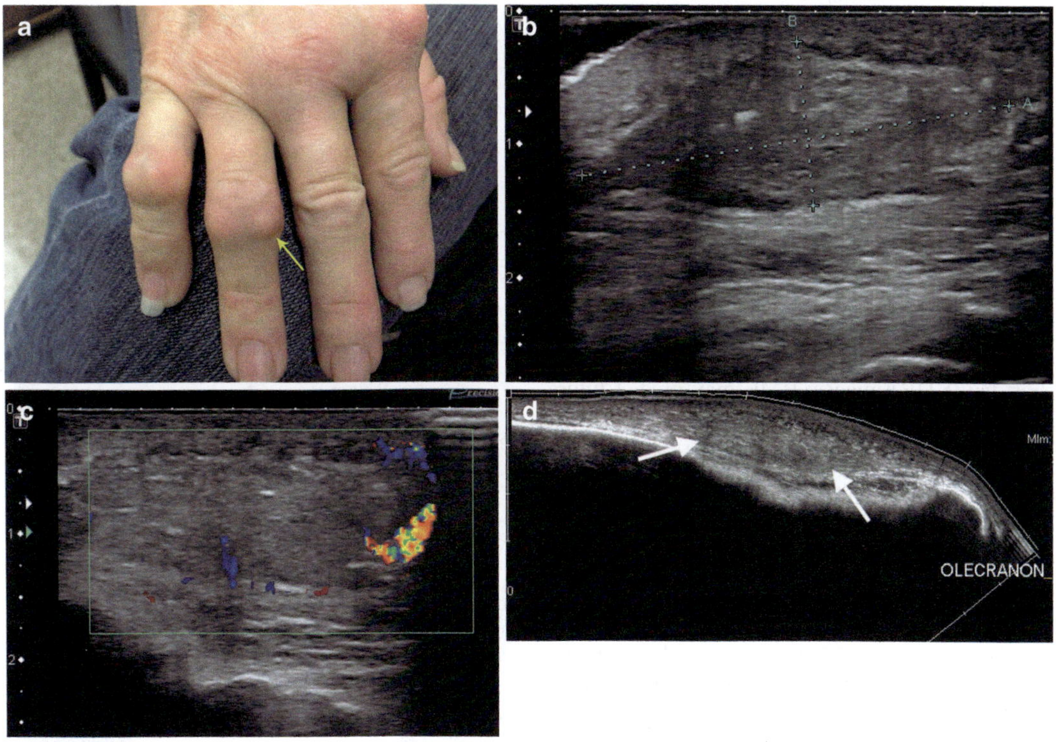

Fig. 5.19 Nodules around PIPJs in 68-year old woman with longstanding seropositive RA. (**a**) Picture right hand of 68-year old woman with longstanding rheumatoid arthritis with soft tissue nodule (Rheumatoid nodule) over the 4th PIP extensor surface (*arrow*) (**b**) same patient with larger rheumatoid nodule on the extensor surface right elbow on ultrasound with (**c**) peripheral flow on colour Doppler. (**d**) Extended field of view noting the olecranon as a bony landmark (rheumatoid nodule demarcated with *arrows*)

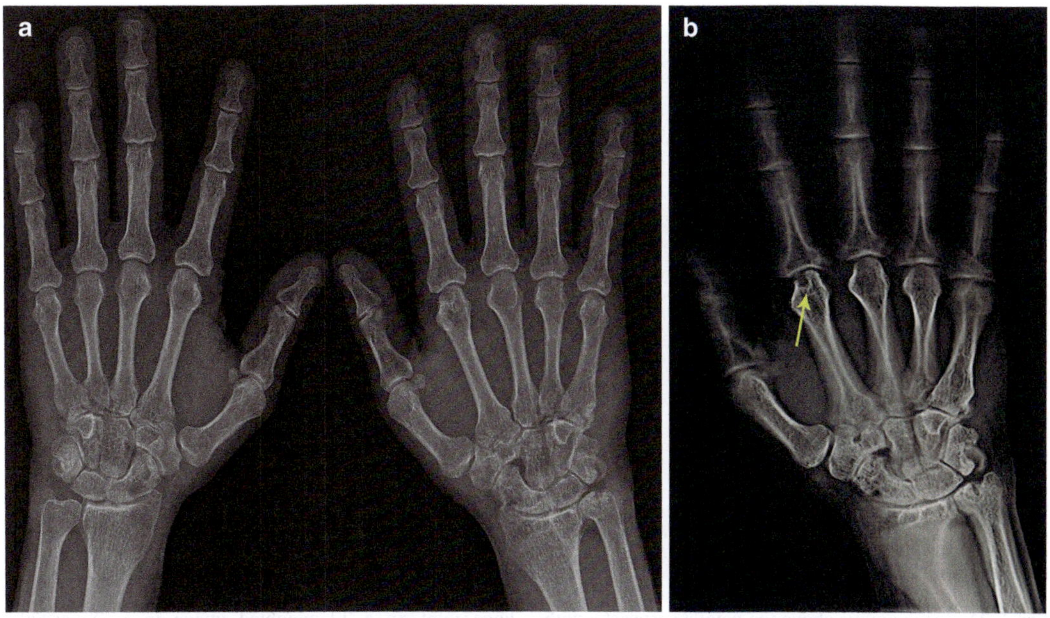

Fig. 5.20 (**a**) Plain radiograph which looks essentially normal in a 38-year-old man with a 1-year history of arthritis symptoms; (**b**) corresponding tomosynthesis image of the same patient taken on the same day showing erosion at second MCP (*arrow*)

Magnetic Resonance Imaging

Magnetic resonance imaging (MRI) (Chaps. 1 and 2) has the advantage of being able to determine synovitis, synovial fluid and bone marrow oedema (which may be an indicator of inflammation), all of which can be seen in early disease in addition to erosions which often occur as the disease progresses. Other imaging modalities cannot determine inflammatory changes within the bone marrow. Bone marrow oedema on MRI is defined as a high signal with irregular borders on T2 fat-suppressed or short tau (STIR) images. BME may predict future erosions. Synovitis has been defined by the OMERACT group as post-gadolinium enhancement of the thickened synovial membrane. On T1-weighted images, erosions appear as focal cortical defects of low signal intensity (SI). Synovitis enhances post-gadolinium. On T2 images, synovitis, bone marrow oedema and synovial fluid have high SI (Figs. 5.21a and 5.22). Active tendon involvement with tenosynovitis also appears high SI.

Using dedicated views of the MCP joints (Fig. 5.23) with coronal STIR, 3D fat-saturated T1 post-gadolinium, axial T2 Fat-Sat images, the pathological processes of tendinosis, joint effusions, synovitis, tenosynovitis and bone marrow

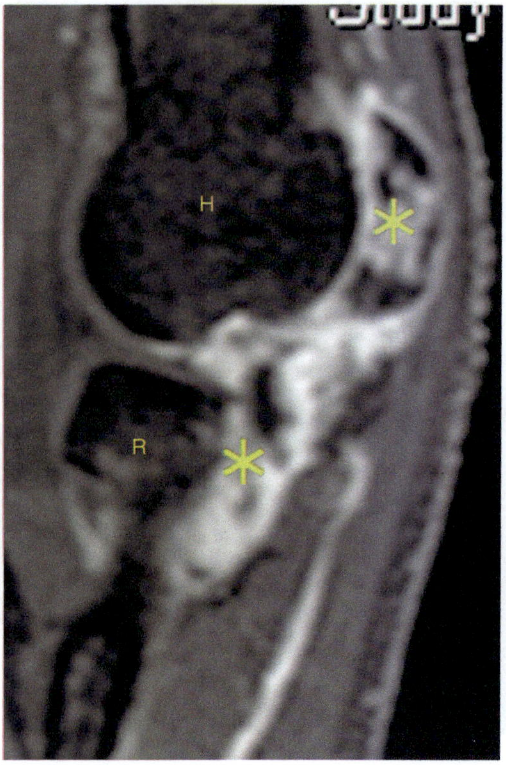

Fig. 5.22 MRI T2 with STIR sequence of the elbow in a 35-year-old woman with inadequately treated RA showing effusion and synovitis (*asterisks*). *H* humerus, *R* radius

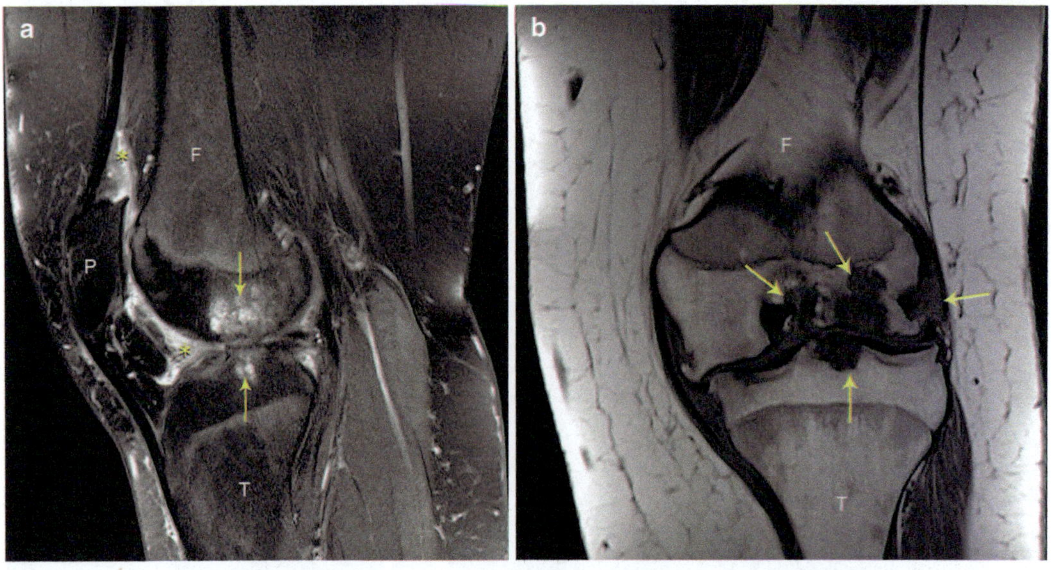

Fig. 5.21 (**a**) Synovitis above the patella (*asterisk*), with bone marrow oedema of the femur and tibia (*arrows*) shown on a T2 Fat-Sat image; (**b**) erosions (*arrows*) of the knee joint on a T1-weighted image in a 28-year-old woman with seropositive, anti-CCP-positive RA diagnosed at the age of 18 years. *F* femur, *T* tibia, *P* patella

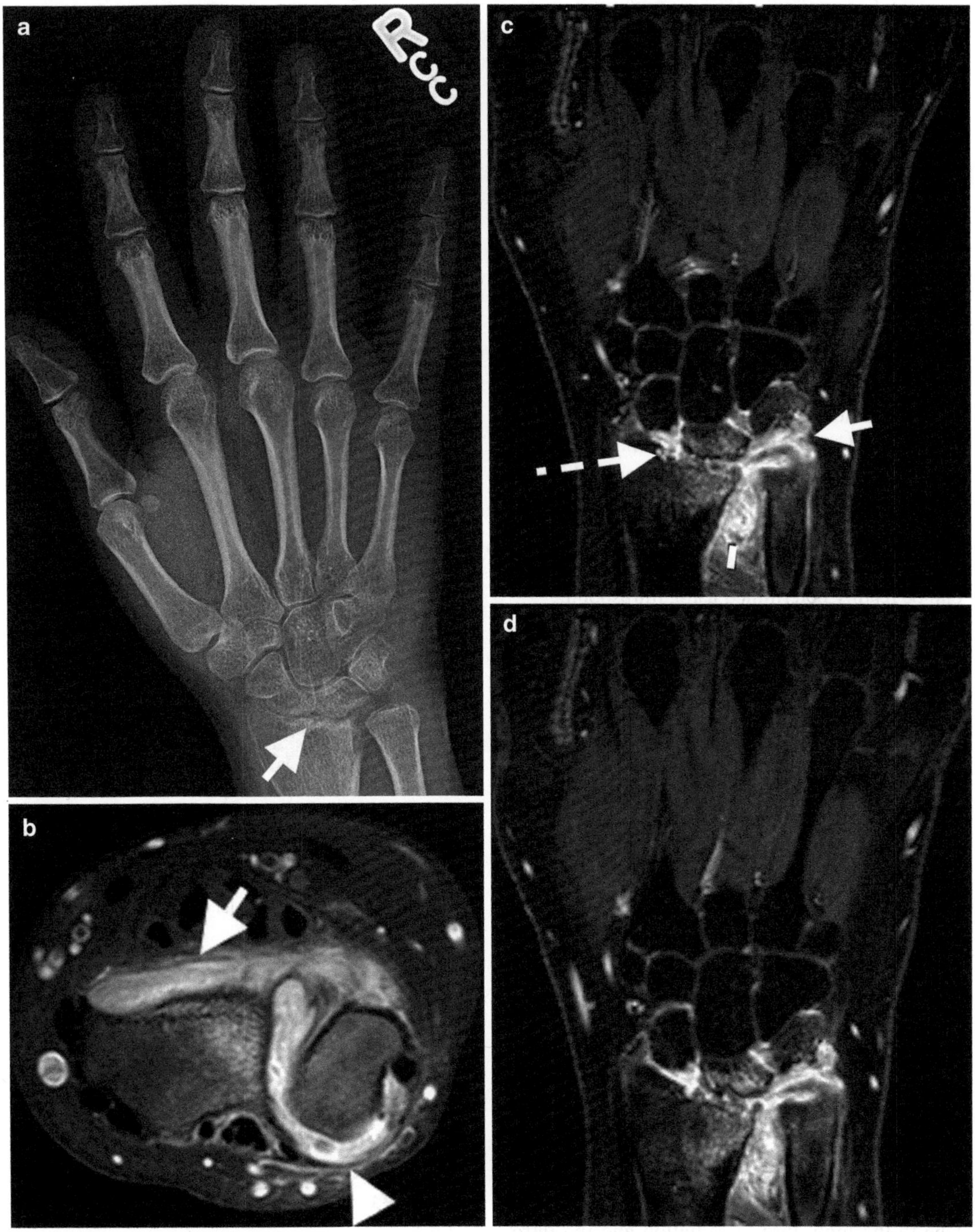

Fig. 5.23 A 23-year-old female with RA and bilateral symmetrical erosive disease wrists. (**a**) AP hand demonstrating periarticular osteopenia, radiocarpal joint space loss and erosions of the lunate and radius (**b**) Axial T2FS MRI of the wrist with high SI fluid vs. synovitis distal radioulnar (*arrowhead*) and radiocarpal joint (*arrow*). (**c**) Cor T1FS PG with extensive synovitis at both joints with marked enhancement and erosions of the ulna and radius (*dashed arrow*), (**d**) without *arrow* overlays

oedema can be detected. Synovial thickening can be differentiated from effusion.

Gadolinium contrast enhancement is often used to better delineate the synovitis; however, recent studies have suggested that with appropriate sequencing, this may not always be necessary. OMERACT scoring is reviewed in Appendix.

Ultrasonography (US)

Ultrasonography has many advantages over other imaging modalities in RA. It is quick, repeatable and relatively inexpensive, enables scanning of multiple joints at the same sitting in real time and, if performed in the rheumatology office, has immediate implications for clinical decision-making.

Pathological changes including synovitis, tenosynovitis, synovial effusions, bone erosions, cartilage thinning and increased synovial vascularity can be readily determined using ultrasound.

Greyscale synovitis with effusion and with increased power Doppler signal representing slow flow in small vessels within the synovium along with break in the bony cortex (erosion) is shown in Fig. 5.24.

OMERACT have developed a standardised scoring method for synovitis, erosions and power Doppler signal. This is described in Appendix.

Computerised Tomography (CT)

This imaging modality is the most sensitive at determining bony structures and erosions. However, CT cannot visualise the inflammatory changes of bone marrow oedema or synovial vascularity and incurs a radiation dose. Given the availability of alternate imaging with ultrasound and MRI, it is not routinely used in RA.

Radioisotope Bone Scan

Due to the high dose of radiation and the introduction of improved high-frequency ultrasound probe technology, the use of this modality for diagnosis and monitoring in RA has reduced significantly over the last decade. If performed, there may be multiple symmetrical joint involvements in a pattern typical of RA (particularly the small joints of hands and feet).

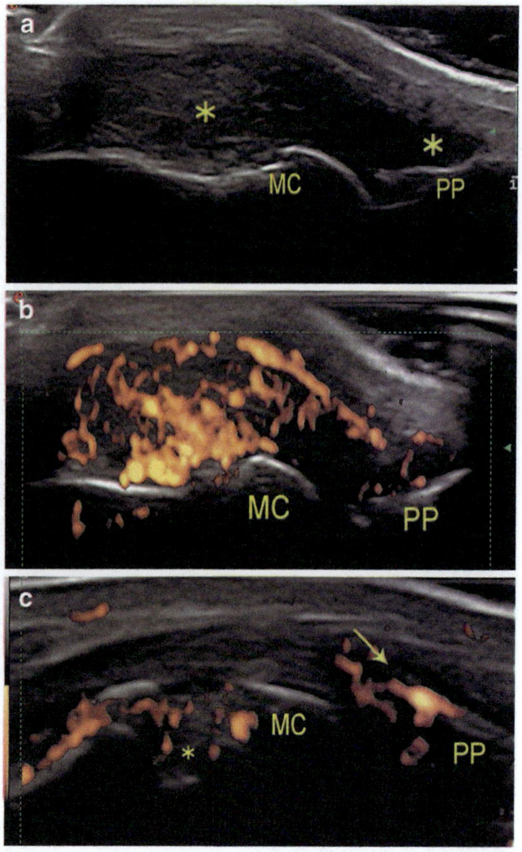

Fig. 5.24 (**a**) Marked synovial thickening (*asterisk*) at MCP joint; (**b**) marked power Doppler signal representing synovial vascularity (*red*) and (**c**) active erosion with power Doppler signal in the bottom of a break in the cortex (*asterisk*). Power Doppler signal in an area of synovial thickening (*arrow*)

Seronegative Spondyloarthropathies: Peripheral Features

Overview

Seronegative spondyloarthropathies (SpA) are a group of chronic autoimmune inflammatory joint diseases predominantly affecting the axial skeleton

Table 5.4 HLA-B27 association and clinical manifestations of each of the SpAs

	AS	PsA	Reactive	Enteropathic
HLA-B27 positive	95 %	60 %	60–80 %	60 %
Sacroiliitis	Usually bilateral; small erosions on iliac side; early ankylosis whole joint	Often unilateral; larger erosions with bony proliferation	Often unilateral	Usually bilateral
Peripheral arthritis	Large joint oligoarticular	Large or small joints, can affect DIPs	Large joint oligoarticular and feet	Large joint oligoarticular, knee and ankle, migratory, nondeforming. More common in males
Extra-articular features	Pulmonary fibrosis (apical), aortic incompetence, uveitis, lens dislocation	Psoriasis	Preceding GI or GU infection, sterile urethritis, conjunctivitis, uveitis, keratoderma blennorrhagicum, circinate balanitis, erythema nodosum, nail changes	Diarrhoea, aphthous ulceration, uveitis, erythema nodosum and pyoderma gangrenosum
Axial involvement (see Chap. 6)	Corner lesions, posterior and lateral involvement	Indistinguishable from AS	Less common	Less common (women > men)

and often accompanied by a peripheral arthritis. This group is composed of ankylosing spondylitis, psoriatic arthritis, reactive arthritis, enteropathic arthritis, juvenile spondyloarthritis and undifferentiated spondyloarthritis. They are all characterised by sacroiliitis (usually bilateral), enthesitis, peripheral arthritis and dactylitis. The axial manifestations including sacroiliitis are reviewed in Chap. 6. It is important to note that axial diseases (inflammatory back pain symptoms and signs) are not necessary to make the diagnosis of a SpA, i.e. SpA may be diagnosed on the basis of relevant clinical findings associated with peripheral arthritis alone (Table 5.4).

The peripheral arthritis of SpA has been defined by several criteria including, most recently, the Assessment of SpondyloArthritis International Society (ASAS) classification criteria and includes asymmetric peripheral arthritis and/or predominant involvement of the lower limb. Dactylitis, soft tissue inflammation in a digit with resulting "sausage shape", and enthesitis, inflammation at the site of tendon, ligament or capsule insertion onto bone, are common features. Extra-articular manifestations common to all of SpAs include anterior uveitis or conjunctivitis, aphthous ulceration, aortic incompetence and an HLA-B27 genetic association. Erythema nodosum and pyoderma gangrenosum are skin manifestations particularly associated with the enteropathic peripheral arthritis. Any of the seronegative SpAs can cause anterior chest wall pathology (most commonly seen in SAPHO syndrome). The pathological processes of the peripheral joint involvement include synovitis and enthesitis.

A well-described pathological finding in the seronegative SpAs is inflammation around the entheseal complex (Fig. 5.25) which may be associated with new bone formation (Figs. 5.27 and 5.28). Entheses commonly involved include the superior and inferior pole of the patella, tibial tuberosity, Achilles tendon and the calcaneal attachment of the plantar aponeurosis (Fig. 5.28).

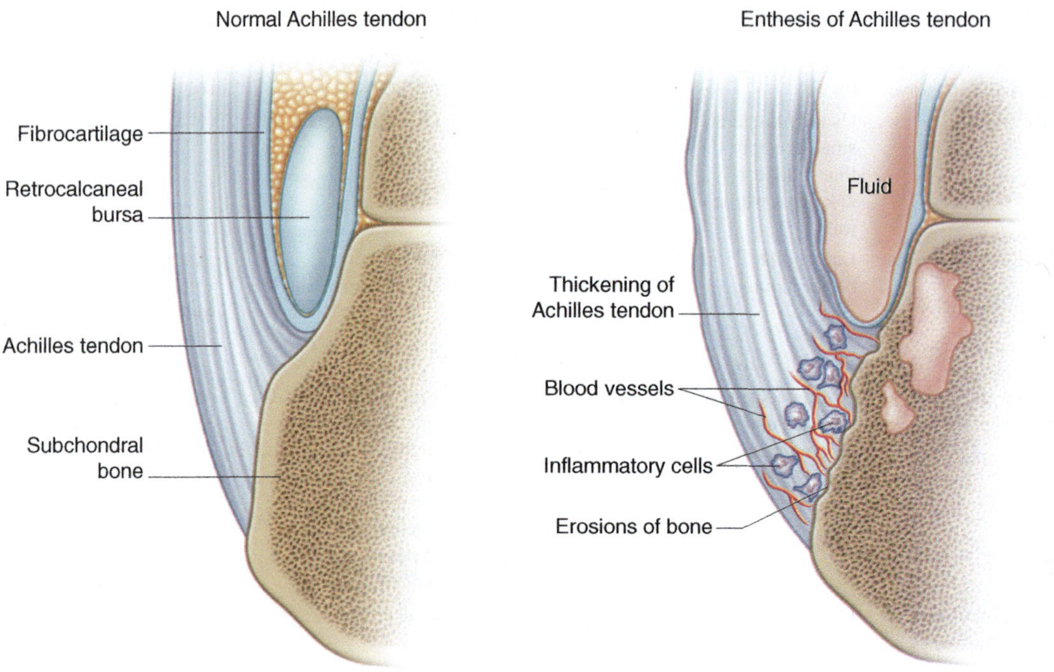

Fig. 5.25 Illustration of normal vs. inflamed enthesis

Common Imaging Features of the Spondyloarthropathies: Peripheral Joints

Radiographs (Figs. 5.26, 5.27, and 5.28)

As described above, the pathological hallmarks of peripheral involvement of the SpAs include synovitis, erosions, enthesitis, new bone formation and dactylitis.

Radiographic features of enthesitis include new bone formation, bone erosions, periarticular sclerosis and cysts, and calcification of ligaments and tendons. New bone formation is suggested by enthesophytes and periostitis. Synovitis will appear like a joint effusion as previously described in RA section. Dactylitis can be observed as diffuse soft tissue swelling throughout a whole digit (see Fig. 5.30).

Common entheseal sites assessed in any of the SpAs are outlined in Table 5.5.

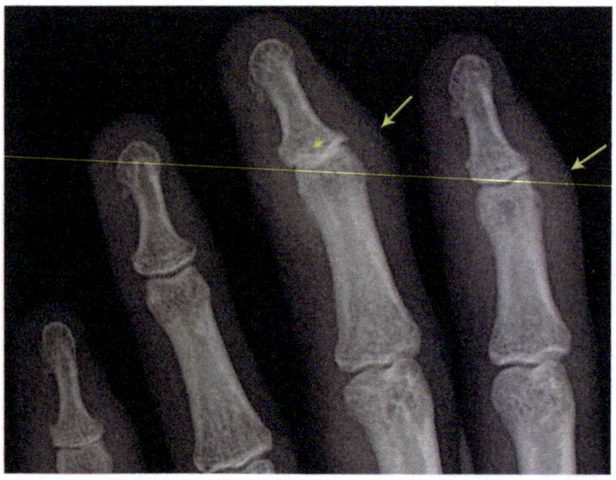

Fig. 5.26 Soft tissue swelling at DIPs (*arrows*) with joint space narrowing (*asterisk*) in a 32-year-old woman with a 6-year history of untreated psoriatic arthritis

The imaging features of each of the individual SpA will be described in detail in the following sections.

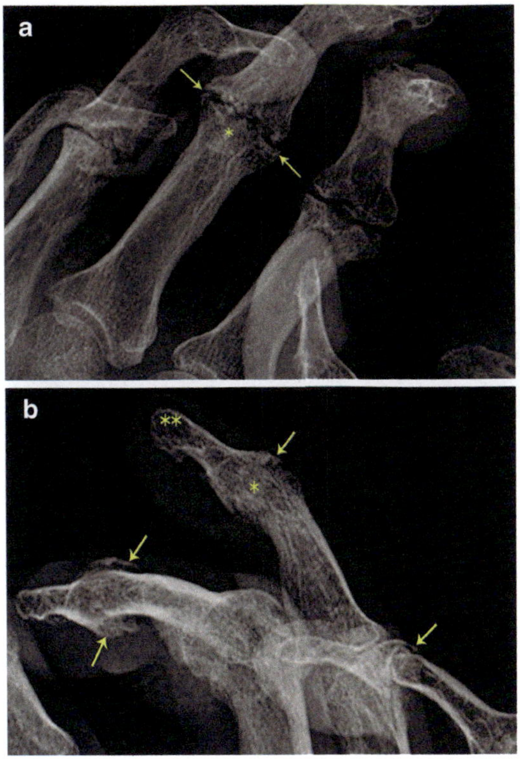

Fig. 5.27 (**a**) Erosions (*asterisk*) and bony overgrowth (*arrows*) at PIP and DIP joints; (**b**) with distal phalangeal tuft resorption (*double asterisk*), central erosions (*asterisk*) and new bone formation (*arrows*) in a 66-year-old man with long-standing psoriatic arthritis

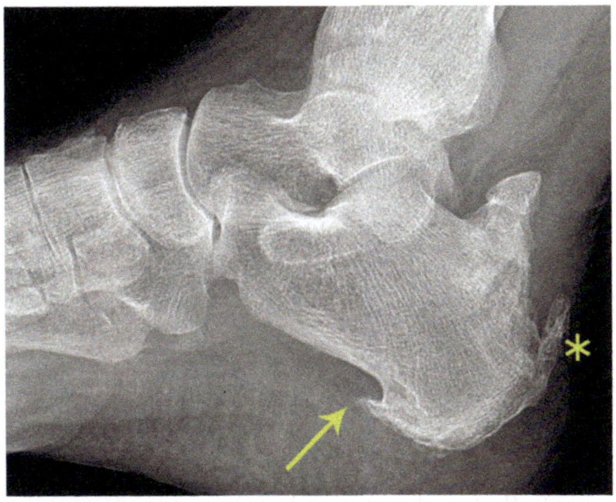

Fig. 5.28 Entheseal bony spur at plantar fascia (*arrow*) and at Achilles insertion (*asterisk*)

Table 5.5 Common entheseal attachments

Common entheseal sites	
Proximal plantar fascia	Distal Achilles tendon
Distal patellar ligament	Proximal patellar ligament
Distal quadriceps tendon	Brachial triceps insertion
Common flexor tendon of forearm	Common extensor tendon of forearm

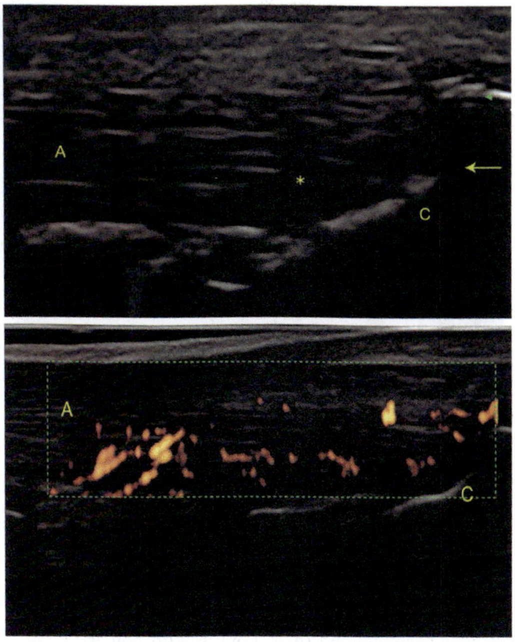

Fig. 5.29 Achilles tendinosis with thickened irregular tendon (*asterisk*), erosions (*arrow*) and increased power Doppler signal within tendon and around tendon insertion. *A* Achilles tendon, *C* calcaneus

Ultrasound

The advantage of US over conventional radiography in the peripheral manifestations of SpA includes the ability to image active inflammatory changes within joints and tendons and at the entheses using greyscale and power Doppler (Figs. 5.29 and 5.30). US may be preferable to MRI in imaging the peripheral manifestations of the SpAs as multiple joints or entheseal sites can be imaged at one session, it can be more comfortable for patients and can aid in more rapid clinical diagnosis.

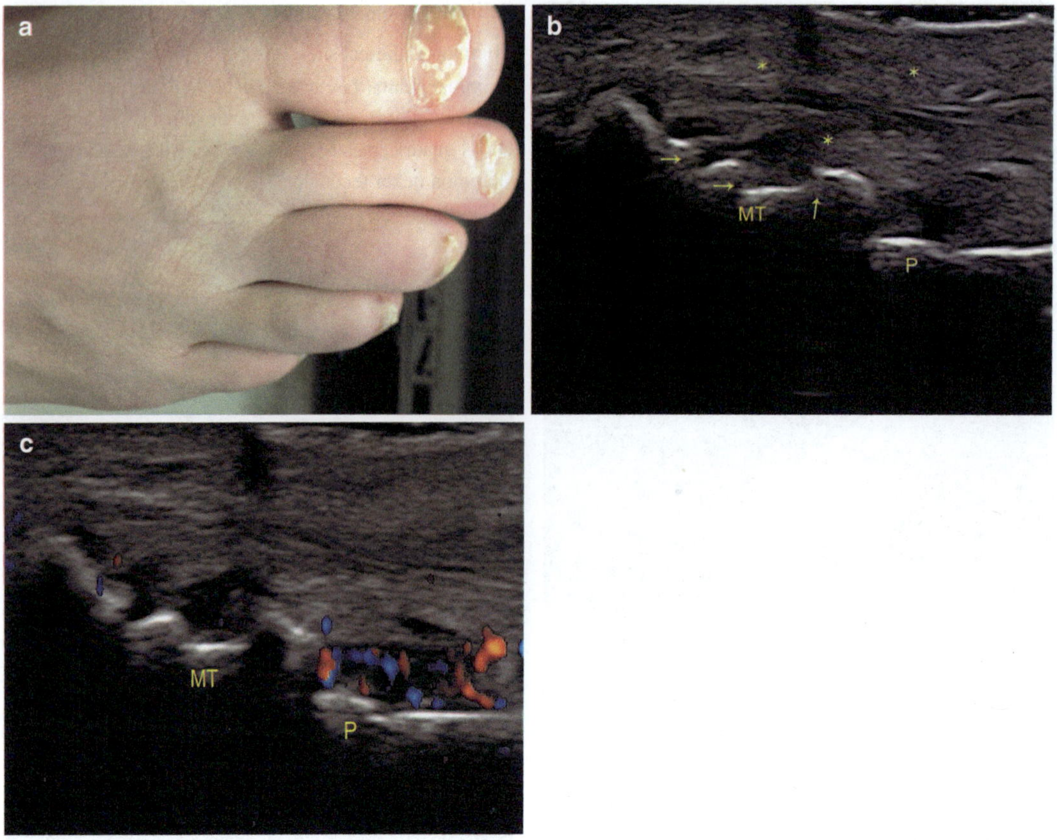

Fig. 5.30 (**a**) Dactylitis of the right third toe in a 31-year-old man with (**b**) soft tissue swelling, synovitis (*asterisks*) erosions (*arrows*) and (**c**) synovitis with power Doppler signal (*blue* and *red colour*). *MT* metatarsal bone, *P* phalanx, *C* calcaneus (Ultrasound images courtesy of Dr. Gurjit Kaeley, University of Florida, Jacksonville, Florida)

Characteristic ultrasound findings of enthesitis include abnormal echogenicity and thickness of tendons with calcific deposits or tears in the tendons, bony erosions, cortical irregularity and enthesophytes (bony overgrowth along the line of the tendon or ligament) (Chap. 3). Bursitis is also a feature of the peripheral involvement of SpA. Two sonographic indices to monitor enthesitis are the Glasgow Ultrasound Enthesitis Scoring System (GUESS) and the Madrid Sonography Enthesitis Index. These indices are primarily used for research purposes and are not routinely used in clinical practice.

Ultrasonographic findings of increased power Doppler signal in the synovium and at the entheses correlate strongly with the histopathological findings of markedly increased vascular infiltration into the synovium of affected joints.

MRI

MRI has several advantages over plain radiography in assessing peripheral arthritis in the SpAs. These include the assessment of synovitis, bone marrow oedema (Fig. 5.31), erosions, enthesitis, dactylitis and tendinopathies. This is a reliable imaging modality to assess peripheral joint involvement at an early stage of disease. MRI reveals that enthesitis and osteitis are intimately related. Fifty percent of patients with plantar fasciitis have associated osteitis. These findings are

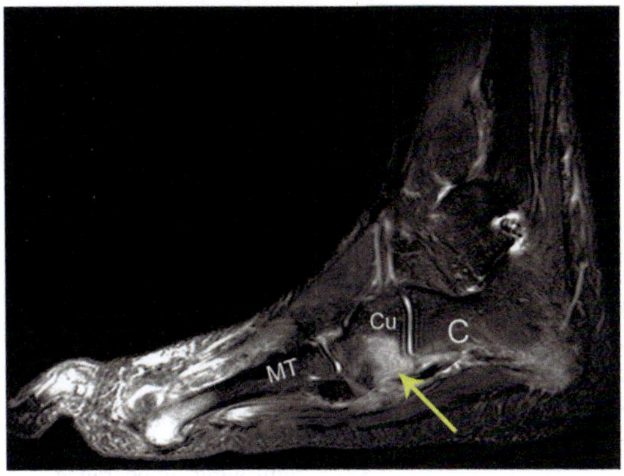

Fig. 5.31 Bone marrow oedema on T2-weighted MRI in cuneiform (*arrow*). *C* calcaneus, *Cu* cuneiform, *MT* metatarsal

best visualised on T2-weighted fat-suppressed sequences. With the aid of MRI, dactylitis is now described as involving the entheseal insertion of the nail, the soft tissues and the flexor tendons.

Bone marrow oedema near the tendons, ligaments and capsules is more marked in HLA-B27-positive individuals.

Psoriatic Arthritis

Overview

Psoriatic arthritis (PsA) is an inflammatory arthritis associated with psoriasis (or a family history of psoriasis in a first-degree relative). It is characterised by synovial proliferation with neovascularisation, enthesitis and bony proliferation. About 20 % of patients with psoriasis will develop PsA within 10 years, and the arthritis rarely develops prior to or in the absence of psoriasis. There are several patterns of joint involvement with PsA:

- Asymmetrical oligoarthritis (≤5 joints) affecting large or small joints (approx. 50 %)
- Predominant DIP involvement (looks like erosive OA) (approx. 40 %)
- Symmetrical small joint polyarticular (looks like RA) (up to 30 %)
- Arthritis mutilans – a destructive, deforming arthritis (rare)
- Spondyloarthritis with sacroiliitis and large joint involvement (up to 30 %) (Chap. 6)

Presentation

In adults, PsA usually presents after the onset of psoriasis, but in children, arthritis frequently predates the skin disease (indeed psoriasis may only be present in a first-degree relative). Patients may present with arthritis along with dactylitis; nail changes such as onycholysis, pitting and ridging; and enthesitis (Table 5.6). They may also present with extra-articular features of PsA including iritis or an overlap with inflammatory bowel disease.

Typically, inflammatory markers are raised, but autoantibodies including RF and anti-CCP are negative.

There are five domains of psoriatic arthritis:

1. Peripheral arthritis
2. Skin/nail changes
3. Axial arthritis
4. Dactylitis
5. Enthesitis

The comparative plain radiographic findings of RA, PsA, OA and erosive OA are outlined in Table 5.7.

Table 5.6 The clinical and imaging features of PsA

Feature	
Articular features	Synovial hypertrophy, erosions, periosteal reactions, sacroiliitis
Joints involved	DIPs (like OA) 40 %, large joints with enthesitis 50 %, MCPJs/PIPJs (like RA) up to 30%, sacroiliitis (like AS) up to 30 %
Other features	Dactylitis, nail changes enthesitis, psoriasis, iritis, aphthous ulceration
Inflammatory markers	Usually raised
Autoantibodies	Usually negative
Imaging changes	See below

Table 5.7 Plain radiographic findings of RA, PsA and OA

RA	PsA	OA	Erosive OA
MCPJs, carpal joints, distal ulna, extensor carpi ulnaris tendon	DIPs, PIPJs, MCPJs, wrist. Extensor tendons of first (ext pollicis brevis and abductor pollicis longus) and second compartments (extensor carpi radialis brevis and longus)	DIPs, PIPJs, 1st CMC	DIPs, PIPJs, 1st CMC
Joint space narrowing – symmetrical	Joint space narrowing – asymmetrical	Joint space narrowing – asymmetrical	Diffuse joint space narrowing
Erosions (marginal)	Erosions (often central) with bony overgrowth	Subchondral cysts and osteophytes	Subchondral erosions with central location creating "gull-wing" appearance
Periarticular osteopenia	Osteopenia uncommon	Subchondral sclerosis	Subchondral sclerosis, occ. joint ankylosis
Soft tissue swelling	Soft tissue swelling including dactylitis	Soft tissue swelling	Absence of marginal erosions, soft tissue swelling or osteopenia

Imaging Peripheral Psoriatic Arthritis

Plain Radiography

Plain radiography is commonly requested in peripheral PsA. The hands are more frequently affected than the feet in PsA. Characteristic features include marked soft tissue swelling, which can affect the whole digit (dactylitis), periosteal reaction on the shaft of the bone ("fluffy" periostitis) and new bone formation (particularly at the site of entheseal insertions resulting in bony spurs), central erosions with osteolysis (creating a "pencil-in-cup" appearance), osteolysis of the tufts of the terminal phalanges, involvement of the DIPs with ankylosis (not seen in RA) and absence of periarticular osteopenia (seen in RA). Unlike RA, new bone formation is characteristic around the site of the erosion, and DIPs are frequently involved (Fig. 5.32).

Ultrasound

The Group for Research and Assessment of Psoriasis and Psoriatic Arthritis (GRAPPA) has recently proposed US indices to assess enthesitis and dactylitis (see Fig. 5.30) including soft tissue changes, synovitis, erosions and osteoproliferation. Nail changes and skin plaque lesions can also be assessed using this technology as it has a resolution of >0.1 mm. However, these are not routinely assessed in the clinical setting. Flexor tenosynovitis is often seen in patients with hand involvement in PsA and is readily imaged using US.

Entheseal insertions which typically become inflamed in PsA include the insertions of the following:

- Quadriceps tendon
- Proximal and distal patellar ligament
- Achilles tendon
- Plantar aponeurosis
- Triceps
- Flexor and extensor tendon of the forearm (Fig. 5.33)

Ultrasonographic scoring systems for enthesitis related to psoriatic arthritis have been described (see Appendix).

MRI

The site of erosion can help differentiate peripheral joint PsA (around entheseal insertions and centrally resulting in "pencil in cup") from RA (marginal). Synovitis is generally the same between the two inflammatory arthritis conditions, but bone marrow oedema may be more prominent and occurs at the bony corners of

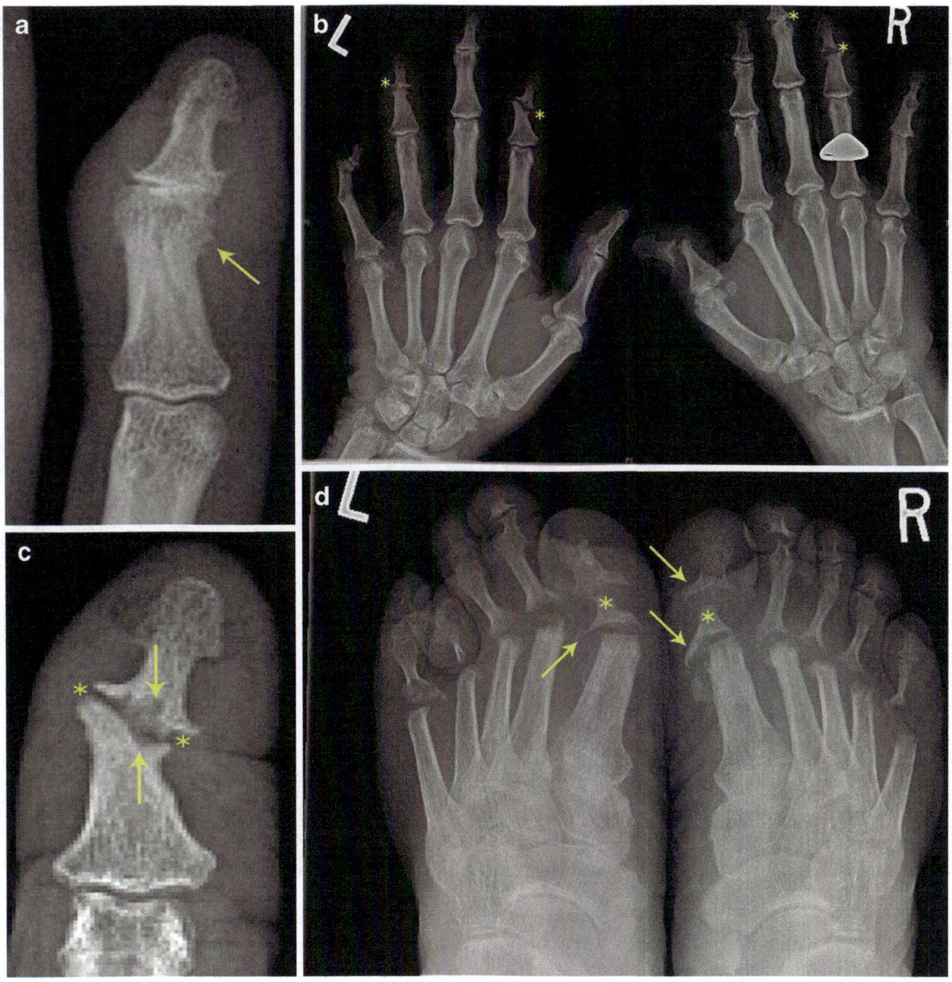

Fig. 5.32 (**a**) Fluffy periostitis (*arrow*) in a 34-year-old woman with untreated PsA; (**b**) central erosions with bony overgrowth (*asterisks*) in the same patient; (**c**) pencil-in-cup deformity with central erosion (*arrow*) and bony overgrowth (*asterisks*) in a 65-year-old man who was treated with intraarticular corticosteroid injections and oral prednisone for many years; (**d**) multiple destructive arthropathy with erosions (*asterisks*) and bony overgrowth (*arrows*) in the same patient as c

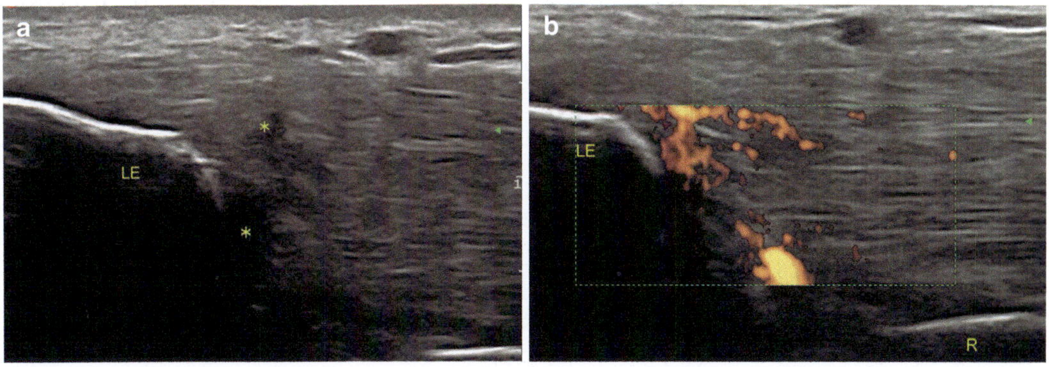

Fig. 5.33 A 28-year-old man with active psoriatic arthritis and enthesitis. Lateral epicondylitis with (**a**) heterogeneity (*asterisks*) in common extensor tendon inserting on lateral epicondyle (*LE*) and (**b**) marked power Doppler signal in that tendon complex as it inserts

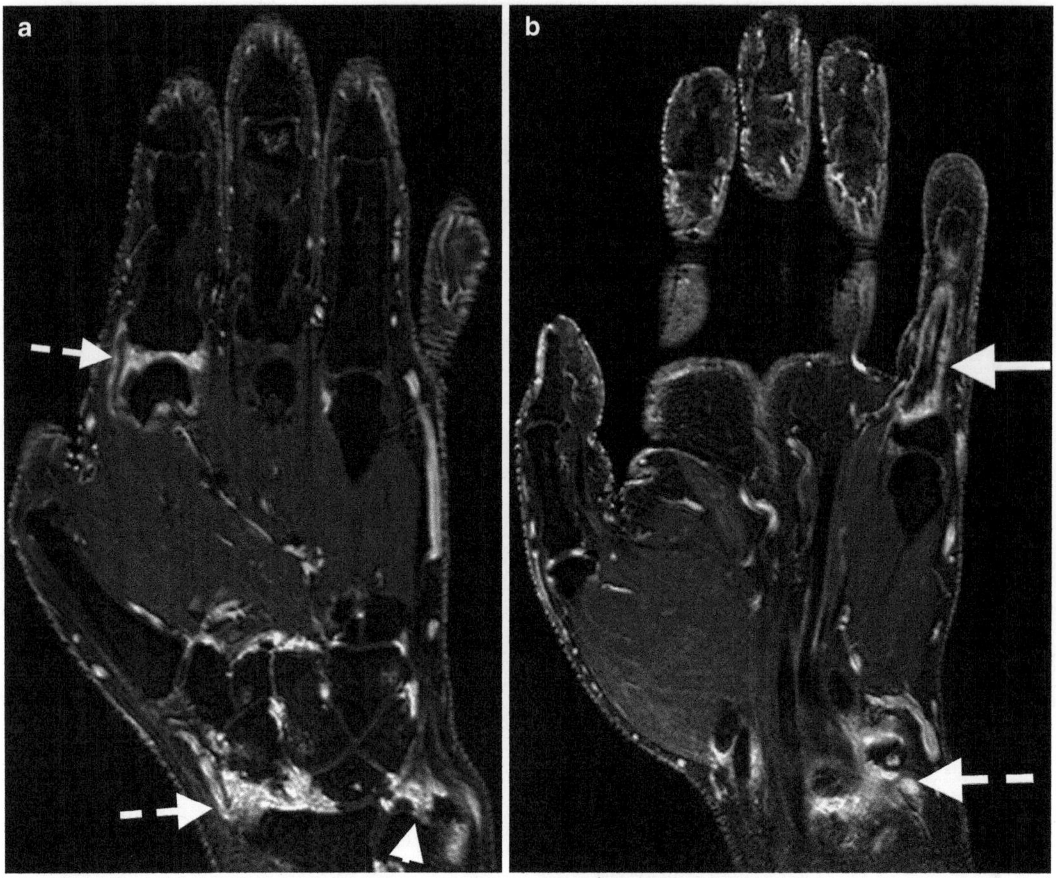

Fig. 5.34 MRI of the right hand in a 37-year-old male with PsA presenting with bilateral asymmetrical arthritis. (**a**) Cor TIFS PG with enhanced synovial tissue at the radiocarpal and second MCP joints (*dashed arrows*) and erosion of the distal ulna (*arrowhead*). Note the adjacent enhanced bone marrow oedema. (**b**) Cor TIFS PG in the same patient with 5th common flexor enhanced tenosynovitis (*arrow*) and radiocarpal synovitis (*dashed arrow*)

joints and at the entheseal sites in PsA (Fig. 5.34a, b). MRI of the peripheral joint may also help differentiate PsA from RA and PsA from OA. Dynamic MRI can also detect increased vascularity compared with RA (this increased vascularity is also seen in biopsy samples of PsA). MRI can clearly depict the enthesitis at the DIPJs which occurs in PsA but not OA. Furthermore, whole body multi-joint MRI can be used to assess the extent of disease in joints and entheses.

The GRAPPA group along with OMERACT have also outlined the utility of MRI in the diagnosis and monitoring of psoriatic arthritis. The PsAMRIS has been proposed for assessing peripheral arthritis in PsA. It is currently used as a research tool and may be adapted for clinical use in the future. This scoring system includes scoring of synovitis, tenosynovitis, periarticular inflammation, bone marrow oedema, erosions and osteoproliferation. An outline of the scoring sheet can be found in the Appendix.

Ankylosing Spondylitis (AS)

Overview

Ankylosing spondylitis is a chronic systemic inflammatory disorder strongly associated with the HLA-B27 genotype. It is characterised by male predisposition and the propensity to cause ankylosis particularly in the sacroiliac joints, the facet joints and the intervertebral discs. The spondylitic features of AS are described in Chap. 6. Extra-axial features include enthesitis, anterior uveitis and large joint synovitis.

Presentation

Adult males in their second and third decades are most commonly affected with a 3:1 male preponderance. The symptoms are often insidious with chronic low back pain and/or buttock pain and stiffness usually beginning in late adolescence or early adulthood. Symptoms are typically "inflammatory" in nature with morning stiffness, pain worse on inactivity and better with movement or stretching. AS can also present with a large joint oligoarthritis, particularly affecting the hip (usually bilateral) and shoulder.

Specific Imaging Features

Radiographs

Typically large joints such as hip, knee, shoulder and elbow are affected in peripheral AS, with synovitis, effusion and enthesitis. Plain radiographic features typical of hip, shoulder and knee joint AS include diffuse cartilage loss (rather than localised as in OA), effusion, erosions (Fig. 5.35a) (particularly on the superolateral humeral head in the shoulder) and significant ankylosis. Patellar tendon enthesitis is also common with bony spurs and irregular bony margins.

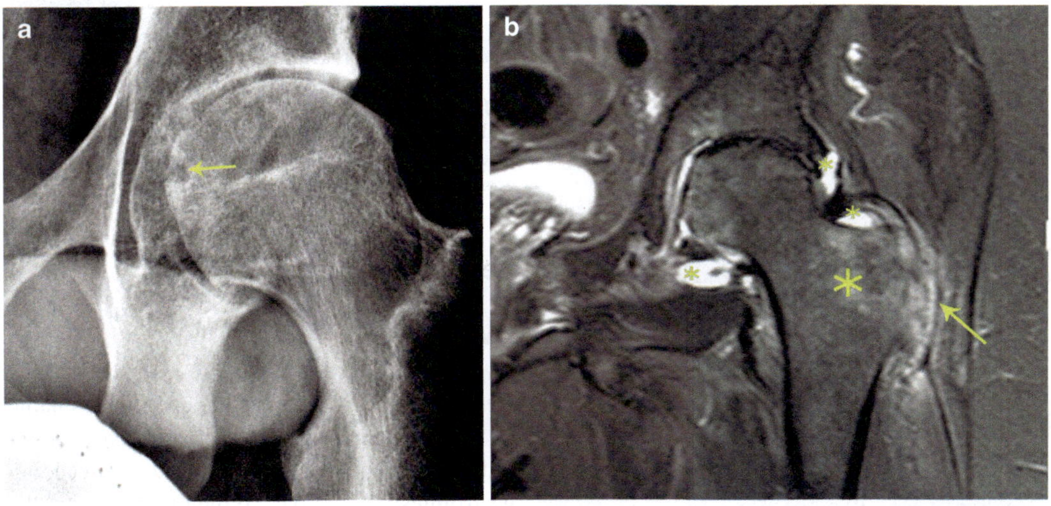

Fig, 5.35 (**a**) Erosion (*arrow*) on plain radiography; (**b**) synovitis (*small asterisk*), BME (*large asterisk*) and trochanteric bursitis and enthesitis (*arrow*) on T2-weighted STIR sequence MRI

Ultrasound

Dactylitis (see Fig. 5.30) and enthesitis, effusions, tendinosis (Fig. 5.36), bursitis, bony proliferation and erosion can be clearly depicted using US. These features are indistinguishable from those of the other seronegative spondyloarthropathies. Ultrasound and MRI are particularly good imaging modalities for detecting enthesitis. Synovitis and enthesitis are found predominantly in the lower limbs, particularly the midfoot, ankle and knee joints.

MRI

Large joint involvement is the most frequent peripheral finding in AS with synovitis, bone marrow oedema, bursitis and enthesitis clearly visualised by MRI particularly of the hip (Fig. 5.35b), shoulder and knee in a symmetric pattern. The arthritis can be erosive or nonerosive, but in both types, bony overgrowth followed by ankylosis is found in end-stage disease. Erosive disease is less frequent and usually causes eccentric erosions in the large joints e.g. humeral head (Fig. 5.37). CT representation of humeral head eccentric erosions.

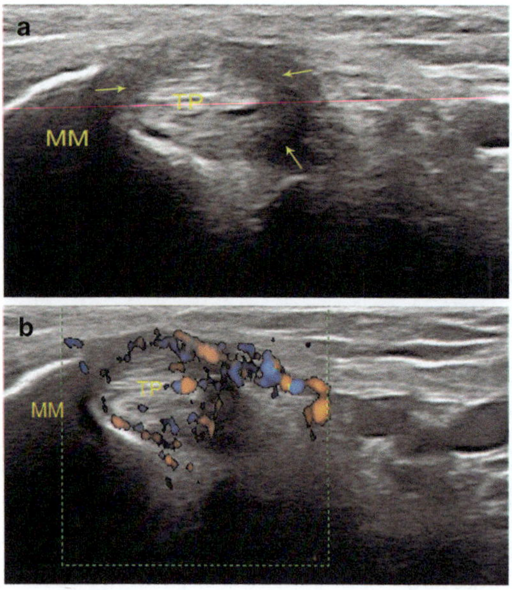

Fig. 5.36 (**a**) Tibialis posterior (*TP*) tenosynovitis (*arrows*), (**b**) in power Doppler. *MM* medial malleolus

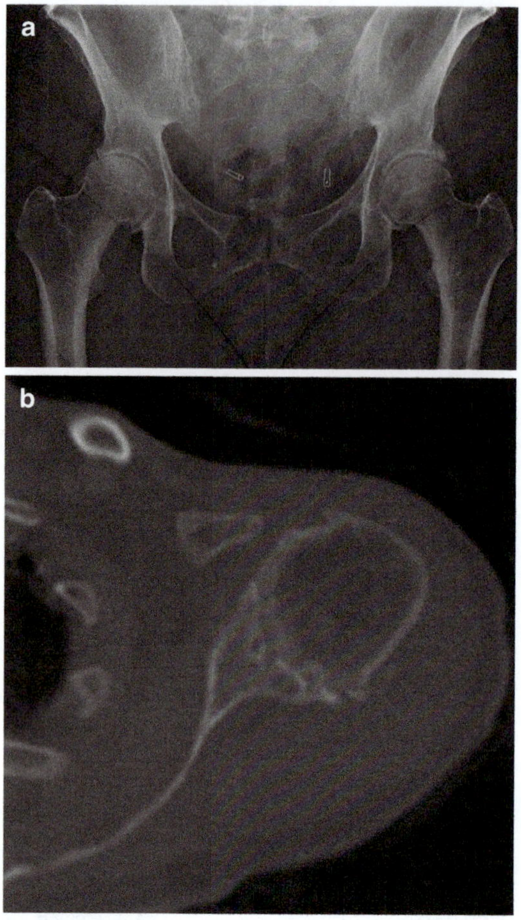

Fig. 5.37 (**a**) AP pelvis in long-standing AS with bilateral hip joint involvement and secondary degenerative disease. (**b**) Axial CT of the left shoulder with multifocal erosions and secondary degenerative disease

Reactive Arthritis

Overview

Reactive arthritis also has the eponymous name of Reiter's syndrome. This is an inflammatory arthritis which occurs in relation to a preceding gastrointestinal (GI), typically *Salmonella*, *Shigella*, *Yersinia*, *E. coli*, *Clostridium difficile* or *Campylobacter*, or genitourinary (GU), particularly *Chlamydia*, infection. Chlamydia pneumonia has also recently been added to this

Table 5.8 Extra-articular features found in reactive arthritis and other seronegative SpAs

Extra-articular features			
Ocular	Anterior uveitis	Conjunctivitis	Episcleritis
Skin	Keratoderma blennorrhagica	Erythema nodosum	
Nails	Ridging and pitting – similar to psoriatic nails		
Mucosa	Aphthous ulceration	Circinate balanitis	
GU	Pelvic pain and dysuria	Urethritis	Cervicitis or prostatitis

list. Aseptic arthritis may develop between 1 week and several months after the antecedent infection. HLA-B27 is a predisposing genetic susceptibility to the development of arthritis following a GU or GI infection, and this genotype may also portend more severe disease with a chronic course.

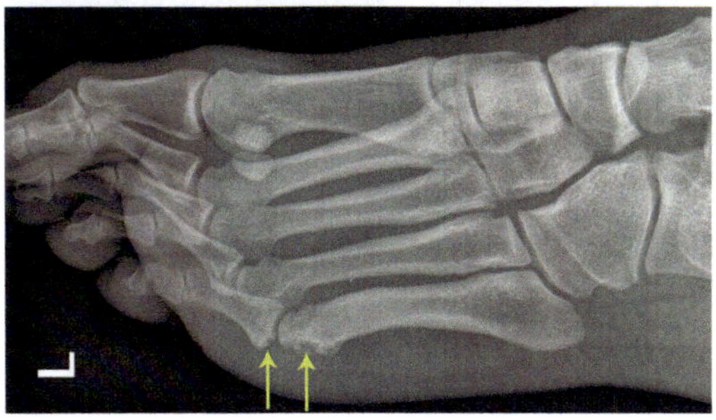

Fig. 5.38 Asymmetrical marginal erosion of the head of MTP5 (*arrows*) in a 25-year-old man with a 2-year history of reactive arthritis

Presentation

Young adults are particularly affected by this type of arthritis occurring within 1–4 weeks after the inciting infection. It is typically a mono- or asymmetrical oligoarticular disease affecting the lower limbs. This is usually a self-limiting arthritis with >50 % resolving within 6 months and the majority resolving within 1 year. The lower extremity joints of the knees, hips and feet (MTPJs and calcaneus) are most commonly affected in reactive arthritis. The sacroiliac joints, hands, wrists, elbows or shoulders are the most commonly involved joints. Extra-articular features occur in around 20 % (Table 5.8).

Specific Imaging Features

Radiographs

Peripheral arthritis associated with reactive arthritis usually involves the lower limbs. Around 26 % of patients with reactive arthritis report swelling or pain in the heel at initial presentation of the disease. This is often due to Achilles tendinosis (widening of the Achilles shadow and obliteration of the normal fat planes), retrocalcaneal bursitis (radiodense shadow displacing the normal fat planes between Achilles tendon and calcaneus, with associated erosion) or plantar fasciitis (calcaneal new bone formation at the plantar aponeurosis insertion). Early in the disease process, soft tissue swelling with dactylitis, periarticular osteoporosis and linear periostitis along the phalangeal shafts are radiographic features. Other soft tissue findings include joint effusion, bursitis and tendonitis. Joint space narrowing is typical in the bones of the carpus and tarsus. Entheseal calcification related to the patellar and Achilles tendons is commonly found. As the disease progresses, marginal erosions develop (Fig. 5.38) (as seen in RA), as well as erosions associated with overlying bursitis, particularly around the calcaneum along with fluffy periostitis causing bony proliferation (as seen in psoriatic arthritis). In reactive arthritis, there is relative sparing of the hands (DIPs in particular) and more frequent axial involvement when compared to PsA.

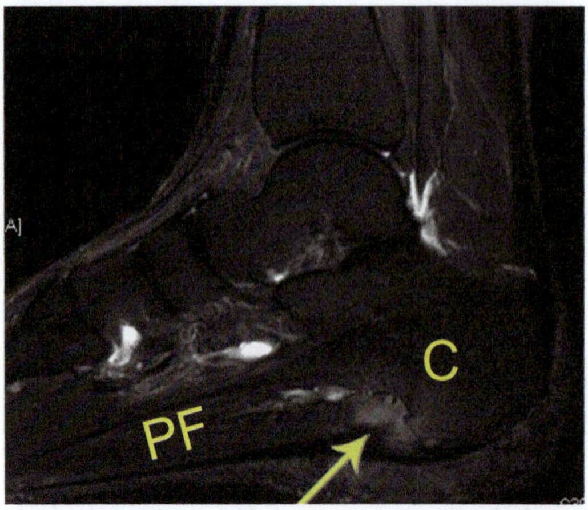

Fig. 5.39 A 31-year-old man with recurrent plantar fasciitis (*arrow*) on gadolinium-enhanced MRI. *PF* plantar fascia, *C* calcaneus

The original term Reiter's syndrome refers to a triad of arthritis, sterile urethritis and conjunctivitis, but these three features are found only in a minority of patients, so the term "reactive arthritis" is preferred.

MRI

In ReA, the relative sparing of the hands and predominance of the lower limb entheses with bone marrow oedema particularly around the calcaneal (Fig. 5.39), tibial and patellar entheseal insertions are typical MRI findings. Otherwise, MRI findings are the same as the other SpAs.

Enteropathic Arthritis

Overview

Enteropathic arthritis relates to inflammatory arthritis associated with ulcerative colitis and Crohn's (the so-called inflammatory bowel diseases). Other diseases with gastrointestinal (GI) manifestations including coeliac disease, Whipple's disease, Behcet's disease, sarcoid, systemic sclerosis, systemic lupus erythematosus and vasculitis and the enteropathic infectious diseases (reactive arthritis) can cause arthritis (inflammation in the joints) or arthralgia (pain in the joints), but these are not considered "enteropathic arthritis".

Presentation

The arthritis associated with inflammatory bowel diseases (IBD) typically causes a picture of spondyloarthritis with a mono- or oligoarticular pattern of peripheral arthritis (polyarticular involvement has been reported) and enthesitis particularly affecting the feet (plantar fasciitis, Achilles tendonitis) and knees (patellar tendonitis). The spondyloarthritic manifestations are discussed in Chap. 6. The arthritis is most commonly preceded by bowel disease but can occur before the onset of clinically apparent IBD in up to 6 % of cases.

The peripheral arthritis without axial involvement associated with IBD may fall into one of two groups – an oligoarticular large joint arthritis mainly affecting the lower limbs which has a self-limiting nonerosive course and often recurs with exacerbations of IBD or a bilateral symmetrical polyarthritis predominantly affecting the small joints of the upper limbs, with a persisting erosive course.

Peripheral arthritis has been reported in around 28 % of patients with Crohn's disease and 13 % of patients with ulcerative colitis. Involvement of the knee, ankle, wrist and elbow is found in 65, 62, 23 and 15 % of cases of peripheral arthritis associated with inflammatory bowel disease, respectively, with the MTPJs and MCPJs being less commonly involved.

Specific Imaging Features

Radiographs

The extra-axial joint involvement is usually nonerosive, although asymmetrical erosions have been described in the feet and hands in Crohn's disease. In a similar manner to the other

SpAs, soft tissue swelling characterised by dactylitis, bursitis, tendonitis and synovitis is commonly found. Enthesitis with bony overgrowth is also a frequent finding.

MRI

Erosive or nonerosive oligoarticular involvement is found in arthritis related to Crohn's disease or ulcerative colitis. Hip involvement is common with synovitis, effusions and trochanteric bursitis (Fig. 5.40). MRI reveals synovitis, BME, enthesitis (Fig. 5.41) and dactylitis (as in the other SpAs).

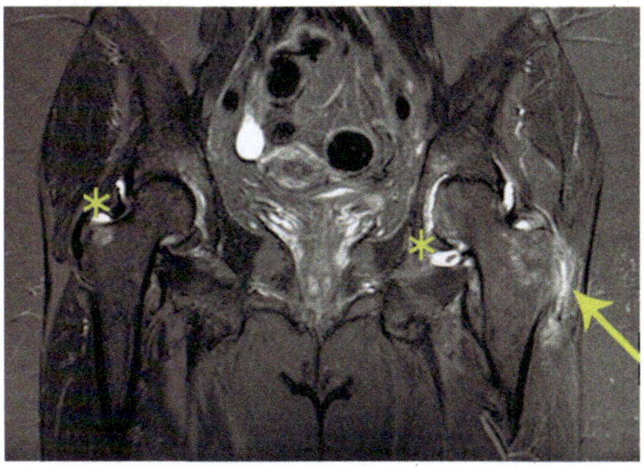

Fig. 5.40 A 53-year-old woman with ulcerative colitis with large hip effusions (*asterisks*) with synovitis and trochanteric bursitis (*arrow*) with BME on T2-weighted MRI

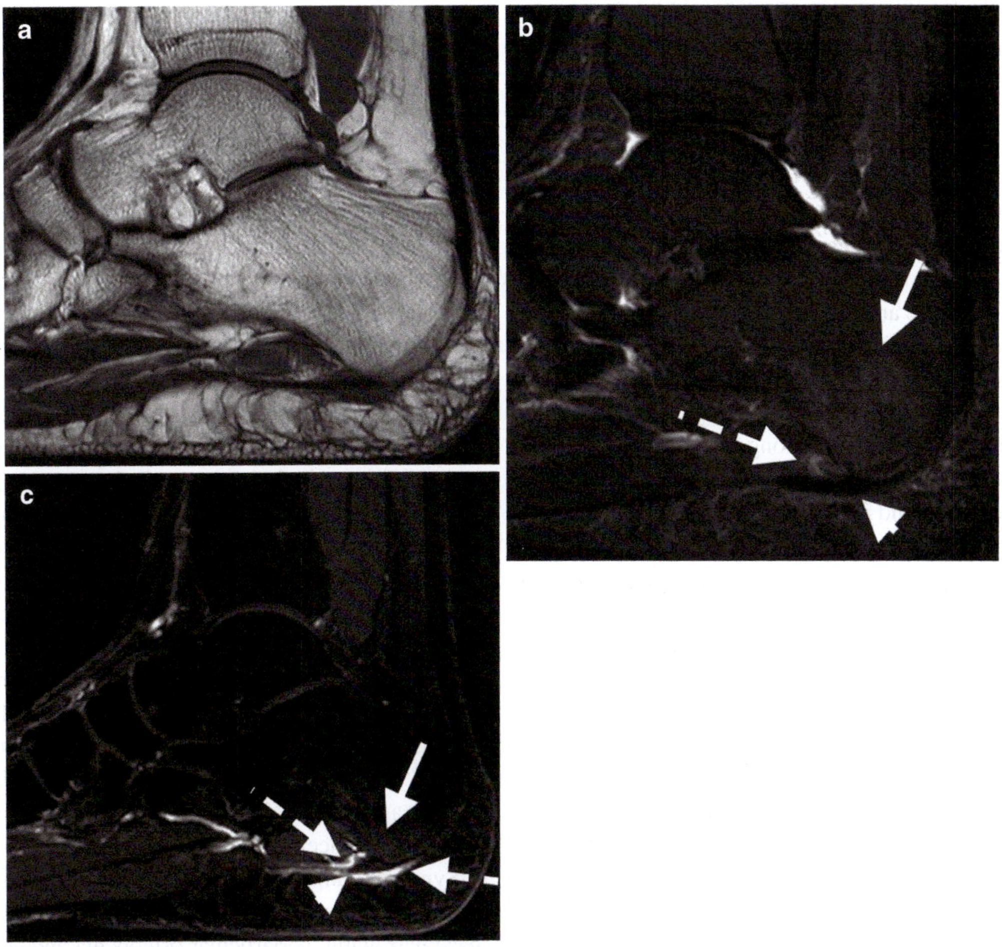

Fig. 5.41 (**a**) Sag T1FS thickened plantar fascia at calcaneal insertion. (**b**) Sag T2FS thickened low signal intensity plantar fascia, perifascial oedema and calcaneal bone marrow oedema. (**c**) Sag T1FS PG demonstrates enhancement of perifascial oedema and mild enhancement of underlying osteitis. Plantar fascia = *arrowhead*, bone marrow oedema = *arrow*, perifascial oedema = *dashed arrow*

SAPHO Syndrome and CRMO

Overview

Synovitis, acne, pustulosis, hyperostosis and osteitis (SAPHO), also referred to in children and adolescents as chronic recurrent multifocal osteomyelitis (CRMO) (Table 5.9), are within the spectrum of the seronegative arthritides and are characterised by sterile osteomyelitis. The two major differential diagnoses include infection and malignancy (particularly in children). In up to 10 % of cases, there is an associated inflammatory bowel disease, and HLA-B27 is frequently positive. Appropriate and timely diagnosis is important as patients may otherwise undergo unnecessary multiple bone biopsies or prolonged courses of antibiotics.

Presentation

SAPHO syndrome can present at any age and is characterised by recurrent episodes of local sterile inflammation. This can occur in any bone but particularly the anterior chest wall including the sternoclavicular joint or the medial clavicle and is associated with dermatological manifestations including acne and pustulosis. In children, it most frequently affects the long bones and clavicles, while in adults, it particularly affects the anterior chest wall and axial spine. It is often multifocal.

Table 5.9 Clinical differences between CRMO and SAPHO

	CRMO	SAPHO
Age (mean)	10 years	28 years
Bones	Long bones metaphyses	Chest wall and pelvis
Extra bony features: rash	Less common	Common
Ossification of ligaments; arthritis and enthesitis	Less common	Common

Adapted from Khanna G, Sato TS, Ferguson P. Imaging of chronic recurrent multifocal osteomyelitis. *Radiographics*. 2009;29(4):1159–77

The associated sacroiliitis is often unilateral and axial involvement is indistinguishable from the spondyloarthropathies (see Chap. 6). It is rare, with an estimated prevalence of around 1 in 10,000, with a slight female predisposition.

The pustulosis found in SAPHO syndrome can resemble palmoplantar pustulosis of psoriasis but can also mimic several other dermatological disorders including Sweet syndrome, hidradenitis suppurativa and severe acne.

Imaging

Plain Radiography

Initial radiographs should evaluate the symptomatic sites. Early in the disease process, lesions tend to be destructive (osteolytic) in appearance, while in later disease, osteoproliferation is more common around the lytic lesion. The radiographic appearance of these lesions can thus vary from purely osteolytic to predominantly sclerotic depending on the duration of the disease. Exacerbations can be determined radiographically by the appearance of new lytic lesions and periosteal reaction.

The medial third of the clavicle is the most typical site with hyperostosis, sclerosis and hypertrophy of the medial ends (Fig. 5.42), followed by lateral extension as the disease progresses.

Axial disease includes corner lesions on vertebral bodies, discitis, sclerosis adjacent to endplate erosions, paravertebral ossification and destructive vertebral lesions (often resulting in bony collapse), along with sacroiliitis (usually unilateral with hyperostosis on the iliac side).

Synovitis, hyperostosis (appears as thickening and enlargement), osteitis and enthesitis can be visualised by plain radiography. Hyperostosis appears as thickening of the cortical bone, while osteitis appears as increased trabecular infrastructure of cancellous bone.

Synovitis can occur in the axial or appendicular skeleton and the arthritis is characterised by joint space narrowing, periarticular osteopenia and erosions. Peripheral arthritis is less common than axial

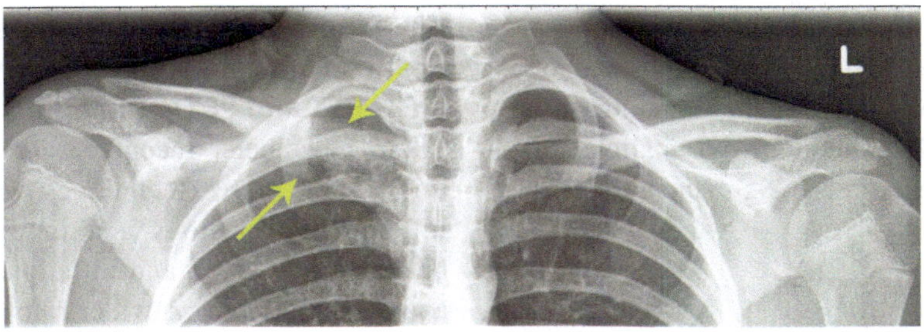

Fig. 5.42 Proximal clavicular expansion and irregularity on plain radiograph in a 13-year-old boy with CRMO (*arrows*)

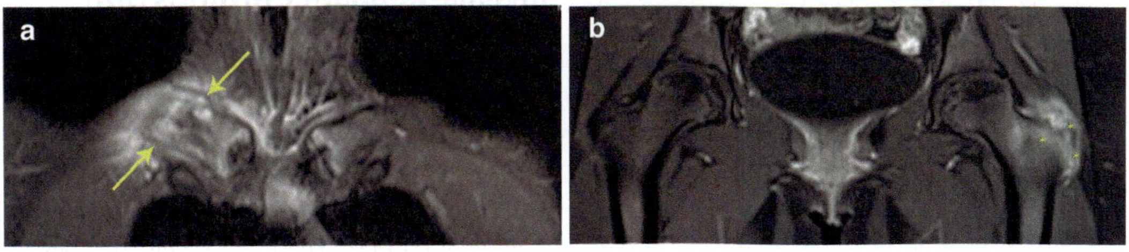

Fig. 5.43 T2-weighted MRI findings of (**a**) expanded, irregular clavicle (*arrows*) with BME in the same patient as Fig. 5.42 and (**b**) BME and enthesitis at the greater trochanter of a 14-year-old girl with CRMO

disease and most often affects hips, knees and ankles: hands and feet are less commonly involved.

Ankylosis may be seen in axial joints such as sternoclavicular and sacroiliac joints, costochondral joints and symphyses, e.g. manubriosternal and pubic.

MRI

If the radiographs are normal in the presence of significant symptoms, MRI should be undertaken to evaluate for BME. MRI is a more sensitive modality than plain radiographs for detecting lesions in SAPHO syndrome. A recent study has shown that radiographs detect only 16 % of lesions found on MRI. Other features best imaged by MRI include soft tissue and bone marrow oedema (Fig. 5.43a), enthesitis (Fig. 5.43b), discitis, vertebral body corner lesions, sacroiliitis and synovitis.

Whole body MRI has been proposed to delineate extent of disease at diagnosis; many lesions up to 67 % are asymptomatic. The multifocal nature of SAPHO syndrome differentiates it from a primary bone tumour or infection. Furthermore, whole body MRI scanning can be useful in monitoring of the disease in terms of differentiating active vs. quiescent lesions and has the advantage over scintigraphy in the lack of ionising radiation.

MRI is useful for determining both the extent of disease and for monitoring. During active disease, MRI might show BME, periostitis, effusions and soft tissue swelling (Fig. 5.43).

CT

CT has the advantage of clearly delineating bony pathology and extent of disease, lytic and sclerotic areas (Fig. 5.44). It has the drawback of not being able to determine the inflammatory changes of bone marrow oedema and carries a significant radiation burden. For those reasons, MRI is generally preferred for diagnosis and monitoring of disease activity.

Whole Body Scintigraphy

Technetium bone scanning typically shows areas of focal increased uptake, allows for whole body bony assessment and is useful in the detection of subclinical lesions. Increased uptake in the sternoclavicular (Fig. 5.45) and sternocostal area with the "bull's head sign" is pathognomonic. However, many of these findings may be difficult to differentiate from malignancy or infection. A bone biopsy is mandatory in these cases.

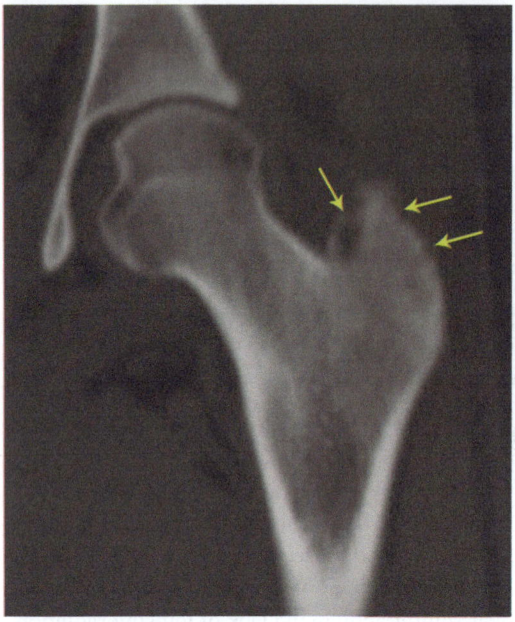

Fig. 5.44 Corresponding CT of irregular bony surface at the greater trochanter (*arrows*)

18F-Fluoro-2-Deoxy-D-Glucose Positron Emission Tomography (FDG-PET and PET/CT Imaging

There have been recent case reports of the utility of these techniques in localising inflammatory lesions and in differentiating between neoplastic and inflammatory lesions and these may have a wider role to play in the future.

Juvenile Idiopathic Arthritis (JIA)

Overview

Juvenile idiopathic arthritides are a group of conditions causing inflammatory arthritis in children under the age of 16 years. The prevalence of JIA is around 1:1,000. There are seven subtypes of JIA based on the International League Against Rheumatism (ILAR) criteria.

- Polyarticular
- Oligoarticular (≤4 joints)
  - Persistent
    - ANA positive
    - ANA negative
  - Oligoarticular

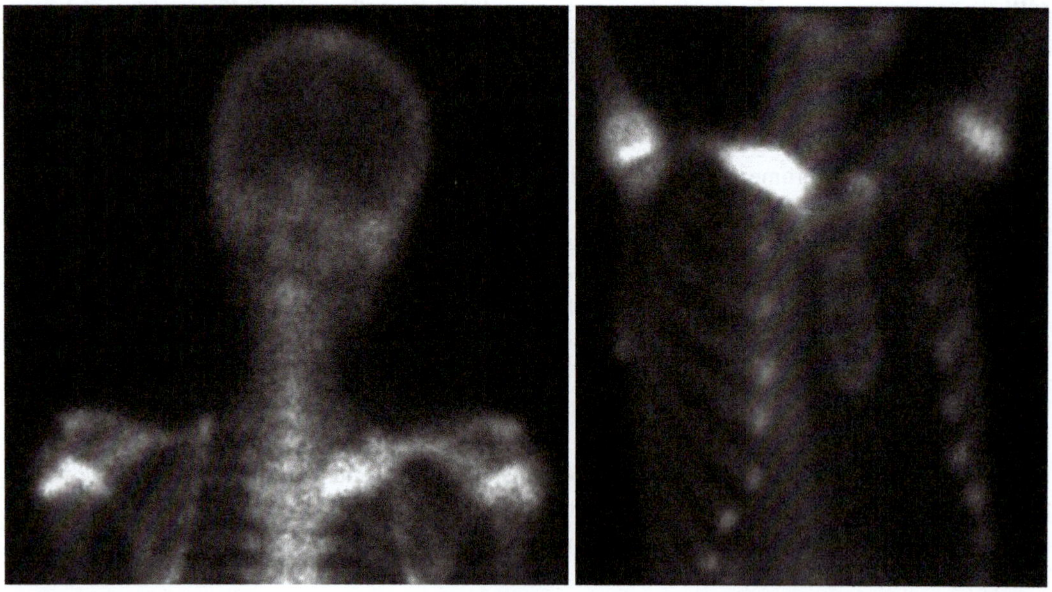

Fig. 5.45 Scintigraphy bone scan showing increased uptake in medial right clavicle

Table 5.10 Clinical and serological features of the subtypes of JIA

	Polyarticular	Oligoarticular	Systemic onset	Enthesitis related	Psoriatic
Frequency	30 %	50 %	Up to 10 %	Up to 10 %	Up to 15 %
Age at onset (years)	2–5, 10–14	2–3	Any age	12–16	6–11
Sex	F>M	F>M	F=M	M>F	F=M
Joints	≥5 joints, mainly small joints of the hands including DIPs and wrists	≤4 joints, often large joints (spares hips)	Any or none	Spine, large joints	Any
Extra-articular manifestations	Rare	Uveitis in 20 %	Fever, weight loss, rash, lymphadenopathy, amyloidosis, macrophage activation syndrome (MAS)	Uveitis, inflammatory bowel symptoms, rash	Psoriasis or first-degree relative with psoriasis. In patients, arthritis often precedes psoriasis
Serology	RF positive in 20 % >10 years	ANA positive in 30 % (highest risk of uveitis)	RF and ANA negative	RF and ANA negative	RF and ANA negative

- Systemic onset
- Enthesitis-related arthritis (ERA)
- Psoriatic
- Undifferentiated

Presentation

Clinical presentation of JIA can be very variable depending on the type of JIA and the age of the child. The presentation and clinical features of JIA are outlined in Table 5.10. Imaging features of the different subtypes of JIA are outlined in Table 5.11.

Imaging

Plain Radiography

Rheumatoid factor-positive polyarticular JIA behaves in a similar fashion to RA and has similar imaging findings including symmetrical soft tissue swelling (Fig. 5.46), periarticular osteopenia, joint space narrowing and erosions. On radiographs there may be additional changes of periostitis of the metaphyses and diaphyses and erosions without cartilage loss.

The growth plates in children are areas of cartilage where new bone is formed. These are areas that are susceptible to damage by injury or arthritis. These growth plates fuse around the time of puberty. There can be distortion with ballooning of the epiphyses and potentially premature fusion of the growth plates causing brachydactyly, or shortening of the digits (Fig. 5.47). In polyarticular JIA, the temporomandibular joint is frequently affected (this is uncommonly affected in RA).

Ultrasound

Ultrasonography is becoming the imaging modality of choice in children with JIA, as multiple joints can be examined for bony, soft tissue, tendon and cartilage abnormalities without ionising radiation.

The ultrasonographic features of JIA are similar to the US features of each of the inflammatory arthritides outlined in previous sections and include synovitis, effusions (Fig. 5.48), tenosynovitis (Fig. 5.49), enthesitis, dactylitis, bony erosions, osteoproliferation and cartilage loss. Cartilage is clearly represented by ultrasonography and the thickness decreases as the bone age of the child increases.

MRI

MRI is a valuable tool in some cases, but small children require sedation in order to lie still enough for adequate quality images. MRI features are typical of any of the inflammatory

Table 5.11 Imaging features of JIA subtypes

	Polyarticular	Oligoarticular	Systemic onset	Enthesitis related	Psoriatic
Soft tissues	Synovial (including tenosynovium) swelling, effusions, nodules (especially if RF positive)	Synovial (including tenosynovium) swelling, effusions	Less common	Synovial (including tenosynovium) swelling, effusions	Synovial (including tenosynovium) swelling, effusions
Bone density	Periarticular osteopenia; periostitis	Periarticular osteopenia; periostitis	Generalised osteopenia	Periarticular osteopenia; periostitis	Periarticular osteopenia; periostitis
Erosions	Particularly in carpal bones often without cartilage loss	Unusual	Unusual	At site of enthesis	With hyperostosis bony reaction
Joint space narrowing	Late	Unusual	Unusual	Unusual	Common
Growth abnormalities	Brachydactyly, micrognathia	Distended epiphyses	Growth retardation (often corticosteroid related)	Spinal ankylosis and growth retardation	Brachydactyly

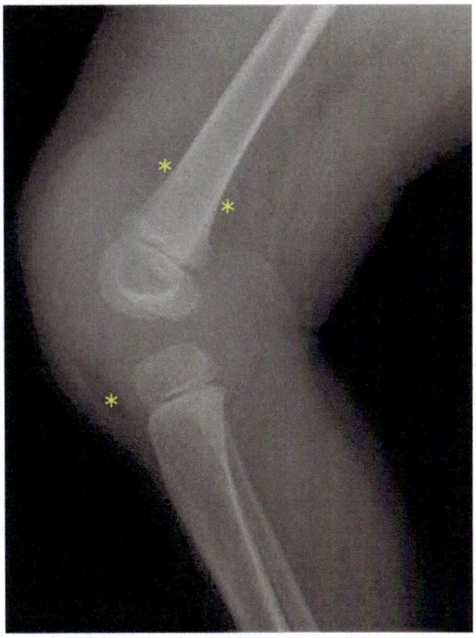

Fig. 5.46 Plain radiograph of a 3-year-old girl with knee effusion (*asterisks*) and soft tissue swelling

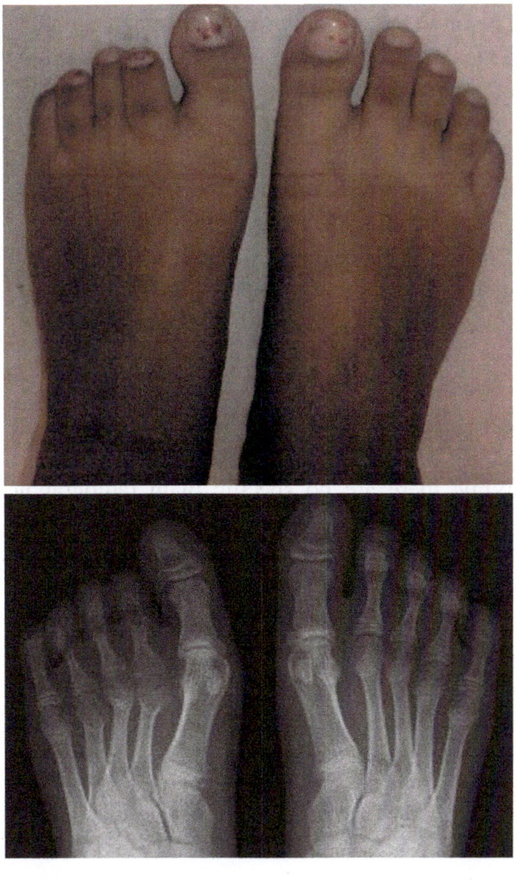

Fig. 5.47 Brachydactyly of L toes 2–5 and corresponding plain film (Photograph courtesy of Dr. Peter Dent, McMaster University, Hamilton ON)

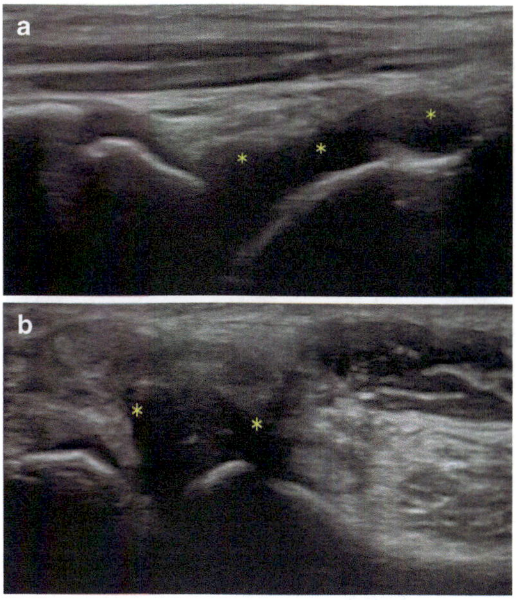

Fig. 5.48 (**a**) Synovial hypertrophy and effusion (*asterisks*) of tibiotalar joint; (**b**) effusion of subtalar joint (Courtesy of Dr. Alessandra Bruns, University of Sherbrooke, Quebec)

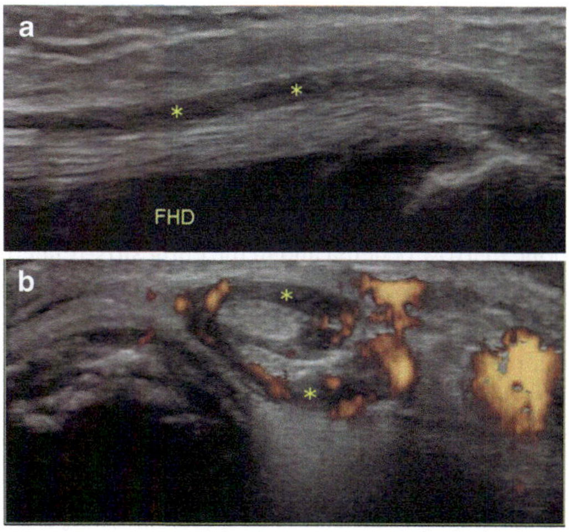

Fig. 5.49 (**a**) Tenosynovitis (*asterisks*) of flexor hallucis digitorum (*FHD*); (**b**) peroneus longus and brevis tenosynovitis in a 9-year-old boy (Courtesy of Dr. Alessandra Bruns, University of Sherbrooke, QC, Canada)

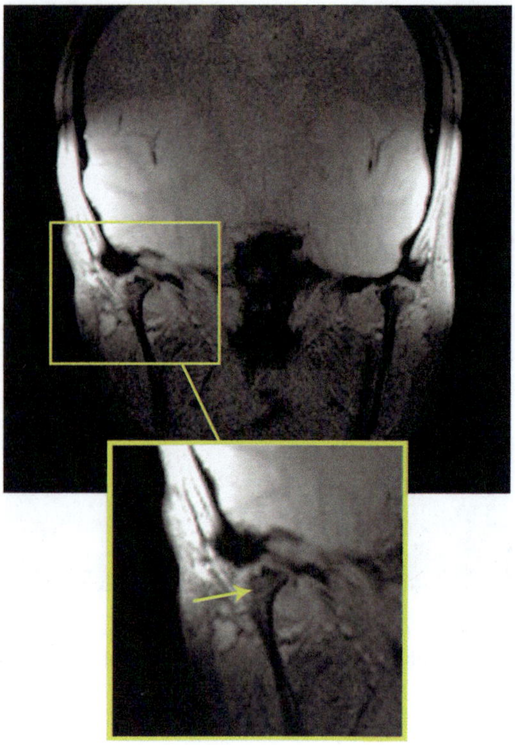

Fig. 5.50 MRI showing flattening and erosions (*inset arrow*) of temporomandibular joint (TMJ) bilaterally in a 21-year-old woman with an 8-year history of JIA affecting TMJ

arthritides and include synovitis, effusions and bone marrow oedema and in the enthesitis-related (ERA) or psoriatic arthritis features of enthesitis including tendonitis, tenosynovitis and bone marrow oedema at the entheseal insertions. MRI is particularly useful at delineating TMJ involvement in JIA (Fig. 5.50).

Remitting Seronegative Symmetrical Synovitis with Pitting Oedema (RS3PE)

Overview

Remitting seronegative symmetrical synovitis with pitting oedema (RS3PE) is a recently described inflammatory arthritis which typically affects the hands and less commonly the feet (and can also affect the wrists, ankles, elbows, shoulders and knees) of older adults (men > women) with a mean age of onset of between 70 and 80 years.

Presentation

It often presents with acute-onset polyarthritis with marked pitting oedema most often in the dorsum of the hand in the context of a negative rheumatoid factor and has a dramatic improvement with steroids. Men are more frequently affected than women (2:1 ratio) with a predilection for the elderly. Remission is expected within 3–36 months following initiation of steroid treatment. It is a diagnosis of exclusion, as other causes of pitting oedema including congestive cardiac failure, hypothyroidism and nephrotic syndrome should be excluded. Furthermore, the differential diagnosis of acute polyarthritis in this age group includes late-onset RA and polymyalgia rheumatic, both of which require more intensive (and longer duration of) immunosuppressive therapy, making this disorder important to diagnose appropriately. It can be associated with underlying malignancy and a thorough search is therefore warranted in this condition. When compared with PMR, systemic features of fever, anorexia and weight loss are much less common (59 % in PMR vs. 9 % in RS3PE).

Imaging

While there are no specific plain radiographic features other than soft tissue swelling, MRI and ultrasonography can clearly image the characteristic marked soft tissue oedema, synovitis and tenosynovitis of flexor and extensor tendons in the hand (Fig. 5.51) and extensor tendons of the feet. The soft tissue swelling is usually diffuse and symmetrical involving the hands and wrists in both flexor and extensor compartments and the feet extensors.

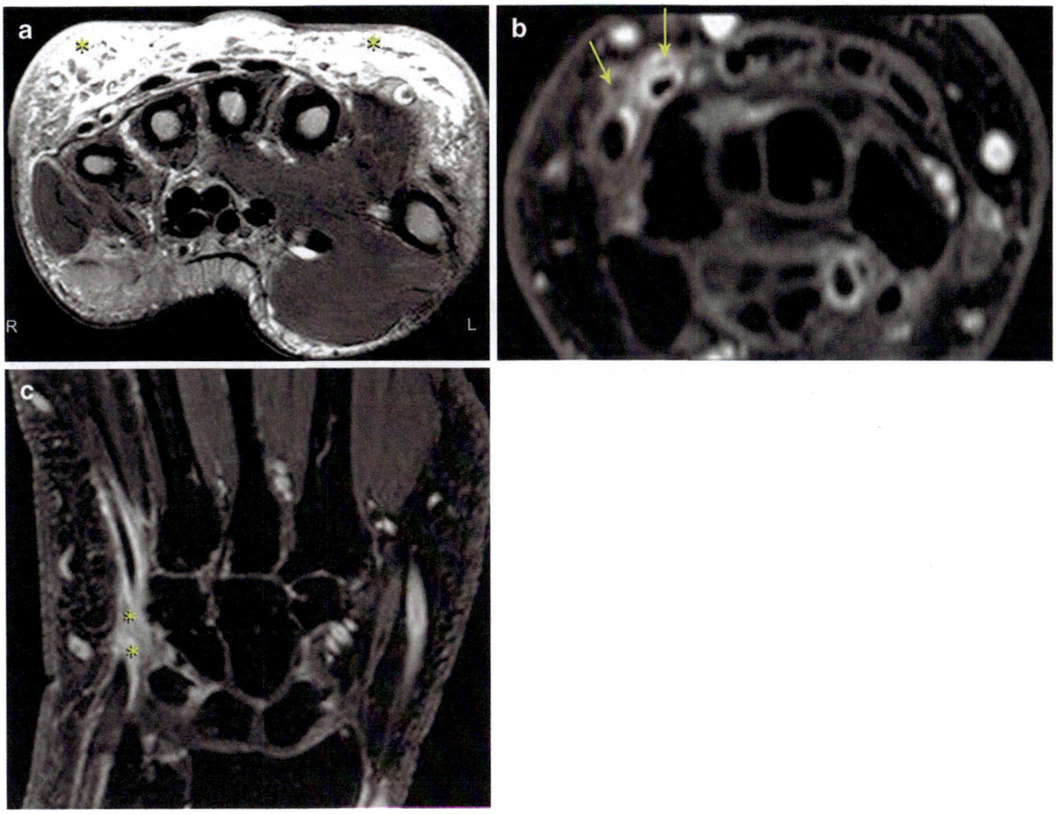

Fig. 5.51 (**a**) Soft tissue oedema on T1-weighted MRI; (**b**) tenosynovitis of extensor pollicis brevis and abductor pollicis longus (*arrows*) and (**c**) synovitis around extensor carpi ulnaris tendon (**b**, **c** are both T2-weighted images in a 75-year-old man with acute diffuse swelling in the hands bilaterally)

Further Reading

Rheumatoid Arthritis

1. Aletaha D, Neogi T, Silman A, Funovits J, Felson D, et al. Rheumatoid arthritis classification criteria: an American College of Rheumatology//European League against rheumatism collaborative initiative. Arthritis Rheum. 2010;62:2569–81. http://www.rheumatology.org/practice/clinical/classification/ra/ratree_2010.asp.
2. Colebatch AN, et al. EULAR recommendations for the use of imaging of the joints in the clinical management of rheumatoid arthritis. Ann Rheum Dis. 2013. doi:10.1136/annrheumdis-2012-203158.
3. MacGregor AJ, Silman AJ. Rheumatoid arthritis: classification and epidemiology. In: Klippel JH, Dieppe PA, editors. Rheumatology. 2nd ed. London: Mosby; 1998.
4. McQueen FM, Ostergaard M. Established rheumatoid arthritis – new imaging modalities. Best Pract Res Clin Endocrinol Rheumatol. 2007;21:841–56.
5. Østergaard M. Can imaging be used for inflammatory arthritis screening? Semin Musculoskelet Radiol. 2012;16(5):401–9.
6. Ostergaard M, Pedersen SJ, Dohn UM. Imaging in rheumatoid arthritis – status and recent advances for MRI, US, CT and conventional radiography. Best Pract Res Clin Rheumatol. 2008;22:1019–44.

Seronegative Spondyloarthropathies (SpA)

7. Amrami KK. Imaging of the seronegative spondyloarthropathies. Radiol Clin North Am. 2012;50(4):841–54.
8. Coates LC, Hodgson R, Conaghan PG, Freeston JE. MRI and ultrasonography for diagnosis and monitoring of psoriatic arthritis. Best Pract Res Clin Rheumatol. 2012;26(6):805–22.
9. Gladman, Chandran. Review of clinical registries of psoriatic arthritis: lessons learned?: value for the future? Curr Rheumatol Reports. 2011;13(4):346–52.

10. Luong AA, Salonen DC. Imaging of the seronegative spondyloarthropathies. Curr Rheumatol Rep. 2000; 2(4):288–96.
11. McGonagle D, Marzo-Ortego H, Benjamin M, Emery P. Report of the second international enthesitis workshop. Arthritis Rheum. 2003;48:896–905.
12. Oostergaard M, McQueen F, Wiell C, Bird P, et al. The OMERACT Psoriatic Arthritis Magnetic Resonance Imaging Scoring System (PsAMRIS): definitions of key pathologies, suggested MRI sequences, and preliminary scoring system for PsA hands. J Rheum. 2009;36(8):1816–24.
13. Orchard TR, Wordsworth BP, Jewell DP. Peripheral arthropathies in inflammatory bowel disease: their articular distribution and natural history. Gut. 1998; 42:387–91.
14. Rudwaleit M, van der Heijde D, Landewé R, et al. The Assessment of SpondyloArthritis International Society classification criteria for peripheral spondyloarthritis and for spondyloarthritis in general. Annal Rheumatic Dis. 2011;70(1):25–31.
15. Yuksel, et al. Peripheral arthritis in the course of inflammatory bowel diseases. Dig Dis Sci. 2011; 56:183–7.

SAPHO and CRMO

16. Colina M, et al. Clinical and radiological evolution of synovitis, acne, pustulosis, hyperostosis and osteitis syndrome: a single centre study of a cohort of 71 subjects. A&R. 2009;61:813–21.
17. Depasquale R, et al. SAPHO: what radiologists should know. Clin Radiol. 2012;67:195–206.
18. Dihlmann W, Dihlmann SW. Acquired hyperostosis syndrome: spectrum of manifestations at the sternoclavicular region. Radiologic evaluation of 34 cases. Clin Rheumatol. 1991;10:250–63.
19. Fritz, et al. Chronic recurrent multifocal osteomyelitis: comparison of whole-body MR imaging with radiography and correlation with clinical and laboratory data. Radiology. 2009;252:842–51.

Juvenile Idiopathic Arthritis (JIA)

20. Cassidy T, Petty R, Laxer R, Lindsley C. Textbook of pediatric rheumatology: expert consult. 6th ed. Philadelphia: Saunders; 2010.
21. Graham TB. Imaging in juvenile arthritis. Curr Opin Rheumatol. 2005;17(5):574–8.

Remitting Seronegative Symmetrical Synovitis with Pitting Edema (RS3PE)

22. McCarty, et al. Remitting seronegative symmetrical synovitis with pitting edema: RS3PE syndrome. JAMA. 1985;254:2763–7.
23. Olivo D, D'Amore M, Lacava R, et al. Benign edematous polysynovitis in the elderly (RS3PE syndrome). Clin Exp Rheumatol. 1994;12:669–73.
24. Sayarlioglu M. Remitting seronegative symmetrical synovitis with pitting oedema (RS3PE) and malignancy. Eur J Gen Med. 2004;1(2):3–5.

6 Spondyloarthropathy

John O'Neill

The seronegative spondyloarthropathies (SpA) are a group of chronic autoimmune inflammatory joint diseases predominantly affecting the axial skeleton and often accompanied by a peripheral arthritis. Seronegative implies that there is no association with rheumatoid factor. Ankylosing spondylitis (AS) is the prototype of the SpA that also includes psoriatic arthritis, reactive arthritis, arthritis associated with inflammatory bowel disease and undifferentiated spondyloarthropathies. Onset of disease commonly occurs in young adulthood, and in many cases, ankylosing spondylitis is a progressive disease.

Presentation

The onset of inflammatory low back pain in these patients is often insidious with periods of relapse and remittance, which often leads to delay in the clinical diagnosis. Using AS as our model for SpA, it has been demonstrated that there can be a significant delay in the diagnosis from onset of symptoms with some studies finding a delay of 9 years from the patient's initial onset of symptoms. This delay in diagnosis has a significant negative impact on the clinical and economic status of the patient. It is essential therefore for patient well-being and, particularly since the advent of effective treatment options with anti-TNF agents, that SpA is diagnosed early in the course of the disease.

AS is more common in men, ratio of 2:1. Men also develop chronic radiographic changes earlier than women. The majority of patients are young or middle aged with 75 % presenting between 20 and 45 years. Twenty percent of patients present before the age of 20 years and 5 % after 45 years.

Pain and stiffness, usually in the lower back and pelvis, are relieved with activity and not by rest. Patients will often wake in the second half of the night with back pain. Symptoms lasting for more than 30 min and present for 3 months or more are characteristic of inflammatory back pain. Clinically the patients demonstrate limited spinal mobility via multiple tests including lateral spinal flexion, the modified Schober test (forward flexion) and chest expansion.

Epidemiology

Prevalence of SpA varies between ethnic populations, highest in those of European ancestry, up to 1.4 %. In some populations, it equals or exceeds the prevalence of rheumatoid arthritis. Current estimates of the prevalence of SpA in the United States are between 0.2 and 0.5 % for

J. O'Neill, MB, BAO, BCh, MRCPI, MSc, FRCR
Associate Professor, Musculoskeletal Imaging,
Diagnostic Imaging, McMaster University/
St Joseph's Healthcare,
Hamilton, ON L8N4A6, Canada
e-mail: joneill2@me.com

J. O'Neill (ed.), *Essential Imaging in Rheumatology*,
DOI 10.1007/978-1-4939-1673-3_6, © Springer Science+Business Media New York 2015

ankylosing spondylitis, 0.1 % for psoriatic arthritis, 0.065 % for enteropathic peripheral arthritis and between 0.05 and 0.25 % for enteropathic axial arthritis, and the overall prevalence of SpA is as high as 1.3 %.

SpA is closely linked with HLA-B27 status, accounting for up to 40 % of total disease risk, and is positive in up to 95 % with AS and in 60–70 % with PsA or IBD-associated spondyloarthropathy. Prevalence of HLA-B27 is linked to the prevalence of AS in the same population. Approximately 5 % of HLA-B27-positive individuals will develop AS. Up to 75 variants of HLA-B27 have been described so far, some of which demonstrate a greater predisposition to AS, e.g. HLA-B*2705 and B*2702 are the primary subtypes in Caucasians with spondylitis, and B*2704 and B*2707 are the primary subtypes in Asians. Primary relatives of patients with AS, who are HLA-B27 positive, have a 12 % risk of developing AS. It is thought that HLA-B27-positive patients interact with an environmental factor(s), likely infectious, stimulating an inflammatory response at the cartilage-bone interface. Other genetic predispositions include ERAP1, endoplasmic reticulum aminopeptidase 1, interleukin 23 and interleukin 1.

Imaging

Imaging of the sacroiliac joint has a primary role in the diagnosis of SpA. In routine clinical practice, radiographic imaging has become an integral part of the investigation of patients with suspected sacroiliitis (SII). While plain X-rays remain the first and most widespread imaging modality employed in the investigation of SII, MRI has a significantly improved sensitivity and specificity for the diagnosis of SII. Unfortunately, the determination of the exact sensitivities and specificities of these imaging modalities is severely hindered by the absence of a 'gold standard' investigation. MRI is the de facto imaging gold standard. Other imaging techniques used to diagnose SII include CT and scintigraphy. Conventional tomography was employed prior to the use of cross-sectional imaging.

Normal Anatomy and Imaging of the Sacroiliac Joints (Fig. 6.1)

Traditionally, the SIJs were considered to consist of a smaller posterosuperior ligamentous compartment and a larger anteroinferior synovial compartment. More recent research has stimulated a debate on whether the articulation is best classified as a symphysis rather than a synovial joint. The articular margins of the sacrum and iliac bones are irregular with interdigitations, which limit mobility and enhance the strength of these joints. The articular surface of the sacrum is C or L shaped, opening dorsally. There are irregular bony pits, dorsal to the articular surface, at the site of ligamentous attachment, the dorsal syndesmosis. The articular surface at the centre of the SIJs has hyaline cartilage with fibrocartilage only at the periphery. The periphery of the cartilage, with the exception of the distal third of the iliac cartilage, blends with the stabilising ligaments as in a symphysis and forms a wide margin of fibrocartilage. A small synovial recess exists at the ventral aspect of the distal third of the iliac aspect of the joint. The SIJs are probably therefore best described as a symphysis with characteristics of a synovial joint being restricted to the ventral aspect of the distal cartilaginous portion at the iliac side.

Under the age of 30 years, the SIJs are usually symmetric in appearance. A higher prevalence of asymmetric non-uniform joint space narrowing and ill-defined subchondral sclerosis has been observed in women, obese and multiparous females than in age-matched males, and individuals of normal weight and non-multiparous, respectively. The width of the normal SIJ varies from 2 to 5 mm. The normal SIJ can demonstrate considerable variability, particularly with increasing age. Prominent sacral irregularities and marrow defects at the attachment of the interosseous

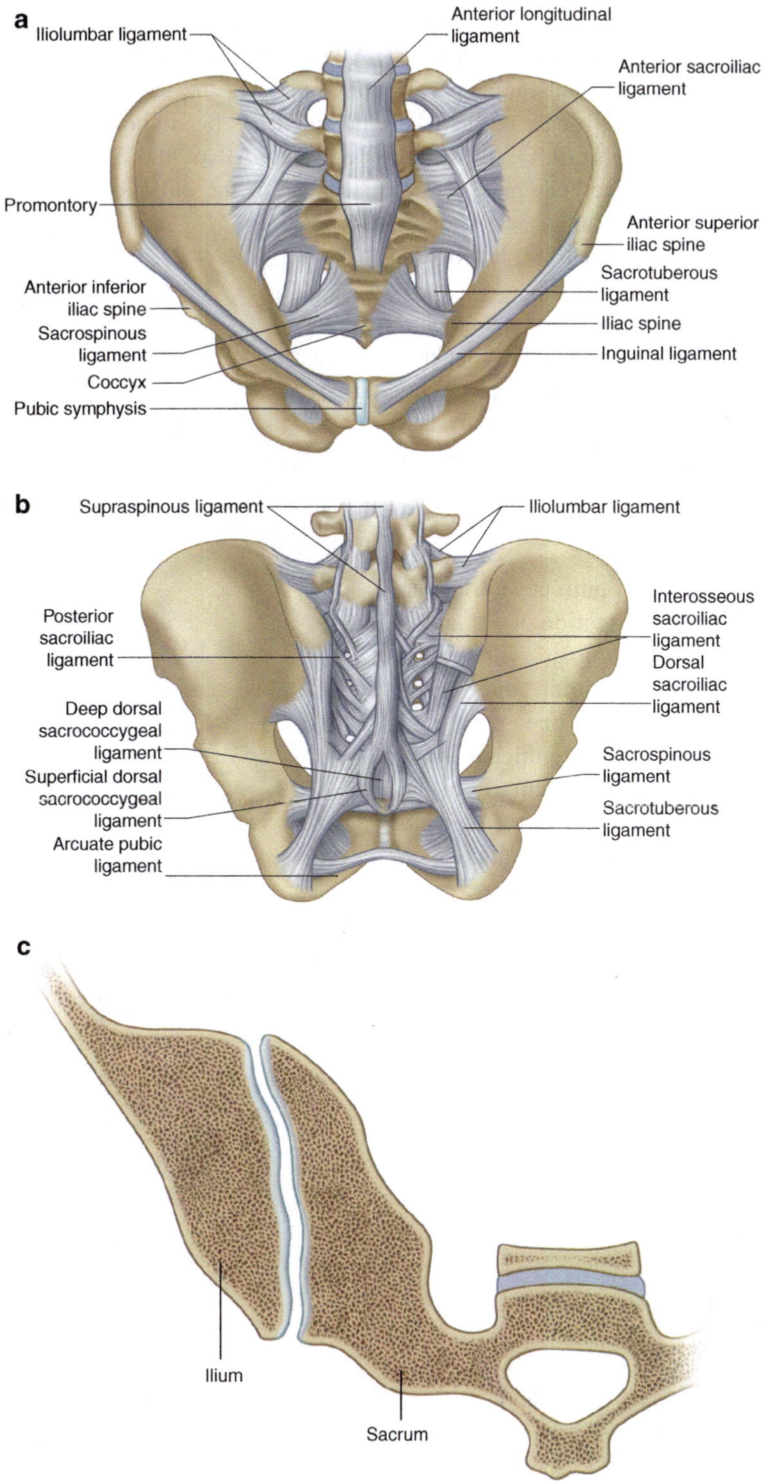

Fig. 6.1 Normal anatomy of the sacroiliac joint, (**a**) anterior and (**b**) posterior ligaments of the sacrum and sacroiliac joint, (**c**) axial through right sacroiliac joint demonstrating normal interdigitations of the articulations

ligaments, termed insertion pits, may be seen in normal subjects. Multiple anatomical variants have been observed in patients undergoing pelvic CT for indications other than disease of the SIJs. These include accessory joints (19 %), 'iliosacral complex' (6 %), bipartite iliac bony plate (4 %), crescent-like iliac bony plate (4 %), semicircular defects at the sacral or iliac side (3 %) and ossification centres (1 %).

There are a number of different imaging techniques used in the diagnosis of SII. They include plain radiographs, conventional tomography, scintigraphy, ultrasound, computed tomography and magnetic resonance imaging. Imaging allows for objective evidence of SII.

Plain Radiography

Plain radiography has and continues to play an important role in the investigation of SII and is an integral part in the diagnosis of AS. The anatomy of the sacroiliac joint, due to its oblique nature and overlap of the sacral and iliac components, has led to significant inter- and intraobserver variations particularly in the interpretation of early SII. Differentiation from normal patients is particularly problematic in women and in older age groups where early degenerative changes may simulate early SII. Plain radiographs of the sacroiliac joint can be performed and include dedicated AP and bilateral oblique views (Fig. 6.2). However, an AP radiograph of the lumbar spine often clearly demonstrates the sacroiliac joints and if fully included has been shown to be as sensitive as dedicated AP of the SIJ (Figs. 6.3 and 6.4). Because of the oblique orientation of the SIJs

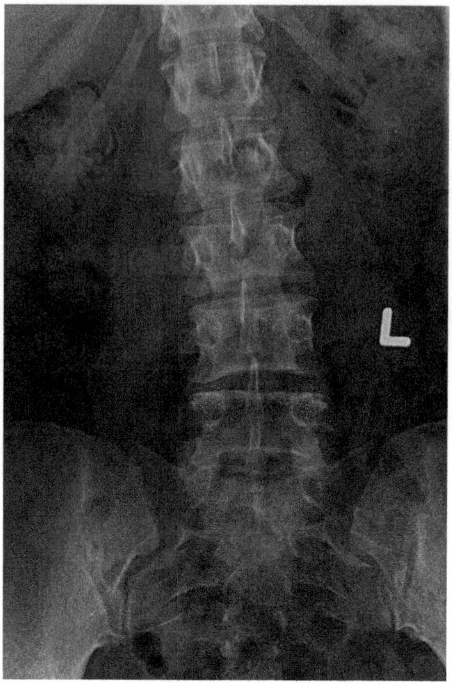

Fig. 6.3 AP radiograph of the lumbar spine which includes normal sacroiliac joints

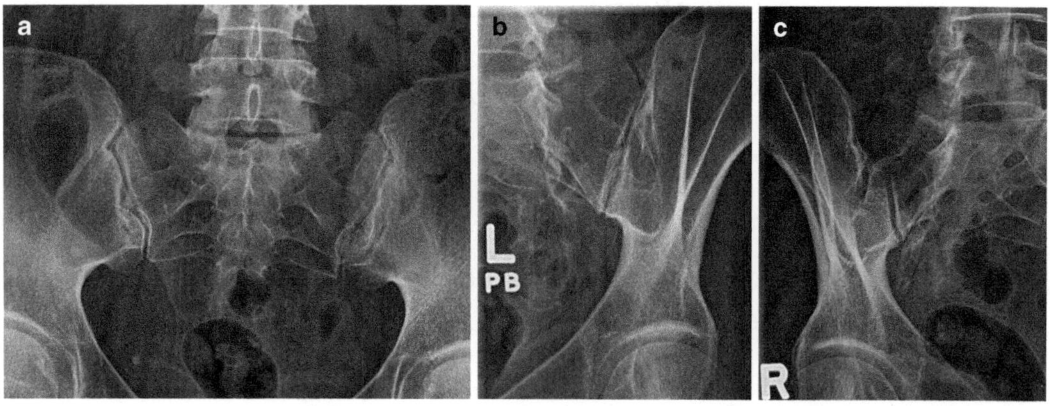

Fig. 6.2 Normal radiographs of the sacroiliac joints, (**a**) AP, (**b**) left oblique and (**c**) right oblique

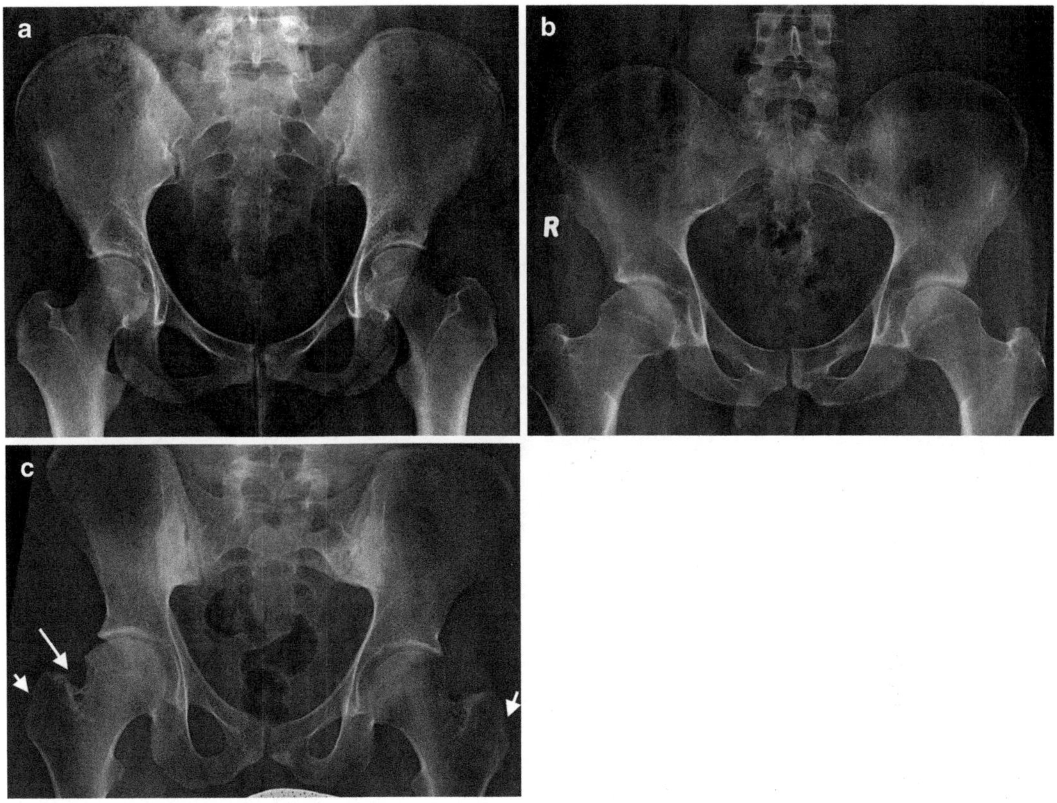

Fig. 6.4 (**a**) AP pelvis with normal SIJs and allows for assessment of hip joints and symphysis pubis, (**b**) a 34-year-old male with AS with symmetrical SIJ space loss, erosions and subchondral sclerosis and bilateral hip involvement, (**c**) a 35-year-old male with AS and similar changes as in fig (**b**) but with additional cortical changes, early erosions (*small arrows*) of the greater trochanter and enthesophyte formation (*large arrow*)

on the frontal radiograph, there is considerable overlap of the joints on plain radiography, and oblique views may be required for further detailed evaluation in selected cases. Some centres advocate a baseline AP pelvis. This allows for assessment of the sacroiliac joints and the hip joints; the latter is involved in up to 25 % of patients with SpA. Plain radiography should be performed as the initial imaging modality.

Radiographic changes include periarticular osteopenia, erosions and initial joint space widening progressing to narrowing joint space in later disease, subchondral sclerosis and finally bony ankylosis. The modified New York criteria include radiographs as a key component in the diagnosis of AS (Table 6.1). Grade 2–4 bilateral disease or unilateral grade 3–4 disease with one clinical criterion was required for the diagnosis

Table 6.1 Modified New York grading criteria

New York modified grading criteria	
Grade 0	Normal
Grade 1	Suspicious change
Grade 2	Minimal abnormality – small localised areas with erosion or sclerosis without alteration in joint width
Grade 3	Definite abnormality – moderate or advanced disease including partial ankylosis
Grade 4	Severe abnormality – total ankylosis

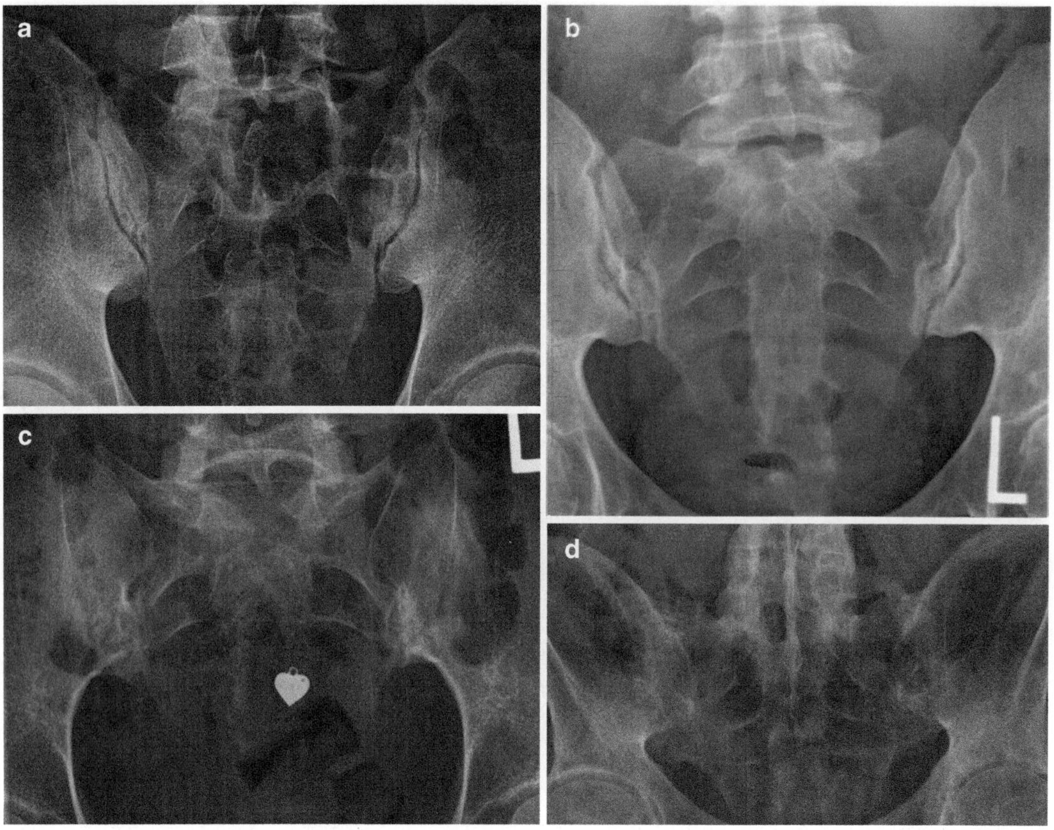

Fig. 6.5 New York modified grading criteria for radiographic sacroiliitis, grade 0 (Fig. 6.2), (**a**) grade 1 with suspicious changes, possible early erosions of the inferior sacroiliac joints bilaterally, (**b**) grade 2 in a 36-year-old female with bilateral erosions and maintained joint space, (**c**) grade 3 in an 18-year-old female with bilateral erosions, joint space loss and partial ankylosis, (**d**) bilateral SIJ ankylosis

(Fig. 6.5). Involvement of the spine was not included in this criteria set.

Conventional Tomography and Tomosynthesis

Conventional tomography is associated with a higher radiation burden than plain radiographs and is no longer used. The newer technique of tomosynthesis holds promise, but our initial evaluation demonstrated a higher radiation burden than low-dose CT and is not indicated until further research is performed to evaluate its position in the investigation of sacroiliitis.

Ultrasound

Ultrasound is not currently utilised in clinical practice in the assessment of SII. Ultrasound can evaluate the posterior portions of the sacroiliac joints with Doppler and has shown in some studies increased vascularisation with decreased resistive indices in this portion of sacroiliac joint in patients with active SII. Further research is warranted to assess what role ultrasound will play in SII.

Nuclear Medicine

Scintigraphy had previously been a commonly used modality in the investigation of SII in clinical practice. It is very sensitive in the detection of early articular inflammatory change but is nonspecific (Fig. 6.6). Radionuclide normally accumulates at the SIJs, and the differentiation of normal uptake and early SII can be difficult. Quantitative analysis of the SIJs has proven more sensitive in this regard. There are limitations however due to the wide range of variation in quantitative evaluation in the normal population. Other factors including age and prominent first sacral spine may all cause difficulties. Scintigraphy has poor sensitivity when compared with MRI in symptomatic spondyloarthropathy patients. Due to the above limitations and given the significant associated radiation dose, scintigraphy is not part of our diagnostic imaging algorithm.

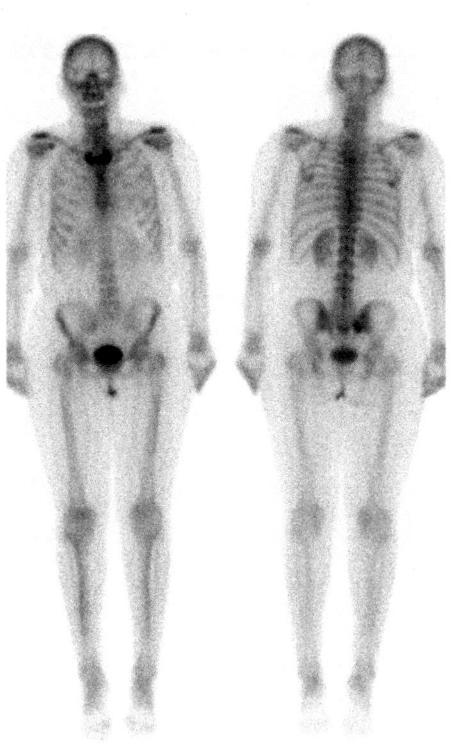

Fig. 6.6 Bone scan in a patient known with asymmetrical sacroiliitis; note increased uptake of the right inferior sacroiliac joint on posterior view. Increased uptake at sternoclavicular joints was related to incidental degenerative disease

CT

CT is excellent in demonstrating the anatomy of the SIJs and allows high-resolution axial acquisition with coronal and sagittal reconstruction (Fig. 6.7). Modern comparative studies between plain radiographs and CT have demonstrated marked advantage of CT in the delineation of chronic changes including erosions, subchondral sclerosis, ankylosis and fat replacement of bone marrow (Fig. 6.8). CT has the advantage that it can also demonstrate new bone formation at entheses. CT does not offer evaluation of acute inflammatory changes, which can be delineated on MRI. In addition CT involves the use of ionising radiation. CT can be useful in delineating alternate pathology, reviewed later in this chapter.

Magnetic Resonance Imaging (MRI)

MRI is the imaging gold standard for sacroiliitis. MRI is nonionising and provides excellent anatomical detail and delineation of both acute and chronic changes of sacroiliitis. We will briefly review the anatomy of the sacroiliac joints on MRI prior to reviewing pathological changes. On MRI, cartilage is well visualised as a zone of intermediate signal intensity on both T1 and T2 weighting bounded on either side by low signal intensity intact cortex of the underlying sacrum or ilium

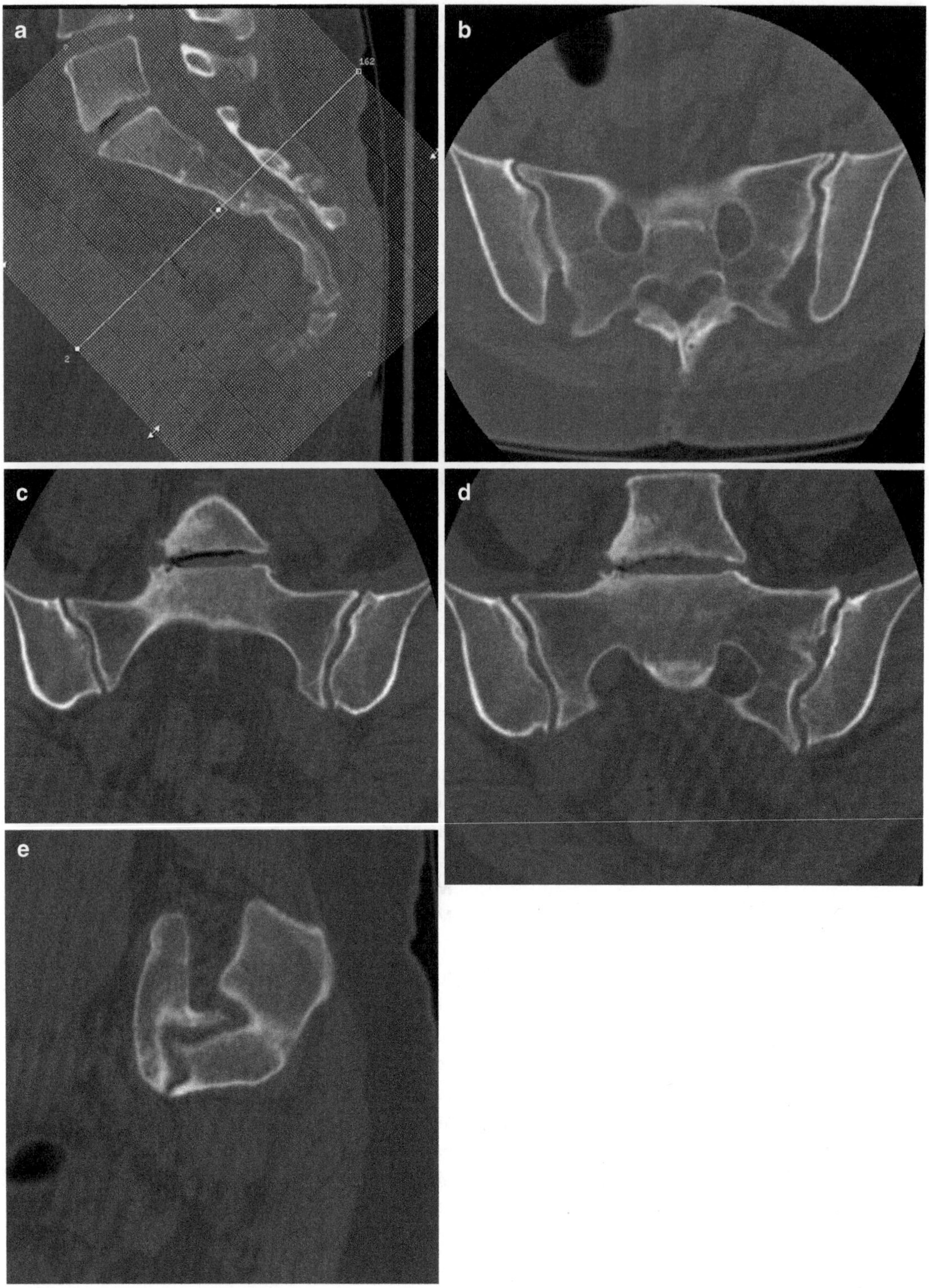

Fig. 6.7 CT of the sacrum and sacroiliac joints, (**a**) localiser image of the sacrum, the scan planes are acquired from this image, the axial line transversing the image is in the true axial plane sacrum. Figs. (**b–d**) are true coronal through the sacroiliac joints and (**e**) is a sagittal reconstruction (usually not required for sacroiliac disease but may be beneficial for other pathology including fracture assessment)

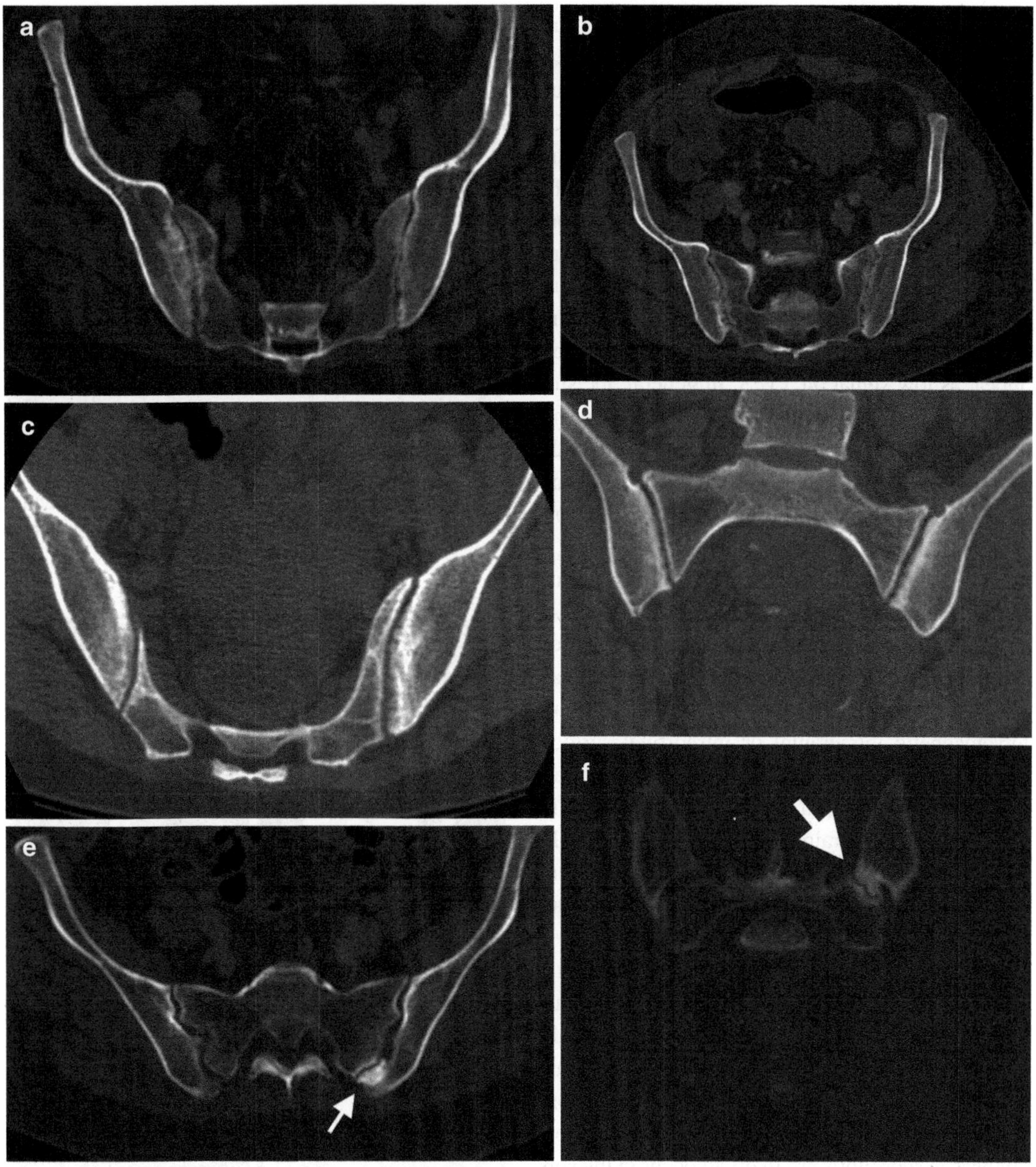

Fig. 6.8 (**a**) A 31-year-old male with ulcerative colitis (UC). CT of the pelvis, bone windows, demonstrates bilateral sacroiliac joint space loss, erosions and mild subchondral sclerosis. CT performed for assessment obstruction (**b**) demonstrates dilated small bowel loops secondary to distal obstruction. (**c**) A different patient, also with UC, demonstrates similar bilateral disease with coronal reformats (**d**). Incidental left accessory facet joint (*arrow*) in another patient on axial (**e, f**) coronal reformat CT

(Fig. 6.9). The combined cartilage has a maximum thickness of 4–5 mm and is slightly thinner anteriorly and inferiorly. It is not possible to differentiate hyaline and fibrous cartilage by signal intensity. On T1FS the cartilage is of intermediate to high signal intensity, and the altered greyscale of the T1FS sequence improves visualisation of the cartilage and adjacent cortical bone. Standard T1 sequences are, however, invaluable in assessing the subchondral bone marrow and, in particular, in differentiating between subchondral sclerosis and fat that may both appear as low signal on T1FS. In general, the subchondral bone marrow has homogeneous intermediate signal intensity on T1. In adults, the subchondral bone may be of heterogeneous signal due to the non-uniform haemopoietic marrow. Assessing the marrow signal intensity at the level of the sacral foramina can serve as baseline for the normal appearance of marrow in individual patients.

The referring clinician needs to be aware of certain contraindications to MRI. These include cardiac pacemakers, cochlear implants and ferromagnetic intracranial or intraorbital surgical clips or foreign bodies. Certain types of hardware elsewhere also are contraindicated. It is best to discuss possible contraindications with your MRI centre. With the advent of short bore MR scanners, claustrophobia is less of a problem but appropriate sedation is still required in some patients.

In the first description of MRI in sacroiliitis, Ahlstrom et al. found striking changes in the subchondral bone marrow. They emphasised the unique ability of MRI to demonstrate abnormalities in subchondral bone and periarticular bone marrow. They concluded that the early inflammatory changes in sacroiliitis are likely to occur in the subchondral structures of the SIJ. This study opened the door for the potential use of MRI in the investigation of SII, and thereafter a multitude of studies confirmed their initial finding and supported the development of MRI in the diagnosis and management of patients with SII. Research on the use of MRI in SII has proliferated with the advent of anti-TNF treatment. Early research concentrated on the quantification of active disease involving the sacroiliac joints with the use of contrast enhancement

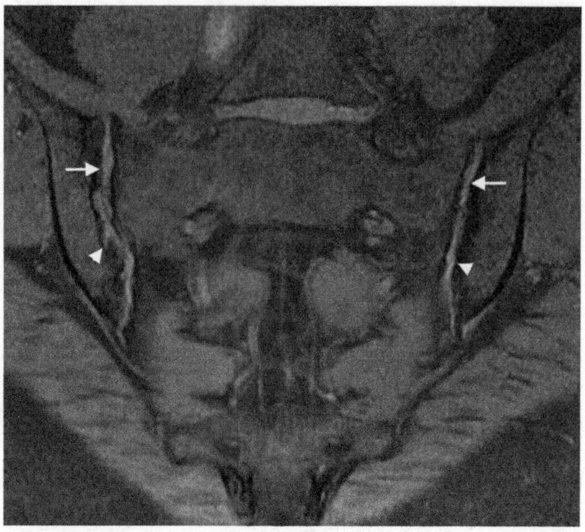

Fig. 6.9 Cor T1FS demonstrates intermediate SI articular cartilage (*arrows*) and early erosive disease (*arrowheads*)

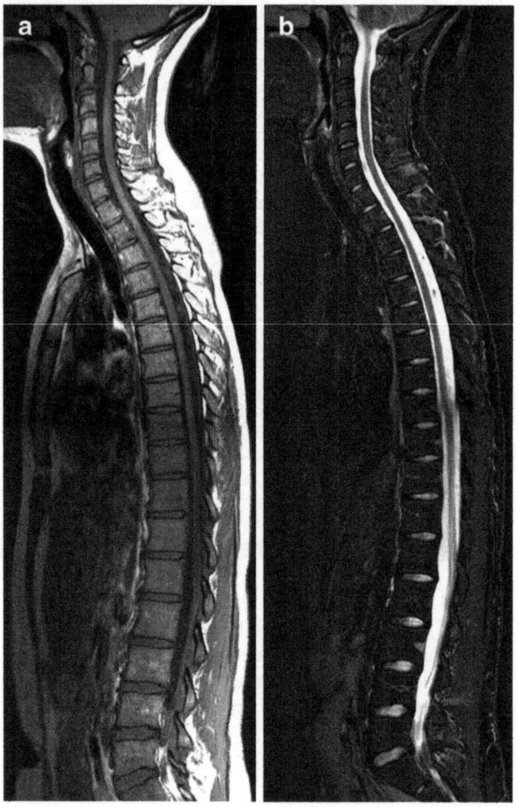

Fig. 6.10 Normal MRI, spondylitis protocol with normal bone marrow signal intensity, (**a**) Sag T1 and (**b**) Sag STIR of the whole spine

and dynamic contrast enhancement. STIR imaging was found to be almost as sensitive as the enhanced examination and was less expensive and time consuming and has become a major imaging sequence for the assessment of active disease. Enhanced studies are now rarely acquired in our clinical practice except in those cases where alternate pathology such as infection or tumour is suspected.

Imaging

Spinal

Spinal changes of SpA usually commence and are most pronounced within the thoracic spine. Spinal disease usually occurs with or after the onset of sacroiliitis, but in a minority of patients, spinal changes are the initial imaging finding on MRI. Spinal changes include spondylitis, Romanus lesions, syndesmophytes, spondylodiscitis, enthesitis and facet and costovertebral arthritis (Figs. 6.10 and 6.11) (Table 6.2).

A *Romanus lesion*, initially described on radiographs as an early spinal change in AS, is an erosion of a vertebral corner at the discovertebral junction (Fig. 6.12). Erosions heal with the development of corner sclerosis, 'shiny corners', occurring at the anterior superior or inferior corners of the vertebral body. This is secondary to new bone formation at the site of prior inflammation and may represent an altered healing response that occurs in AS. With MRI, inflammatory changes can be identified prior to any radio-

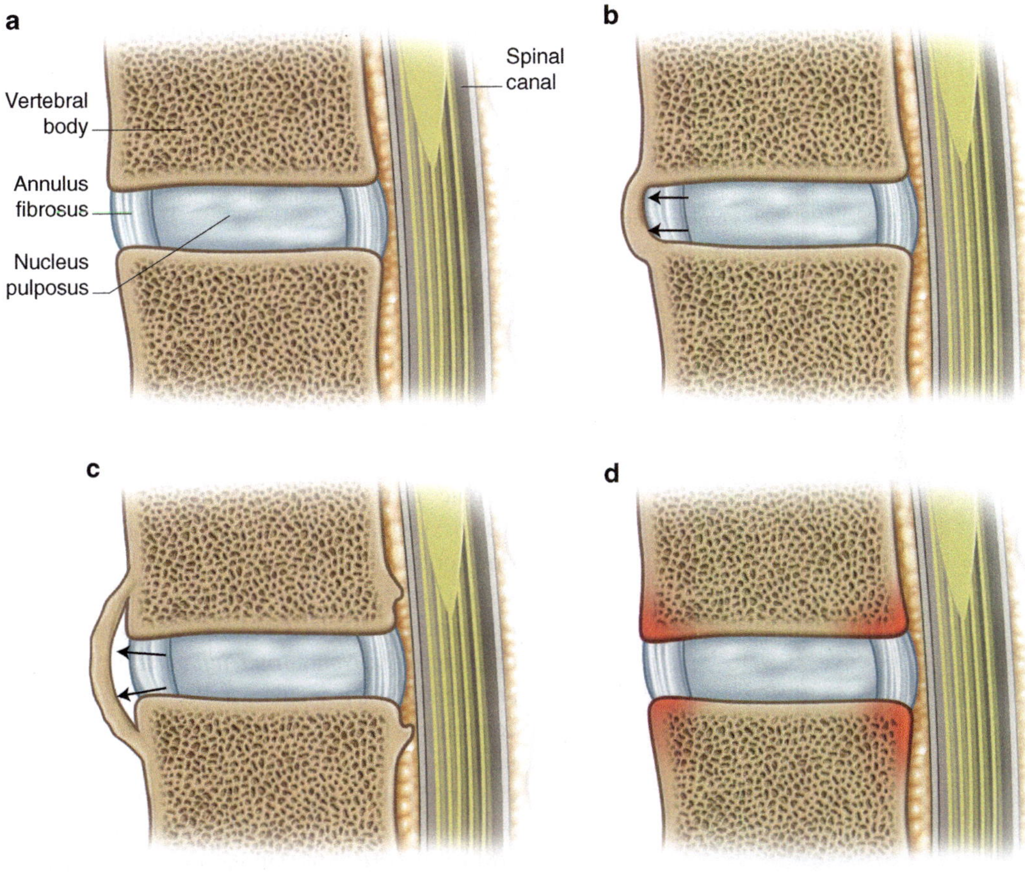

Fig. 6.11 Spinal changes SpA, (**a**) normal, (**b**) syndesmophyte formation in ankylosing spondylitis and (**c**) in psoriasis and Reiter's (**d**) vertebral osteitis (outlined in *red*)

Table 6.2 Spinal changes in spondylitis

Spinal pathology	Radiograph	MRI
Romanus lesion	Anterior vertebral body corner erosion. May heal with sclerosis, the shiny corner	Focal osteitis, high SI on STIR, low T1, anterior corners of the vertebral body. Chronic lesions are depicted as foci of fat signal intensity, high on T1 and T2
Andersson lesion/spondylodiscitis	Types 1, 2 and 3. Localised or generalised discovertebral destruction with surrounding ill-defined sclerosis. Fractured posterior elements in type 3	Irregularity to frank erosion of cortical endplate, adjacent osteitis of increased SI on STIR vertebral body, low SI disc and sclerosis deep to osteitis. Assess for posterior element fracture
Spondylitis	Anterior (Romanus) or posterior vertebral body corner erosion. May heal with sclerosis, the shiny corner	Corner or non-corner osteitis vertebral body, high SI STIR, low on T1. Chronic lesions are depicted as foci of fat signal intensity, high on T1 and T2
Facet joint arthritis	Erosions, subchondral sclerosis and eventually joint ankylosis	Erosions, osteitis pedicles, subchondral sclerosis and eventually joint ankylosis
Costovertebral arthritis	Erosions, sclerosis and fusion. Difficult to detect on radiographs	Erosions, subchondral osteitis, subchondral sclerosis and eventually joint ankylosis, involves costotransverse and costovertebral joints
Enthesitis	May be normal or erosion and osteopenia, reactive sclerosis	High SI within ligament and osteitis at bony attachment, may develop erosion and sclerosis, commonly seen in posterior element involvement
Syndesmophytes	New bone formation within the outer fibres of the annulus fibrosis of the intervertebral disc commencing at the juncture with the vertebral body, eventually bridging between vertebral bodies	May be difficult to identify on MRI, radiographs are more sensitive. Non-bridging bone following marrow SI on all imaging sequences
Ankylosis	Bony fusion, partial or complete, across a joint space	Bony fusion, partial or complete, across a joint space. May have bone marrow SI (easier to identify on MRI) or be sclerotic and low SI on all sequences

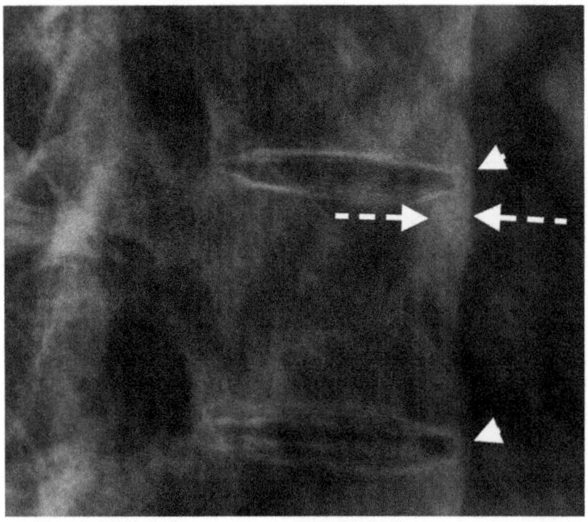

Fig. 6.12 Magnified lateral lower thoracic spine radiograph with anterosuperior corner vertebral sclerosis (*dashed arrow*) in keeping with a healed Romanus lesion. Note syndesmophytes (*arrowheads*) and early squaring of the anterior vertebral body

graphic change. MRI can demonstrate focal *osteitis*, high SI on STIR, low on T1, at the anterior corners of the vertebral body in the acute stage (Fig. 6.13). This is also termed a *corner inflammatory lesion*. These may occur anteriorly or posteriorly. *Non-corner inflammatory lesions* are identified as osteitis parallel to the endplate centrally. When osteitis involves the more lateral margins of the vertebral body, at the level pedicles and beyond, it is termed a *lateral inflammatory lesion*. Osteitis at the costovertebral and costotransverse articulations may occur and is thought to be a more sensitive indication of SpA (Figs. 6.14). Inflammation may also involve the posterior elements of the vertebra including the facet joints (including capsule, facets and peri-facet soft tissues), posterior ligaments and related

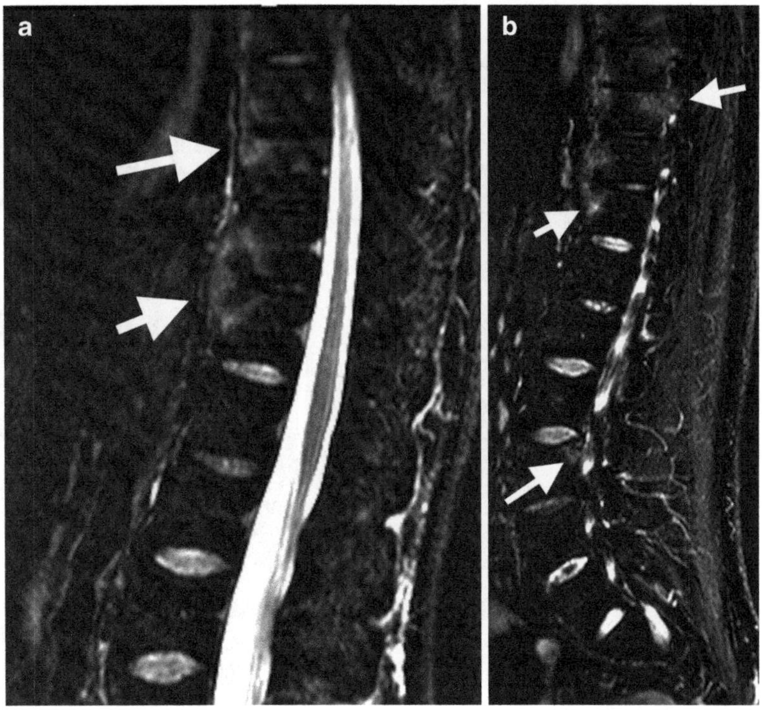

Fig. 6.13 (**a**) Anterior corner osteitis (*arrows*) of the lower thoracic spine on Sag STIR and MRI, note the bridging bone, syndesmophyte, at the lower level also of high SI in keeping with active disease, (**b**) the same patient with additional posterior corner osteitis

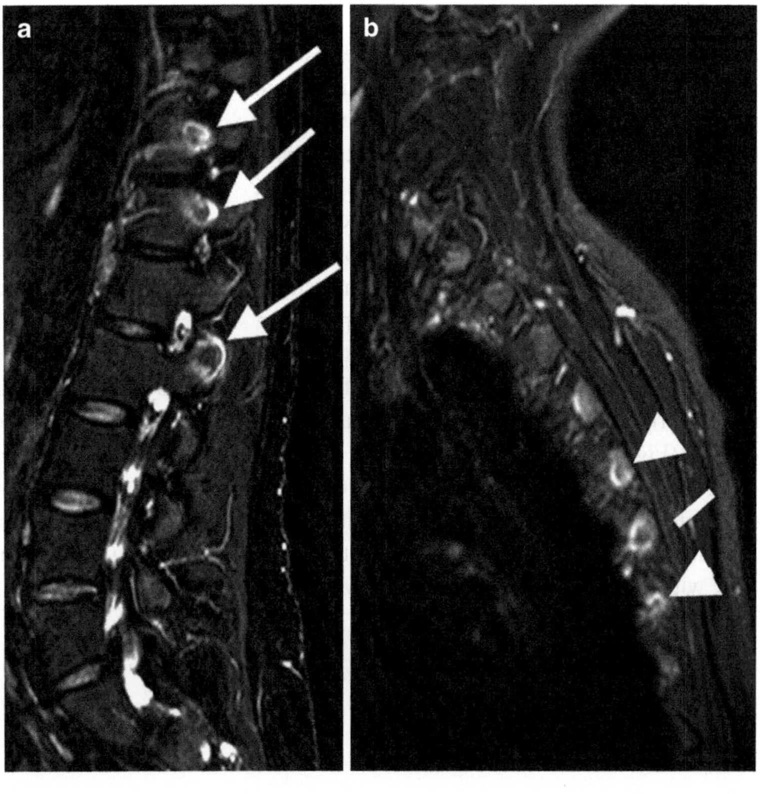

Fig. 6.14 (**a**) Sag STIR image and MRI image of the lower thoracic spine with costovertebral (*upper 2 arrows*) and costotransverse (*lower arrow*) osteitis and (**b**) the same patient with the osteitis rib adjacent to the costotransverse joint (*arrowheads*)

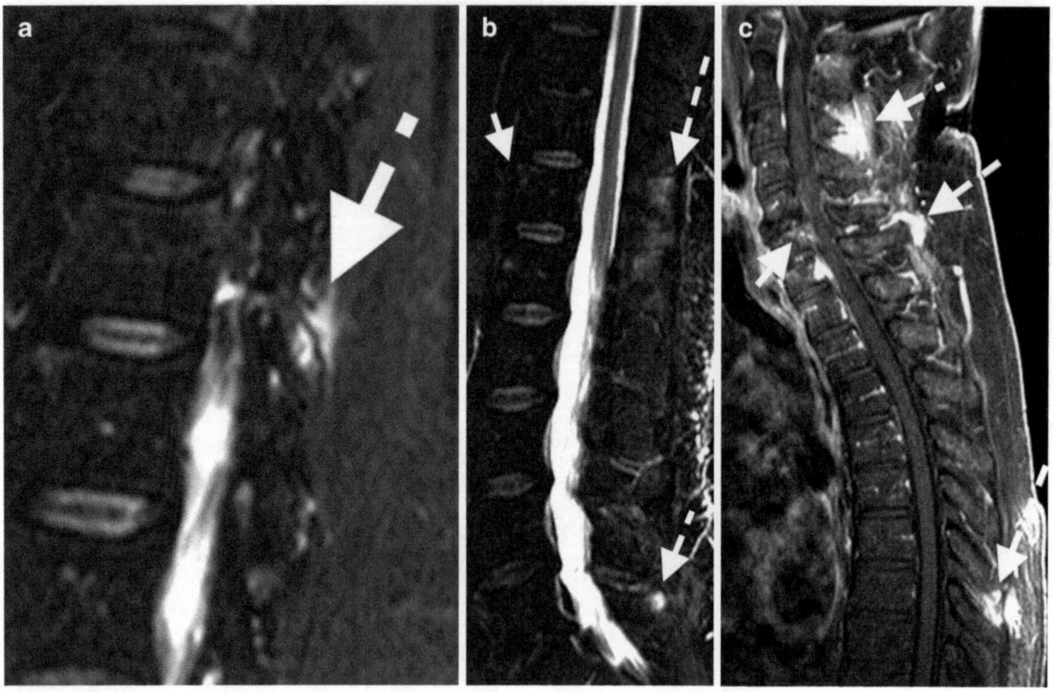

Fig. 6.15 Posterior element involvement, (**a**) Sag STIR T11–12 facet joint with osteitis and pericapsular oedema (*arrow*); (**b**) interspinous (*upper dashed arrow*) and supraspinous ligament oedema at the insertion spinous process (enthesitis), note also the anterior corner osteitis (*arrow*); (**c**) Sag T1FS PG (contrast not usually required in imaging SpA, given in this case for alternate clinical indication) demonstrates multifocal posterior ligamentous enhancement and enthesitis at ligament insertion (*dashed arrows*) and enhancing posterior corner osteitis (*arrow*)

enthesis (Fig. 6.15). When the acute osteitis resolves, the normal haemopoietic tissue within the marrow is no longer present, and the marrow is predominantly of fat signal intensity. These post-inflammatory fat accentuation (PIFA) foci appear as high SI on both T1 and T2 sequences (Fig. 6.16). *Spondylitis* is inflammation of the vertebral body. It encompasses corner osteitis both anterior, the Romanus lesion, and posterior, non-corner osteitis and posterior element involvement. *Squaring* of the vertebra is loss of the normal anterior concavity due to vertebral corner erosion (Fig. 6.17).

A *syndesmophyte* is new bone formation within the outer fibres of the annulus fibrosis of the intervertebral disc commencing at the juncture with the vertebral body, Sharpey's fibres (Fig. 6.18). Bone growth eventually forms a bridge between the involved vertebral bodies. They are most pronounced at the anterior and lateral margins of the vertebral body. This is a late finding in the disease; approximately 25 % of patients will demonstrate syndesmophytes by 10 years and 65 % by 20 years of disease. They need to be differentiated from DISH where the anterior longitudinal ligament is ossified and extends over the vertebral body. Endplate osteophytes are more triangular in nature and grow outwards. Psoriasis- and Reiter's-related paravertebral ossification begins proximal to the juncture of the intervertebral disc and vertebra. Radiographs are more sensitive than MRI in identifying syndesmophytes.

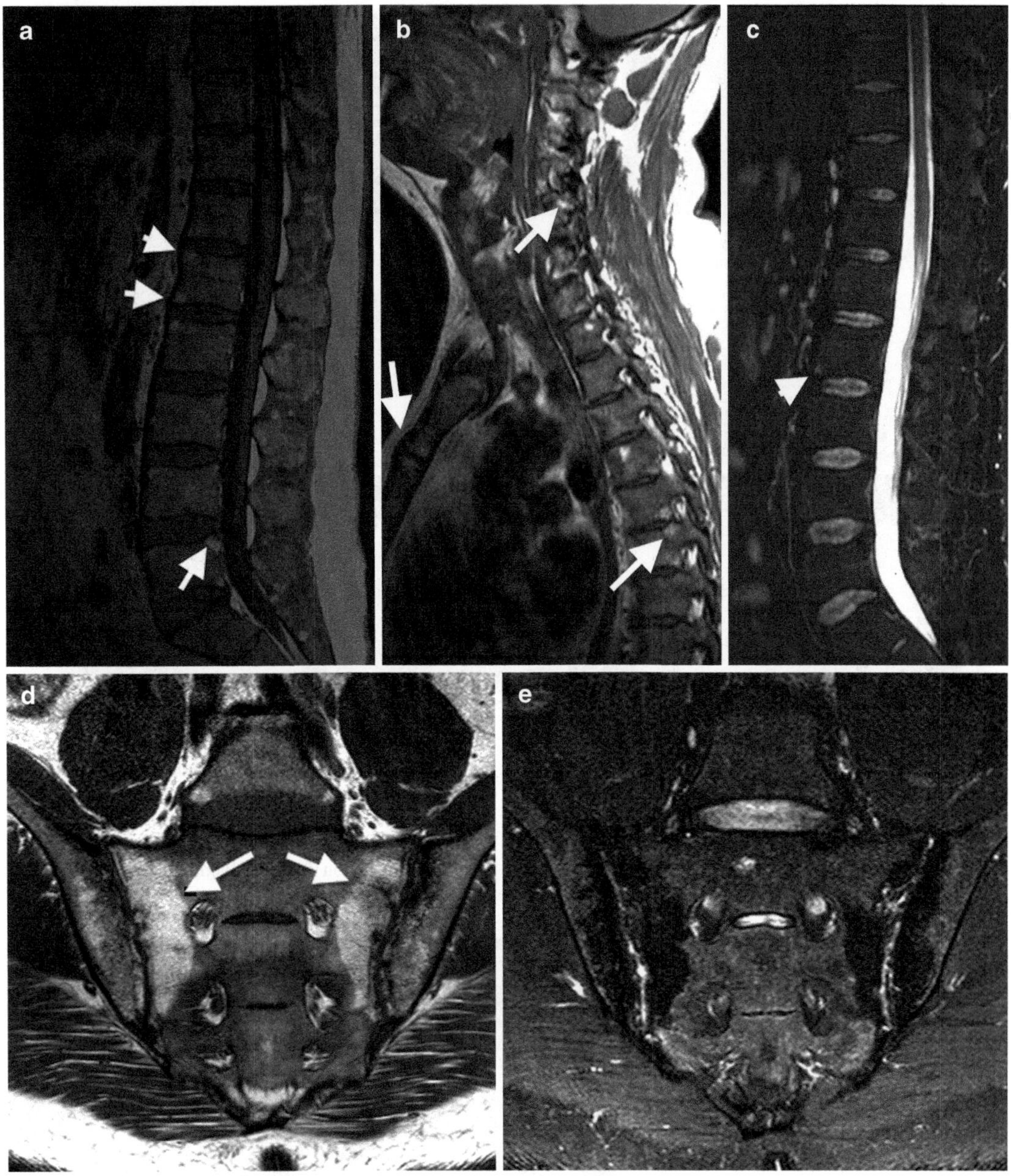

Fig. 6.16 MRI in a 45-year-old male with chronic AS, (**a**) Sag T1 of the lower spine with multiple corner post-inflammatory fat accentuation, PIFA (*arrows*); (**b**) Sag T1 of the upper spine with similar changes with additional PIFA related to the manubriosternal joint and cervical facet joint; (**c**) Sag T2 of the lower spine with loss of SI from PIFA lesions and single anterior corner osteitis of L2 (*arrow*); (**d**) Cor T1 SIJ PIFA of the bilateral sacral aspect of SIJs with fat saturation and loss of SI on (**e**) Cor STIR. Note also joint space loss, erosions and sacroiliac joints without active sacroiliitis

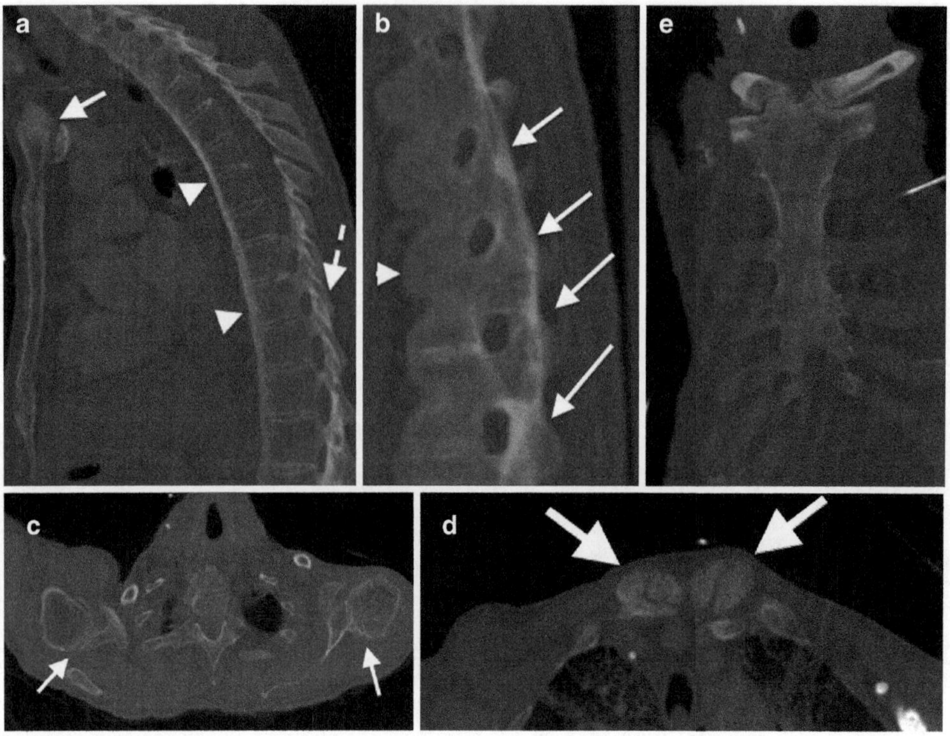

Fig. 6.17 CT chest in a patient with chronic AS demonstrating typical chronic changes; (**a**) Sag reformatted image with extensive thoracic syndesmophyte formation (*arrowheads*), facet joint fusion (*dashed line*) and sternoclavicular joint erosion and subchondral sclerosis (*arrow*); (**b**) magnified from (**a**) with syndesmophyte formation (*arrowhead*), facet joint fusion (*arrows*), (**c**) bilateral glenohumeral joint involvement (*arrows*) with joint space loss, erosions and osteophytes; (**d**) similar changes at sternoclavicular joints, note also upper lobe pulmonary fibrosis; and (**e**) Cor reformatted image with fused manubriosternal joint, ossification of the first costochondral junction and involvement of the sternoclavicular joints

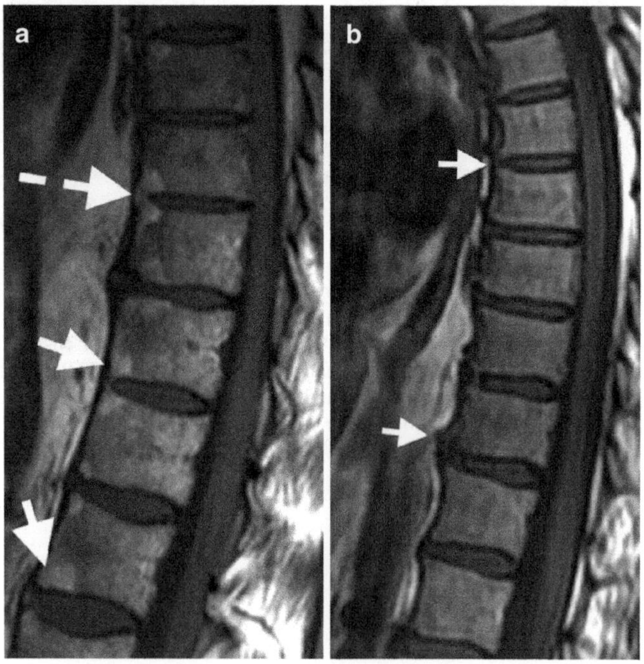

Fig. 6.18 (**a**) MRI syndesmophytes on Sag T1 with ossification of outer annulus fibrosis (*dashed arrow*) and anterior corner PIFA, (**b**) early syndesmophyte formation on Sag T1 (*arrows*), (**c**) a different patient with history of psoriatic SpA, lateral radiograph of the cervical spine with multiple syndesmophytes (*arrows*) and facet joint fusion (*dashed arrows*), (**d**) magnified view of same patient

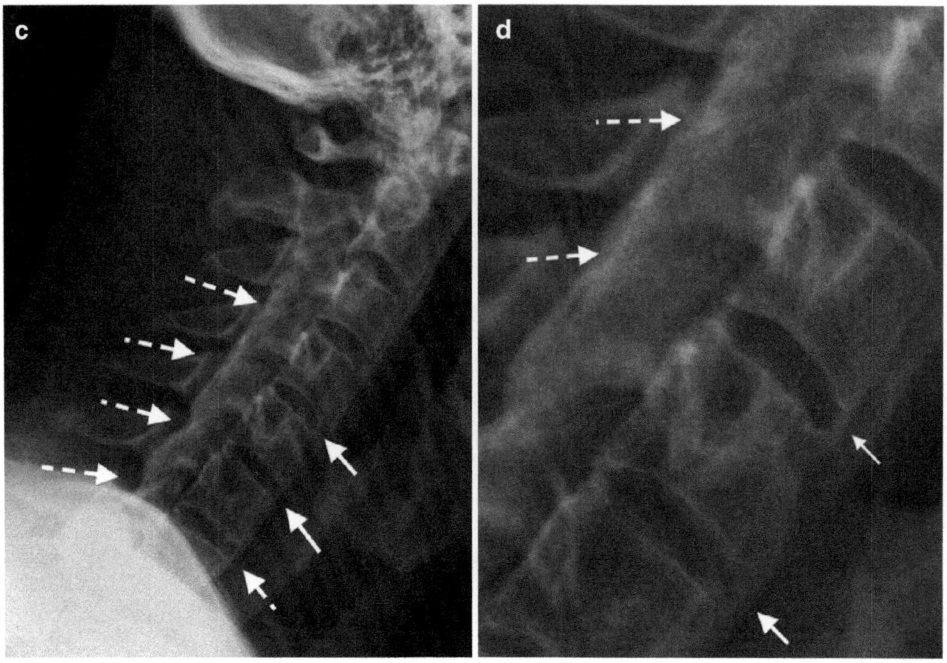

Fig. 6.18 (continued)

Spondylodiscitis or *Andersson lesion* is the occurrence of discovertebral erosions in patients with SpA (Figs. 6.19 and 6.20). Lesions may be localised or diffuse. The localised lesion may be central or peripheral. The diffuse or generalised involves the whole discovertebral junction and can be subdivided into those with and without fractured posterior elements. It is a noninfected heterogeneous entity that has two major aetiologies, inflammatory and traumatic. Localised lesions occur more commonly in the non-ankylosed spine and may relate to inflammation, secondary osteoporosis and herniation of disc contents through the weakened endplate. Radiographs demonstrate localised destruction or erosion of the vertebral endplate with radiolucent foci and surrounding sclerosis. MRI demonstrates irregularity to frank erosion of the cortical endplate, adjacent osteitis of increased SI on STIR within the vertebral body, low SI disc and sclerosis deep to osteitis. The posterior elements should be closely evaluated for fracture. The generalised lesion is more common in chronic disease with a fused spine. The chronic ankylosed spine is more prone to both traumatic acute fracture and stress fracture. Intact posterior elements have unfused facet joints, and the lesion is transdiscal. Posterior element fracture can be associated with both transdiscal and transvertebral lesions. The generalised lesion will result in a pseudoarthrosis and may be associated with a secondary kyphotic deformity. Radiographic changes are dependent on the acuity of an associated fracture. A fracture through the disc may be invisible on radiographs but can be suspected by fracture of a syndesmophyte if present at that level. This progresses to generalised destruction of the vertebral endplates with surrounding sclerosis. There may be narrowing of the intervertebral height. Kyphosis with loss of anterior vertebral body height may be present.

Erosions, osteitis, capsulitis, enthesitis, reactive subchondral sclerosis and joint ankylosis occur at the apophyseal joints and costovertebral joints (Figs. 6.21 and 6.17). Erosions may also occur at the atlantoaxial articulation. Ligamentous ossification is common in chronic disease. The *dagger sign*, a linear band of

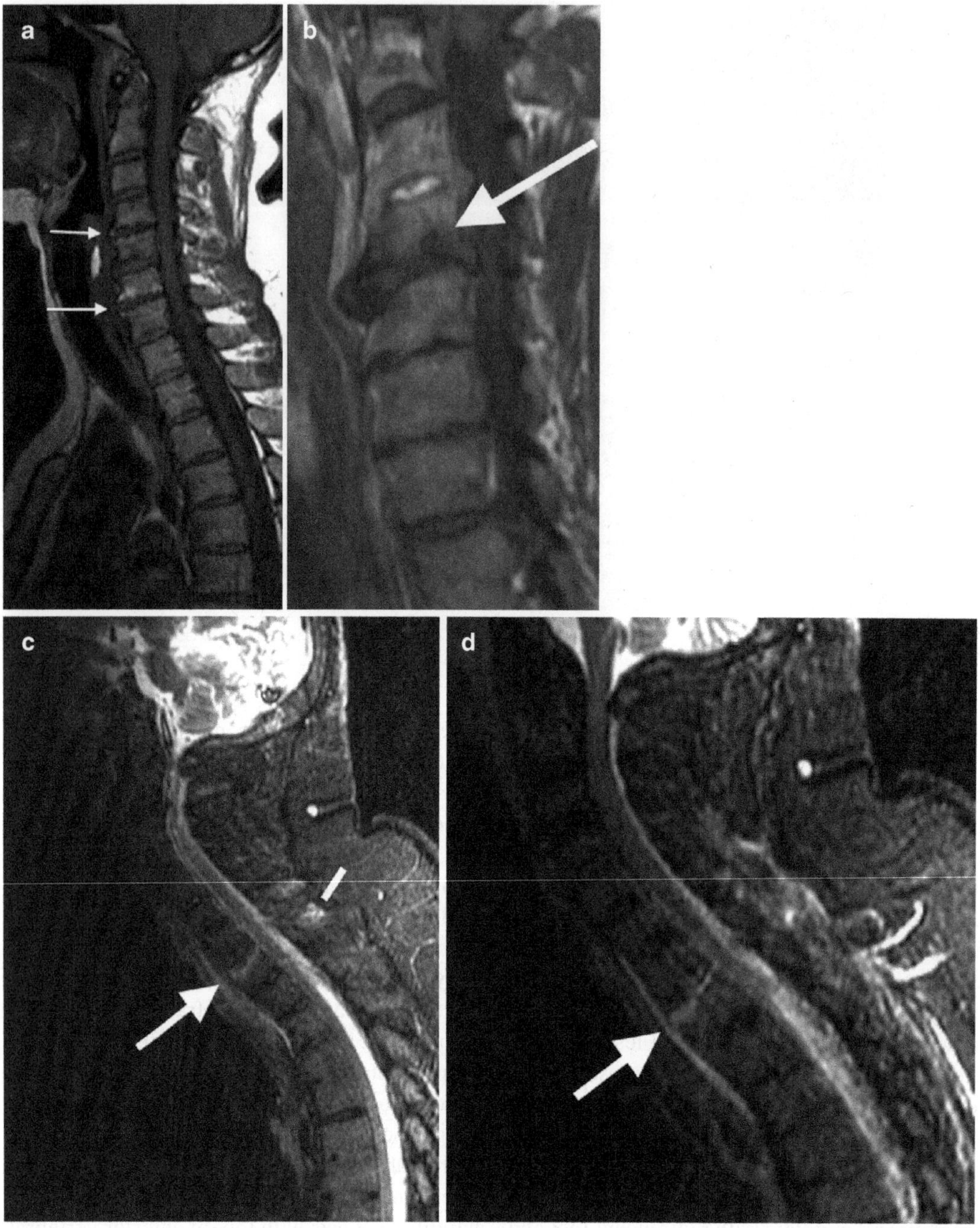

Fig. 6.19 (**a**) Sag T1 of the upper spine with C4–5 and C6–7 endplate erosions, (**b**) C4–5 endplate erosion with early kyphosis, (**c**, **d**) acute fracture T1 on Sag T2FS, image degradation due to patient motion, oedema noted at the posterior soft tissues without posterior element fracture, note also prevertebral oedema. This predisposes to development of traumatic Andersson lesion

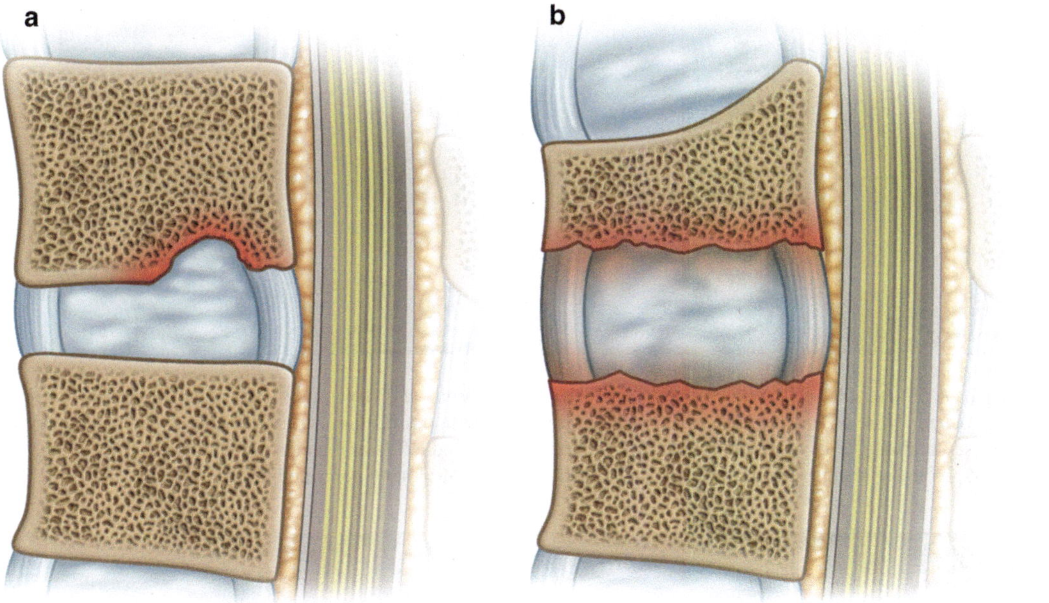

Fig. 6.20 Illustration of Andersson lesions (**a**) localised with endplate erosion, (**b**) posttraumatic with endplate erosions and loss of height vertebra anteriorly with secondary kyphosis

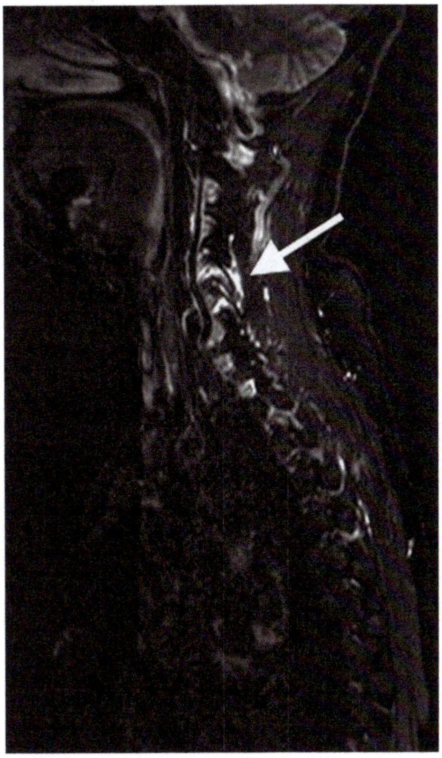

Fig. 6.21 Sag T2FS in a 52-year-old female with psoriatic spondyloarthropathy demonstrating facet joint distension, capsulitis and extensive osteitis

radiodensity, white band, on frontal radiograph, is secondary to ossification of the supraspinous and interspinous ligaments (Fig. 6.22). When there is additional apophyseal capsule ossification, a *trolley track sign* can be seen on frontal radiographs as three bands of radiodensity superimposed over the spine (Fig. 6.22). These changes are usually more evident within the lumbar region. Discal calcification occurs in chronic disease and may appear ballooned with disc endplate convexity. This is likely secondary to osteoporosis, common in chronic disease (Fig. 6.23). BMD assessment of the spine may be inaccurate due to paravertebral ossification as described above, and thus lateral spinal assessment is more accurate than AP. In addition non-spinal sites without evidence of disease involvement on radiographs should be assessed. Assessment of the sternoclavicular joints and manubriosternal articulation is also often possible when assessing the upper spine and should be reviewed for active disease (osteitis, joint effusion and capsulitis at the sternoclavicular joint and osteitis at the manubriosternal articulation) and chronic changes including fusion

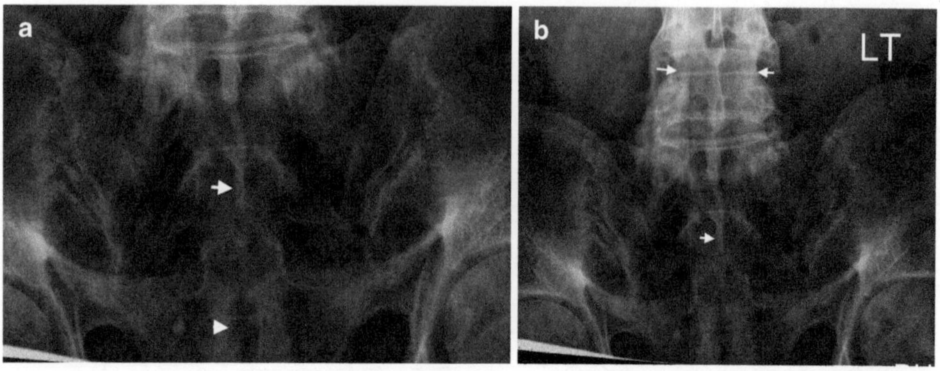

Fig. 6.22 A 59-year-old male with chronic AS, (**a**) dagger sign (*arrow*) on AP radiograph, SIJs with central radiodense band due to ossification of the supraspinous and interspinous ligaments, note erosions of the symphysis pubis, and (**b**) trolley track sign, the same patient as (**a**) with ossification across the apophyseal joints causing right and left lateral bands of radiodensity with respect to the central band described in (**a**)

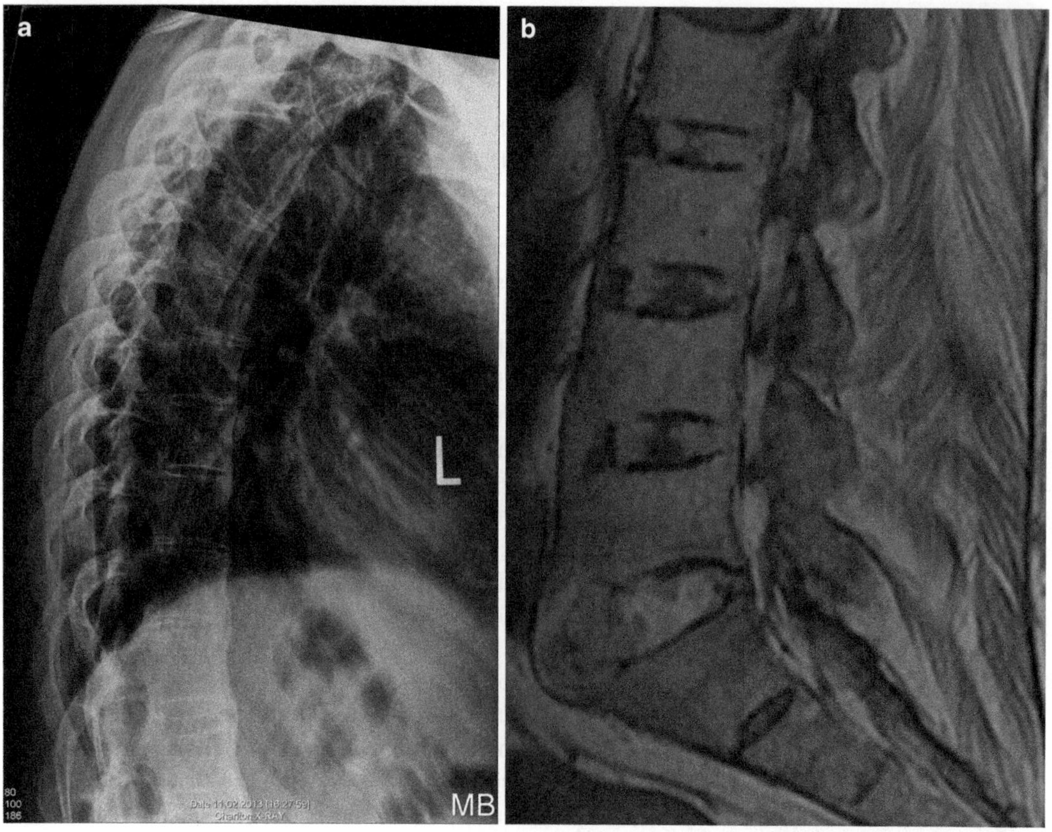

Fig. 6.23 (**a**) Lateral thoracic spine in a patient with long-standing AS demonstrating osteopenia and syndesmophyte formation, (**b**) MRI lumbar spine, Sag T1, with widened intervertebral discs and mild endplate convexity

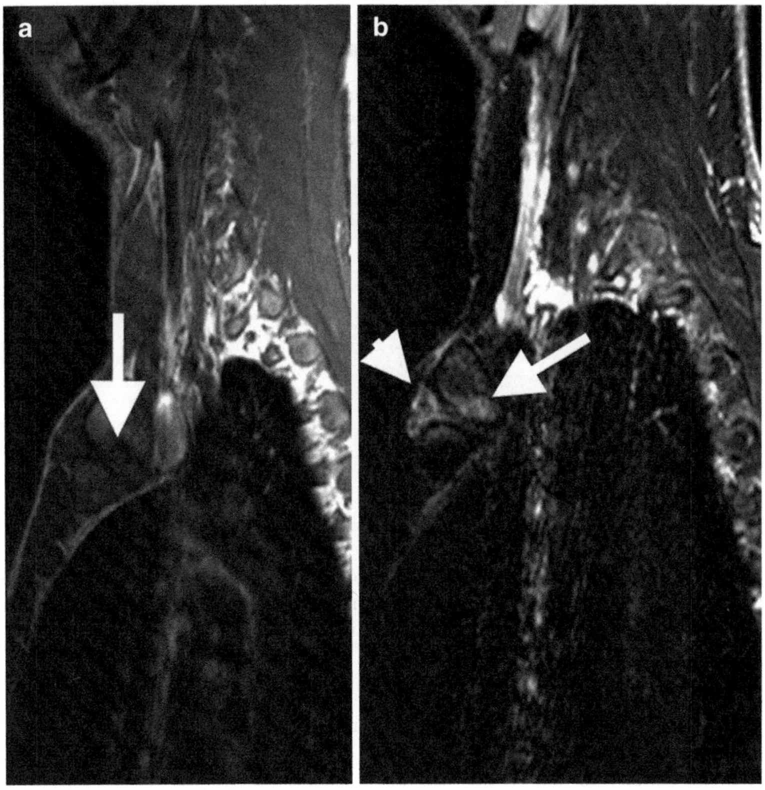

Fig. 6.24 A 30-year-old male with known AS, (**a**) Sag T1 and (**b**) STIR of the cervical and upper thoracic spine demonstrate erosion (*arrow*) and joint distension (can be either effusion or synovitis on this unenhanced study) of the left sternoclavicular joint

manubriosternal articulation and erosions at the sternoclavicular joint (Fig. 6.24).

Sacroiliac Joints

The sacroiliac joints are primarily involved in SpA. Acute and chronic changes occur with acute changes identified on MRI and chronic changes on MRI, CT and radiographs with varying sensitivity and specificity. Acute changes include osteitis, synovitis, capsulitis and enthesitis (Fig. 6.24). Subchondral sclerosis, erosions, periarticular fat deposition, bony bridging and ankylosing are chronic changes (Fig. 6.25) (Table 6.3). Subchondral *bone marrow oedema* usually occurs first on the iliac aspect of the joint, thought to be due to the thinner cartilage on the iliac side. When extensive bone marrow oedema is present on MRI, the diagnosis of acute sacroiliitis is straightforward in the correct clinical context (Fig. 6.26). Likewise when osteitis is completely absent, the absence of acute sacroiliitis is confirmed. Difficulty arises in the cases where there is mild subchondral bone marrow oedema, particularly when a thin linear focus is present (Fig. 6.27). Assessing other concomitant changes of acute or chronic changes of SpA in the spine and sacroiliac joint is essential in order to achieve the correct diagnosis. In addition alternate pathologies that may cause bone marrow oedema such as degenerative disease (usually mild thin linear subchondral oedema), insufficiency fractures and infection should be excluded. ASAS classification criteria require the presence of acute sacroiliitis for the diagnosis of SpA and requires, focal subchondral osteitis, lesion should be present on two adjacent MRI slices or, if more than one

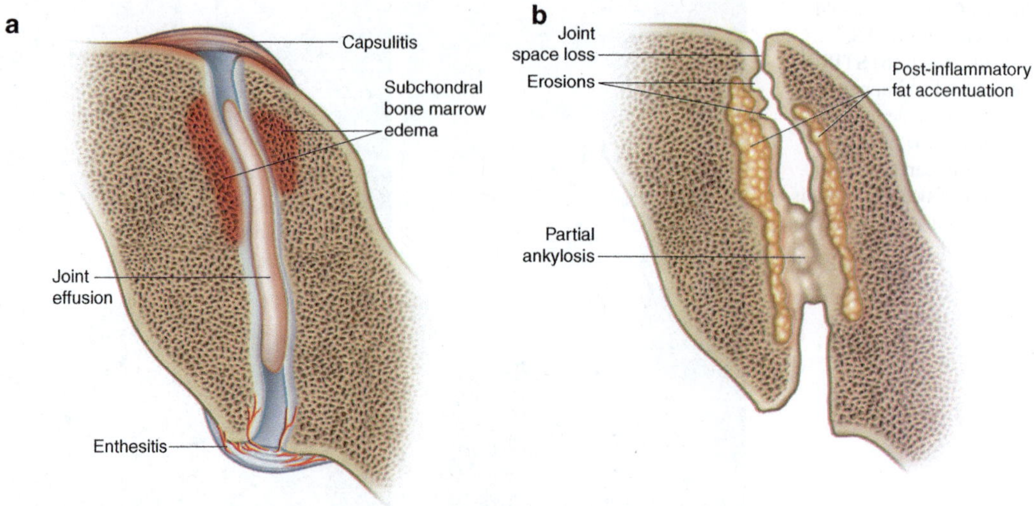

Fig. 6.25 Illustration demonstrating features of (**a**) acute superior capsulitis, enthesitis within posterior compartment and subchondral bone marrow oedema on both aspects of the joints and (**b**) chronic sacroiliitis with erosions of the joint surface, joint space loss, areas of ankylosis and subchondral fat infiltration

Table 6.3 Sacroiliac changes in spondyloarthropathy

Sacroiliac pathology	Radiograph	MRI
Oedema (osteitis)	ND	Periarticular high signal intensity on STIR or contrast-enhanced T1FS
Enthesitis	ND	High signal intensity on STIR or contrast-enhanced T1FS at site ligament or tendon attachment to bone
Synovitis	ND, may be associated with joint space widening	Intra-articular high signal intensity on contrast-enhanced T1FS
Effusion	ND, may be associated with joint space widening	Intra-articular high signal intensity on STIR, no enhancement on contrast-enhanced T1FS
Capsulitis	ND	Capsular high signal intensity on STIR or contrast-enhanced T1FS. May extend medially or laterally into periosteum as an enthesitis
Erosions	Yes	Cortical defect within cartilaginous compartment joint. Low signal intensity on all imaging sequences. In active erosions may be high signal intensity within, active synovitis, or deep to erosion, osteitis
Fat deposition	ND	Periarticular high signal intensity on T1, low signal intensity on T1FS and STIR
Sclerosis	Subchondral area of high attenuation, appears 'white'	Periarticular low signal intensity on T1, low signal intensity on T1FS and STIR
Ankylosis	Partial or complete bony fusion across joint. Discernable joint space is lost	Partial or complete bony fusion across the joint. Discernable joint space is lost. Follows bone marrow signal intensity on all imaging sequences

ND not detectable

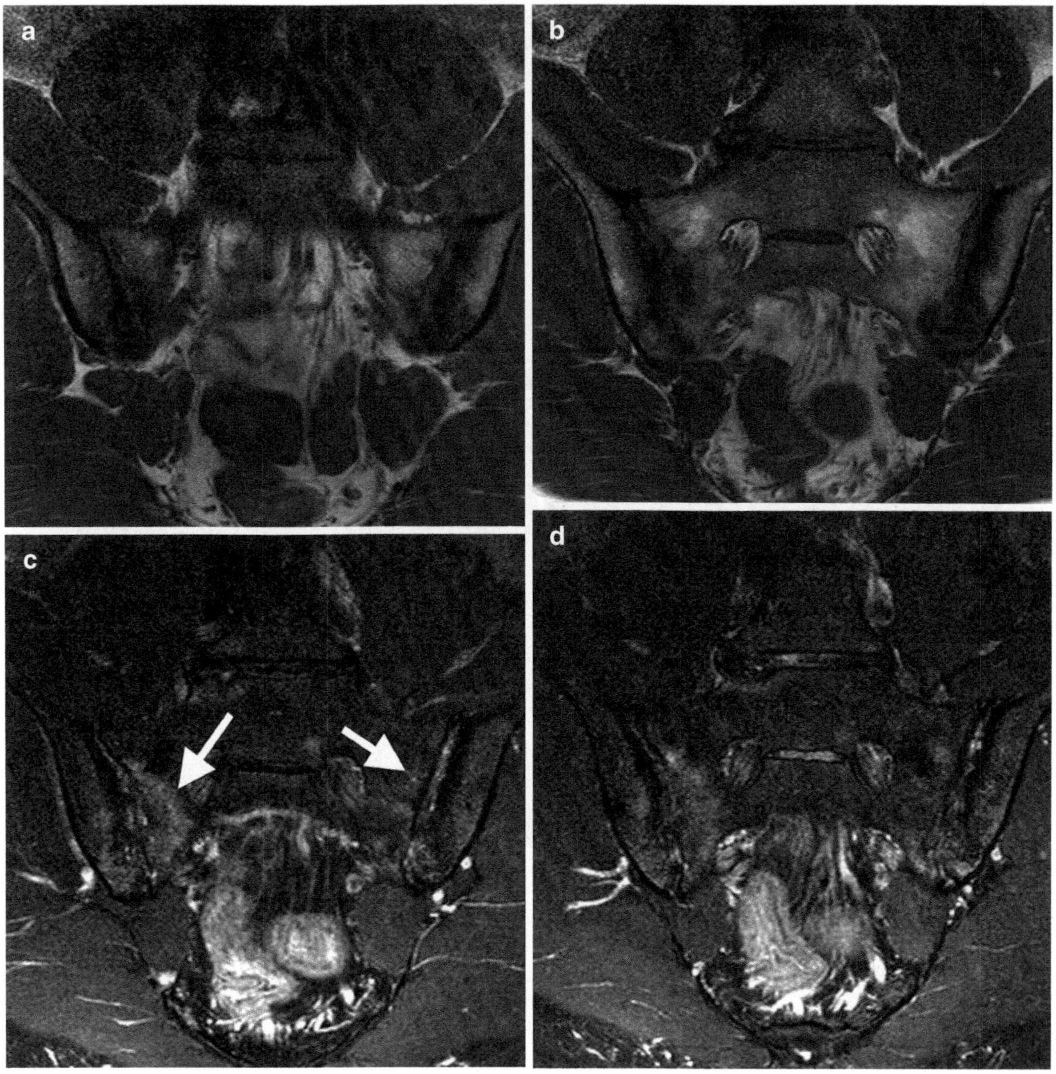

Fig. 6.26 A 39-year-old male patient on initial presentation with a 20-year history of low-grade inflammatory back pain, MRI SIJs, (**a**, **b**) Cor T1 demonstrate bilateral erosions, iliac subchondral sclerosis and (**c**, **d**) Cor STIR active osteitis (*arrows*), joint space loss and erosions

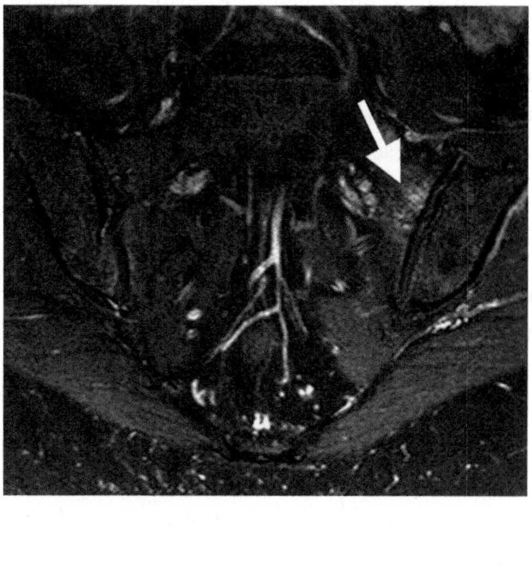

Fig. 6.27 Mild subchondral bone marrow oedema (*arrow*) on the sacral aspect of the left sacroiliac joint on Cor STIR image thought to be related to early degenerative disease. Remainder SIJs and spine negative for SpA but did have lower lumbar degenerative disc disease. Imaging findings should be reviewed in clinical context and other positive or negative findings on remainder of the imaging study

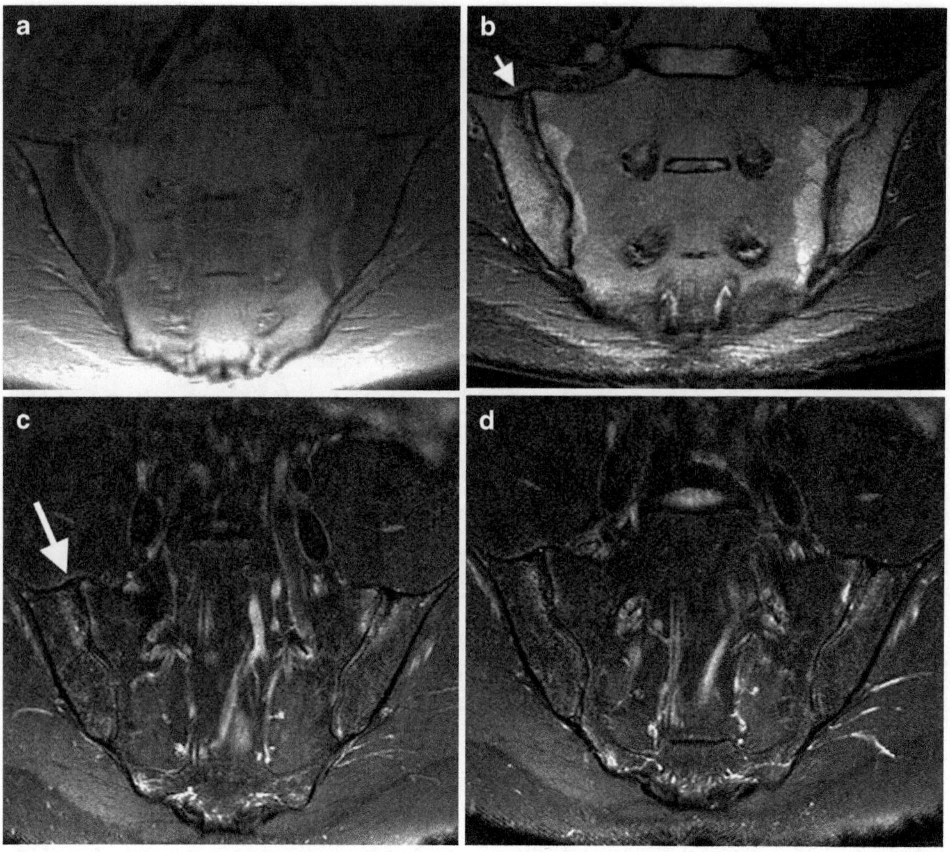

Fig. 6.28 Capsulitis, (**a**) pre- and (**b**) post-contrast Cor T1FS SIJ demonstrating post-contrast enhancement on both sides of SIJs in keeping with osteitis and capsular enhancement of the right superior SIJ (*arrow*), (**c**, **d**) a different patient with Cor STIR high right capsular SI in keeping with capsulitis (*arrow*) on a background of acute or chronic sacroiliitis with joint space loss, small erosions and periarticular osteitis

lesion, they may be on the same or a different slice. Unfortunately the definition remains limited, as there is no precise definition to the size of a lesion. ASAS criteria do not include acute spinal changes or other acute or chronic changes of the sacroiliac joints and are therefore limited in their use as a diagnostic criterion for individual patients at this time. This is expanded upon further in the section on diagnosis of SpA.

Capsulitis is acute inflammation of the joint capsule and is only identifiable on MRI (Fig. 6.28). Capsular high signal intensity is noted on STIR or contrast-enhanced T1FS and may extend medially or laterally into the periosteum as an enthesitis. *Enthesitis* is identified as high signal intensity on STIR or contrast-enhanced T1FS at the site of ligament or tendon attachment to bone (Fig. 6.29). It is best visualised in the entheseal compartment. Active *synovitis* is similar to joint effusion on T2FS sequence, appearing as high SI, but can be differentiated on contrast-enhanced T1FS where synovitis enhances and demonstrates intra-articular high signal intensity (Fig. 6.30). Joint effusion does not enhance. Contrast-enhanced studies are more sensitive in diagnosing both capsulitis and enthesitis and are required for differentiating joint effusion from active synovitis.

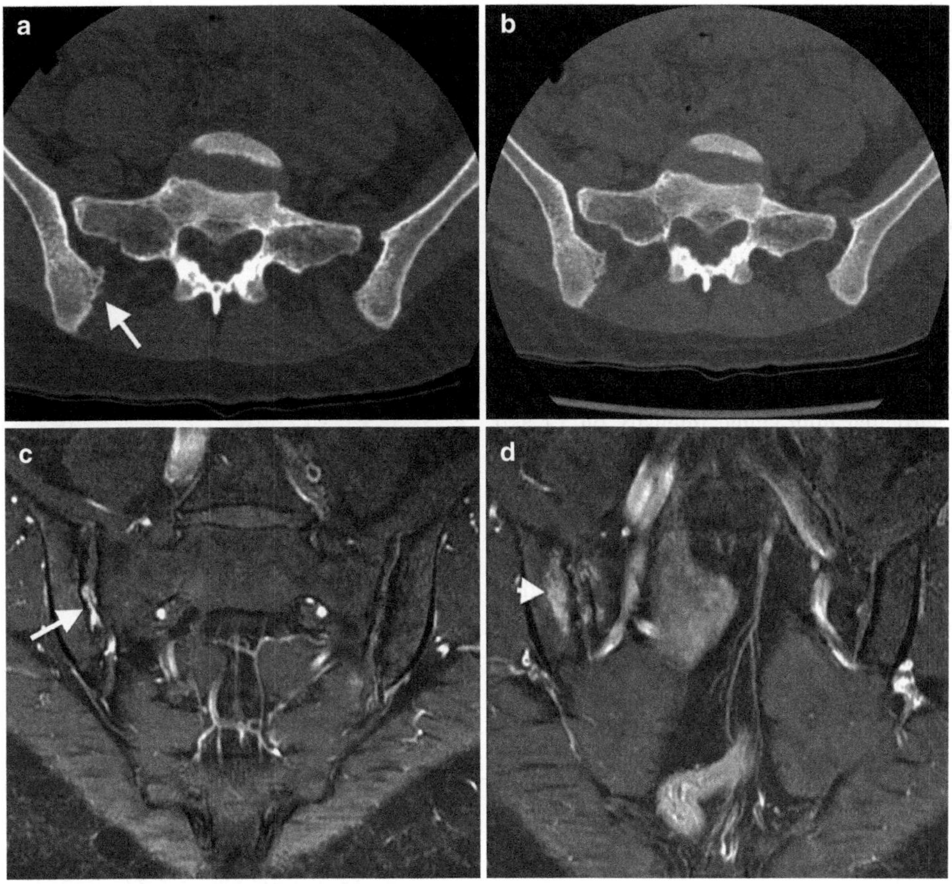

Fig. 6.29 (**a**, **b**) A 32-year-old female with ulcerative colitis demonstrating enthesitis with cortical irregularity and new bone formation, whiskering (*arrow*), right superior entheseal compartment, (**c**) a different patient Cor T1FS post-gadolinium demonstrating enhancement in the right entheseal compartment and (**d**) also enhancing right iliac osteitis

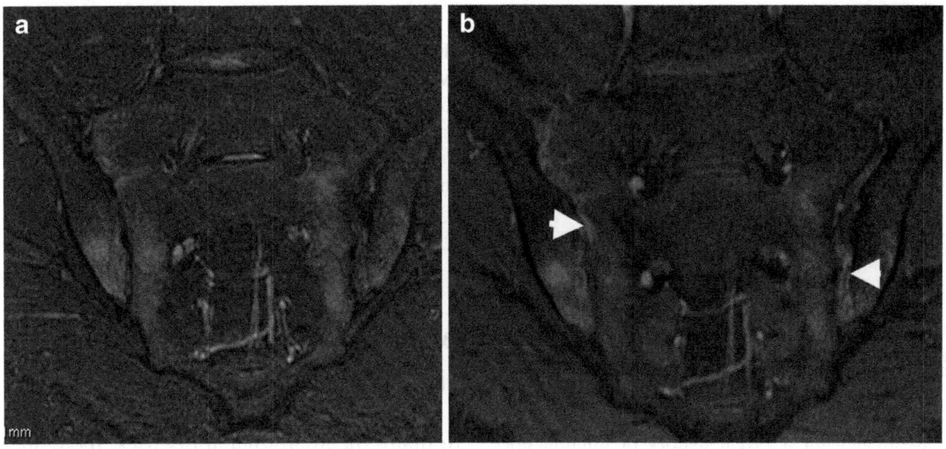

Fig. 6.30 MRI of active bilateral SII. A 24-year-old male patient presenting with inflammatory low back pain. (**a**) Coronal STIR MRI demonstrates bilateral relatively symmetrical subchondral high signal intensity, bilateral moderate loss of joint space with early erosive changes and subtle increased signal intensity in the left sacroiliac joint of joint effusion or synovial proliferation. STIR cannot differentiate between the latter, which requires gadolinium enhancement. (**b**) Coronal T1 fat saturated post-gadolinium demonstrates bilateral enhancement within the joint space, consistent with synovial proliferation (*arrowheads*), bilateral enhancement of subchondral regions and loss of joint space, right greater than left with loss of cortical definition and subtle cortical erosions

Chronic changes include *erosions*, focal cortical defects within the cartilaginous compartment joint (Fig. 6.31). Inactive erosions are low signal intensity on all imaging sequences. In active erosions there may be high signal intensity within, active synovitis, or deep to erosion, osteitis. Cor T1FS is sensitive for erosions but will not demonstrate related osteitis or synovitis. *PIFA*, post-inflammatory fat accentuation, or *fat deposition* is the presence of fat at the site prior inflammation. Since osteitis in SpA is periarticular, so too is the fat deposition. PIFA is identified as periarticular high signal intensity on T1 and low signal intensity on T1FS and STIR (Fig. 6.32). The normal bone marrow signal intensity is assessed at the level of the sacral neural foramina and serves as a reference when assessing the periarticular region. Subchondral *sclerosis* is non-specific and is of low signal intensity on all imaging sequences (Fig. 6.32). Bony bridging and *ankylosis* occur late in the disease (Fig. 6.33). Partial or complete bony fusion occurs across the sacroiliac joint. Discernable joint space is lost, and the bridging new bone follows bone marrow signal intensity on all imaging sequences.

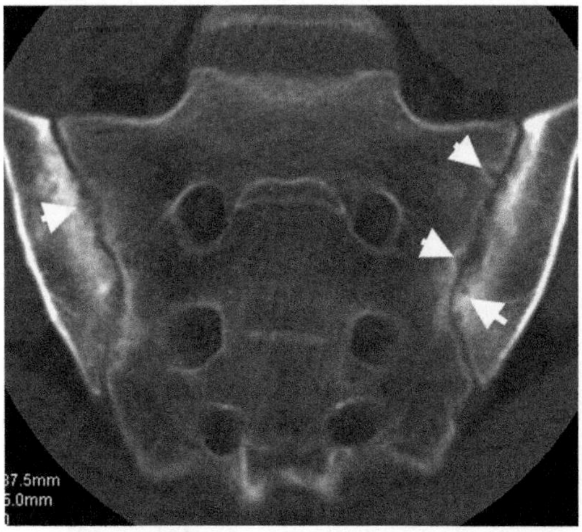

Fig. 6.31 Bilateral SII in a 34-year-old male patient being investigated for a 2-year history of inflammatory low back pain and with a clinical suspicion of SII. Axial CT demonstrates bilateral SII, which is relatively symmetrical with early loss of joint space, subchondral sclerosis, marked erosions (*arrowheads*) and poor definition of the cortical outline

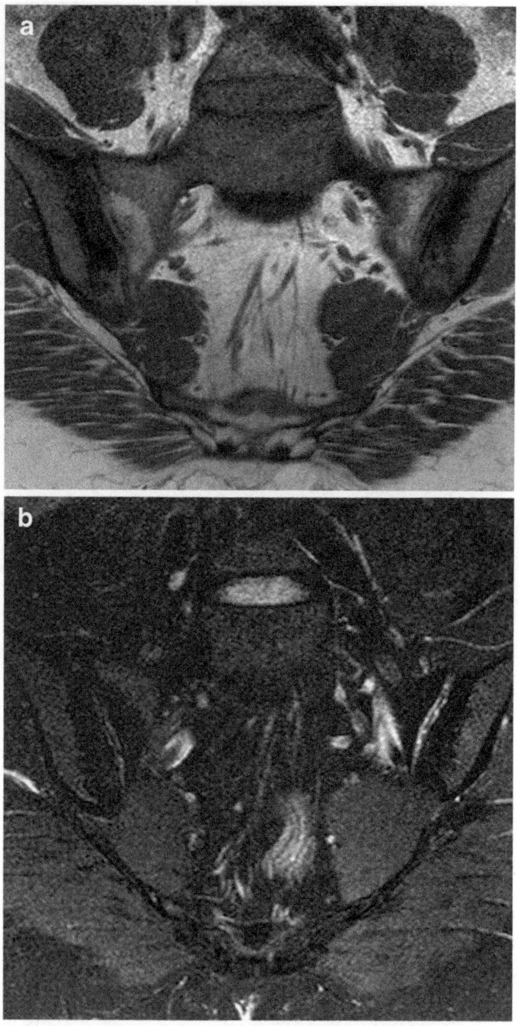

Fig. 6.32 MRI SIJ in a 24-year-old female, HLA positive, (**a**) Cor T1 and (**b**) Cor T2FS demonstrate bilateral post-inflammatory fat accentuation (PIFA) and subchondral sclerosis on the sacral and iliac aspect, respectively. Note the fat is high signal on T1 and becomes low signal on T2FS, whereas the subchondral sclerosis remains low signal on all sequences

Diagnosis of Axial Spondyloarthropathy

In many rheumatological diseases, there are well-established classification criteria but less well-formed diagnostic criteria. This holds true for SpA. Classification criteria allow for the systematic arrangement of similar entities on the basis of cer-

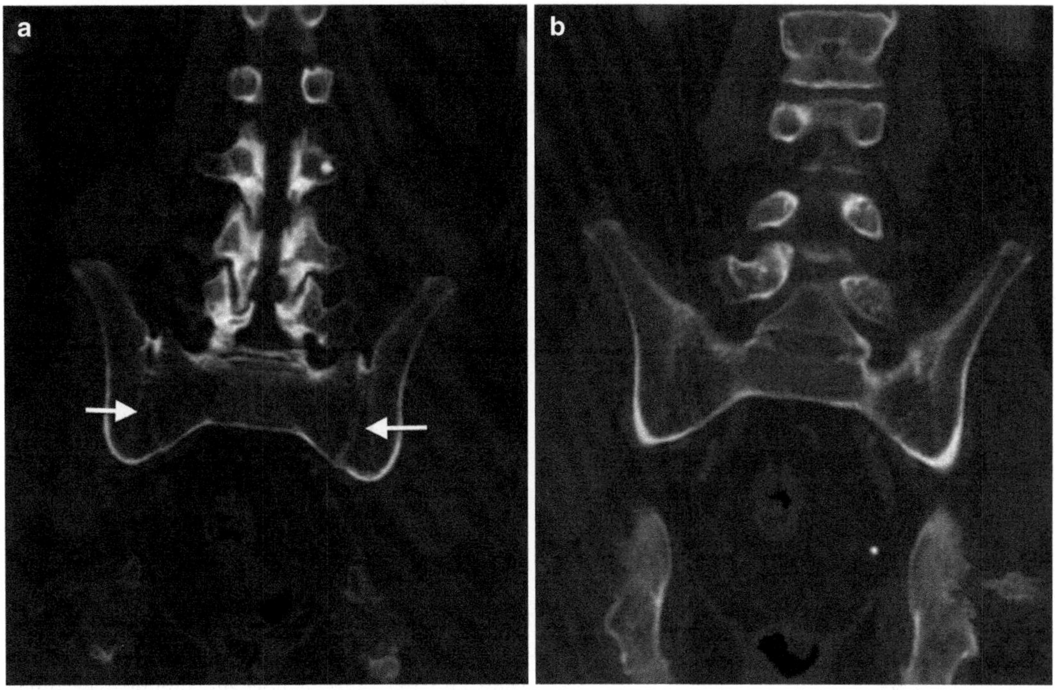

Fig. 6.33 (**a**, **b**) Fused SIJs (*arrows*) in a patient with long-standing paraplegia on coronal reformatted CT

tain differing characteristics creating a homogeneous group with a high specificity but low sensitivity for the disease. Classification criteria are often used in clinical research in patients with a known disease. Classification criteria however have low sensitivity for early disease and do not automatically apply to the general population. Criteria applied to date for axial spondyloarthropathy are classification criteria. This includes the modified New York (Table 6.4), Amor, ESSG (European Spondyloarthropathy Study Group) and the ASAS (Assessment of SpondyloArthritis International Society) criteria. The ASAS criteria include MRI, the gold standard in imaging SpA, which is not present in the other criteria (Tables 6.5 and 6.6). However it has significant limitations. MRI findings are based solely on the presence of active sacroiliitis as described above in the imaging findings section. Active sacroiliitis by ASAS definition has been documented in 7 % of normal control subjects and 23 % patients with non-specific back pain. The ASAS criteria, at this time, exclude all other MRI changes related to acute and chronic

Table 6.4 Modified New York criteria for ankylosing spondylitis (1984)

1. Clinical criteria
A. Low back pain present for at least 3 months not relieved by rest and improves with exercise
B. Limited lumbar spine motion in sagittal and frontal planes
C. Limited chest expansion[a]
2. Radiological criteria
Sacroiliitis: grade 2 bilaterally or unilateral grade 3–4
Ankylosing spondylitis if radiological criteria plus one clinical criteria

[a]Relative to normal values for sex and age

Table 6.5 ASAS criteria for inflammatory back pain: symptoms must be present for 3 months. Considered positive if four out of five symptoms

Insidious onset
Age of onset < 40 years
Improvement with exercise
Pain at night, improved on getting up
No improvement with rest

Table 6.6 ASAS classification criteria for axial spondyloarthropathy

In patients with ≥3 months back pain with age of onset <45 years
Sacroiliitis on imaging[a] plus ≥1 SpA clinical feature
Or
HLA-B27 positive plus ≥2 other SpA clinical features
Clinical features:
Inflammatory back pain (ASAS criteria)
Dactylitis (sausage digit)
Psoriasis
Positive family history of SpA (first- or second-degree relative with any of the following: AS, psoriasis, uveitis, reactive arthritis, IBD)
Good response to NSAIDs (24–48 h post full-dose back pain absent or significantly improved)
Enthesitis (heel)
Arthritis[b]
Crohn's/colitis disease[b]
Elevated CRP in presence of back pain without alternate cause
HLA-B27 positive
Uveitis[b]

MRI: Active inflammatory lesions of the SIJ with definite bone marrow osteitis/osteitis suggestive of sacroiliitis associated with spondyloarthritis
[a]Radiographs: bilateral grade 2–4 or unilateral grade 3–4
[b]Past or present acute synovitis diagnosed by a physician

disease of the sacroiliac joints and the spine. It does however include the New York radiographic changes of unilateral grade 3–4 or bilateral grade 2 disease. As such the ASAS criteria are limited when assessing the individual patient.

A diagnostic criterion allows for the identification of a disease and allows the separation of those patients with the disease from the general population. Diagnostic criteria have a high sensitivity but lower specificity and are used in the diagnosis of the individual patient. Ideally diagnostic criteria would allow for the identification of patients throughout the spectrum of the disease but in doing so will inadvertently include patients without the disease. The gold standard for diagnosis of SpA is the expert opinion of a rheumatologist of the clinical and imaging findings.

There are many proposed clinical MRI grading systems for sacroiliitis. These usually require dividing the sacroiliac joints into segments, assessing acute and chronic changes within those segments and assigning a score. Some scoring systems require the use of intravenous contrast. There is however no agreed upon scoring system that is in wide use in clinical practice. Current work is ongoing in the development of an international grading system that will be available for use both in clinical studies and in individual patient management. Peripheral spondyloarthropathy is reviewed in detail in Chap. 5.

Imaging Algorithm

The wide availability of conventional radiography and the marked cost advantage over other imaging modalities make it the screening examination of choice in the investigation of SII. The main disadvantages of conventional X-rays are the lack of sensitivity in detecting early SII, the false-positive rate, the use of ionising radiation and the high inter- and intraobserver variation. If radiographs are diagnostic, then no further imaging may be required.

MRI is the imaging gold standard and allows for detection of pre-radiographic changes of SpA and can serve as a biomarker for active disease. Indications for MRI include those with normal or equivocal plain radiographic findings. In addition, patients who demonstrate positive findings on plain radiographs can also be considered for MRI if a baseline assessment of the extent of acute and chronic changes with the sacroiliac joints and spine is required. In patients who are unresponsive to treatment regimes and with ongoing clinical uncertainty, MRI may be beneficial in assessing whether there is ongoing inflammatory change and to exclude alternate pathologies.

CT and MRI in Alternate SIJ Pathology

Osteitis condensans ilii (OCI) is more common than SpA affecting up to 2.5 % of the population. It is a benign pathology presenting usually in young to middle-aged adults with bilateral subchondral sclerosis related to the sacroiliac joints. It is most common in multiparous females but is also identified in males and nulliparous females. It is thought to be a reactive change with bone remodelling with lamellar bone secondary to mechanical stress at the sacroiliac joints. Patients may be symptomatic or it may be identified as an incidental finding on imaging. Symptoms, if present, are usually of a chronic mechanical low back pain. Inflammatory markers are negative, and there is no association with HLA-B27. Radiographs demonstrate subchondral sclerosis anteroinferiorly with a triangular configuration most pronounced within the ilium. It is usually bilateral and symmetrical, but unilateral involvement has been described. There is no joint space narrowing and no erosions. If there is classical appearance on radiographs in asymptomatic individuals, no further follow-up is required. CT demonstrates the same findings albeit in greater detail (Fig. 6.34). On MRI sclerosis is low signal intensity on both T1 and T2. There is no bone marrow oedema, erosions or post-inflammatory fat accentuation.

CT is useful in diagnosing *SIJ infection* and may identify unilateral changes suggesting the diagnosis. Review of the examination on soft tissue windows is essential lest soft tissue abnormalities be missed. Changes involving the sacroiliac joint include widening of the joint cleft with erosions, thinning of the periarticular fatty tissue layer, increase in size of adjacent muscles and abscess formation. CT however may appear normal in the early course of the disease. Therefore in the relevant clinical setting, more sensitive imaging modalities in the acute phase including MRI should be employed (Fig. 6.35). Anterior and/or posterior subperiosteal infiltrations of juxtaarticular muscle layers are characteristics of septic SII on MRI and could be used to differentiate septic arthritis from SII in spondyloarthropathy. Fluoroscopic or CT-guided joint aspiration may also be beneficial in confirming the diagnosis and may be crucial in planning appropriate antimicrobial therapy.

CT and MRI may be invaluable in assessing and staging tumours at or about the SIJ. Bone destruction and soft tissue masses can be readily identified. The differentiation between benign and malignant bone lesions is usually possible. CT has a well-established role in the management of patients with pelvic trauma. It is the preferred imaging modality for assessing bone injury. CT and MRI may be invaluable in the diagnosis of insufficiency fractures. These fractures most commonly occur in elderly females with osteoporosis (Fig. 6.36). The osteopenia makes assessment of plain X-rays difficult. The diagnosis can be confirmed by CT, which demonstrates patchy sclerosis, often with fissure-like fractures and no associated soft tissue mass. The absence of an associated mass makes it possible to differentiate an insufficiency fracture from a metastatic lesion, which is often a clinical dilemma in these patients. Other pathologies that may be associated with joint resorption should also be considered in the differential diagnosis, including renal osteodystrophy and hyperparathyroidism (Fig. 6.37), as well as erosive arthropathies such as rheumatoid arthritis. Degenerative disc disease and transitional vertebrae are common aetiologies for low back pain and may be associated with degenerative changes in the sacroiliac joints. Both entities are reviewed in detail in Chap. 15.

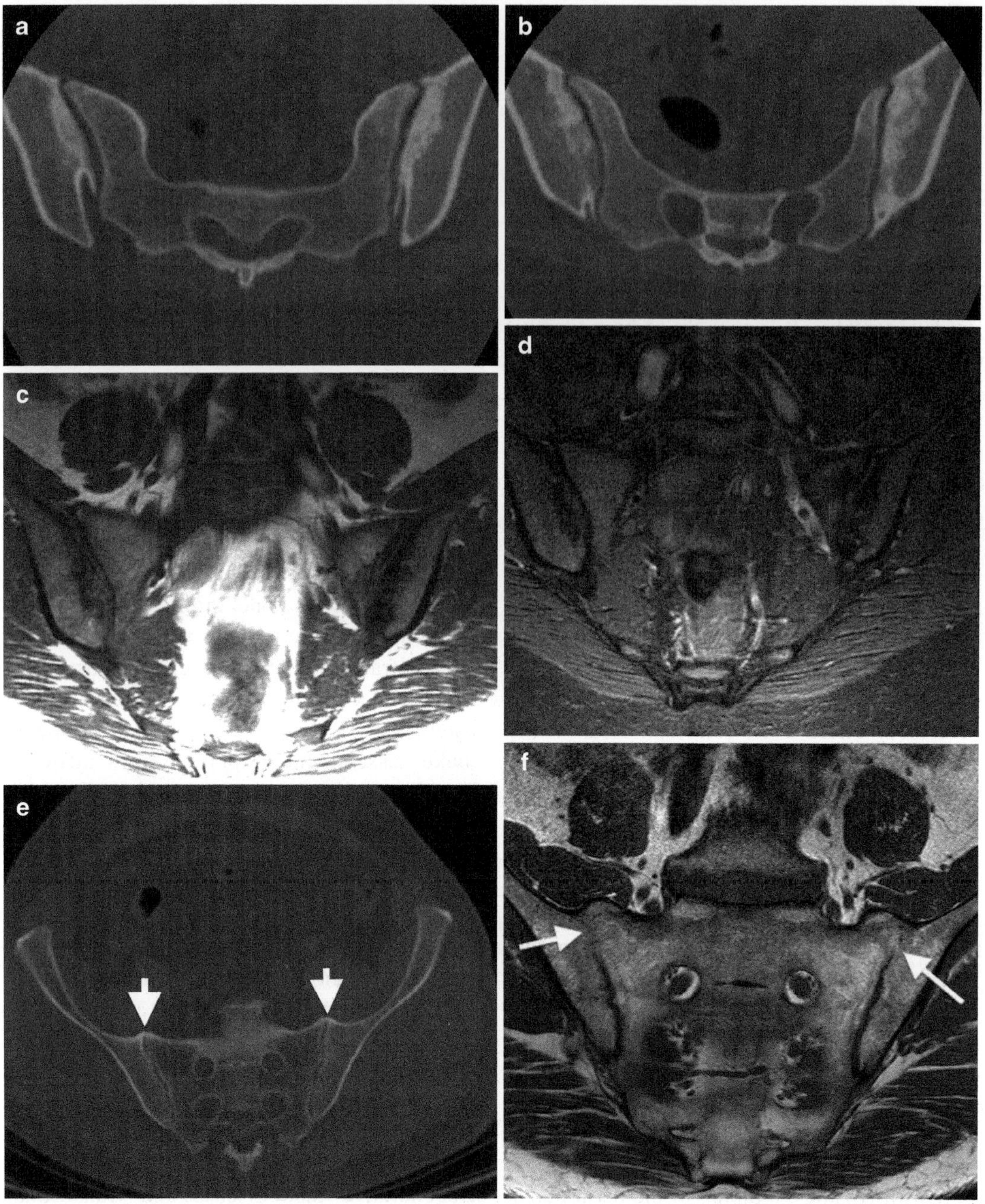

Fig. 6.34 (**a**) & (**b**) OSI in a 34-year-old female with subchondral sclerosis without joint space loss or erosions on axial CT, (**c**) Cor T1 and (**d**) Cor T2FS MRI with bilateral subchondral iliac sclerosis in keeping with OCI, (**e, f**) DISH in a 66-year-old female with ossification of the anterior SIJ capsule and ligaments (*arrows*), note ossification is more extensive superiorly with a normal inferior SIJ, (**e**) Cor T1 MRI in a patient with DISH with ossification of the superior SIJs and normal inferior joint space

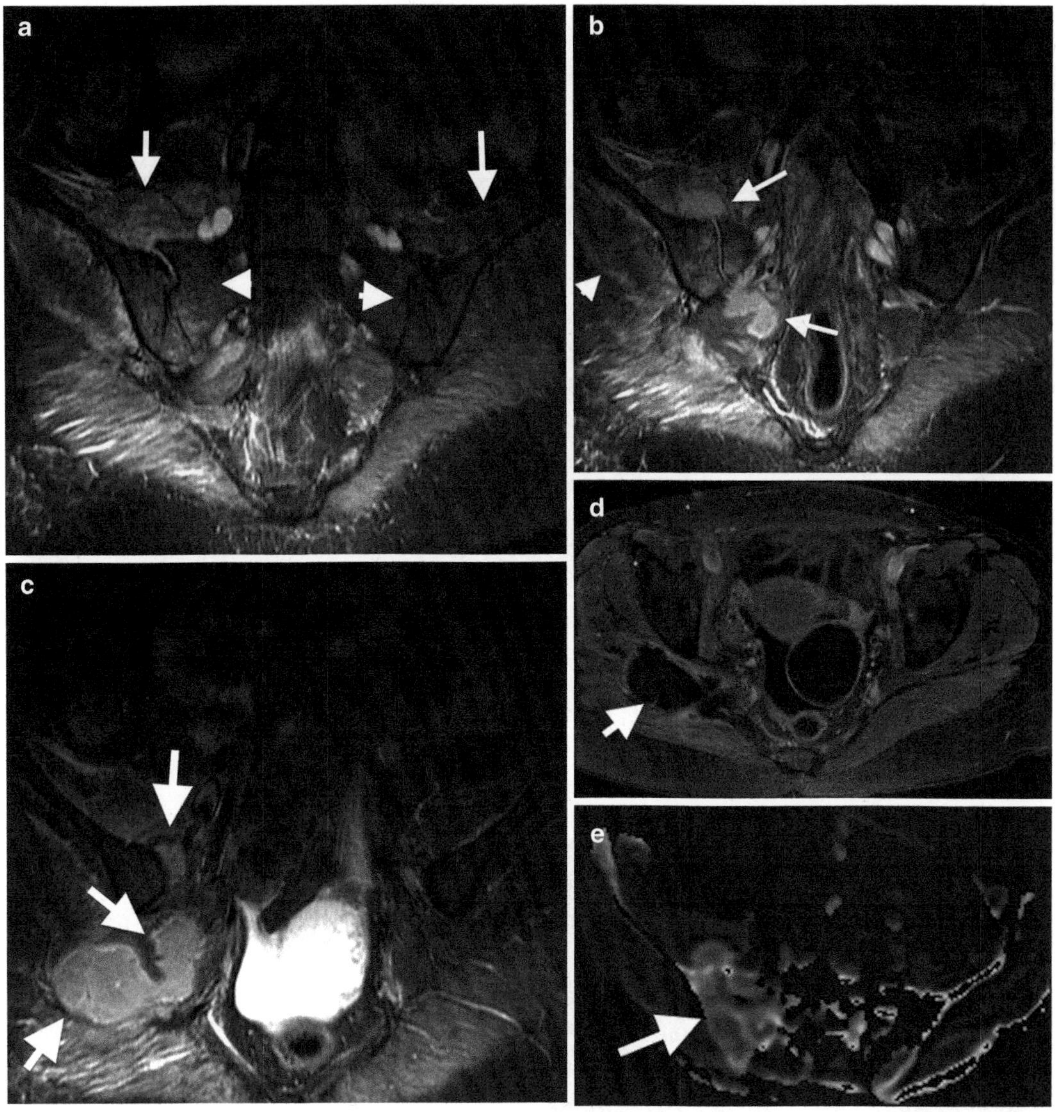

Fig. 6.35 A 35-year-old female with SLE on steroids developed acute onset of right sacroiliac joint pain with limited range of motion and fever, (**a**) Cor T2FS demonstrates periarticular right SIJ osteitis (*right arrowhead*) and surrounding myositis (*right arrow*), note normal contralateral side, (**b**) Cor T2FS with periarticular high SI collections (*arrows*) extending superiorly and inferiorly from right SIJ and surrounding myositis (*arrowhead*), (**c**) more anterior image from (**b**), (**d**) periarticular collection is low SI on this axial T1FS PG with thin rim enhancement (*arrow*), (**e**) ADC and (**f**) exponential diffusion demonstrate restricted diffusion (low SI ADC and high SI on exponential) within periarticular collections in keeping with pus (*arrow*). (**g**) AP SIJ on 6-month follow-up with chronic right SIJ changes including joint space loss, erosions and subchondral sclerosis and (**h**) corresponding Cor T1 image

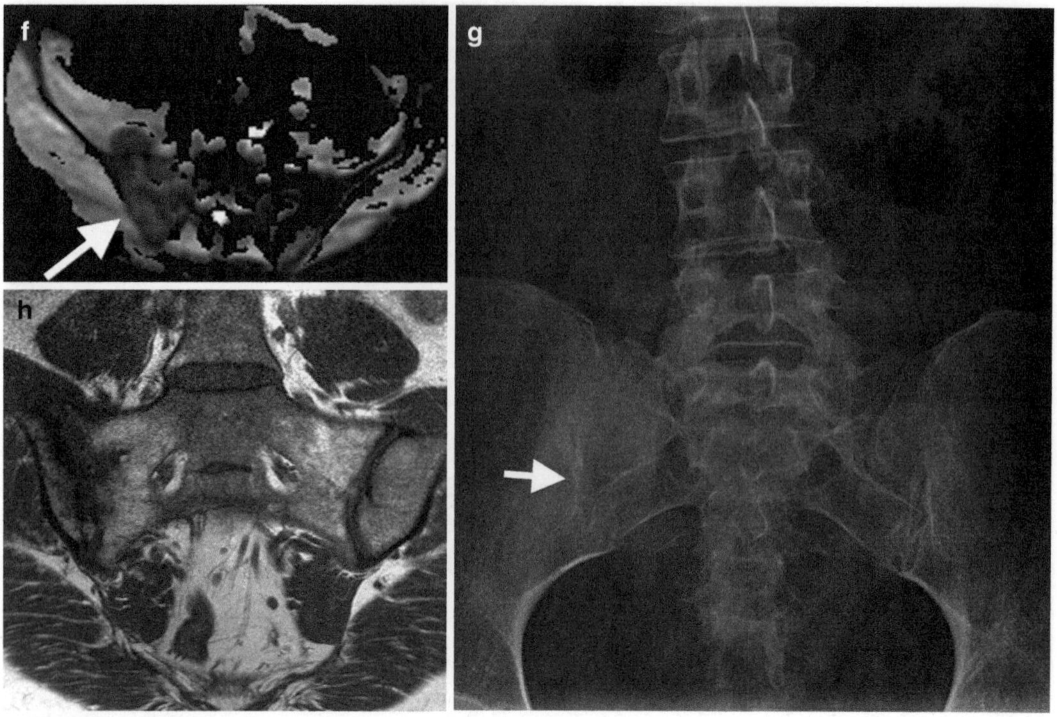

Fig. 6.35 (continued)

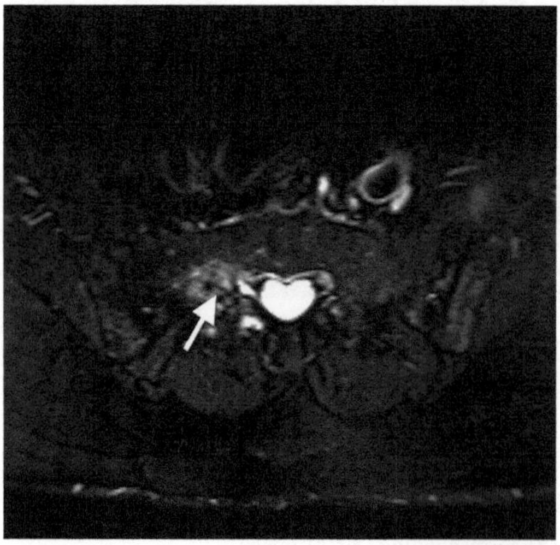

Fig. 6.36 A 55-year-old female with inflammatory back pain, superior sacral insufficiency fracture (*arrow*) with surrounding oedema on axial T2 STIR performed as part of spondylitis MRI protocol

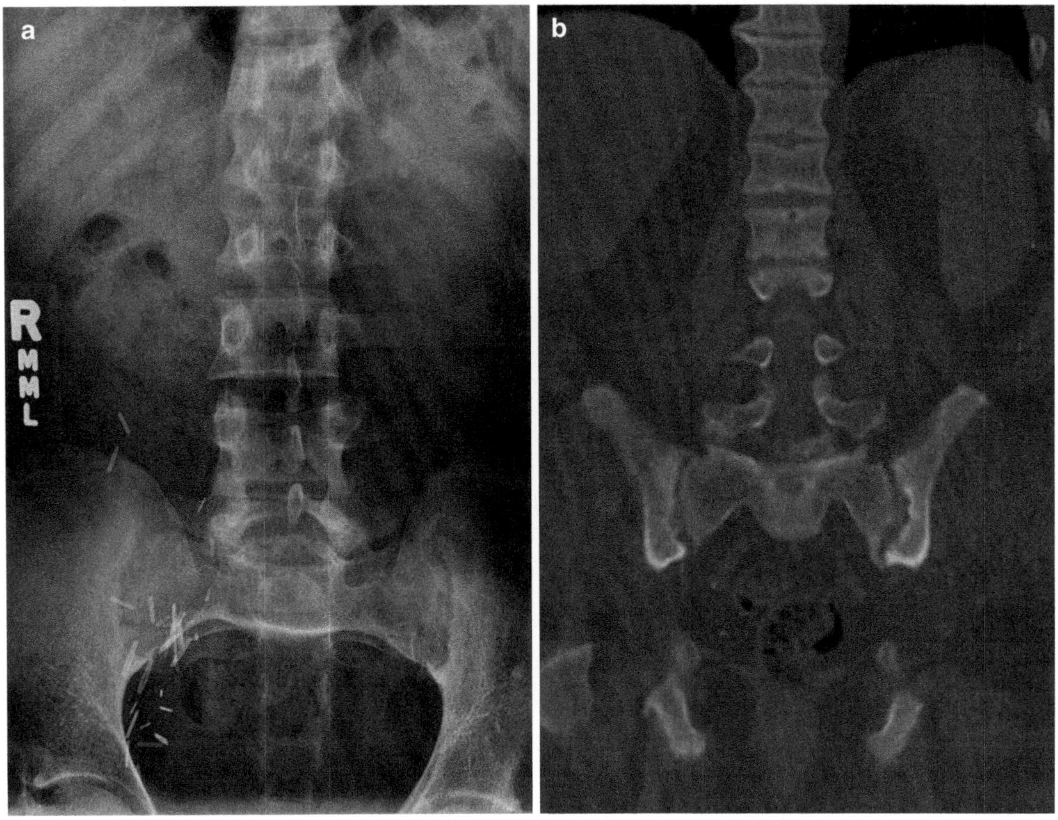

Fig. 6.37 AP lumbar spine demonstrates multiple surgical clips of the right iliac fossa in keeping with history of renal transplant in a 25-year-old male patient. Note the widened sacroiliac joints with pronounced inferior resorption secondary to hyperparathyroidism. (**b**) A 44-year-old male with chronic end-stage renal failure with renal osteodystrophy, resorption of SIJ on Cor reformatted CT

Further Reading

1. Ahlstrom H, Feltelius N, Nyman R, Hallgren R. Magnetic resonance imaging of sacroiliac joint inflammation. Arthritis Rheum. 1990;33(12):1763–9.
2. Ehrenfeld M. Spondyloarthropathies. Best Pract Res Clin Rheumatol. 2012;26(1):135–45.
3. Muche B, Bollow M, Francois RJ, et al. Anatomic structures identified in early and late stage sacroiliitis and spondyloarthritis. A detailed analysis by contrast-enhanced magnetic resonance imaging. Arthritis Rheum. 2003;48(5):1374–84.
4. Navallas M, Ares J, Beltrán B. Sacroiliitis associated with axial spondyloarthropathy: new concepts and latest trends. Radiographics. 2013;33(4):933–56.
5. Puhakka KB, Jurik AG, Egund N, et al. Imaging of sacroiliitis in early seronegative spondyloarthropathy. Acta Radiol. 2003;44:218–29.
6. Puhakka KB, Melsen F, Jurik AG, et al. MR Imaging of the normal sacroiliac joint with correlation to histology. Skeletal Radiol. 2004;33:15–28.
7. Resnick D. AS. In: Resnick D, editors. Diagnosis of bone and joint disorders. 4th ed. Philadelphia: WB Saunders Co. Ltd. p. 1023–81.
8. Reveille JD. Epidemiology of spondyloarthritis in North America. Am J Med Sci. 2011;341(4):284–6.
9. van Tubergen A, Weber U. Diagnosis and classification in spondyloarthritis: identifying a chameleon. Nat Rev Rheumatol. 2012;8(5):253–61.
10. Weber U, Lambert RG, Østergaard M. The diagnostic utility of magnetic resonance imaging in spondyloarthritis: an international multicenter evaluation of one hundred eighty-seven subjects. Arthritis Rheum. 2010;62(10):3048–58.

7 Connective Tissue Disease

Leilani Famorca and John O'Neill

Systemic Lupus Erythematosus

Overview

Systemic lupus erythematosus (SLE) is a multiorgan autoimmune disease arising from dysregulation in the immune system. The disease process begins when a genetically susceptible individual is exposed to an environmental trigger, i.e., infection, which in turn triggers the process of antinuclear antibody production. This process starts the deposit of immune complex materials in various organs that can initiate an inflammatory process. Furthermore, B- and T-cell abnormal signaling promotes this immune activation.

Due to its multisystem involvement, there is related significant morbidity and mortality. SLE affects women nine times more than men, and the severity differs between ethnic groups.

Diagnosis is based on clinical history, physical examination, laboratory testing, biomarkers, imaging of the involved organs, and biopsy. Identified autoantibodies correlated to this disease include antinuclear antibodies (95 %), anti-double-stranded DNA, anti-SM, anti-RNP in correlation with mixed connective tissue disease, anti-SSA/anti-SSB for Sjogren-related lupus, and anti-ribosomal P in neuropsychiatric lupus.

The ACR (American College of Rheumatology) criteria aid in the classification of SLE. It may have its inherent weaknesses due to the myriad of symptoms of this disease. A recently new classification criterion, the SLICC (Systemic Lupus International Collaborating Clinics Classification Criteria), has been developed (Table 7.1) due to the complex multiorgan involvement in this disease process. We will separately review each involved system below.

Musculoskeletal System

Musculoskeletal involvement is one of the most common manifestations of SLE with an incidence ranging from 65 to 95 %. Arthritis is characterized as migratory, with associated swelling almost similar to that of rheumatoid arthritis involving the wrists, metacarpophalangeal (MCP), interphalangeal, (IP) and knee joints. Generally they are nondeforming and nonerosive; however, about 5–15 % may develop a deforming arthropathy (Fig. 7.1).

Jaccoud's arthropathy is a classic example of a deforming arthropathy related to ligament and tendon laxity resulting from capsular and periarticular

L. Famorca, MD (✉)
Division of Rheumatology, McMaster University, Cambridge, ON N3H4L5, Canada
e-mail: leilani.famorca@medportal.ca

J. O'Neill, MB, BAO, BCh, MRCPI, MSc, FRCR
Associate Professor, Musculoskeletal Imaging, Diagnostic Imaging, McMaster University/
St Joseph's Healthcare,
Hamilton, ON L8N4A6, Canada
e-mail: joneill2@me.com

J. O'Neill (ed.), *Essential Imaging in Rheumatology*,
DOI 10.1007/978-1-4939-1673-3_7, © Springer Science+Business Media New York 2015

Table 7.1 Clinical and immunologic criteria for SLICC

Clinical criteria	Immunologic criteria
1. Acute cutaneous lupus	1. ANA
2. Chronic cutaneous lupus	2. Double-stranded DNA
3. Oral or nasal ulcers	3. Anti-SM
4. Non-scarring alopecia	4. Antiphospholipid antibody
5. Arthritis	5. Low complement (C3, C4, CH50)
6. Serositis	6. Direct Coombs test (do not count in the presence of hemolytic anemia)
7. Renal	
8. Neurologic	
9. Hemolytic anemia	
10. Leukopenia	
11. Thrombocytopenia	

From Petri M, Orbai AM, Alarcon G et al. Derivation and Validation of the Systemic Lupus International Collaborating Clinics Classification Criteria for Systemic Lupus Erythematosus. *Arthritis and Rheumatism* 2012:64:8:2677–2686

Requirements >4 criteria (at least one clinical and one laboratory or biopsy proven lupus nephritis with (+) ANA or anti-dsDNA)

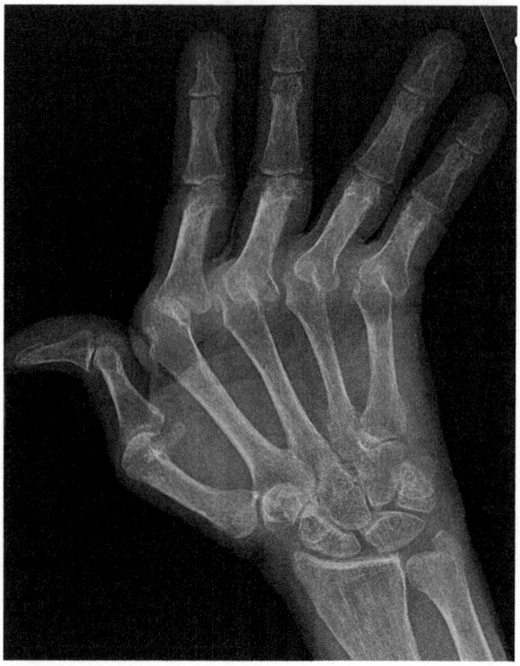

Fig. 7.1 A 49-year-old female with systemic lupus erythematosus, AP radiograph shows subluxations at the second to fifth MCPJs and Jaccoud's arthropathy. Features were bilateral and symmetrical. Note also swan neck deformity thumb, periarticular prominence of a generalized osteopenia. This patient also had clinical features of rheumatoid arthritis; note the periarticular erosion on the radial margin second metacarpal head. Erosions are rarely reported in SLE, and if present an alternate diagnosis or a second arthritis should be considered as in this case

fibrosis and synovial vasculitis. The interplay of inflammatory cells and the presence of cytokines such as IL1 and IL6 play a role in its pathogenesis. Radiographic feature reveals joint deviation with MCP joint subluxation and ulnar deviation without erosions involving the second to fifth MCPJ. This was initially described in patients post-rheumatic fever but is now more commonly seen in SLE and mixed connective disease. In addition, reversible swan neck deformity of the thumb may be present, hyperextension at the IP joint, and flexion at the MCP joint.

In patients with erosive features, this may be related to Rhupus syndrome whereby the patient has clinical features of SLE overlapping with rheumatoid arthritis (Fig. 7.1). Rhupus patients initially present with characteristics that of rheumatoid arthritis (RA) but later on present with clinical and laboratory features of SLE. Hormonal factors may play a role in its pathogenesis. Biomarkers of RA such as rheumatoid factor and anti-CCP (anti-citrullinated peptide) are also noted. Rhupus arthropathy is a symmetrical polyarthritis which could lead to debilitating deformities. Radiographic features may show marginal erosions similar to that in rheumatoid arthritis. Dystrophic soft tissue calcification (Fig. 7.2) may occur with skin and periarticular deposition. Imaging findings are reviewed in detail in Chap. 16. Ultrasound features include synovial hypertrophy, joint effusion, and erosions. Tenosynovitis and tendinosis may be present and is related to an increased risk of tendon rupture (Fig. 7.3). Magnetic resonance imaging (MRI) provides optimal images for bone edema, erosions, and soft tissue involvement such as capsular swelling, synovial hypertrophy, and tenosynovitis (Fig. 7.4).

Osteonecrosis is defined as "bone death" resulting from arterial blood supply compromise. It affects about 13 % of patients, usually involving the femoral head, humeral head, tibial plateau, and scaphoid. The patient may be asymptomatic or may develop vague pain on joint movement or

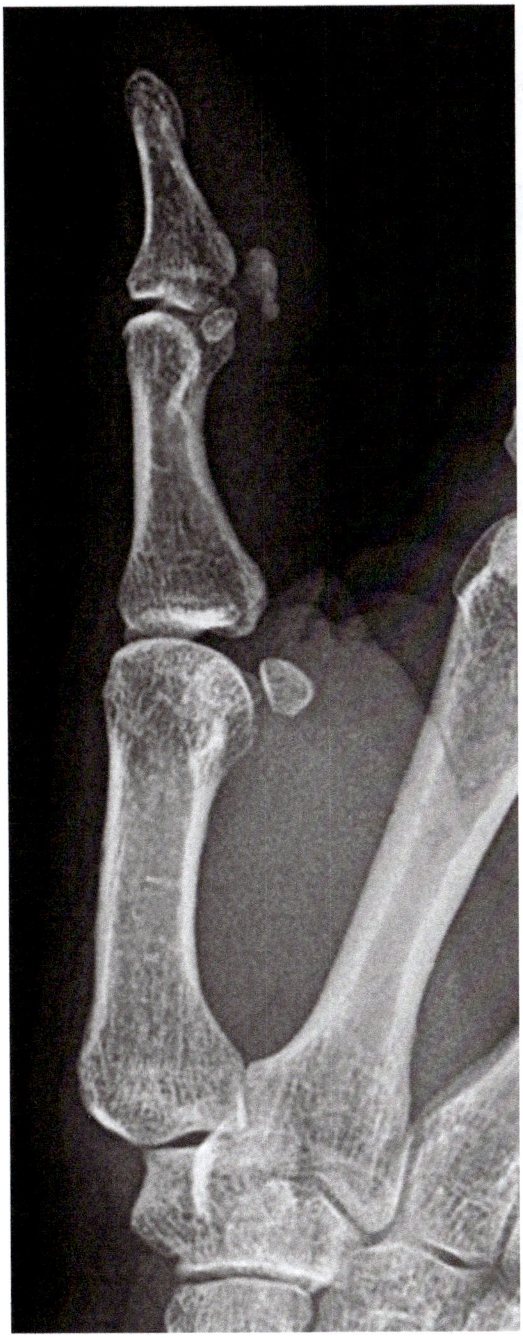

Fig. 7.2 A 34-year-old female systemic lupus erythematosus demonstrating soft tissue calcification on the volar aspect on the 1st interphalangeal joint

sudden severe pain over the affected joint due to collapse. Corticosteroid use may be the most common etiology; however, vasculitis, embolic phenomenon, and antiphospholipid syndrome are

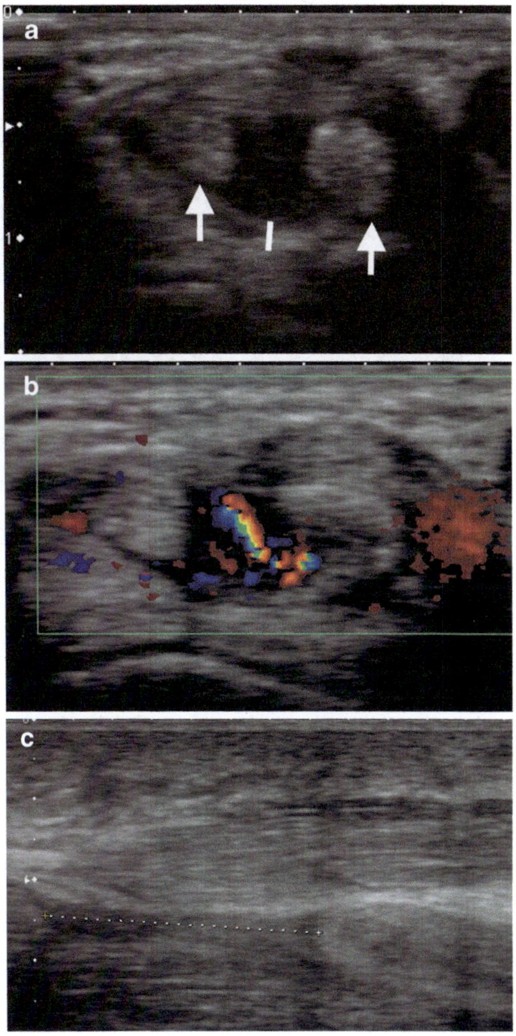

Fig. 7.3 A 42-year-old female with long-standing SLE presenting with acute tenosynovitis, (**a**) transverse ultrasound dorsal wrist, fourth extensor compartment, with enlarged tendons with heterogeneous echotexture (*arrows*) and tendon sheath distension (*line*); (**b**) marked increased flow within the tendon sheath in keeping with active synovitis; and (**c**) different patient with rupture flexor pollicis longus tendon, separated tendon ends indicated by a *dashed line*

possible etiologies. Imaging features of osteonecrosis are reviewed in Chap. 12.

Myalgia is a common manifestation of SLE. Myositis is less common, 7–15 %. Proximal muscle weakness is the usual manifestation associated with elevated muscle enzymes, and EMG findings of spontaneous fibrillations, positive potentials, small amplitude, polyphasic potentials,

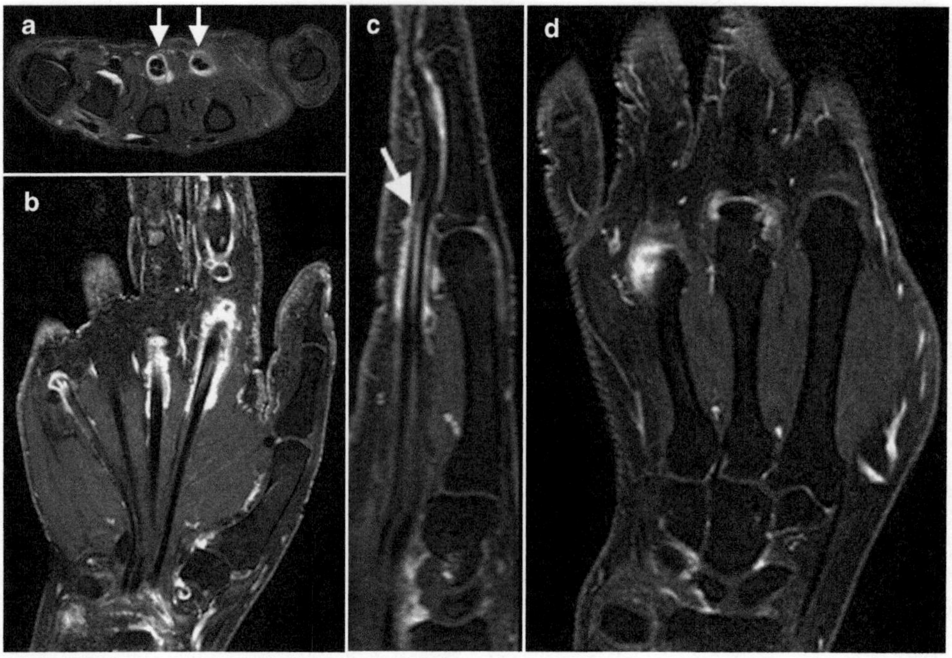

Fig. 7.4 A 62-year-old female with systemic lupus erythematosus presenting with persistent left hand pain. Multiplanar MRI imaging sequences including post-gadolinium study. (**a**) Axial T2FS reveals diffuse to moderate second and third common flexor tenosynovitis (*arrows*) and mild effusion at the fourth metacarpophalangeal joint. (**b**) Cor T1FS PG demonstrates enhancement of the second, third, and fifth common flexor sheath (tenosynovitis) and (**c**) third flexor tenosynovitis (*arrow*) on Sag T1Fs. (**d**) Cor T1FSPG demonstrates active synovitis at the third and fourth MCPJs and periarticular erosion of the third metacarpal head

and repetitive high frequency potentials are seen similar to patients with polymyositis. Biopsy findings include interstitial inflammation, fibrillar necrosis, and degeneration. MRI findings reveal hyperintense signal in myositis on T2, which may enhance post gadolinium.

Central Nervous System (CNS) and Peripheral Nervous System (PNS)

CNS and PNS involvement in SLE may present in different patterns which includes seizures, psychosis, aseptic meningitis, stroke, myelopathy, and neuropathy. Diagnoses and treatment has been a challenge, and determining the immunopathology of neuropsychiatric systemic lupus erythematosus (NPSLE) is restricted due to reluctance in doing brain biopsies. Biopsies however have been the gold standard with pathology demonstrating necrosis of the vasculature, disruptions of the elastic lamina, with inflammatory cell infiltration, and the presence of thrombi. Diagnosis is based on clinical presentation, spinal fluid analysis, serum biomarkers, as well as imaging. I will be outlining more of the neurologic rather than the psychiatric imaging in NPSLE.

Magnetic Resonance Imaging (MRI)

Magnetic resonance imaging is more sensitive and the most useful imaging for both cerebrovascular and spinal pathologies. Small vessel cerebrovascular involvement in NPSLE shows white matter lesions and periventricular hyperintensities on T2. T2 FLAIR provides greater conspicuity of lesions. T1-weighted sequences may be normal or demonstrate subtle hypointensity. Periventricular lesions are noted to be associated with antiphospholipid syndrome (APS). This however may mimic many other white matter diseases, and findings have to be reviewed in the correct clinical context (Fig. 7.5). Enhanced studies may be

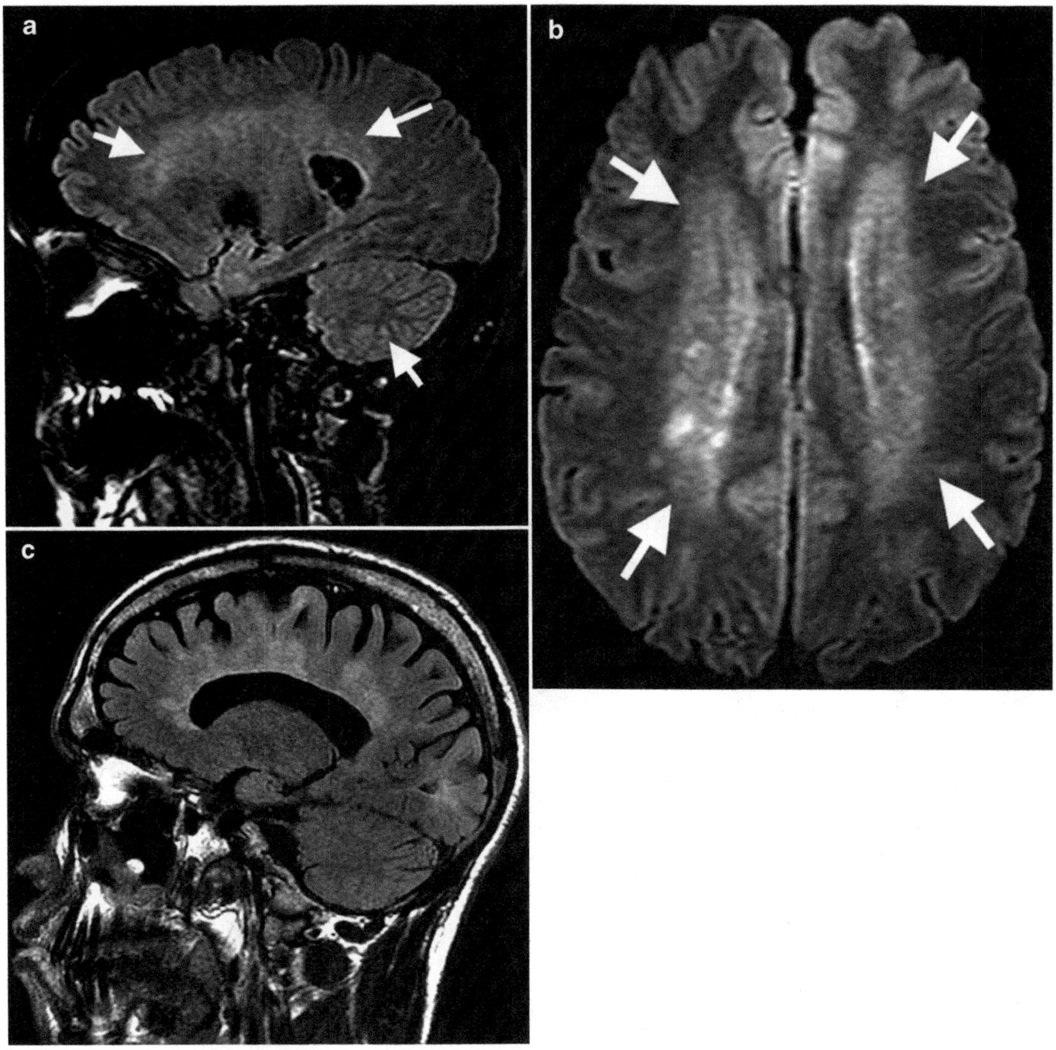

Fig. 7.5 A 29-year-old female with SLE cerebral vasculitis (**a**) sagittal and (**b**) axial T2 FLAIR demonstrates periventricular and deep white matter high signal intensity (*arrows*). Note that imaging findings need correlation with clinical picture. Similar findings in patient with multiple sclerosis (**c**)

beneficial in differentiating between acute and chronic lesions. Due to rapid reversibility of some of these lesions at times, prompt timing of imaging is crucial. Reversible neurologic deficits may also be present in SLE and may reveal T2-weighted sequences of demyelination in the periventricular areas, corpus callosum, and cerebellar area. Hemorrhage may also occur. Large vascular infarcts are less common and occur in a vascular territory. MRI best delineates the extent of involvement with high SI on T2 and restricted diffusion in the acute stage. PRES, posterior reversible encephalopathy, present with hypertension, headaches, and neurologic symptoms related usually to the posterior circulation. MRI is the diagnostic study of choice and demonstrates reversible high SI lesions of the parietal and occipital lobes (Fig. 7.6). Occasionally infarction may occur. Patients with antiphospholipid syndrome in particular may develop venous thrombosis of the venous sinuses and deep cerebral veins.

About 1–2 % of patients develop transverse myelitis. This presents with a rapid onset of motor, sensory, and autonomic dysfunction. This

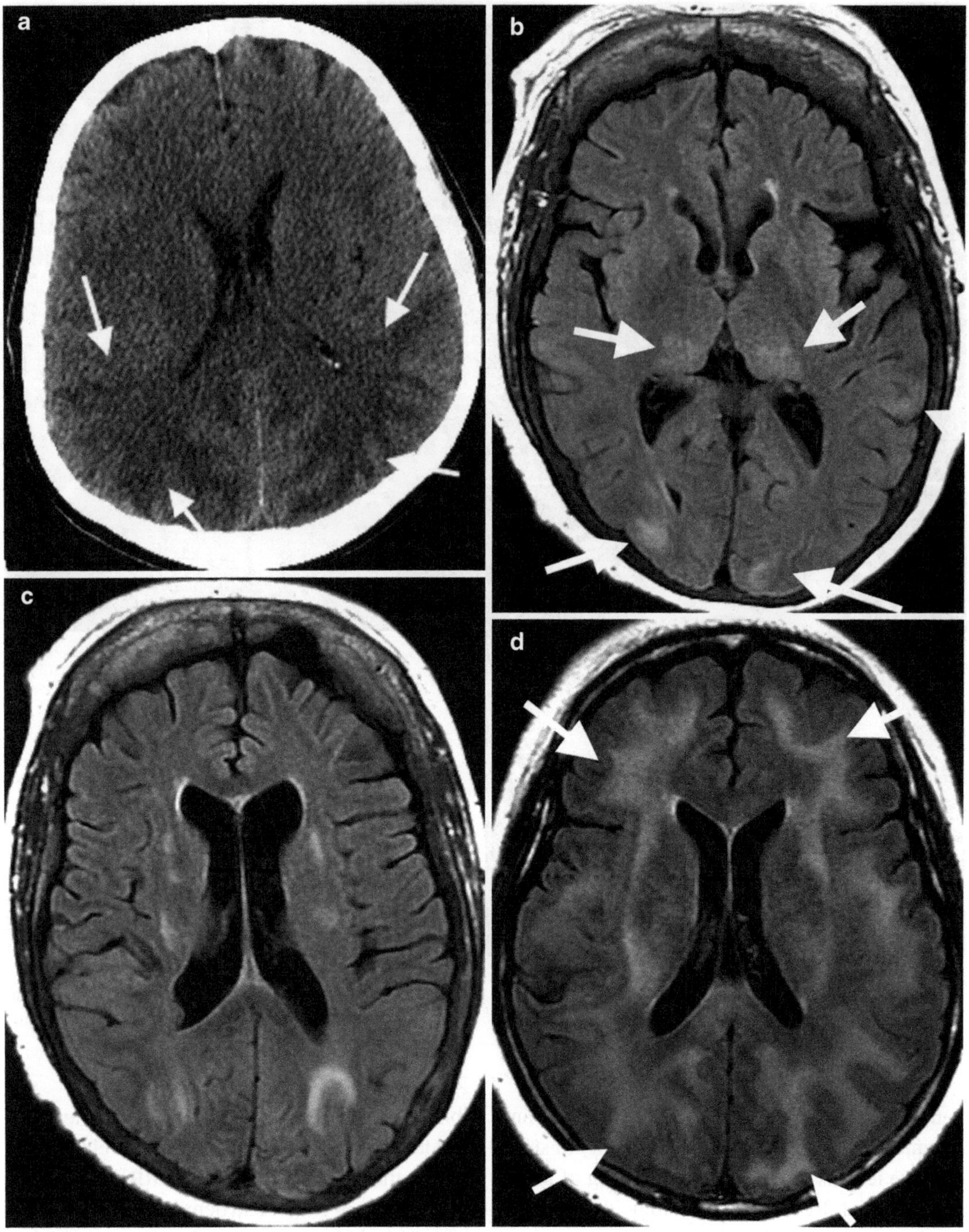

Fig. 7.6 Axial CT of a 25-year-old female with history of SLE with features of PRES on (**a**) axial CT with extensive posterior circulation deep white matter low attenuation and (**b**, **c**) a different patient on axial T2 FLAIR MRI with posterior circulation high signal intensity (*arrows*). (**d**) Chronic lupus cerebritis with superimposed hypertensive crisis and PRES on axial T2 FLAIR (*arrows*) (Kindly submitted by Dr. Judith Coret-Simon, St. Joseph's Healthcare, Hamilton, Ontario, Canada)

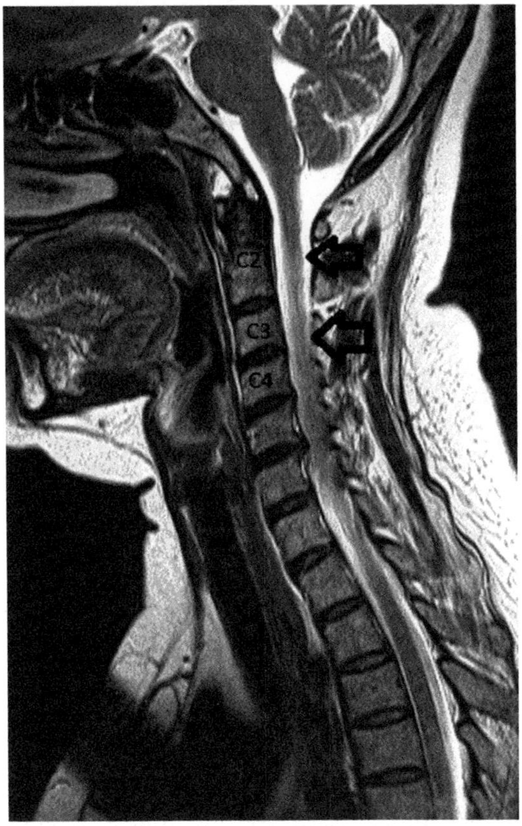

Fig. 7.7 A 56-year-old female with systemic lupus erythematosus presenting with numbness of all extremities, left arm weakness, and ataxia. MRI of the cervical spine revealed a high T2 signal abnormality contiguously affecting *C1–C4* segments of the cervical cord consistent with transverse myelitis (*black arrows*)

is usually correlated with positive antinuclear antibodies and anti-double-stranded DNA. Edema and a hyperintense signal in the spinal cord are present on T2 MRI (Fig. 7.7).

Magnetic Resonance Spectroscopy (MRS)

MRS is a noninvasive imaging procedure that involves biochemical metabolites or neuronal markers such as N-acetylaspartate (NAA), creatine/phosphocreatine, and choline which are quantified in the brain. In the majority of NPSLE, decreased NAA is noted. However these findings are seen in degenerative brain pathologies. Reversibility after treatment would distinguish this from the latter. MRS may be utility as well in monitoring progression of NPSLE. At present, it's more a clinical tool for research.

Single-Photon Emission Computed Tomography (SPECT) and Positron Emission Tomography (PET)

SPECT measures cerebral perfusion using radiolabeled tracers. There has been conflicting data however about its utility. Patchy diffuse hypoperfusion is characteristic of this disease. Focal lesions are noted in patients with a longer duration of disease usually noted in the parietal and temporal lobe and occasionally in the basal ganglia. SPECT could detect abnormalities long before the development of irreversible impairment. PET measures the metabolic activity including glucose uptake and oxygen utilization. In SLE, the most frequent finding is hypometabolism in the parietal area and parieto-occipital area. PET may demonstrate widespread regional increases and decreases in brain glucose uptake. This imaging device has been advocated to be more sensitive than MRI especially with subtle changes in NPSLE. Limitations of PET include cost and the duration of the test. Further clinical studies are required to evaluate its position in the imaging algorithm in clinical practice.

CAT Scan (CT)

The role of CT remains to be unclear in NPSLE. It is usually performed in the acute presentation of neurologic deficits to exclude infarction or intracranial hemorrhage. CT however is significantly less sensitive than MRI for the assessment of white matter lesions.

Angiogram

Central nervous system vasculitis in SLE is a secondary type of vasculitis. The role of angiogram may be valuable if findings are present such as typical stenosis or occlusion "beading pattern" of the vessels. However magnetic resonance angiography has superseded formal angiograms.

Pulmonary and Cardiovascular System

Pulmonary involvement in SLE can present in varying degrees involving the respiratory vasculature, airways, pleura, parenchyma, and surrounding including the diaphragm. Pleural effusions and pericardial effusion are common. *Acute pneumonitis* is an uncommon manifestation of SLE that may present with a clinical picture of dyspnea with productive cough plus or minus hemoptysis, tachypnea, and basal crepitations. Diagnostic investigation through bronchioalveolar lavage is key in ruling out infection. Pathology shows diffuse interstitial lymphocytic infiltration, bronchiolitis, hyaline membrane formation, alveolar hemorrhage, arterial thrombi, and interstitial edema. Furthermore, immune complex deposition may be found. Chest radiographs may demonstrate migratory pulmonary infiltrates, diffuse acinar infiltrates with predilection to the bases, or pleural effusions. Cavitary infiltrates and consolidation are unusual features in SLE pneumonitis. CT shows a ground glass appearance due to alveolitis and honeycombing and subpleural thickening in pulmonary fibrosis in chronic disease (Fig. 7.8). Gallium scintigraphy involves measuring damage through alveolar membrane permeability in a slope time activity curve from the dynamic lung imaging. Increase uptake may be noted.

Pulmonary hypertension involving the pulmonary vasculature can be a life-threatening complication with prevalence between 0.5 and 14 %. Its pathogenesis is thought to be related to recurrent pulmonary embolism, particularly in antiphospholipid syndrome, or chronic pulmonary fibrosis. Manifestations can be nonspecific such as dyspnea, chest pain, nonproductive cough, and jugular venous distension. Radiographic findings can initially be normal. Advanced findings can reveal enlarged central pulmonary arteries with pruning of the distal arteries and enlargement of the right ventricle on both radiographs and CT (Fig. 7.9).

Interstitial lung disease may be in the form of nonspecific interstitial with fibrosis or organizing pneumonia. Clinical presentation may again be nonspecific with fever and a cough usually acute or insidious in onset. Plugs of fibrous tissue are noted in the respiratory bronchioles and alveolar ducts associated with inflammatory infiltrates involving the bronchioles and interstitial tissue. Although radiographic features may show evidence of interstitial lung disease, high-resolution CT better defines the different patterns. Organizing

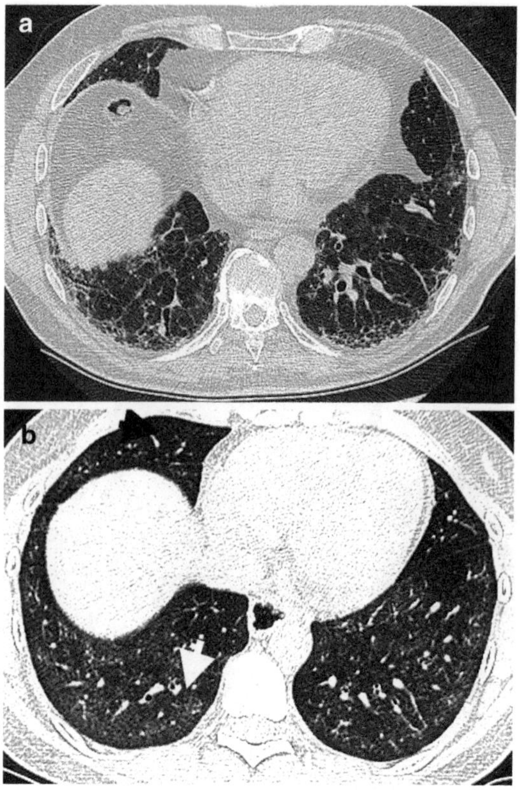

Fig. 7.8 High-resolution CT chest (HRCT) in SLE. (**a**) Chronic fibrosis with honeycombing, subpleural thickening, and mild ground glass attenuation of alveolitis and traction bronchiectasis. (**b**) Different patient with features of NSIP on this axial high-resolution image with bilateral symmetrical ground glass opacities (*arrow*), more pronounced at the lung bases and sparing the subpleural zones

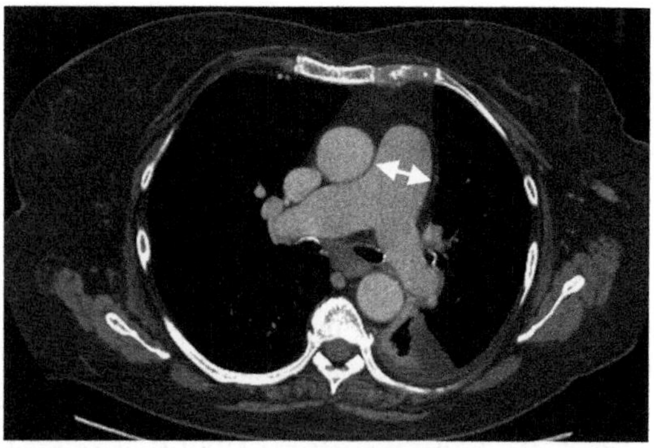

Fig. 7.9 A 52-year-old female with chronic SLE and pulmonary hypertension. Axial-enhanced CT level pulmonary artery bifurcation demonstrates enlargement pulmonary trunk with a transverse diameter of 34 mm (*arrows*) and small left-sided effusion

pneumonia manifests with bilateral ground glass opacities or airspace consolidation with any lung zone being affected. Bilateral airspace consolidation with lymphadenopathy or pleural effusion may also be present. Nonspecific interstitial pneumonia with fibrosis presents as both ground glass appearance and irregular linear opacities, usually bibasilar (Fig. 7.8).

Pulmonary hemorrhage in SLE may present acutely with dyspnea, hypoxemia, and occasionally hemoptysis. A classic triad of hemoptysis, rapid fall in hemoglobin, and new in radiographic infiltrates is highly suspicious of diffuse alveolar hemorrhage. Diffusing capacity carbon monoxide (DLCO) monitoring is highly sensitive for ongoing alveolar hemorrhage. Identification of hemosiderin-laden macrophages through bronchioalveolar lavage is diagnostic. Bilateral alveolar infiltrates are noted on chest radiographs. CT allows for full assessment extent of parenchymal hemorrhage.

Neuromuscular disease and diaphragmatic dysfunction is a rare complication of SLE. The term shrinking lung syndrome has been correlated due its radiographic findings. It may cause significant morbidity and occasional mortality. The etiology is still controversial whether or not it is secondary to diaphragmatic dysfunction secondary to a myopathy, chest wall restriction, or phrenic nerve injury. It manifests as progressive dyspnea, pleuritic chest pain, and fever. Elevated hemidiaphragms are common in chest radiographs. Subsegmental atelectasis and ill-defined opacities above the diaphragm have also been noted. High-resolution CT scans may reveal no parenchymal involvement, elevation of the hemidiaphragms, and atelectatic bands. Pleural effusion may be present.

Cardiovascular manifestation of SLE may be either coronary or non-coronary. Non-coronary manifestation of SLE would involve the valves, endocardium, myocardium, pericardium, and sinoatrial tract causing conduction abnormalities. The prevalence of cardiovascular involvement in SLE can be as high as 50 %.

Libman–Sacks endocarditis also known as "atypical verrucous endocarditis" is the most typical valvular disease. The clinical picture is nonspecific including fever, anemia, tachycardia, and presence of the murmur in either mitral or aortic valve which are generally involved. Patients may be asymptomatic with a new murmur being the only manifestation. A hypothesis of antiphospholipid antibodies and anti endothelial antibodies binding to the endothelial cells causing platelet aggregation and thrombus formation with deposition of these immune complexes into the valvular lining is presently the known pathophysiology. The vegetations could either be active consisting of fibrin clumps and inflammatory cells or healed lesions. Transesophageal echocardiogram is more sensitive in detecting the lesions compared to transthoracic echocardiogram (50–60 % vs 40–50 %). Echocardiogram reveals thickened leaflets with or without regurgitation. Although rare, sequelae of this type of endocarditis include embolic events and chordae tendineae rupture.

Pericardial involvement in SLE is around 26 % as a common manifestation of SLE (Fig. 7.10). Patients complain of a sharp pericardial pain and dyspnea with findings of a pericardial rub, typical ECG findings, and cardiomegaly with well-defined margins on chest radiograph. Echocardiogram is the standard method utilized for diagnosing and quantitating the pericardial effusion. CT scan and MRI may also demonstrate effusion and have an advantage of providing a larger view distinguishing simple fluids from blood, assessing thickness of the pericardium and better characterization of the surrounding struc-

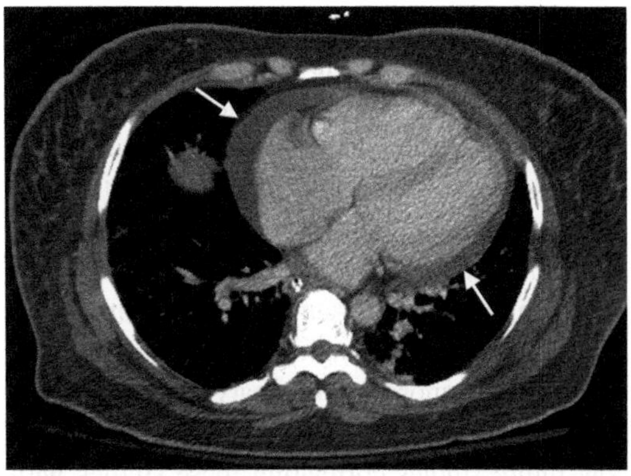

Fig. 7.10 Same patient as in Fig. 7.6 with pericardial effusion (*arrows*) on axial-enhanced CT

tures. Transudative effusions have low signal intensity on T1-weighted images, while hemorrhagic or exudative effusions have medium to high signal intensity on T1 sequences. Cardiac tamponade and constrictive pericarditis are known complications.

Myocarditis in SLE is about 7–10 % of cases likely due to initiation of immediate immunosuppressant therapy. Clinical manifestations are similar to other causes of myocarditis (i.e., infectious or toxic) and would range from resting tachycardia, overt heart failure, or conduction abnormalities. There are some reports showing an association of myocarditis and anti-SSA antibodies. Histologic findings reveal fibrinoid necrosis and infiltration on lymphocytic and plasma cells. Echocardiography is a tool used in assessing cardiac function such as segmental wall abnormalities and ejection fraction. A breakthrough in imaging is the use of cardiac MRI, which is able to detect subtle changes in the myocardium. Increase in T1 and T2 relaxation time of the myocardium is demonstrated in SLE myocarditis. An increase in T2 SI may be an indicator of active myocarditis in the absence of clinical features.

Systemic lupus erythematosus is an independent risk factor for *coronary artery disease*. It has been shown that the relative risk of having a myocardial infarction is 10.6 and that women between 35 and 44 have more chances of a coronary ischemic event. The basis of this phenomenon is accelerated atherosclerosis leading to a thrombotic event usually correlated with corticosteroid use and or the presence of antiphospholipid antibody. Rarely, intimal weakening can lead to aneurysmal dilatation and dissection. The gold standard for evaluating flow limiting arterial lesions is an angiogram with the most common sites involved are the left anterior descending artery and the least affected is the left main artery. Different noninvasive techniques have been proposed such as thallium scintigraphy or sestamibi which evaluates for perfusion defects, CT angiogram assessing for calcification, but moreover coronary calcium scoring has been more predictive for coronary events, and now future studies correlating these studies with SPECT would be valuable in managing these patients. Intravascular ultrasound is also used in assessing for coronary plaque features (stability) with intima–media involvement.

Gastrointestinal System

Different manifestations of gastrointestinal involvement in SLE include pseudo-obstruction, vasculitis, and thrombosis. A few may present with cholecystitis and pancreatitis. Nonspecific abdominal pain may be an initial presentation together with laboratory findings of anemia, leukocytosis, and elevated inflammatory markers. Pathogenesis is drawn from immune complex deposition and immune complex vasculopathy.

Vasculitis in the gastrointestinal tract may result in bowel ischemia, perforation, or hemorrhage. The mesenteric vessels are commonly involved with an evolved term of *lupus mesenteric vasculitis* (LMV). Radiographic findings may include the thumbprint sign indicating submucosal edema or hemorrhage. Furthermore, pneumatosis intestinalis and free air can be noted. CT scan is superior to radiographic imaging in such cases revealing focal or diffuse wall thickening with abnormal enhancement known as "target sign." Other findings include ascites and stenosis with vessel engorgement "comb sign."

Pseudo-obstruction secondary to a SLE is a rare condition secondary to visceral smooth neuromuscular dysfunction as well as autonomic dysfunction. Pathogenesis is unknown, but a vasculitic process may play a role. *Chronic intestinal pseudo-obstruction* (CIPO) is a rare condition as sequelae of loss of peristaltic motility. It can be part of a triad called generalized megaviscera of lupus (GML) with components of CIPO, ureterohydronephrosis, and megacholedochus defined as hepatobiliary hollow viscera dilatation. Radiographic features reveal dilated bowel loops which are further assessed and confirmed through CT scan.

Pancreatitis in SLE has an annual incidence of 0.4–1.1/1,000 lupus patients based on the literature. This condition may be life threatening requiring

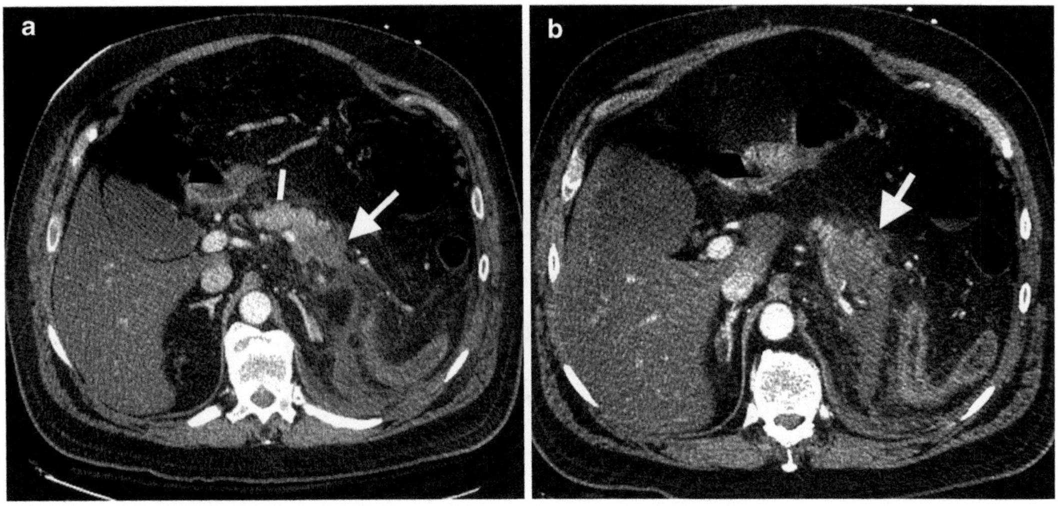

Fig. 7.11 Acute necrotic pancreatitis on axial arterial phase CT through pancreas, (**a**, **b**) note normal pancreatic enhancement proximal body (*line*) and diminished enhancement mid and distal body pancreas (*arrows*). Note also surrounding inflammatory changes

immediate diagnosis and intervention. Ultrasound is usually the first line of investigation and may be normal or demonstrate a hypoechoic pancreatic gland with intra-abdominal fluid. Contrast-enhanced CT is the most useful which helps assess for severity of pancreatitis and its sequelae such as necrosis, peripancreatic collections, and secondary infected collections (Fig. 7.11). MRI would demonstrate similar findings. *Acalculous cholecystitis* in SLE responds well to steroid treatment. Ultrasound demonstrates gallbladder wall thickening and hyperemia without gallbladder calculi. Contrast-enhanced CT may show gallbladder wall enhancement, pericholecystic fluid attenuation, and fat stranding.

Renal System

Renal involvement is a serious complication and a major predictor of poor prognosis. Its incidence and prevalence is higher among Asian, Hispanic, and African ancestry. An immune complex microvascular injury secondary to dsDNA antibody immune complexes and imbalance of cytokine homeostasis plays an important role in its pathogenesis. Renal infarction from renal artery or vein thrombosis may be seen in patients with antiphospholipid syndrome. Renal Doppler ultrasound demonstrates compromised blood flow into the kidneys, and CT scan may reveal lack of contrast medium opacification within the thrombosed vessel and presence of collaterals in chronic cases.

Antiphospholipid Syndrome

One of the manifestations of systemic lupus erythematosus is antiphospholipid syndrome. Antiphospholipid syndrome (APS) is defined as thrombotic and obstetrical complications associated with persistent antiphospholipid antibodies. These thrombotic complications may affect different organ systems involving arterial, venous, and microvascular structures (Fig. 7.12). Recurrent early miscarriages secondary to intraplacental thrombosis are a possible hypothesis leading to fetal loss. These criteria however lack specificity. Placenta-mediated complications are also noted in obstetrical antiphospholipid syndrome. Coagulation assays include the presence of nonspecific inhibitor or immunologic assays that include anticardiolipin antibody or anti-beta 2 glycoprotein that have to be positive in two occasions 12 weeks apart.

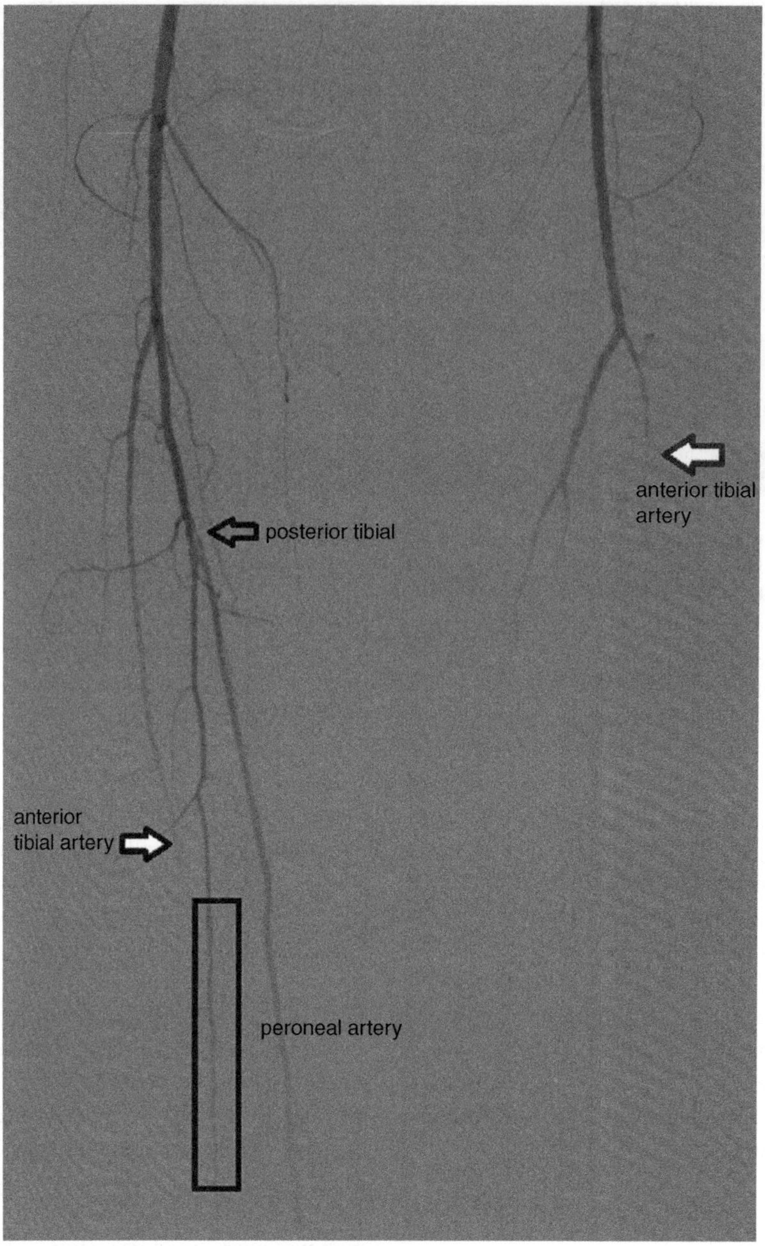

Fig. 7.12 A 36-year-old female with antiphospholipid syndrome presenting with a second left ischemic toe and right foot ulcer. Aortogram with runoffs reveals an intraluminal filling defect from the origin of the right posterior tibial artery consistent with an intravascular thrombus (*outlined black arrow*). Within the mid distal thirds of the right calf, the peroneal artery shows a small caliber with subtle corkscrewing (within black rectangle). Furthermore, right anterior tibial artery shows an abrupt occlusion in the mid-calf area (*black arrow* with *white fill*). The left anterior tibia abruptly occludes within the mid third of the calf (*red arrow*)

Clinical manifestations in patients with systemic lupus erythematosus may vary from stroke-like syndromes, pulmonary embolisms (Fig. 7.13), or deep venous thrombosis and as mentioned obstetrical complications as defined above. Imaging routinely used are CT angiograms showing the occluded segment. Treatment includes lifelong anticoagulation.

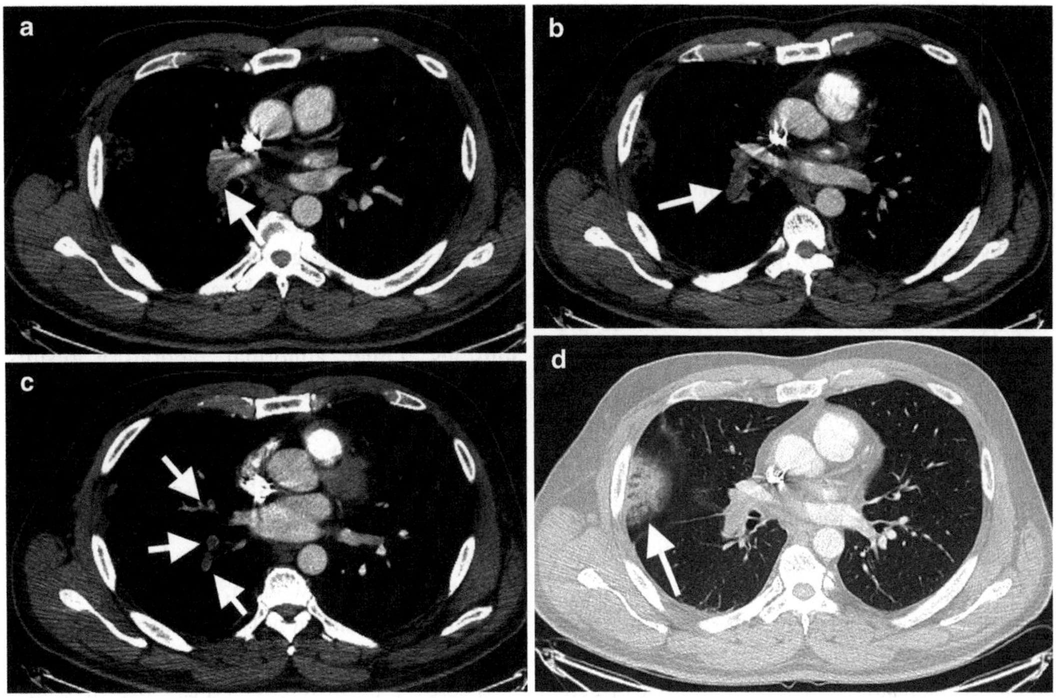

Fig. 7.13 Acute pulmonary embolism in a 28-year-old female with antiphospholipid syndrome. (**a**, **b**, **c**) Axial arterial phase-enhanced CT with acute filling defects (*arrows*) distal right pulmonary artery, right interlobar artery segmental branches, respectively, and (**d**) peripheral parenchymal infarct on lung windows

Mixed Connective Tissue Disease (MCTD)

Mixed connective tissue disease has been defined based on its features of four overlapping disease entities including systemic lupus erythematosus, polymyositis/dermatomyositis, scleroderma, or rheumatoid arthritis plus the presence of a high U1 RNP titer. Mixed connective tissue disease being a distinct disease entity is still controversial. It may involve both children and adults with predominance in women and prevalent in the third decade of life. The most common symptoms on disease onset is Raynaud's 93 % and swollen hands 74 %. Interestingly, through time sclerodactyly replaces the edema phase in the hands. Joint involvement may be similar to that of rheumatoid arthritis with the presence of erosions on imaging. Other clinical features include hypomotility of the esophagus, pulmonary involvement, pleuritis or pericarditis, pulmonary hypertension in 20–30 % of patients, and proximal muscle weakness due to myositis. Radiographic findings of pulmonary involvement are similar to that of systemic sclerosis or polymyositis/dermatomyositis showing an interstitial pattern with peripheral and basal involvement. Furthermore, CT scan findings reveal ground glass opacities or honeycombing with disease progression. Serologic features besides the presence of the RNP antibody may include leukopenia, thrombocytopenia, elevated creatine kinase, and positive anti-dsDNA, anti-SM, anti-SCL-70, anti-citrullinated peptide, and anti-SSA antibodies. Treatment is usually symptom based and may require immunosuppressants.

Inflammatory Myopathies

Overview

Inflammatory myopathies include a spectrum of diseases such as polymyositis, dermatomyositis, and inclusion body myositis. There are various possible etiologies including infectious, toxic, or even drug-induced myositis. In this chapter we will focus on polymyositis (PM) and dermatomyositis (DM), which are, classified as idiopathic inflammatory myopathies. These are rare disorders with an annual occurrence of ten new cases per million persons. An incidence rate of 1.52 per 100,000 person-years for polymyositis and 1.70 for dermatomyositis. An annual prevalence was noted at 20.62–25.32 per 100,000. Female preponderance is 3:1 to males for both dermatomyositis and polymyositis. Dermatomyositis has a close relationship with malignancies. Immune self-reactivity where T lymphocyte reacts to myocytes with increased expression of MHC (major histocompatibility complex) is the basis of its pathogenesis. In polymyositis, CD8+ T cells together with macrophages express spike-like projections in normal muscle fibers which compress and displace the fibers. Furthermore, damage is then augmented by a cytotoxic effector mechanism through the perforin pathway.

Muscle weakness is a characteristic similar to both groups with proximal muscles being more involved than the distal musculature and the lower extremity being more affected than the upper extremity. Some studies have found that polymyositis patients are weaker compared to those with dermatomyositis. Hip flexors, extensors, abductors, neck flexors, and shoulder abductors are the muscle groups with greatest weakness. There are distinguishing clinical features between polymyositis and dermatomyositis.

Patients with dermatomyositis have skin manifestations such as Gottron's papules, which are erythematous eruptions usually, found symmetrically in the metacarpophalangeal and interphalangeal joints. A heliotrope rash is a violaceous eruption on the eyelids; shawl's sign, a diffuse erythematous patch on the neck and anterior chest; and erythroderma, an erythematous rash on the forehead. One common skin manifestation in both idiopathic inflammatory arthropathies is "mechanic's hands" described as cracking or roughening of the skin.

The Dalakas diagnostic criteria have been developed as a tool in the diagnosis (Table 7.2). It has a 77 % sensitivity and 99 % specificity compared to other proposed criteria and emphasized on the importance of histopathology and immunopathology.

Laboratory investigations include utilizing muscle enzymes, and the most commonly performed test is creatine kinase (CK). Besides being a tool for diagnosis, it is used for monitoring disease activity. A more specific isoenzyme of CK is CK MB found in skeletal muscles. Other abnormal laboratory results include aldolase, lactate dehydrogenase, myoglobin, and transaminases (ALT and AST). Furthermore, leukocytosis, elevated erythrocyte sedimentation rate (ESR), C-reactive protein (CRP), and elevated immunoglobulins are other markers of inflammation. CK levels may be higher in men than women, in blacks compared to Caucasians, and in polymyositis compared to dermatomyositis.

There are different types of myositis-associated antibodies in which 50 % of these are found in these inflammatory myopathies (Table 7.3). Its correlation helps predicts future outcomes.

Electromyographic features include short-duration low-amplitude polyphasic motor units and high-frequency repetitive discharges. Biopsy demonstrates perivascular lymphocytic infiltration and endomysial inflammation associated with necrosis and fiber degeneration and regeneration. In dermatomyositis, CD+ 4 T cells and B cells invade the perivascular as well as perifascicular regions with associated perifascicular atrophy. On the other hand, CD+ 8 infiltration of the endomysial region is seen in polymyositis.

Imaging

Magnetic resonance imaging (MRI) is the imaging of choice for inflammatory myopathies and is extremely useful in selecting the appropriate area for biopsy.

MRI sequences include axial, short tau inversion recovery (STIR), or fat-suppressed T2-weighted

Table 7.2 Dalakas diagnostic criteria

	Polymyositis		Myopathic dermatomyositis		Amyopathic dermatomyositis
Criterion	Definite	Probable	Definite	Probable	Definite
Muscle weakness	Yes	Yes	Yes	Yes	No
Electromyographic findings	Myopathic	Myopathic	Myopathic	Myopathic	Myopathic or nonspecific
Muscle enzymes	High (up to 50× normal)	High (up to 50× normal)	High (up to 50× normal) or normal	High	High (up to 10 times normal) or normal
Muscle biopsy findings	Primary inflammation, with CD8/MCH1 complex and no vacuoles	Ubiquitous MHC 1 expression, but no CD8 positive infiltrates or vacuoles	Perifascicular, perimysial, or perivascular infiltrates; perifascicular atrophy	Perifascicular, perimysial or perivascular infiltrates; perifascicular atrophy	Nonspecific or diagnostic for dermatomyositis (subclinical myopathy)
Rash or calcinosis	Absent	Absent	Present	Not detected	Present

Reprinted from *Lancet*, 362/9388, Dalakas M, Hohlfeld R., T Polymyositis and dermatomyositis, 971–982, Copyright 2003, with permission from Elsevier

Table 7.3 Myositis-associated antibodies

Autoantibodies	Clinical association
Anti-SRP (signal recognition particle)	High serum CKs and necrotizing myopathy
	Severe PM and cardiac involvement
	Steroid response poor
Anti-Mi-2	Found in classic DM
	Good prognosis with therapy
Anti-synthetase antibodies (anti-Jo, PL7, anti-PL 12, EJ, OJ, and KS)	Polymyositis associated with interstitial lung disease Raynaud's phenomenon, mechanic's hands, polyarthritis, and fever (antisynthetase syndrome)

images in the axial and coronal plane of the involved region, usually the lower pelvis and proximal thighs. STIR sequences are preferred to fat-suppressed T2-weighted images as it provides a more homogenous fat suppression. Post-gadolinium T1 fat-saturated sequences can detect muscle inflammation similar to that of STIR, or T2-weighted sequences however are usually not required. MRI is of value in both diagnosing, assessing therapeutic response, and determining the area where a biopsy would yield a positive pathologic finding for either dermatomyositis or polymyositis.

Both polymyositis and dermatomyositis initially show muscle inflammation without atrophy or fatty infiltration compared to another type of myositis known as inclusion body myositis and usually involve distal muscles. MRI detects muscle edema, muscle atrophy, fatty replacement, and stage of myositis (Fig. 7.14). Severe fascial edema is usually seen in dermatomyositis. Objective scoring systems are being developed based on muscle inflammation, soft tissue edema, and perifascicular inflammation.

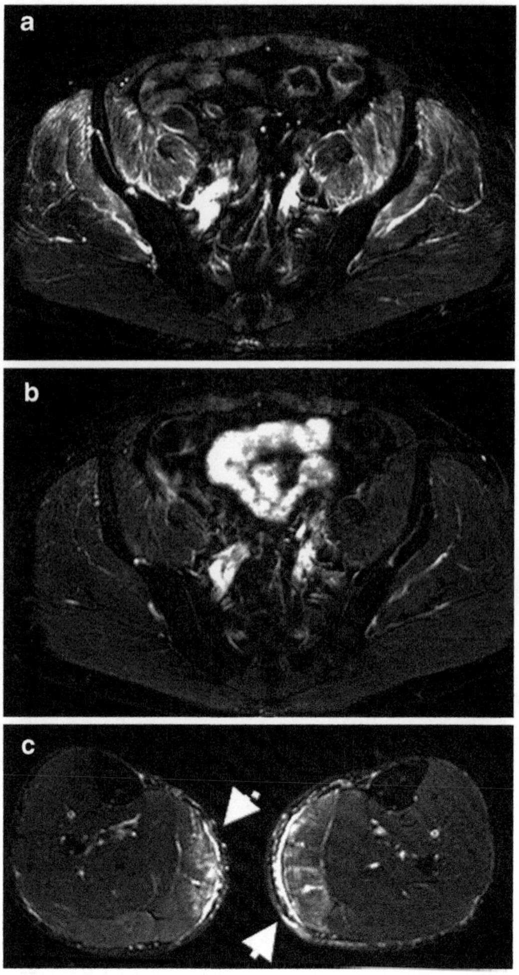

Fig. 7.14 A 53-year-old male presenting with proximal muscle weakness over the lower extremity with biopsy-proven idiopathic polymyositis. (**a**) Axial T2FS MRI proximal pelvis demonstrates bilateral extensive myositis, high signal intensity (*arrows*) with (**b**) full response to treatment. (**c**) Axial MRI bilateral calves in a 62-year-old male with dermatomyositis demonstrating bilateral myositis medial gastrocnemius and subcutaneous edema

Ultrasound may appear normal or demonstrate subtle changes in echogenicity muscles and fascial edema. It is helpful in localizing the correct anatomical site for biopsy when correlated with pathology on MRI. CT and nuclear medicine studies are not indicated. Evaluation of interstitial lung disease associated with inflammatory myopathies includes radiographs, and HRCT (high-resolution CT scan) scans showing heterogeneous basilar infiltrates demonstrating consolidation with linear platelike subpleural patterns that can progress to frank fibrosis.

Systemic Sclerosis

Overview

Systemic sclerosis (Ssc), scleroderma, is a multiorgan chronic connective tissue disease with significant morbidity and mortality due to vascular malfunction, inflammation, and significant fibrosis. Different studies have presented divergent estimates in both prevalence and incidence influenced by geographical factors. Among the different countries, an incidence may vary from ten or greater per one million per year and a prevalence of less than 150 per one million. There is a female preponderance with a ratio of 1:7–8. Age of onset is usually between 30 and 50 years.

The pathogenesis of systemic sclerosis is still unknown although as in any connective tissue disease both genetic and environmental factors play a role leading to loss of self-tolerance. It is known that vascular injury is an inciting event involving loss of integrity of the endothelial lining, perivascular cell infiltration leading to microvascular obliteration, and in the long run paucity of small blood vessels. T cell plays a role in secretion of profibrotic cytokines in systemic sclerosis specifically in interstitial lung disease that stimulates collagen secretion. Fibrosis in scleroderma initially involves the reticular dermis with accumulation of fibrillar collagen. Immune activation and inflammation with differentiation of these fibroblasts to myofibroblasts precedes this process. Furthermore, hypoxia itself serves as a potent stimulus for activation of fibroblast and progression of fibrosis. There is support that cytomegalovirus and parvovirus B19 may contribute to the etiopathogenesis of this disease through innate and adaptive processes.

CREST syndrome is a variant of systemic sclerosis with its own acronym defined as calcinosis, Raynaud's, esophageal dysmotility, sclerodactyly, and telangiectasia. They are noted to have a positive ANA with an anticentromere pattern. Treatment is symptom based and may include surgical intervention for some with severe calcinosis.

Presentation

The multiorgan involvement of systemic sclerosis leads to unwanted destructive sequelae. There are two main subtypes, limited systemic sclerosis and diffuse systemic sclerosis. Initial disease presentation includes Raynaud's phenomenon (RP), which is the most prominent hallmark, caused by reversible spasm of arteries. Raynaud's phenomenon is defined as color changes in the peripheral extremities, mainly fingers and toes, but may be seen in other parts of the body (i.e., tongue). The color changes include blanching or whitish discoloration followed by bluish discoloration then eventually hyperemia on rewarming associated with discomfort over the affected area.

Non-RP manifestations depend on the organ system involved, and its onset may occur 2–5 years from the initial RP. The clinical picture may also include digital joint synovitis, muscle weakness, sclerodactyly, tendon friction rubs, and skin manifestations. Dermatologic findings include skin thickening without tethering (comparing to eosinophilic fasciitis), presence of telangiectasias which are spiderlike lesions usually noted in the face and chest, digital ulcers, calcinosis, and dilated capillaries in the nail beds. Other organ manifestations are summarized in Table 7.4. In one systematic review severe organ

Table 7.4 Organ system involvement and clinical features

Organ system	Clinical features
Musculoskeletal	Sclerodactyly, joint synovitis, tendinitis, flexion deformity, and contractures
Cardiovascular	Pericardial effusion, pericardial effusion, myocarditis, right-sided heart failure due to secondary pulmonary hypertension, arrhythmias
Respiratory	Interstitial lung disease and pulmonary hypertension
Gastrointestinal	Gastroesophageal reflux, esophageal dysmotility, malabsorption, diarrhea, fecal incontinence
Renal	Renal crisis
Neurologic	Cranial nerve involvement
Hematologic	Anemia

complications occurred in 15 % of cases, and the prevalence of pulmonary hypertension was 15 %. A severe life-threatening complication includes a renal crisis presenting with malignant hypertension, rapidly deteriorating renal function, and microangiopathic hemolysis.

Recently, new classification criteria (Table 7.5) have been developed since the 1980 American College of Rheumatology classification criteria for systemic sclerosis lack sensitivity for early Ssc and limited cutaneous Ssc.

The criteria are not applicable to patients with the finger skin thickening sparing the fingers or to patients who have a scleroderma-like disorder that better explains their manifestations (e.g., nephrogenic sclerosing fibrosis, generalized morphea, eosinophilic fasciitis, scleroderma diabeticorum, scleromyxedema, erythromyalgia, porphyria, lichen sclerosis, graft-versus-host disease, diabetic cheiroarthropathy). The sensitivity of the new classification criteria is 91 % and specificity is 92 %. Poor prognosis is noted in advanced age, diffuse skin involvement, other organ involvement, and (+) Scl 70.

Imaging Features

Musculoskeletal System (Figs. 7.15 and 7.16)

Musculoskeletal manifestations of Ssc occur in approximately 61 % of patients and present with pain and the presence of synovitis over the joints in both hands and feet usually involving the wrists, metacarpophalangeal joints, and proximal and distal interphalangeal joints with symmetrical presentation. There is still a debate if it is a sole manifestation of the disease or an overlap with another inflammatory arthritis such as rheumatoid arthritis, and that it could be underestimated due to skin involvement. There is no doubt that skin thickening due to fibrosis may be a contributing factor to impaired joint mobility. Furthermore, peritendinous sclerosis leading to tendon shortening and associated tendon friction rubs contribute to functional disabilities mainly due to loss of handgrip capabilities. An erosive arthropathy can be seen in about 21 % of patients. There may be associated joint space narrowing, and periarticular osteopenia or demineralization (23 %) usually

Table 7.5 The American College of Rheumatology /European League Against Rheumatism criteria for the classification of systemic sclerosis

Item	Subitem (s)	Weight/score[a]
Skin thickening of the fingers of both hands extending proximal to the metacarpophalangeal joints (sufficient criterion)	–	9
Skin thickening of the fingers (only count higher score)	Puffy fingers	2
	Sclerodactyly of the fingers (distal to the metacarpophalangeal joints but proximal to the proximal interphalangeal joints)	4
Fingertip lesions (only count the higher score)	Digital tip ulcers	2
	Fingertip pitting scars	3
Telangiectasia	–	2
Abnormal nail fold capillaries	–	2
Pulmonary arterial hypertension and/or interstitial lung disease (maximum score 2)	Pulmonary arterial hypertension	2
	Interstitial lung disease	2
Raynaud's phenomenon	–	3
SSc-related autoantibodies (anticentromere, anti-topoisomerase I (anti-Scl 70), anti-RNA polymerase III) (maximum score 3)	Anticentromere	3
	Anti-topoisomerase I	
	Anti-RNA polymerase III	

From Van den Hoogen F, Khanna D, Fransen J et al. 2013 Classification Criteria for Systemic Sclerosis. *Arthritis and Rheumatism* 2013:65:11:2737–2747

[a]The total score is determined by adding the maximum weight (score) in each category. Patients with a total score of ≥9 are classified as having definite Ssc

correlated with systemic inflammation and arthritis. Occasionally changes such as a pencil cup deformity, involvement of the DIP and PIP joints simulates both erosive osteoarthritis and psoriatic arthropathy. Phalangeal tuft resorption or acro-osteolysis is one of the most characteristic features of Ssc and is associated with digital ulcers due to compromised blood flow. This can lead to a "penciling" deformity and may lead to total digital destruction. Synovitis with joint effusion, erosions, as well as tenosynovitis may be verified by ultrasound. The presence of synovitis is corre-

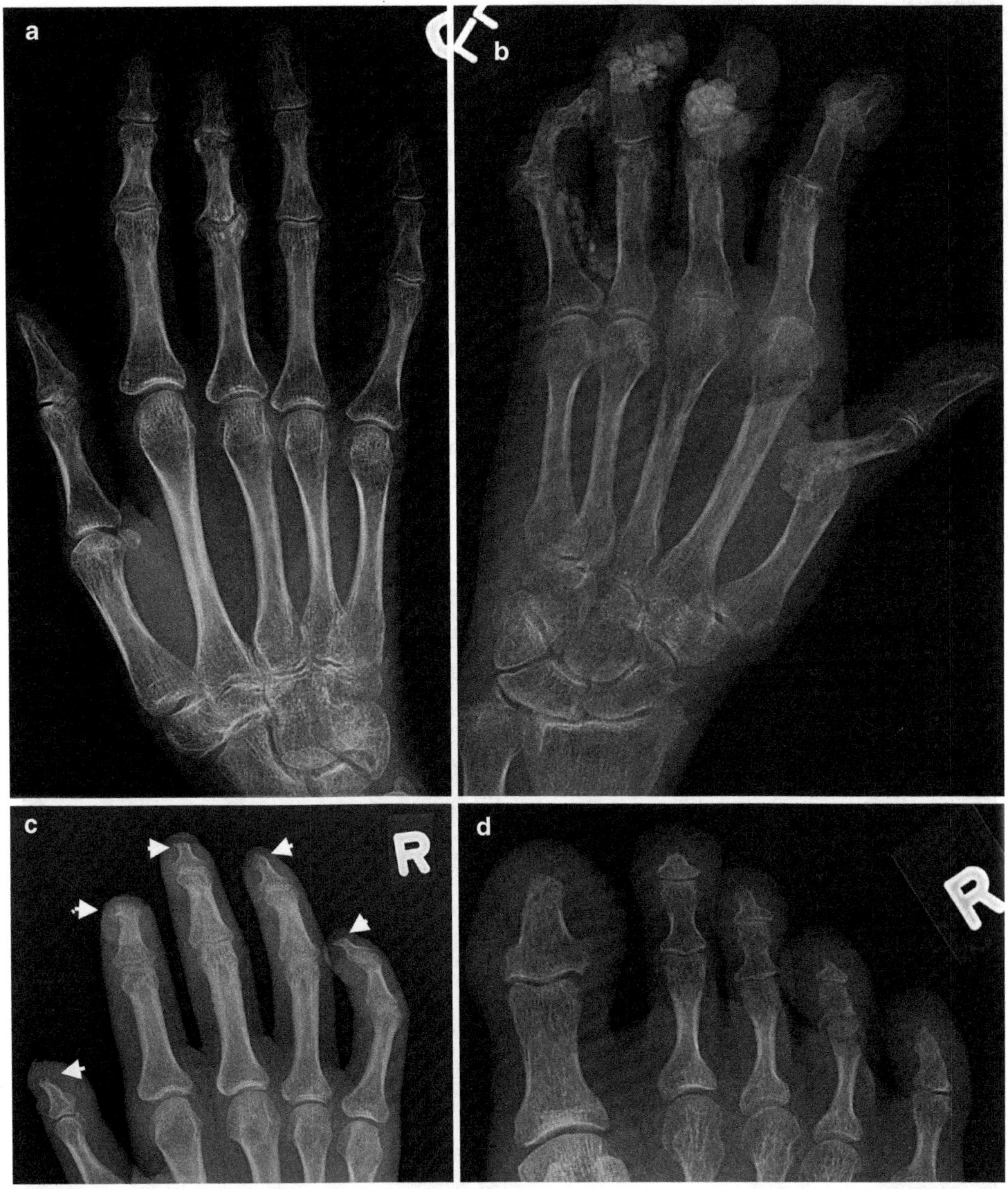

Fig. 7.15 (**a**) A 68-year-old female with systemic sclerosis on prednisone and methotrexate. Anterior posterior radiograph of the right hand shows generalized osteopenia, (**b**) patient with scleroderma and PsA, (**c**) 36-year-old female with systemic sclerosis, with severe Raynaud's requiring prostacyclin infusion. AP radiograph shows acro-osteolysis (*arrows*) of the distal tufts of the right hand and (**d**) similar changes on the right foot. (**e**) Different patient with extensive calcinosis at the first digit

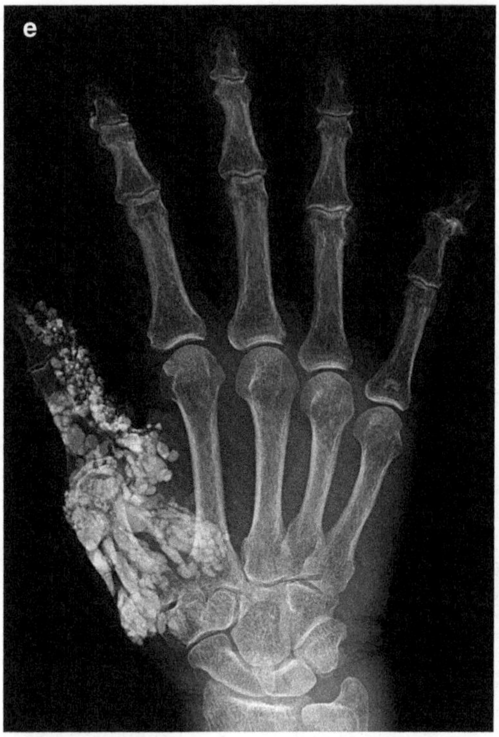

Fig. 7.15 (continued)

lated with high C-reactive protein levels. These main findings may also be assessed by magnetic resonance imaging, and choice of imaging may depend on local expertise.

Flexion contracture as a consequence of non-articular manifestations such as tenosynovitis associated with diffuse cutaneous involvement is another hallmark of Ssc. This can be found in about 27 % of patients and can be seen in the late course of the disease due to synovial fibrosis.

One of the radiographic findings in patients with Ssc is calcinosis and may be associated with digital ulcers. Usually the dominant hand or areas of chronic stress are involved. There is no difference in the presence between limited and diffuse cutaneous systemic sclerosis.

Pulmonary and Cardiovascular System

Pulmonary hypertension (PH) and interstitial lung disease (ILD) are the two most common cardiopulmonary manifestations of Ssc leading to death. Interstitial lung disease is seen about 40 % of patients with Ssc and associated more with dif-

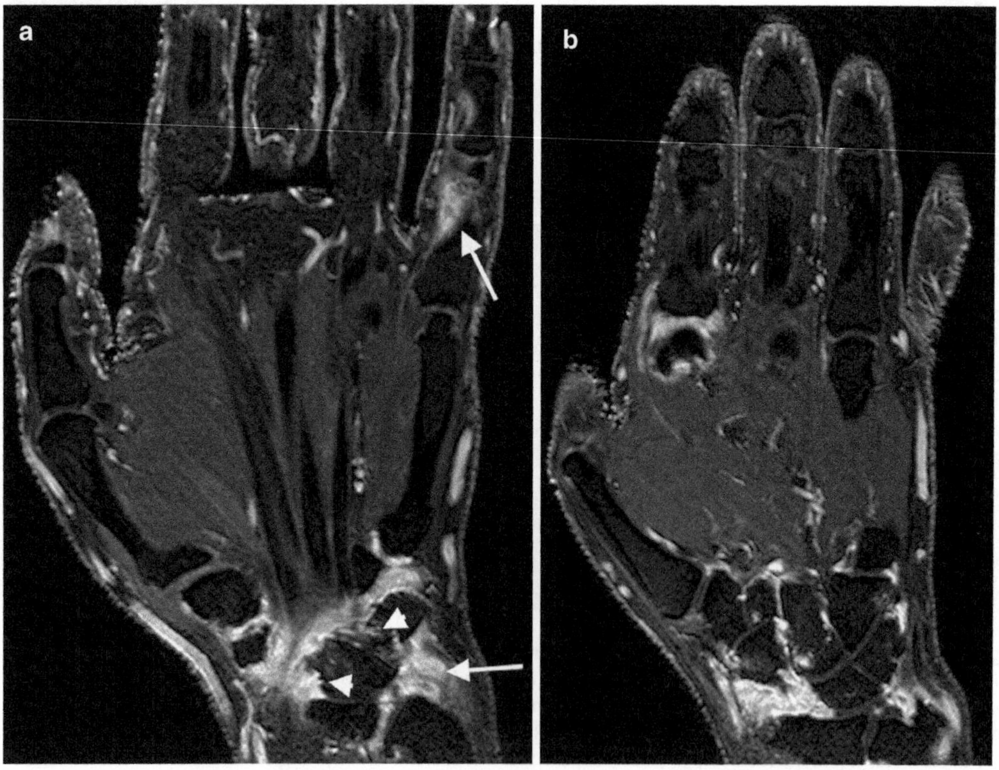

Fig. 7.16 MRI in patient with scleroderma (**a**, **b**) Cor T1FS PG images with active synovitis at the (*arrows*) wrist and second and fifth MCPJs with early carpal erosions (*arrowheads*)

fuse skin involvement, African-American ethnicity, hypothyroidism, cardiac involvement, and elevated creatine kinase levels. Clinical manifestations include dyspnea, fatigue, nonproductive cough, as well as chest pain. Inspiratory crackles described as Velcro crackles at the lung bases are characteristic of this disease. Initial diagnostic interventions include a pulmonary function test as well as imaging. Pulmonary function test aids in evaluating mainly a decrease in diffuse capacity of carbon monoxide (DLCO), which correlates with severity of interstitial lung disease. There are different types of ILD; however, nonspecific interstitial pneumonia 75 % corresponds more to Ssc. Although an insensitive test, chest X-ray is one of the required screening tests to determine the presence of interstitial lung disease but may be normal in early disease. Bibasal reticulonodular interstitial lung changes progressing to honeycombing and low lung volumes are observed (similar features to Fig. 7.8).

High-resolution CT scan (HRCT) offers more defined and subtle changes especially in early disease such as ill-defined subpleural crescents and ground glass attenuation in the posterior lobes. As the disease progresses, honeycombing with traction bronchiectasis, ground glass, and reticular patterns are observed and in later stages pulmonary fibrosis. Mediastinal adenopathy is common. Bronchoalveolar lavage, thoracoscopy/mediastinoscopy, and biopsy can be supplementary diagnostic interventions to further evaluate disease burden and to rule out any other possible etiology.

Pulmonary hypertension (PH) is usually associated with patients with limited scleroderma, female preponderance, late onset of the disease, and disease duration greater than 10 years. Chest X-ray reveals enlarged pulmonary arteries with oligemic lung fields. HRCT helps define the presence or absence of ILD. Prognosis is poor in patients with PAH.

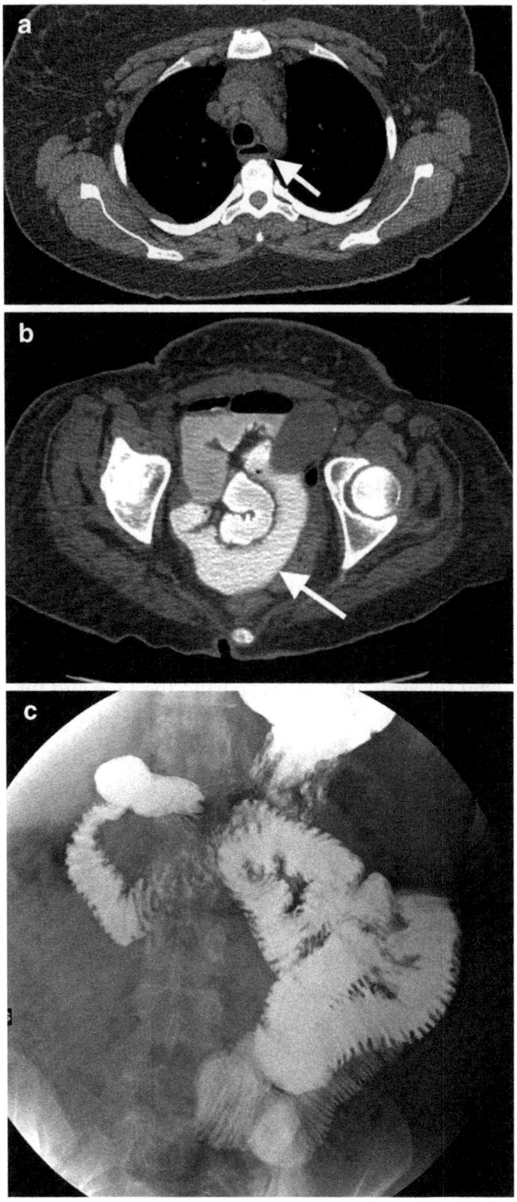

Fig. 7.17 Gastrointestinal manifestations of scleroderma. (**a**) Axial CT with esophageal dilatation in scleroderma patient, (**b**) dilated small bowel loops (*arrow*) with hypomotility on axial CT, (**c**) hidebound pattern on a barium follow-through study in a different patient

Gastrointestinal System (Fig. 7.17)

Gastrointestinal manifestation of Ssc includes dysphagia, acid reflux, constipation or diarrhea, and pseudo-obstruction. Unfortunately, the presence of these symptoms is usually seen in severe disease and is usually hard to treat. Malnutrition secondary to malabsorption syndrome is a poor prognostic factor. Esophageal involvement is the most common gastrointestinal manifestation with an incidence of about 70–90 % which includes dysphagia, acid reflux, dyspepsia, substernal chest pain with nausea, food regurgitation, and earlier satiety. Motility problems are a main factor in these different manifestations at which chronic esophagitis may lead to esophageal stricture that may be seen on barium studies. Furthermore due to loss of lower esophageal tone, dilatation of the esophagus may be present. Endoscopy is usually performed for assessment for esophagitis and to rule out any Barrett's esophageal metaplasia or carcinoma. Small bowel follow-through studies demonstrate dilatation bowel with crowding of the mucosal folds, termed a hidebound pattern and is characteristic of scleroderma. Pseudodiverticula are common in both small and large bowel.

Eosinophilic Fasciitis (Fig. 7.18)

One of the differential diagnoses of systemic sclerosis is eosinophilic fasciitis. It is a rare disease with clinical features of progressive skin induration with symmetrical involvement of the distal forearm and calves sparing the face and fingers. Compared to systemic sclerosis, the fascia is edematous, thickened, fibrotic, and may be tethered, and the superficial skin can still be wrinkled. The typical peau d'orange hue may also be noted. Pathophysiology is still unknown; however, its onset may be seen following trauma or extreme physical effort. There may be some correlation with exposure to Borrelia species, tryptophan exposure, or toxic oils. It is emphasized that it may be a paraneoplastic manifestation and that age-appropriate malignancy screen should be considered. Eosinophilia may be a feature but may be absent in 20 % of untreated cases. Furthermore, hypergammaglobulinemia may be noted together with an elevated erythrocyte sedimentation rate. Biopsy usually shows eosinophilic and mononuclear infiltrates in the fascia. Imaging may play a role in distinguishing it from systemic sclerosis. High-frequency ultrasound reveals less subcutaneous compressibility compared to that of systemic sclerosis or normal skin, but more studies are needed. Magnetic resonance imaging demonstrates diffuse fasciitis, thickening of the fascia, hyperintense signal within the fascia on fluid-sensitive sequences, and enhancement on contrast. Prednisone is the mainstay of treatment.

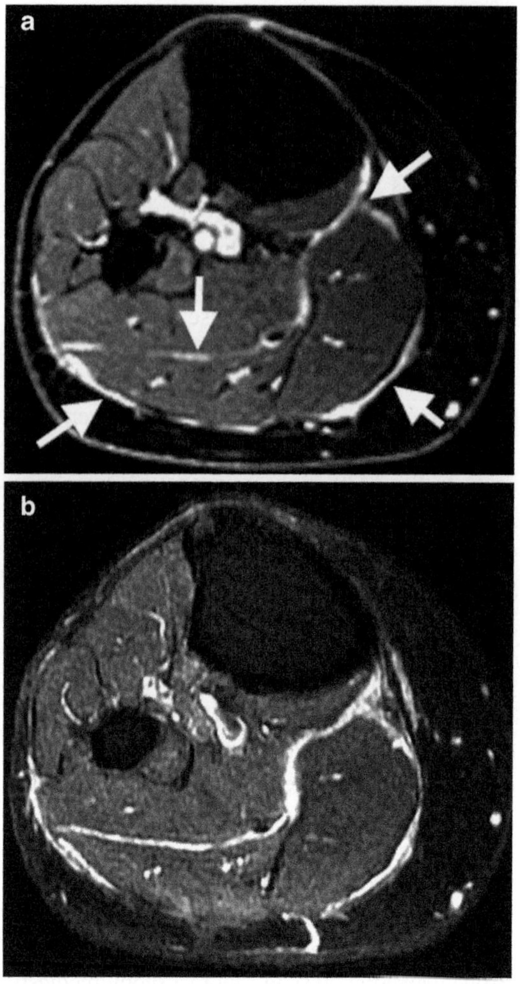

Fig. 7.18 Eosinophilic fasciitis on MRI, (**a**) axial T2FS calf demonstrating high SI thickened fascia (*arrows*) and (**b**) with marked enhancement on axial T1FS post-gadolinium

Vasculitis

Overview

Vasculitis is a rare inflammatory disorder characterized by blood vessel necrosis with complications such as thrombus formation leading to ischemic events, infarction of involved organ tissues, hemorrhage, aneurysm formation, and vessel rupture. Recently, the 2012 Chapel Hill Nomenclature has been established, while a diagnostic and classification study in vasculitis is ongoing (Table 7.6).

Table 7.6 Revised International Chapel Hill consensus conference nomenclature of the vasculitides 2012

Large vessel vasculitis (LVV)	Takayasu's arteritis (TAK) and giant cell arteritis (GCA)
Medium vessel vasculitis (MVV)	Polyarteritis nodosa (PAN) and Kawasaki disease (KD)
Small vessel vasculitis (SVV)	ANCA-associated vasculitis (AAV) including: microscopic polyangiitis (MPA), granulomatosis with polyangiitis (Wegener's) (GPA), and eosinophilic granulomatosis with polyangiitis (Churg–Strauss) (EGPA)
	Immune complex SVV including: anti-GBM disease, cryoglobulinemic vasculitis, IgA vasculitis (Henoch–Schönlein) (IgAV), and hypocomplementemic urticarial vasculitis (anti-C1q vasculitis) (HUV)
Variable vessel vasculitis (VVV)	Behçet's disease (BD) and Cogan's syndrome (CS)
Single organ vasculitis (SOV):	Cutaneous leukocytoclastic angiitis, cutaneous arteritis, primary CNS vasculitis, and isolated aortitis
Vasculitis associated with systemic disease	Lupus vasculitis, rheumatoid vasculitis, and sarcoid vasculitis
Vasculitis associated with probable etiology	Hepatitis C virus-associated cryoglobulinemic vasculitis, hepatitis B virus-associated vasculitis, syphilis-associated aortitis, serum sickness-associated immune complex vasculitis, drug-associated immune complex vasculitis, drug-associated ANCA-associated vasculitis, and cancer-associated vasculitis

From Jennette JC, Falk DJ, Bacon A. 2012 Revised International Chapel Hill Consensus Conference Nomenclature of Vasculitides. *Arthritis and Rheumatism* 2012:1–11

Large Vessel Vasculitis (Giant Cell Arteritis and Takayasu's Arteritis)

Giant Cell Arteritis (Fig. 7.19)

Giant cell arteritis (GCA) is a clinical syndrome that has a spectrum of symptoms. It has a prevalence of 1,400–16,000 per million and incidence of 100–300 per million of population in people greater than 50. Age is one of the main risk factors with the mean age of onset at 70 years old with females being three times more affected than males. Furthermore, Caucasians are more predisposed, and smokers are at higher risk of developing the disease. About 50 % of patients with GCA develop polymyalgia rheumatica (PMR), and about 10 % of patients with PMR develop GCA. Headache is the most common initial manifestation usually localized to the temporal area; however, the occipital arteries may likewise be involved and may present with increased sensitivity or discomfort on combing or brushing their hair. Characterization of the type of headache may range from a dull headache to a sharp or shooting discomfort. Jaw claudication can occur up to two thirds of patients with GCA and is presumably secondary to vascular insufficiency. Throat pain, tingling sensation in the tongue, and even loss of taste may occur.

The most dreaded complication is ocular involvement leading to partial or total visual loss. Ophthalmologic findings reveal anterior ischemic optic neuropathy although the posterior aspect may be involved as well. Early diagnosis and medical intervention is crucial in preventing these irreversible sequelae.

Extracranial manifestation of giant cell arteritis involving the aortic arch and its tributaries may lead to dilation and eventually rupture or dissection. It is the leading cause of inflammatory aortitis, which unfortunately often goes undetected. The axillary arteries are commonly involved compared to the subclavian or brachial arteries. Different imaging techniques have evolved through the years in detecting aortic involvement before structural abnormalities occur. Temporal artery biopsy remains the gold standard for diagnosing cranial involvement. However, only about 15 % of biopsies are positive, and lengths may be a factor for negative biopsies as well as the presence of skip lesions. Furthermore, some patients may present only with aortic involvement.

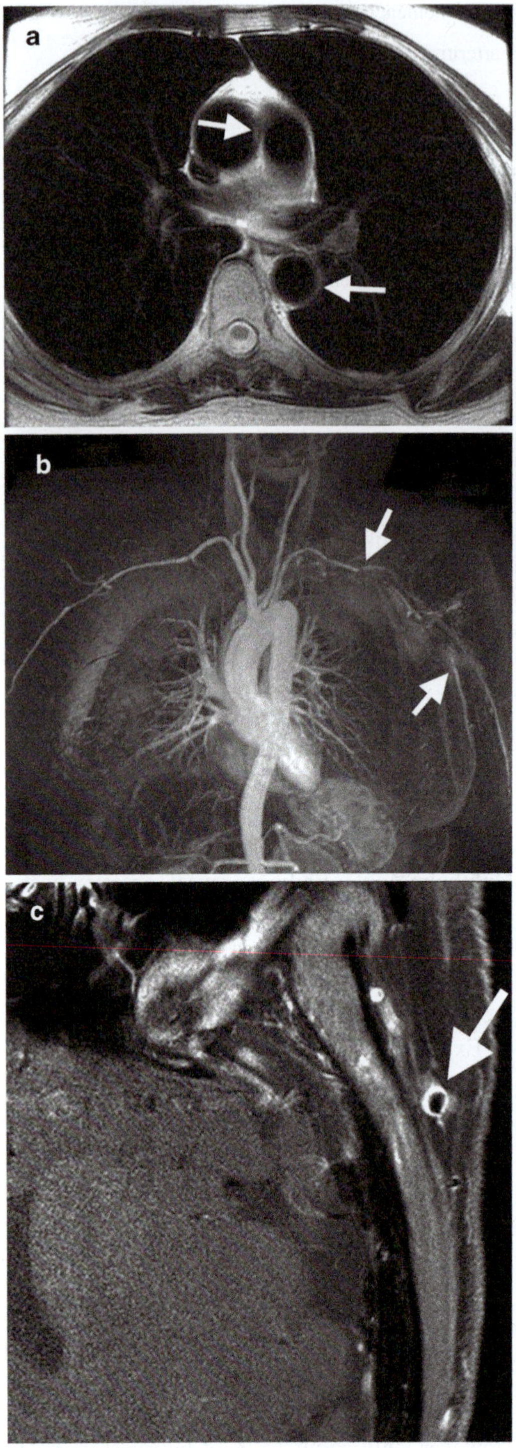

Fig. 7.19 Giant cell arteritis in a 72-year-old female. (**a**) Axial MRI demonstrates left eccentric wall thickening ascending and descending aorta (*arrows*) and (**b**) MRA demonstrating long segment tapering stenosis (between *arrows*) of 50 % distal left subclavian extending into axillary artery. (**c**) High-resolution axial T1FS PG demonstrating wall thickening and enhancement of superficial temporal artery (*arrow*)

Imaging

Ultrasound and MRI (Fig. 7.20)

Doppler ultrasound may be valuable in evaluating GCA especially with cranial involvement. Hypoechoic edematous wall swelling is noted in

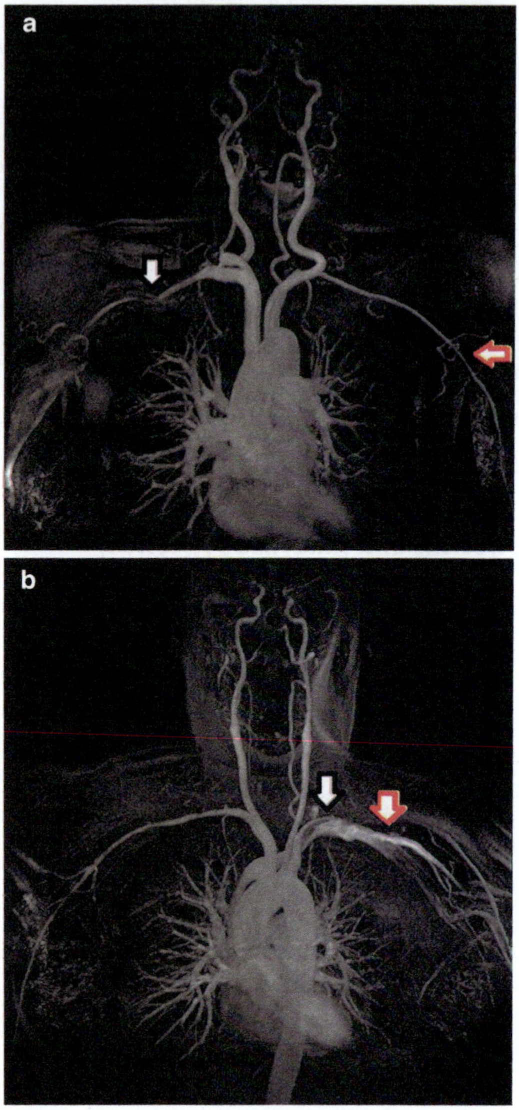

Fig. 7.20 A 78-year-old female with Giant Cell arteritis presenting with upper arm claudication. MRI subclavians with runoffs reveal a short segment stenosis of the proximal third of the right subclavian artery (*black arrow*); furthermore, noted is the tapering of the left subclavian artery to the midaxillary artery (*red arrow*). (**b**) A 57-year-old female presenting with both cranial and large vessel vasculitis. MRI angiogram reveals a high-grade stenosis of the left subclavian, distal to the origin of the left vertebral artery (*black arrow*), and high-grade stenosis of the left subclavian at the junction of subclavian and axillary portions (*red arrow*)

acute temporal arteritis as well as short segments of stenosis that increased maximum systolic blood flow velocity. Ultrasound is helpful in localizing areas of involvement for biopsy. Correlation with biopsies in one meta-analysis shows a sensitivity of 87 % and specificity of 96 %. In aortic and tributary involvement, ultrasound findings reveal wall swelling of greater than >1 mm and findings similar to that of temporal artery as described above. Reliability of this diagnostic procedure is operator dependent as well as dependent on the quality of equipment. Furthermore, these findings may disappear with steroid therapy. Differentiating against atherosclerosis, the vessel wall looks more inhomogeneous with less circumferential involvement and the presence of atherosclerotic calcifying plaques.

Magnetic resonance imaging (MRI)/magnetic resonance angiography (MRA) is another valuable diagnostic imaging tool in both cranial and aortic arteritis. Promising data is evolving in MRI of temporal and occipital arteries showing enhancement of the vessel wall with contrast. Involvement of extracranial vessels demonstrates wall thickening on T1 and T2 images and post-gadolinium enhancement. Furthermore, vessel wall stenosis is noted with active vasculitis. However it is noted that these changes may persist despite both clinical and laboratory remission and thus may not be a great tool for monitoring patients.

Positron emission tomography (PET) combined with CT, CT-PET, has an advantage in detecting both structural and active inflammation (Table 7.7). When inflammatory cells become activated, they undergo a "respiratory burst" at which these cells use more glucose. It is becoming a popular diagnostic imaging tool in large vessel vasculitis with a sensitivity of 77–92 % and a specificity of 89–100 %. Furthermore, vascular uptake correlates with both clinical and laboratory parameters especially with C-reactive protein. PET/CT identifies active inflammation in the arterial wall. Some studies suggest PET has a role in assessing prognosis, but further studies are required.

Both PET/CT and MRI/MRA are both evolving diagnostic and prognostic imaging tools in giant cell arteritis, and there are ongoing studies to better define their role.

Table 7.7 The major features of PET/CT versus MRI/MRA in patients with GCA

Features	MRI/MRA	PET/CT
Detection of vascular inflammation	++	+++
Detection of vascular structural changes	+++	++
Spatial resolution	<1 mm	>4 mm
Visualization of temporal arteries	Yes	No
Location of large arteries visualized	Head, neck, thoracic regions	Whole body
Outcome treatment measure	No proven role	Possible role
Radiation exposure	No	Yes
Presence of renal failure	Contraindicated	No issue
Cost of procedure	+	+++

Adapted from Clifford, A et al. Positron Emission Tomography/Computed Tomography for the Diagnosis and Assessment of Giant Cell Arteritis: When to Consider It and Why, *J Rheumatol*. 2012;39(10):1909–11, Table 1, p. 1910

Angiography and Computed Tomography

Angiography, although not commonly used due it being an invasive procedure, shows long areas of regular circumferential stenosis with either occlusions or dilations. While eccentric thickening of the wall with post-contrast enhancement is noted in computed tomography. Furthermore, circumferential thickening more than 3 mm is indicative of arteritis.

Polymyalgia Rheumatica

Polymyalgia rheumatica (PMR) is an inflammatory disease with clinical features of pain and stiffness mainly in the shoulders, hip girdle, or neck. PMR is known to coexist with giant cell arteritis at which 10–15 % of them may develop this type of vasculitis. It is commonly seen above the age of 50, with peak incidence from 70 to 79 years with female predominance initially by with equal sex distribution with increasing age. Diagnosis is both clinical and based on elevated inflammatory markers. Recently, the 2012 EULAR (European League against Rheumatism)/ACR (American College of Rheumatism) classification criteria have been developed involving a scoring algorithm with components of age greater or equal to 50 and bilateral shoulder achiness with abnormal ESR or CRP. Its sensitivity 92.6 % however with new criteria including the option of utilizing ultrasound of the shoulders or hips increases its specificity to about 91.3 %. Clinical criteria include morning stiffness for more than 45 min, hip pain or limited range of motion, absence of rheumatoid factor or anti-CCP, and absence of other joint pain. Ultrasound criteria include at least one shoulder revealing subdeltoid bursitis and or biceps tenosynovitis, glenohumeral synovitis, and at least one hip with synovitis and or trochanteric bursitis. To date, steroids have been the standard of treatment.

Table 7.8 1990 ACR criteria diagnostic criteria for Takayasu's arteritis

Age of disease onset less than 40 years old
Claudication of extremities
Decrease of brachial artery pulse
Blood pressure difference of >10 mmHg
Bruit over subclavian artery and aorta
Arteriogram abnormality
At least three of the six criteria has to be met to make a diagnosis

From Arend WP, Michel BA, Bloch DA, Hunder GG, Calabrese LH, Edworthy SM, Fauci AS, Leavitt RY, Lie JT, Lightfoot RW Jr, et al. The American College of Rheumatology 1990 criteria for the classification of takayasu arteritis. *Arthritis Rheum.* 1990;33(8):1129–34

Takayasu's Arteritis

Takayasu's arteritis (TA) is a large vessel vasculitis with similar histopathology to that of GCA. It involves the aorta and its branches but never involves the temporal arteries. Disease onset is usually less than 40 years of age, and disease duration is longer. It is prevalent in Asian and Middle Eastern countries with female and male ratio different in each country. Clinical symptoms may be constitutional in nature (fever, fatigue, and weight loss), and TA may only be considered the physical absence of blood pressure or pulse deficit in an affected. Table 7.8 outlines the ACR classification criteria with a 90 % sensitivity and specificity. No blood test is specific for TA; however, inflammatory markers such as erythrocyte sedimentation rate (ESR) and C-reactive protein (CRP) are often used to monitor disease.

Large vessels are involved as a panarteritis. The aorta, subclavian, and carotids are most commonly affected (60–90 %). Imaging features as outlined above for giant cell arteritis are similar in TA (Fig. 7.21). MRI/MRA and PET scan are again evolving diagnostic tools.

Medium Vessel Vasculitis

Polyarteritis nodosa (PAN) is the most common medium vessel vasculitis. PAN is a necrotizing medium vessel vasculitis and is one of the rarest types of vasculitis. It is usually a primary vasculitis but may be associated with hepatitis B. The most common clinical manifestations are generalized constitutional symptoms (93 %), neurologic manifestations (79 %) (mononeuritis multiplex the most frequent) and skin manifestations (49 %), and uncommonly gastrointestinal symptoms. Occasionally a nonerosive migratory polyarteritis may occur. Predictors of mortality include older age onset, recent onset of hypertension, and gastrointestinal manifestations requiring surgery. Furthermore, hepatitis B-related PAN has a higher mortality rate but lower relapse rate. Laboratory investigations are nonspecific with elevated inflammatory markers, and ANCA is negative.

Contrast angiography is an important diagnostic procedure in PAN. A positive abdominal angiography is part of the ACR criteria, sensitivity of 82 % and specificity of 86 % (Table 7.9).

Arterial occlusions and aneurysms are the usual findings (Fig. 7.22). The superior mesenteric artery is commonly involved. MRI/MRA and CT/CTA are other possible imaging tools. CT/CTA findings may show wedge-shaped areas of infarctions in affected organs, hematomas from aneurysmal ruptures, and small microaneurysms. Microaneurysms are more difficult to evaluate

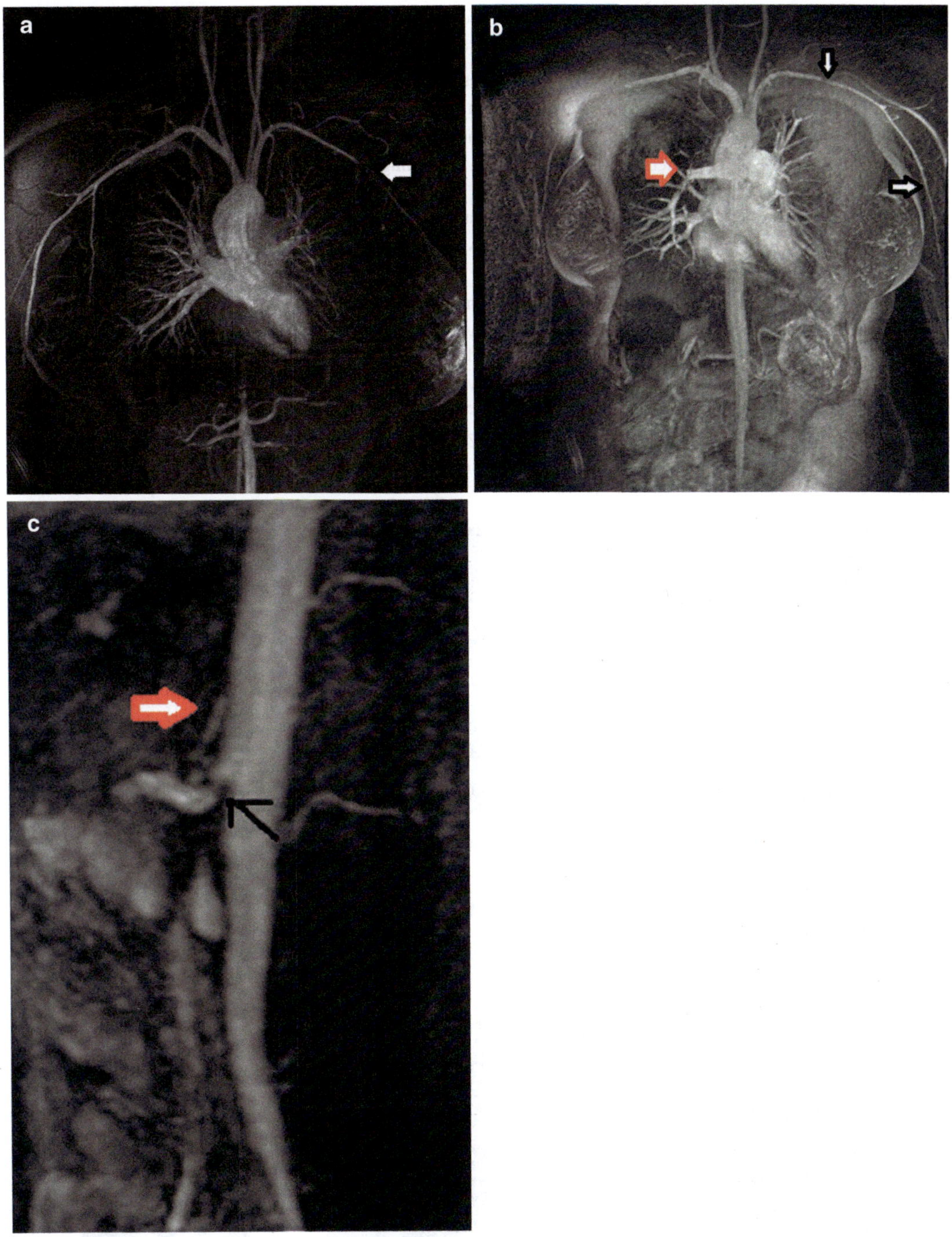

Fig. 7.21 (**a**) A 22-year-old female with Takayasu's arteritis presenting with fatigue and anemia and absence of blood pressure and weak pulses in the left upper extremity. MRI/MRA subclavians with runoffs show at the junction of the left subclavian and axillary arteries, and there is a long string-like stenosis or occlusion (*black arrow*). (**b**) A 30-year-old female with Takayasu's arteritis presenting with fatigue and shortness of breath. MRI/MRA aorta reveals a luminal irregularity in the distal left subclavian and axillary artery (*black arrows*). There is complete obliteration of the truncus anterior and severe stenosis in the interlobar artery of the right pulmonary artery (*red arrow*). (**c**) Same patient as above, MRI/MRA aorta reveals that the superior mesenteric artery is occluded proximally (*black arrow*) and moderate to severe stenosis of the celiac artery (*red arrow*)

Table 7.9 American College of Rheumatology 1990 criteria for the classification of polyarteritis nodosa (PAN). Classified as PAN if at least three of these 10 criteria are present

1.	Weight loss >4 kg: loss of >4 kg body weight since illness began, not related to dieting or other factors
2.	Livedo reticularis: mottled reticular pattern over the skin of portions of the extremities or torso
3.	Testicular pain/tenderness: pain or tenderness of the testicles, not due to infection, trauma, or other causes
4.	Myalgias, weakness, or leg tenderness: diffuse myalgias (excluding shoulder or hip girdle) or weakness of muscles or tenderness of leg muscles
5.	Mono- or polyneuropathy: development of mononeuropathy, multiple mononeuropathies, or polyneuropathy
6.	Diastolic BP >90 mmHg: development of hypertension with the diastolic BP higher than 90 mmHg
7.	Elevated BUN or creatinine: elevation of BUN >40 mg/dl or creatinine >1.5 mg/dl, not due to dehydration or obstruction
8.	Hepatitis B virus: presence of hepatitis B surface antigen or antibody in serum
9.	Arteriographic abnormality: arteriogram showing aneurysms or occlusions of the visceral arteries, not due to arteriosclerosis, fibromuscular dysplasia, or other noninflammatory causes
10.	Biopsy of small- or medium-sized artery containing polymorphonuclear cells: histologic changes showing the presence of granulocytes or granulocytes and mononuclear leukocytes in the artery wall

From Lightfoot RW Jr, Michel BA, Bloch DA, Hunder GG, Zvaifler NJ, McShane DJ, Arend WP, Calabrese LH, Leavitt RY, Lie JT, et al. The American college of rheumatology 1990 criteria for the classification of polyarteritis nodosa. *Arthritis Rheum.* 1990;33(8):1088–93

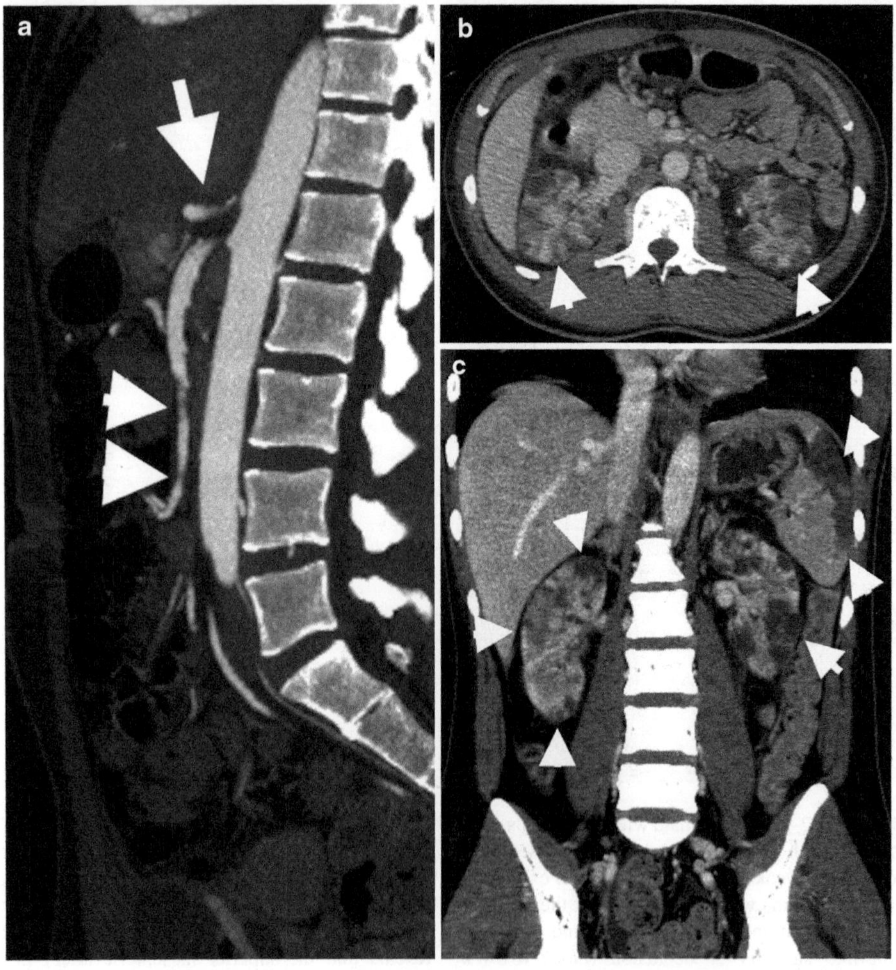

Fig. 7.22 PAN in a 45-year-old male patient, CT findings, (**a**) CT angiogram reconstructed sagittal image with stenosis proximal celiac artery (*arrow*) and multifocal stenosis and wall irregularity of the SMA (*arrowheads*) and (**b**) multiple bilateral renal and (**c**) splenic infarct (*arrowheads*) denoted as peripheral low attenuation foci and (**d**) multiple right hepatic artery aneurysms (*arrows*)

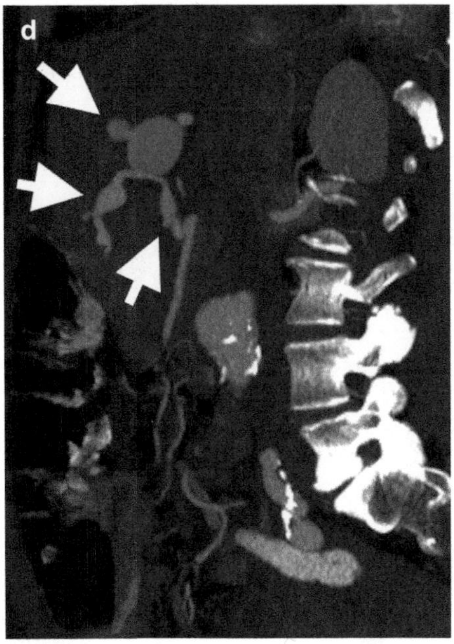

Fig. 7.22 (continued)

with this type of imaging. Furthermore, some of the non-arteriographic findings are nonspecific and can be seen as well in other diseases. To date, angiography is the suggested diagnostic imaging tool.

Primary Angiitis of the Central Nervous System (PACNS) Vasculitis (Fig. 7.23)

Primary angiitis of the central nervous system vasculitis (PACNS) is a rare vasculitis with 2.4 cases per one million person-years affecting more men with a median age of 50. It has a variable clinical presentation. Headache is the most common manifestation; however, this not a specific symptom and could be seen as well with one of the most common mimicker of PACNS such as reversible cerebral vasoconstriction syndrome (RCVS) with thunderclap headache being the most common. Other symptoms include stroke-like syndromes, cognitive impairment, seizures, and myelopathy plus or minus constitutional symptoms. A proposed diagnostic criterion has been suggested by Calabrese et al. (Table 7.10).

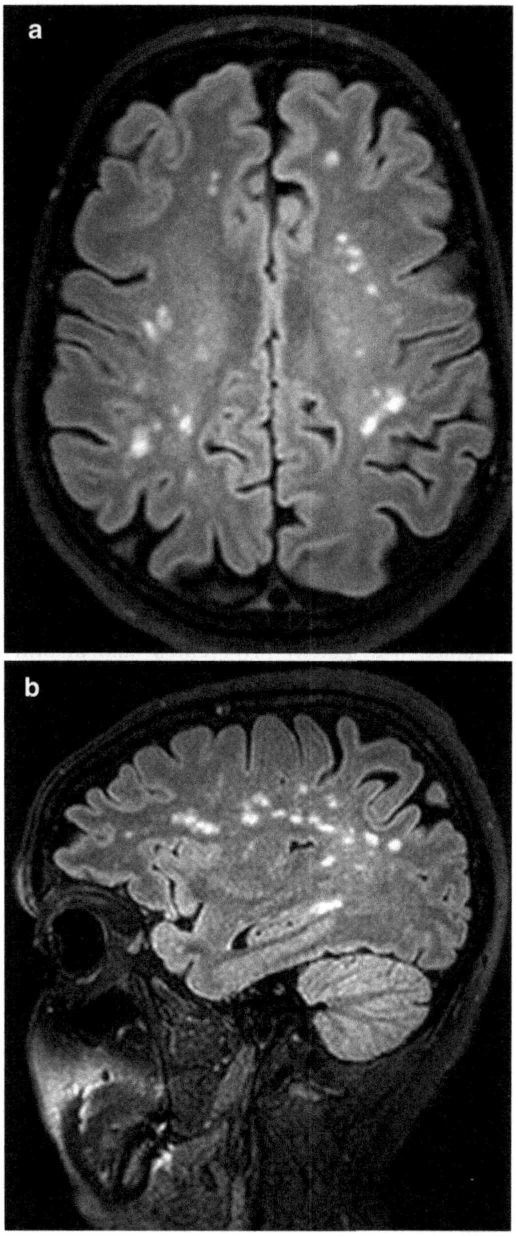

Fig. 7.23 PACNS vasculitis in a 52-year-old male presenting with headache. (**a**) Axial and (**b**) sagittal T2 FLAIR demonstrating nonspecific high SI foci within deep white matter cerebral hemispheres

Unfortunately, there is no single laboratory test to aid the diagnosis of PACNS. ESR and CRP, ANA and ANCA, may be normal in most situations. Cerebrospinal fluid analysis is the most valuable test, which aids in obtaining a

Table 7.10 Proposed criteria for the diagnosis of PACNS

The presence of unexplained neurologic deficit
Evidence of either classic angiographic or histopathologic features of angiitis within the central nervous system
No evidence of systemic vasculitis or any other condition that could elicit the angiographic or pathologic features

Adapted from *Autoimmunity Reviews*, 12/4, Hajj-Ali R, Calabrese L, Primary Angiitis of the central nervous system, 463–466, Copyright 2013, with permission from Elsevier

diagnosis and ruling out other possible etiologies. This should be performed in all patients. A modest pleocytosis and elevated protein levels, with normal glucose with a negative infectious workup, are some of the findings. Brain biopsy is still the gold standard showing lymphocytic infiltration, granulomas, and fibrinoid necrosis in the vascular bed. However, a negative biopsy can be obtained with patchy involvement and inability to access the involved region. Furthermore, it cannot help distinguish between PACNS and a secondary vasculitis. A brain biopsy may be useful in ruling out potential infectious and malignant etiologies.

Neuroimaging is nonspecific, and findings can be seen in other ischemic and demyelinating conditions.

Magnetic resonance imaging (MRI) is a sensitive imaging tool that shows multiple ischemic abnormalities in both white and gray matter and meningeal thickening with symmetrical involvement in T1-weighted sequences. Chronic petechial hemorrhages in T2-weighted imaging can be seen due to vessel breakdown and can be a surrogate marker in the diagnosis of PACNS.

Angiography has limited sensitivity and specificity. Magnetic resonance angiography (MRA) uncovers vascular abnormalities such as intramural vascular inflammation both in the wall and lumen and segmental arterial wall narrowing with poststenotic dilatation (beading or string of pearls) with bilateral cerebral involvement. Conventional angiography with its invasive procedure predisposing to interventional complications may have similar findings as MRA but has better resolution for smaller vessels. Other diagnostic imaging such as magnetic resonance spectroscopy may be useful in ruling out neoplasms. Both diagnosis and treatment of PACNS remain to be a challenge; hence, a thorough workup and multidisciplinary team involvement is always advised.

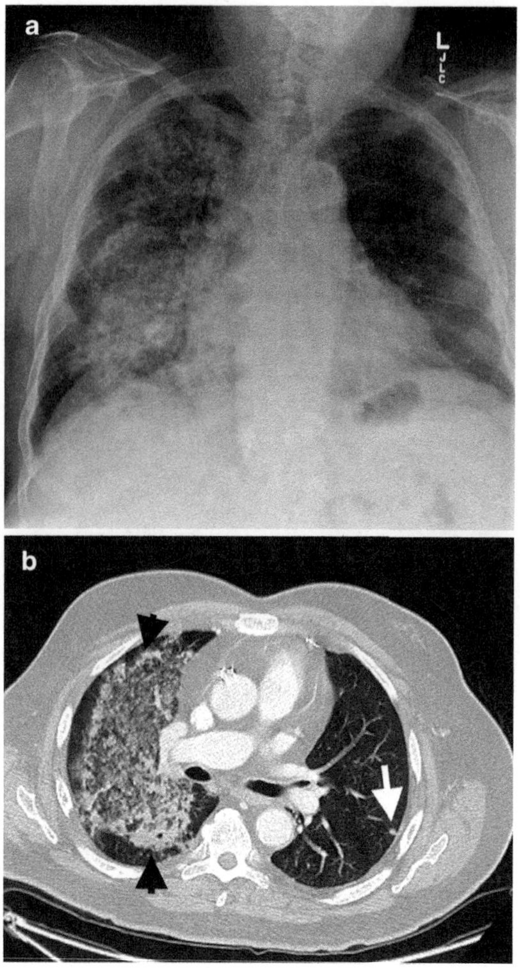

Fig. 7.24 Patients with known GPA presenting with acute hemoptysis. (**a**) PA CXR with new parenchymal opacification right lung and (**b**) axial CT lung windows with diffuse right-sided airspace opacification (*black arrowheads*) in keeping with acute hemorrhage in this case, note subpleural nodule left lung (*arrow*)

Granulomatosis with Polyangiitis (Formerly Known as Wegener's)

(Fig. 7.24)

Granulomatosis with polyangiitis (GPA) is one of the ANCA (antineutrophilic cytoplasmic antibody)-associated vasculitis (AAV) and part of the small vessel vasculitides. The other two ANCA-associated vasculitides are microscopic polyangiitis and eosinophilic granulomatosis with polyangiitis (formerly known as Churg and Strauss).

GPA is a multisystem vasculitis mainly affecting the upper and lower respiratory tract as well as the kidneys. The prevalence of AAV is about 300 per 100 million and an annual incidence rate 9.8 per one million. The median age group affected is about 55 years old with equal sex distribution. There are two subtypes defined, limited GPA and severe GPA, the former with excellent long-term survival. Diagnosis is based on clinical, laboratory, or serologic pathology as well as biopsy. Pulmonary involvement may lead to patchy alveolar infiltrates, hemorrhage, and cavitating lesions seen on routine chest X-rays and better defined with CT scan. Musculoskeletal manifestations include arthralgias sometimes with synovitis which rarely lead to erosive changes on X-rays.

Early diagnosis and therapeutic intervention has influenced the survival of patients with GPA. Through the years, present and previous trials have compared the role of different immunosuppressants in the remission induction and maintenance.

Further Reading

1. Aringer M, Steiner G, Smolen J. Does mixed connective tissue disease exist? Yes. Rheum Dis Clin N Am. 2005;31:411–20.
2. Bossert M, Prati C, Balblanc JC, et al. Aortic involvement in giant cell arteritis: current data. Joint Bone Spine. 2011;78:246–51.
3. Dasgupta C, Cimmino M, Kremers H, et al. Provisional classification criteria for polymyalgia rheumatica. Arthritis Rheum. 2012;2012(64):943–54.
4. Del Grande F, Carrino J, Del Grande M, et al. Magnetic resonance imaging of inflammatory myopathies. Top Magn Reson Imaging. 2011;22:39–43.
5. Gabba A, Piga M, Vacca A, et al. Joint and tendon involvement in systemic lupus erythematosus: an ultrasound study of hands and wrists in 108 patients. Rheumatology. 2012;51:2278–85.
6. Goh YP, Naidoo P, Ngian GS. Imaging of systemic lupus erythematosus. Part I: CNS, cardiovascular, and thoracic manifestations. Clin Radiol. 2013;68:181–91.
7. Goh YP, Naidoo P, Ngian GS. Imaging of systemic lupus erythematosus. Part II: gastrointestinal, renal, and musculoskeletal manifestations. Clin Radiol. 2013;68:192–202.
8. Kissin EY, Garg A, Grayson C, et al. Ultrasound assessment of subcutaneous compressibility, a potential adjunctive diagnostic tool in eosinophilic fasciitis. J Clin Rheumatol. 2013;19(7):382–5.
9. Schmeiser T, Pons-Kuhnemann J, Ozden F, et al. Arthritis in patients with systemic sclerosis. Eur J Int Med. 2012;23:e25–9.
10. Schmidt W. Imaging in vasculitis. Best Pract Res Clin Rheumatol. 2013;27:107–18.

Crystal-Related Disease

8

John O'Neill

Gout

Overview

Gout, a chronic recurrent systemic crystal depositional disease, is the commonest inflammatory arthritis in men over the age of 40 years. It affects 1 % of adults and up to 7 % of men over the age of 65 years. It is uncommon in premenopausal women and has a male to female ratio of 4:1 for primary gout. It is secondary to an inflammatory response incited by the deposition of monosodium urate crystals (MSU) in soft tissues, joint space and marrow. Aetiology can be divided into primary (90 %) and secondary (10 %), related to urate under-excretion or overproduction, respectively. Urate under-excretion pathologies include idiopathic, association with renal dysfunction and drugs including diuretics, ASA and cyclosporine. Urate overproduction includes increased cell turnover in myeloproliferative diseases, related to chemotherapy in treatment of malignancies and increased purine intake, e.g. alcohol.

Gout has likely been present throughout much of human history. The first written description was by the Egyptians in 2640 BC, describing acute arthritis of the first metatarsophalangeal joint, podagra. Hippocrates referred to it as the "the unwalkable disease" and noted that podagra was an arthritis of the rich, whereas rheumatism was an arthritis of the poor. The first radiographic description was by Huber in 1896, which is quite remarkable since the first x-ray was produced only the year before. Polarised light microscopy allows definitive diagnosis by demonstrating strongly negative birefringence needle-shaped crystals in the synovial fluid or tophi. However, it should be noted that sensitivity is dependent on the reader's experience. The European League Against Rheumatism (EULAR) task force developed, via evidence-based recommendations, an approach for the diagnosis and management of gout, which will be adopted in this chapter.

Presentation

Gout may present in multiple ways (Table 8.1). Patients with hyperuricemia may be asymptomatic for years before becoming symptomatic, and indeed many will never develop gout. During this phase, there is deposition of MSU crystals in soft tissues and joints. This deposition incites an acute inflammatory response, acute gouty arthritis,

Table 8.1 Different phases of gout

Asymptomatic hyperuricemia	Acute arthritis	Intercritical phase	Chronic tophaceous gout

J. O'Neill, MB, BAO, BCh, MRCPI, MSc, FRCR
Associate Professor, Musculoskeletal Imaging, Diagnostic Imaging, McMaster University/
St Joseph's Healthcare,
Hamilton, ON L8N4A6, Canada
e-mail: joneill2@me.com

J. O'Neill (ed.), *Essential Imaging in Rheumatology*,
DOI 10.1007/978-1-4939-1673-3_8, © Springer Science+Business Media New York 2015

which is usually oligoarticular, involving the lower limb, commonly the first metatarsophalangeal joint. Clinically there is acute onset of severe pain, swelling, tenderness and erythema around a joint. With the first episode, clinical features are sensitive but not specific for gout and other crystal depositional diseases, CPPD, and infection should also be considered. Diagnosis is confirmed with identification of MSU crystals on aspiration.

The patient may then enter the intercritical phase, an asymptomatic phase between attacks of gout. The length of this phase is variable, from months to years. During this phase, the patient may have normal blood levels of uric acid.

Chronic tophaceous gout has become less common with adequate treatment. Tophi, extracellular deposits of MSU surrounding giant cells and mononuclear cells, take many years to develop. These deposits can be within the periarticular soft tissues such as ligaments or bursa, within the joint involving the capsule, synovium, cartilage or subchondral marrow or be distant from any joint such as the helix of the ear. Uncommonly tophi may cause significant local mass effect and compress adjacent structures, e.g. carpal tunnel syndrome with compression of the median nerve or tendon rupture. Tophi, although uncommon, may calcify.

Imaging

Radiographs (Figs. 8.1, 8.2, 8.3, and 8.4)

Radiographic changes of gout are usually delayed by up to 10 years from the first clinical onset of gout. Initially gout is usually oligoarticular but may progress to an asymmetric polyarticular involvement. The lower limb is more often affected. The feet, hands, wrist, elbows and knees are the commonest joints to be involved. The first tarsometatarsal joint is involved in up to 75 % at some time during the course of the disease. The tarsometatarsal and intertarsal joints in the feet, the distal and proximal interphalangeal joints in the hand and less commonly the metacarpophalangeal joints, all compartments in the wrist, the olecranon process at the elbow, the patella, medial and lateral tibia and femur in the knee are most often involved.

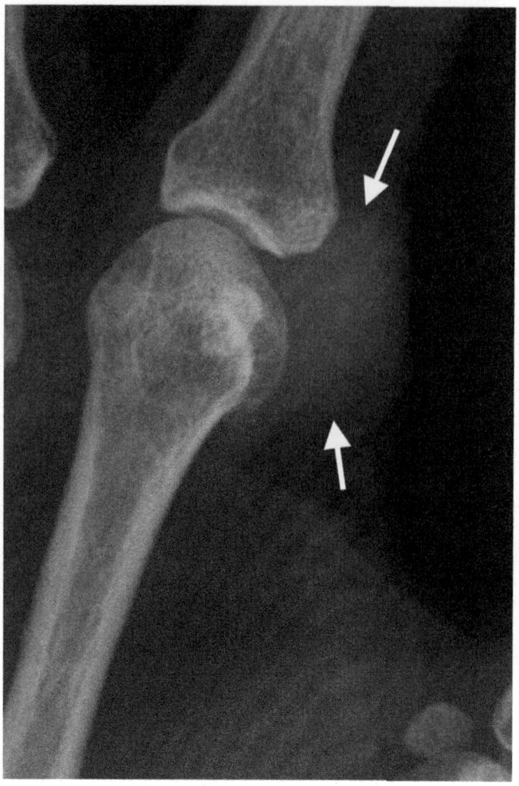

Fig. 8.1 Periarticular tophus, magnified left 2nd MCPJ from AP radiograph of the hand demonstrating soft tissue swelling (*arrows*) with subtle central calcification

Radiographic changes can be divided into early, intermediate and late. In the early stage, corresponding to acute gouty arthritis clinically, radiographs may demonstrate no bony abnormality and may show only periarticular soft tissue swelling. With progression into the intermediate phase, soft tissue tophi deposition occurs which may be visible as nodular soft tissue thickening, of slightly increased attenuation when compared to adjacent normal soft tissue. The adjacent periosteum may develop a lacelike appearance, which may progress to an erosion. Classically these extra-articular erosions have a punched-out appearance with a sclerotic margin and an overhanging edge. The sclerotic margin represents the osteoblastic response to the slowly developing erosion.

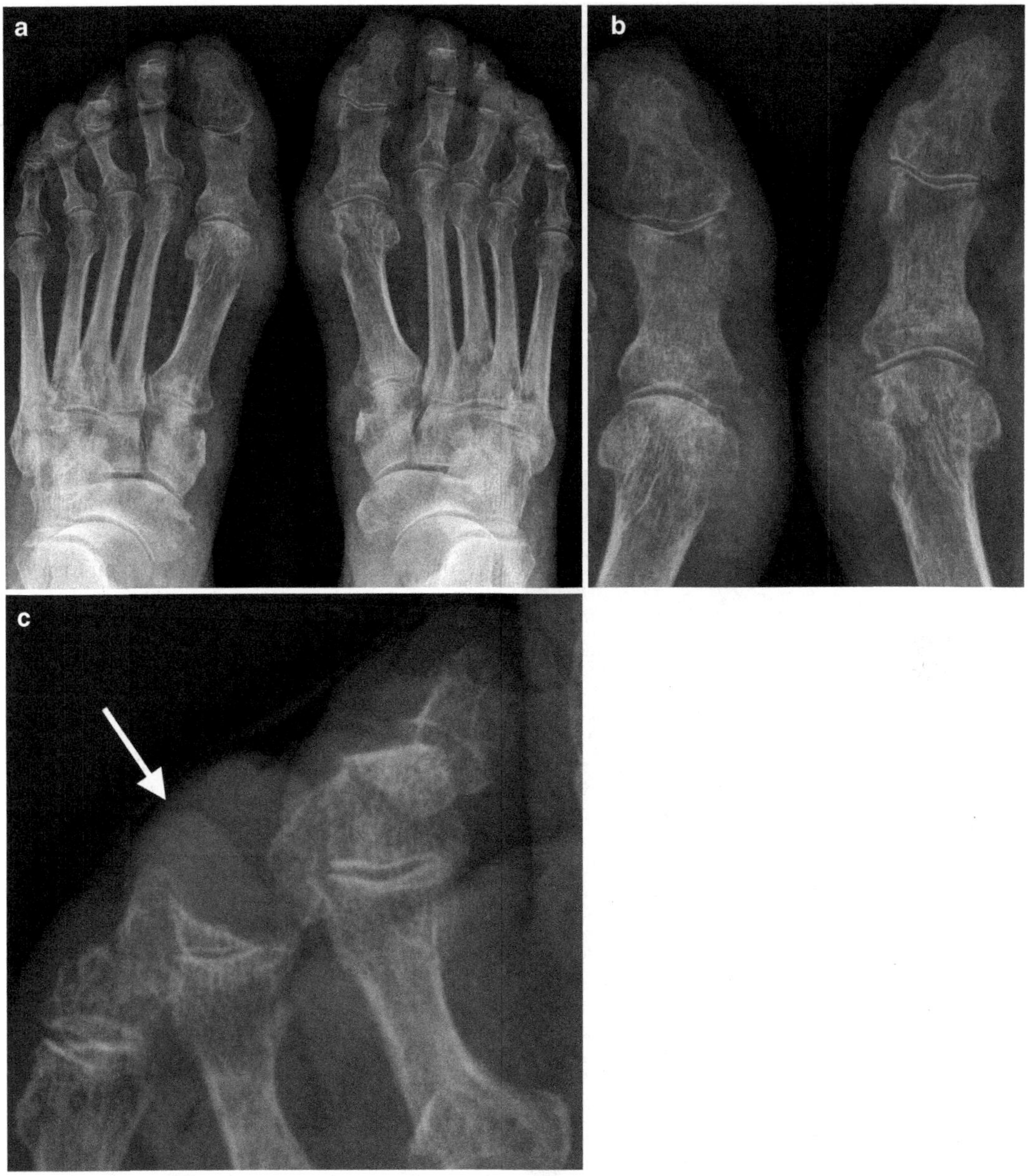

Fig. 8.2 An 87-year-old male with bilateral polyarticular gout of the feet. (**a–c**) AP radiographs of the bilateral feet demonstrating extensive chronic radiographic changes of gout with periarticular erosions, some with overhanging edges. Note the sclerosis on the osseous margins erosions. Marginal erosions, partially calcified gouty tophi and intra-osseous gout deposition with secondary bone loss (*arrow*)

Erosions in gout may be intra-articular or para-articular or occur distant from the joint margin. Those distant from the joint are as described above. Articular erosions start marginally and progress centrally, whereas para-articular erosions are usually deep to soft tissue tophus.

Joint space is maintained in the early and intermediate stages of the disease. Bone density is normal although in acute attacks there may be associated mild periarticular osteopenia. Reactive new bone proliferation may cause localised bone enlargement or mushrooming. Subchondral

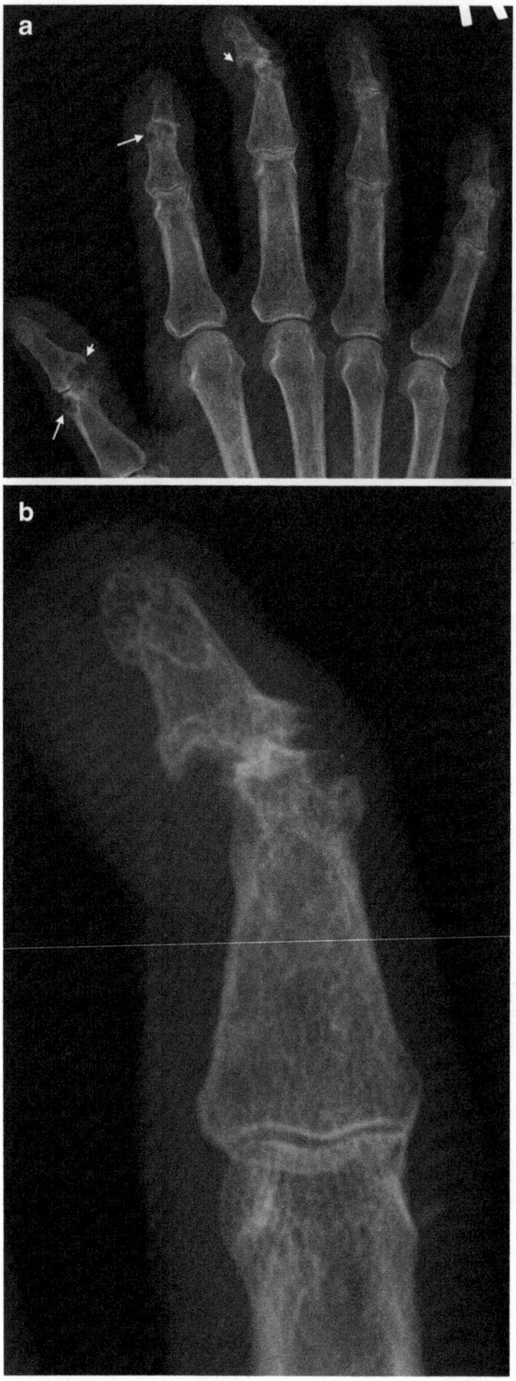

Fig. 8.3 An 80-year-old male with polyarticular gout of the hands. (**a**) AP radiograph, magnified, of the right hand and (**b**) magnified AP 3rd DIPJ demonstrating marginal erosions (*small arrows*) and subchondral cysts in keeping with intra-osseous gout deposition (*long arrows*)

tophi are seen as lucent relatively well-defined foci. Because of the reabsorption of supporting trabeculae, the bone is weakened in these areas, and osteochondral compressions, essentially collapse of the overlying cortical bone into subchondral tophi, can occur. In the late radiographic stage, which is now rarely seen, the soft tissue tophi become confluent and calcify, and joint space is lost with secondary degenerative changes developing. Progressive tapering deformities of the phalangeal shafts may develop. Rarely joint subluxation or ankylosis may occur.

A modified Sharp/van der Heijde scoring method for rheumatoid arthritis was developed as a radiographic damage index in chronic gout. This scoring system assesses erosions and joint space narrowing in the hands and feet, including the distal interphalangeal joints, and is able to discriminate between early and late disease. In addition it strongly correlates with hand function.

Ultrasound (Fig. 8.5)

Ultrasound has a role in acute gout, intercritical periods, chronic tophaceous gout and asymptomatic hyperuricemia. Ultrasound has significant advantages over radiographs as it can identify pathology before radiographic changes. MSU crystals can be identified within both soft tissues and joints. Crystals, as described above, may aggregate in tendons, ligaments, bursae, soft tissues, synovium, cartilage and bone. MSU crystals deposit on the surface of cartilage and can be identified as a linear hyperechoic (bright) contour upon the normal underlying hypoechoic (dark) cartilage forming the "double contour sign"; CPPD crystals deposit within the substance of the cartilage and can thus be differentiated.

Synovial deposition, where MSU crystals are deposited within the synovial lining, incites an acute synovitis. The thickened synovium may have a heterogeneous appearance with hyperechoic micro-foci within representing the crystals. Intra-articular tophi appear hyperechoic with a surrounding hypoechoic rim or halo of inflammatory cells. Extra-articular tophus has a similar imaging appearance. Occasionally calcification

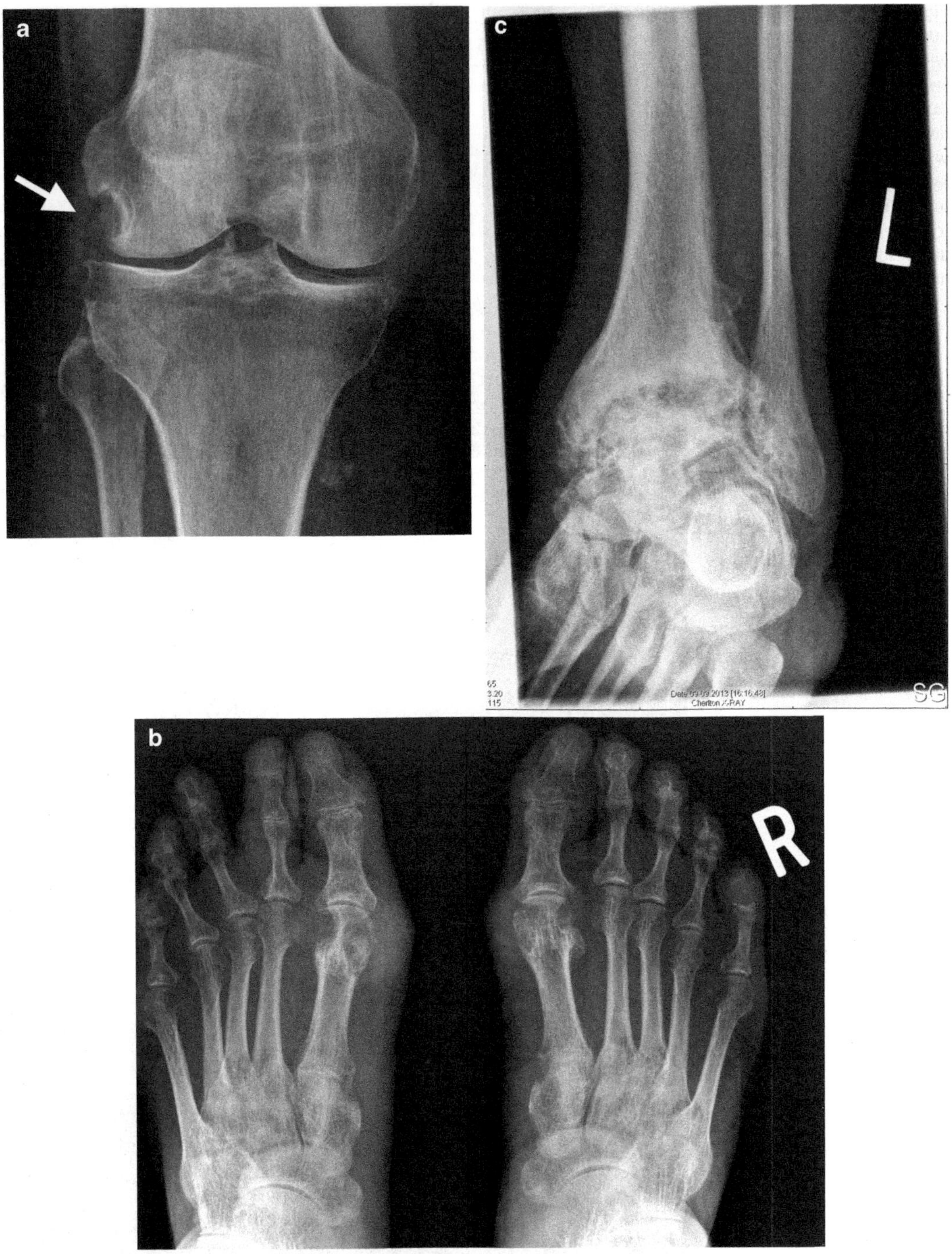

Fig. 8.4 Radiographic changes of gout in different patients. (**a**) AP knee periarticular large erosion (*arrow*) of the lateral femoral condyle with overhanging edge and sclerotic margin, (**b**) another example of polyarticular gout, bilateral AP radiograph of the feet, (**c**) AP ankle with extensive central and marginal erosions, secondary degenerative change with subchondral sclerosis and joint space loss

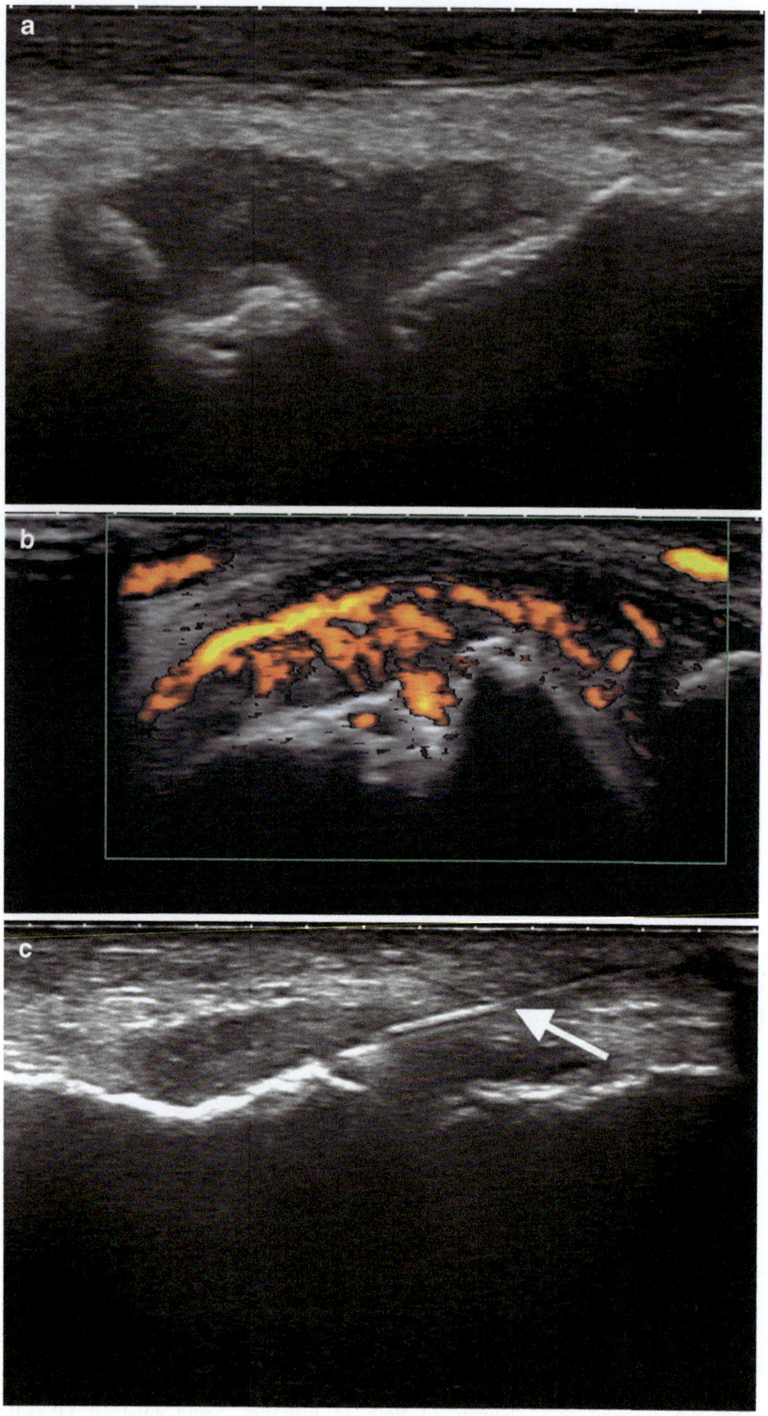

Fig. 8.5 Ultrasound gout of a 50-year-old male presenting with acute left 1st MTPJ pain, swelling and erythema, (**a**) longitudinal ultrasound demonstrating joint distension with soft tissue and minute hyperechoic foci within and underlying cortical irregularity, (**b**) with colour Doppler demonstrating marked internal flow and (**c**) ultrasound-guided aspiration with linear hyperechoic needle (*arrow*)

may occur within the tophus, appearing hyperechoic with posterior acoustic shadowing. The tophus may be more diffuse in appearance. Erosions, focal pathological cortical disruption, should be confirmed in orthogonal planes. Erosions represent chronic disease. A tophus may be identified at the site of the erosion.

Acute gout usually presents as a monoarthritis with localised soft tissue oedema, joint effusion and acute synovitis. One should assess the synovium carefully for hyperechoic foci as described above as well as for tophi and the cartilage double contour sign. Intercritical periods and chronic gout show similar findings excluding the soft tissue oedema. There may be a low-grade chronic synovial thickening present. Tophi size and volume can be measured and may involute and disappear with therapy. Similar changes with decreased cartilage crystal deposition occur particularly if serum urate levels below 6 mg/dl can be achieved.

CT (Fig. 8.6)

Conventional CT is excellent in demonstrating bony anatomy in fine detail and hence in the detection and measurement of erosions. CT is less efficient in evaluating the musculoskeletal

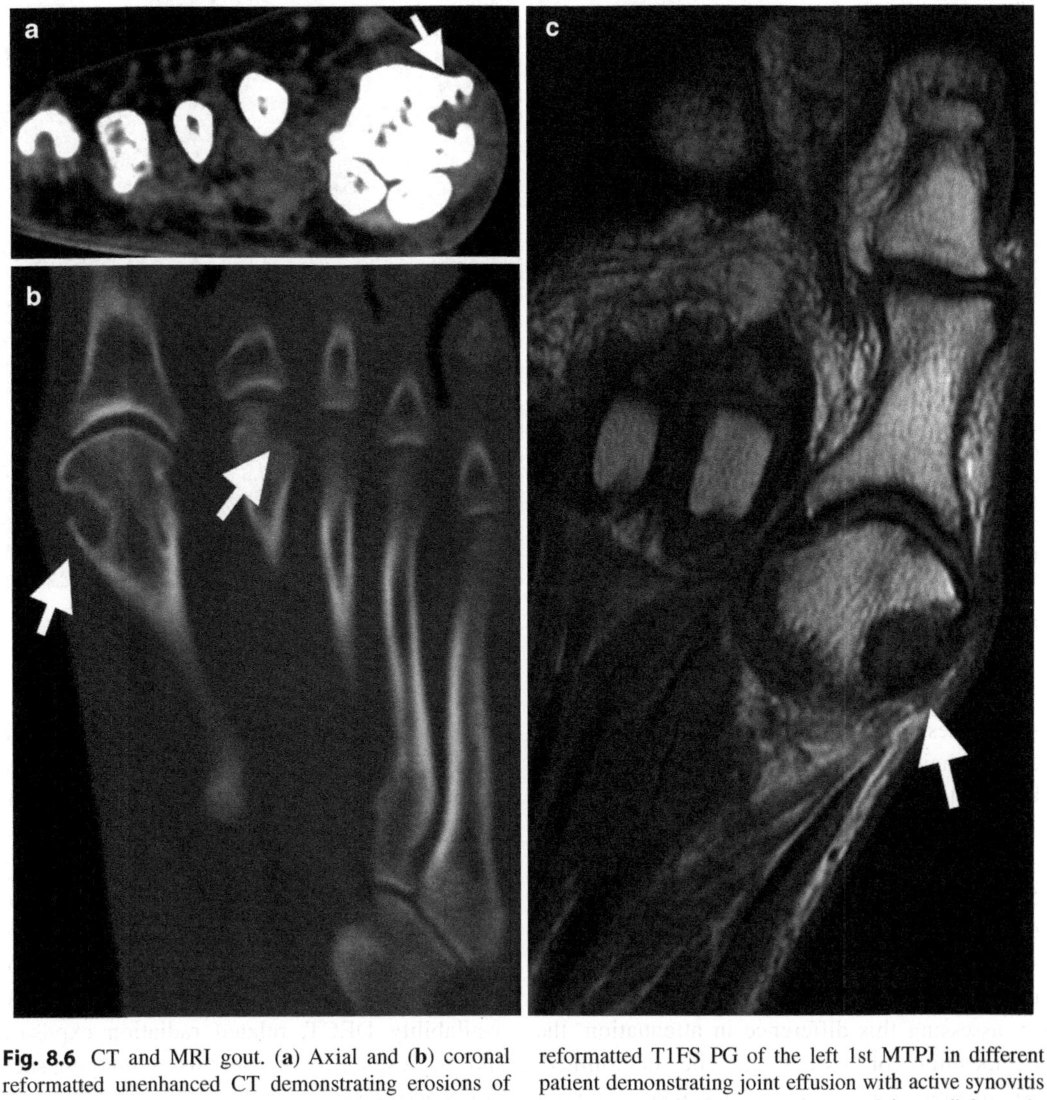

Fig. 8.6 CT and MRI gout. (**a**) Axial and (**b**) coronal reformatted unenhanced CT demonstrating erosions of the 1st and 2nd MTPJs (*arrows*) with sclerotic margin and overhanging edge. (**c**) Cor T1, (**d**) Cor T2FS and (**e**) Sag reformatted T1FS PG of the left 1st MTPJ in different patient demonstrating joint effusion with active synovitis (*arrow* in **e**) and pre-erosive change of the medial margin metatarsal head (*arrow* in **c**)

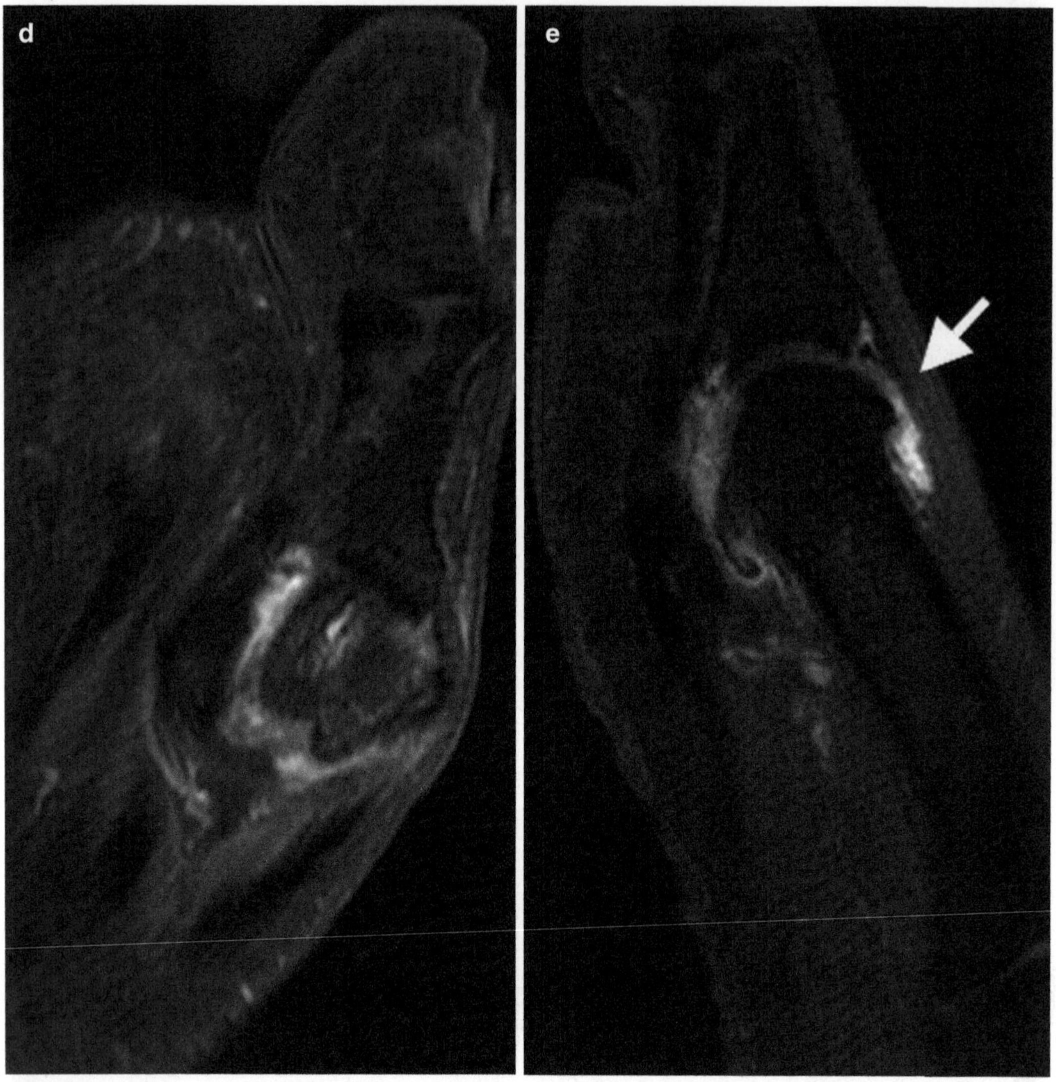

Fig. 8.6 (continued)

soft tissues but can identify tophi from soft tissue due to their intrinsic higher attenuation. Tophi have attenuation values of approximately 170 HU, whereas soft tissues including tendon and muscle have an attenuation of 100 HU and 50 HU, respectively. Dual-energy CT (DECT) uses two x-ray tubes and detectors, exposing tissues to two different x-ray energies. Different tissues will attenuate the x-rays differently, and by assessing this difference in attenuation, the composition of tissues can be determined. Attenuation values can be assigned a colour chart, and MSU crystals can be identified with high sensitivity and specificity. DECT is most commonly used in clinical trials where the volume of MSU deposition can be assessed against different therapeutic options. DECT is at early stages of use in clinical practice and usually confined to cases with a usual clinical picture where alternate imaging has not helped. Limitations of DECT in general practice are related to limited availability DECT, related radiation exposure and the availability of nonionising imaging such as US and MRI.

MRI (Fig. 8.6)

MRI is an excellent imaging modality with the ability to image both osseous and soft tissue structures. MRI can assess both intra- and extra-articular pathology such as joint effusion, synovitis, tophus, cartilage erosion, bone marrow oedema and tendon pathology. A classical erosion and tophi are the best discriminating factors from alternate pathologies. MRI is significantly more sensitive in the detection of erosions than plain radiographs; in one study erosions were detected in 56 % of patients with normal radiographs. Typical gout erosions are as described above. In gout there is usually limited bone marrow oedema related to erosions than what can be seen in other erosive arthropathies. If extensive bone marrow oedema is present, a superimposed infection should be considered.

Tophi on MRI have a variable imaging appearance due to varying fluid and calcific composition. On T2 tophi are usually heterogeneous and of intermediate to low signal intensity but may be diffusely of high or low signal intensity. On T1 there is less variability with tophi usually of low to intermediate signal intensity. Post-gadolinium enhancement is again variable but is usually mild to moderate and homogeneous. In acute gouty arthritis, joint effusion, enhancing synovitis, bone marrow oedema and periarticular oedema can be seen, although nonspecific, but may be helpful when combined with the clinical presentation. Tophi and/or typical erosions are the most helpful in differential diagnosis.

Calcium Pyrophosphate Deposition (CPPD)

Overview

CPPD is a crystal depositional disease. CPPD crystals are deposited in articular and periarticular tissues including hyaline cartilage, fibrocartilage, synovium, ligaments and tendons. Cartilage deposition usually occurs first. The exact pathogenesis is unclear, but it is thought that crystals are deposited in susceptible individuals in areas of cartilage degeneration related to ageing or prior trauma (Table 8.2). Crystals may then accelerate degenerative changes or can be shed into the joint inciting an inflammatory response. Both men and women are affected equally. CPPD is rare under 50 years and doubles every decade thereafter. Presentation in younger patients should raise the possibility of predisposing familial or metabolic disorder. Definitive diagnosis is achieved by confirming CPP crystals in synovial fluid. On polarised light microscopy, CPP crystals are rod shaped and smaller than urate crystals and demonstrate weakly positive birefringence. It is the third commonest inflammatory arthritis and may coexist with other arthropathies in up to 25 % cases.

Table 8.2 Risk factors for CPPD

Risk factors for CPPD
Ageing
Osteoarthritis
Trauma
Haemochromatosis
Hyperparathyroidism
Hypomagnesaemia
Familial

Table 8.3 European League Against Rheumatism (EULAR) terminology and diagnosis of CPPD

Asymptomatic CPPD	OA with CPPD	Acute CPP crystal arthritis (previously pseudogout)	Chronic CPP crystal inflammatory arthritis

There is considerable variation in the terminology for CPPD disease and its varied clinical presentation. The European League Against Rheumatism (EULAR) task force developed, via evidence-based recommendations, a unified terminology and diagnosis for CPPD. This forms the foundation for the approach adapted in this chapter (Table 8.3).

Presentation

As outlined above, CPPD may have variable clinical presentations. Occult CPPD, where the patient is asymptomatic and is discovered incidentally, is likely the commonest. Chondrocalcinosis with or without osteoarthritis may be identified

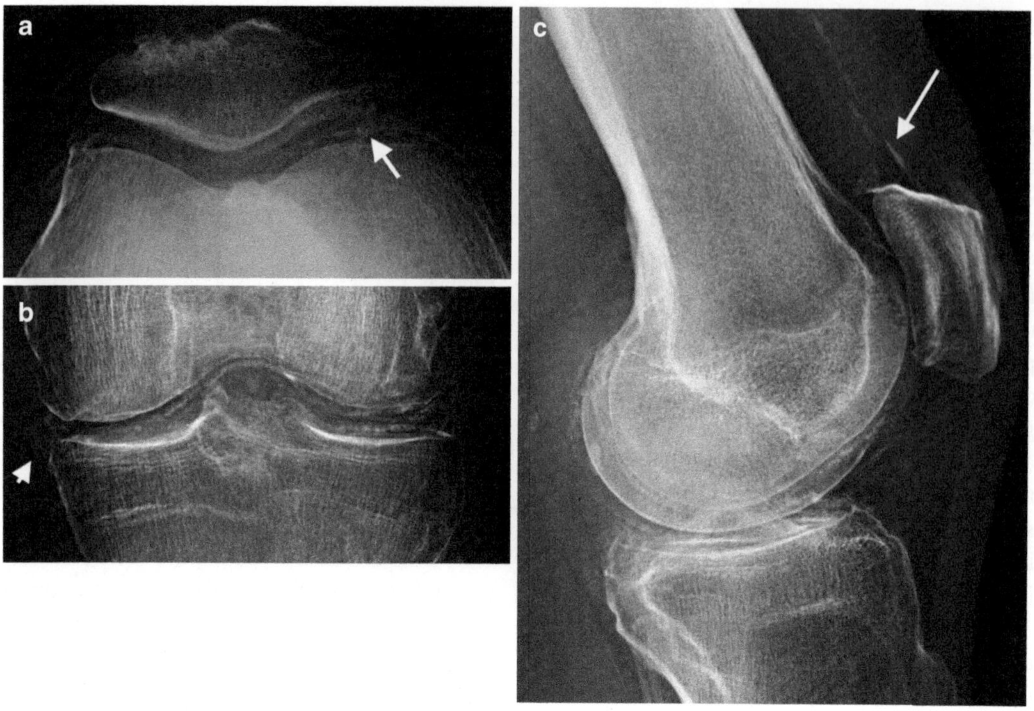

Fig. 8.7 A 70-year-old male with CPPD with osteoarthritis on left knee radiographs. (**a**) Extensive calcification articular cartilage patellofemoral joint (*arrow*) and (**b**) medial and lateral tibiofemoral joints, note also chondrocalcinosis of an extruded medial meniscus (*arrowhead*) and (**c**) lateral demonstrating calcification within the distal quadriceps tendon (*long arrow*)

on radiographs. CPPD may present with features of osteoarthritis with a recurring low-grade inflammatory component. Acute CPP arthritis, previously termed pseudogout, presents nonspecifically as an acute onset self-limiting arthritis with swelling, pain, tenderness and effusion. The differential diagnosis at presentation includes gout and infection. Chronic CPP inflammatory arthritis usually presents as a chronic oligoarthritis with low-grade chronic inflammation and may have a superimposed acute arthritis.

Imaging Features

Radiographs (Figs. 8.7, 8.8, 8.9, and 8.10)

Chondrocalcinosis (CC), calcification of hyaline or fibrocartilage, is best identified on radiographs, with the knees, wrists and symphysis pubis being the commonest sites (Table 8.4). Radiographs of all three areas may serve as a useful screening for

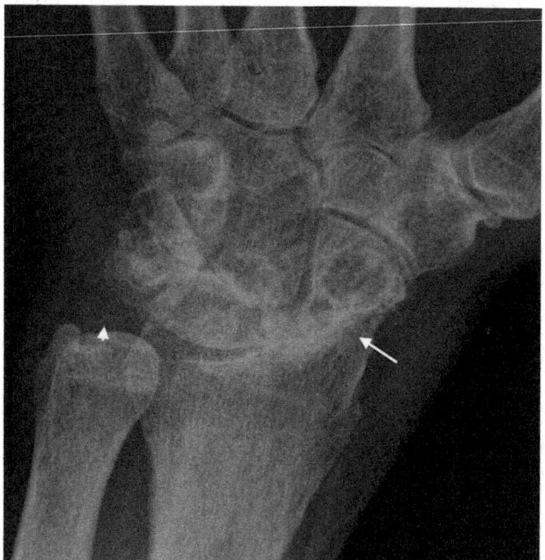

Fig. 8.8 A 70-year-old male with CPPD wrist arthropathy on AP wrist radiograph with chondrocalcinosis of the TFC, complete radiocarpal joint space loss (*arrow*) with subchondral sclerosis and prominent subchondral cysts within the scaphoid. Note the lack of erosions

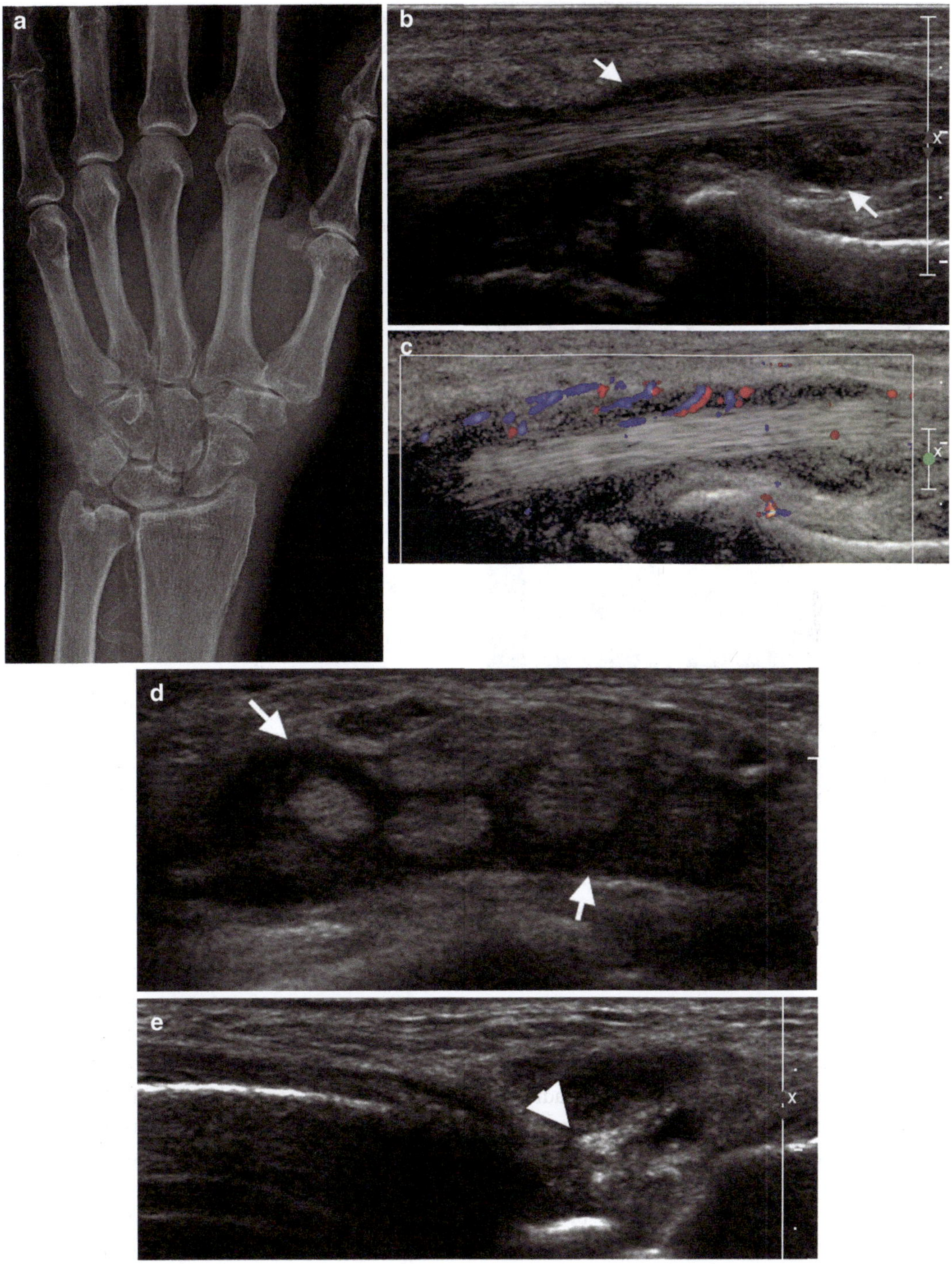

Fig. 8.9 Acute CPPD arthritis and tenosynovitis in a 65-year-old male presenting with acute swelling, erythema and severe pain of the left hand with limited range of motion. Clinical differential of infection versus acute CPPD arthritis. (**a**) AP radiograph demonstrates diffuse soft tissue swelling, chondrocalcinosis and mild radiocarpal degenerative changes, (**b**) longitudinal ultrasound image and (**c**) colour Doppler demonstrating 4th extensor tendon compartment marked tenosynovitis (*short arrows*) extending around normal-appearing tendons, note the hyperechoic foci within the tendon sheath in keeping with CPPD crystals, (**d**) axial ultrasound tenosynovitis (*arrows*) and central hyperechoic tendons, (**e**) longitudinal ultrasound of the radiocarpal joint space with internal hyperechoic crystals (*arrowhead*) and joint effusion and (**f**) axial and (**g**) Cor T1FS PG of the wrist with active enhancing synovitis (*arrow*) without erosions

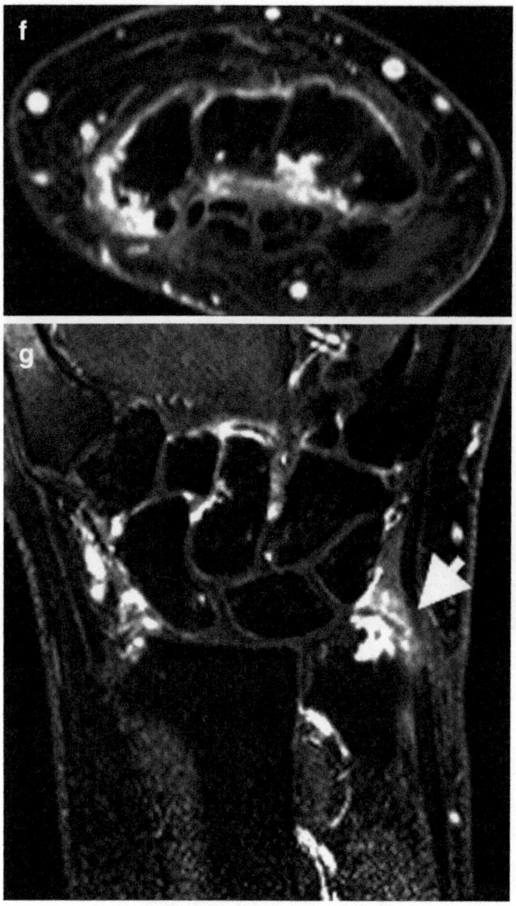

Fig. 8.9 (continued)

CPPD. The knee is affected in up to 8.5 % of the population. CC may be an isolated finding and is not always related to CPPD (Table 8.5).

Osteoarthritis and CPPD are associated, with increased prevalence of CPPD in those who have osteoarthritis. Atypical osteoarthritis distribution should raise suspicion for CPPD (radiocarpal, scaphotrapeziotrapezoidal ((triangular)), metacarpophalangeal, patellofemoral, shoulder and elbow joints). Osteophytes, joint space narrowing and subchondral cysts are present in both; however, distribution differs, for example, at the wrist the radiocarpal joint space is preferentially narrowed in CPPD. In addition, subchondral cysts are more pronounced than in OA. Chondrocalcinosis may not be evident radiographically in the involved joint, and if clinically suspected, a radiographic screen of the wrists (PA), knees (AP) and symphysis pubis (AP) can be performed. There may be significant progression of disease at the wrist joint with development of a SLAC wrist, scapholunate advanced collapse, with widened scapholunate interval, scaphoid rotation, proximal migration capitate and degenerative changes.

Acute CPP crystal arthritis presents as an acute onset of swollen, tender joint (Fig 8.9). Radiographs may demonstrate soft tissue swelling and an effusion. Chondrocalcinosis and changes related to CPPD arthropathy may be present. There may be increased attenuation of joint fluid related to CPP crystals within the joint fluid and synovium. Ultrasound, as discussed below, may be beneficial in further assessment. Chronic CPP crystal inflammatory arthritis may simulate rheumatoid arthritis, and both conditions may coexist in up to 30 %. Features typical of CPPD degeneration are present, but there is notable lack of erosions and periarticular osteopenia that are typically seen in rheumatoid arthritis.

CPPD will occasionally cause a rapidly destructive arthropathy that simulates a neuropathic joint. There is progressive destruction of the articular surface with eventual collapse and multiple intra-articular osseous loose bodies. Soft tissue CPP crystal deposition may involve ligaments, tendons and periarticular soft tissues. The lunotriquetral ligament and the Achilles and supraspinatus tendons are commonly involved. Spinal involvement is underestimated as it is often asymptomatic. Calcification may involve the intervertebral disc, ligamentum flavum, joints, capsules and paraspinal ligaments. There is increased incidence of disc degeneration, loss of disc height and endplate vertebral sclerosis. Degenerative changes in joints with collapse and a pseudo-infective spondylodiscitis may occur. The transverse ligament at the atlantoaxial articulation is commonly involved and may become thickened and degenerate. Chondroid metaplasia with periodontoid soft tissue thickening may encroach upon the spinal canal with secondary canal stenosis and myelopathy. This is more common in elderly women. There may be associated erosion of the odontoid process. This is thought to be a pressure-related erosion as CPPD arthropathy is non-erosive. The crowned dens syndrome is acute neck pain related to calcified periodontoid

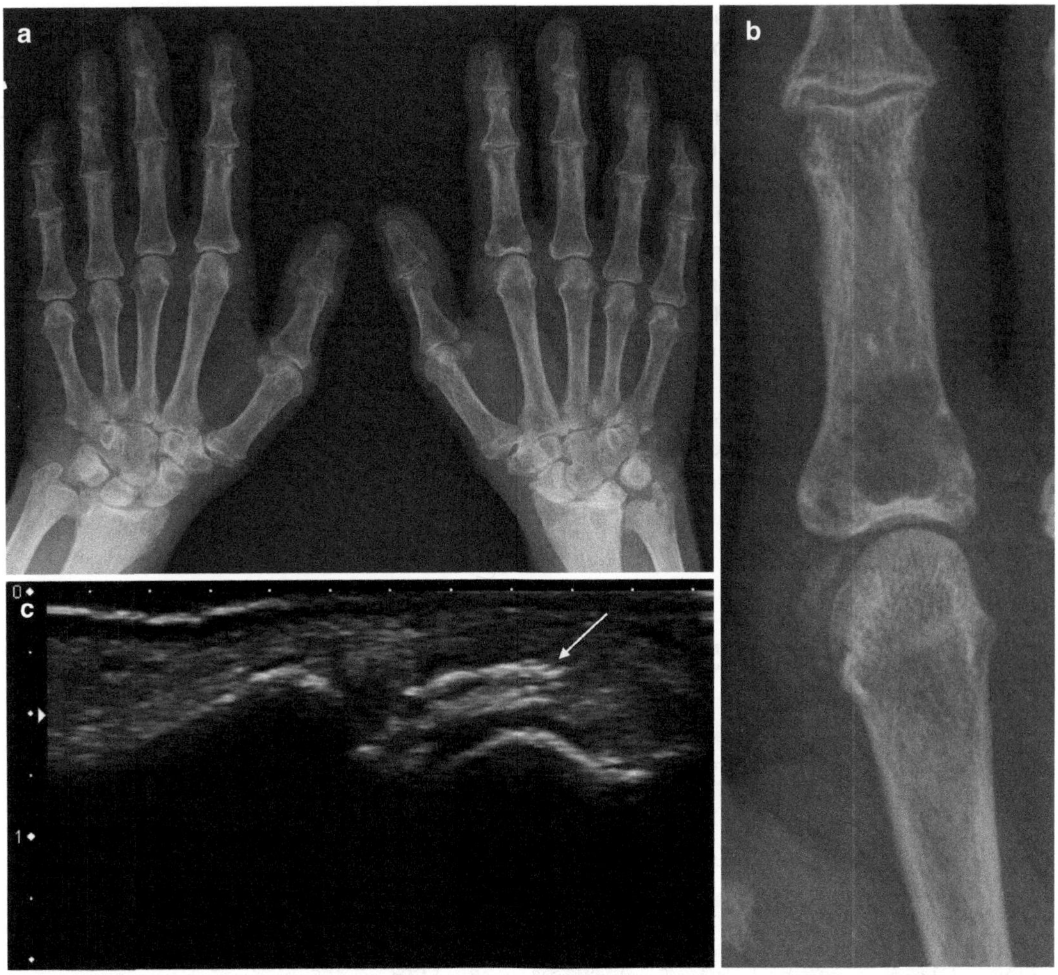

Fig. 8.10 Chronic CPP arthritis in a 55-year-old female. (**a**) Bilateral AP radiographs demonstrating right TFC chondrocalcinosis and bilateral degenerative changes of radiocarpal joints, SLAC wrists, joint space loss and mild osteophytic lipping at the MCPJs without evidence of erosions, (**b**) magnified right 2nd MCPJ with capsular and intra-articular calcification, joint space loss, large subchondral cyst of the proximal phalanx and mild soft tissue swelling, (**c**) longitudinal image of the same joint demonstrating hyperechoic crystals (*arrow*) within the joint

Table 8.4 Chondrocalcinosis aetiology

Chondrocalcinosis
CPPD
Dicalcium phosphate dihydrate
Calcium hydroxyapatite

soft tissue and may be related to CPPD or hydroxyapatite crystal depositional disease.

Table 8.5 Common sites of chondrocalcinosis on radiograph

Chondrocalcinosis	Commonest sites
Wrist	Triangular fibrocartilage Lunotriquetral ligament Scapholunate ligament
Knee	Menisci Hyaline cartilage
Symphysis pubis	Fibrocartilage
Hip	Acetabular labrum

Ultrasound (Fig. 8.9)

High-resolution ultrasound is developing a role in the diagnostic algorithm and assessment of CPPD. Ultrasound can identify both intra-articular and soft tissue involvement. The limitations of ultrasound including assessment of deep structures, inaccessible portions of joints and the experience of the operator have already been discussed in detail. CPPD crystals can be visualised as hyperechoic aggregates and demonstrate a sparkling reflectivity. In hyaline cartilage, crystal aggregates can be identified within the cartilage as subtle hyperechoic foci to extensive deposits. This differs from gout where no intra-articular cartilage deposits are present and crystals aggregate on the surface of articular cartilage. Within fibrocartilage, hyperechoic amorphous deposits are seen. In synovial fluid, hyperechoic floating crystal aggregates with typical reflectivity are noted. In periarticular soft tissue, there may be deposition of amorphous hyperechoic tissue. In tendons, e.g. Achilles tendon, deposition is usually distal, close to calcaneal attachment, linear configuration and may be extensive.

CT and MRI (Fig. 8.11)

CT has a very limited role to play in CPPD. Often incidental articular or soft tissue calcification is noted on examinations carried out for other clinical reasons, e.g. acetabular labral chondrocalcinosis may be seen in patients having a CT of the pelvis. CT does have a role in the investigation of patients with crowned dens syndrome or neurological symptoms related to periodontoid mass. CT can identify soft tissue calcification that may not be visualised on radiograph or is not seen on MRI as the low signal intensity of cartilage may be blended within the low signal intensity of the periodontoid soft tissue mass. MRI however has the advantage of demonstrating in exquisite detail the spinal cord, canal stenosis and any myelopathic changes.

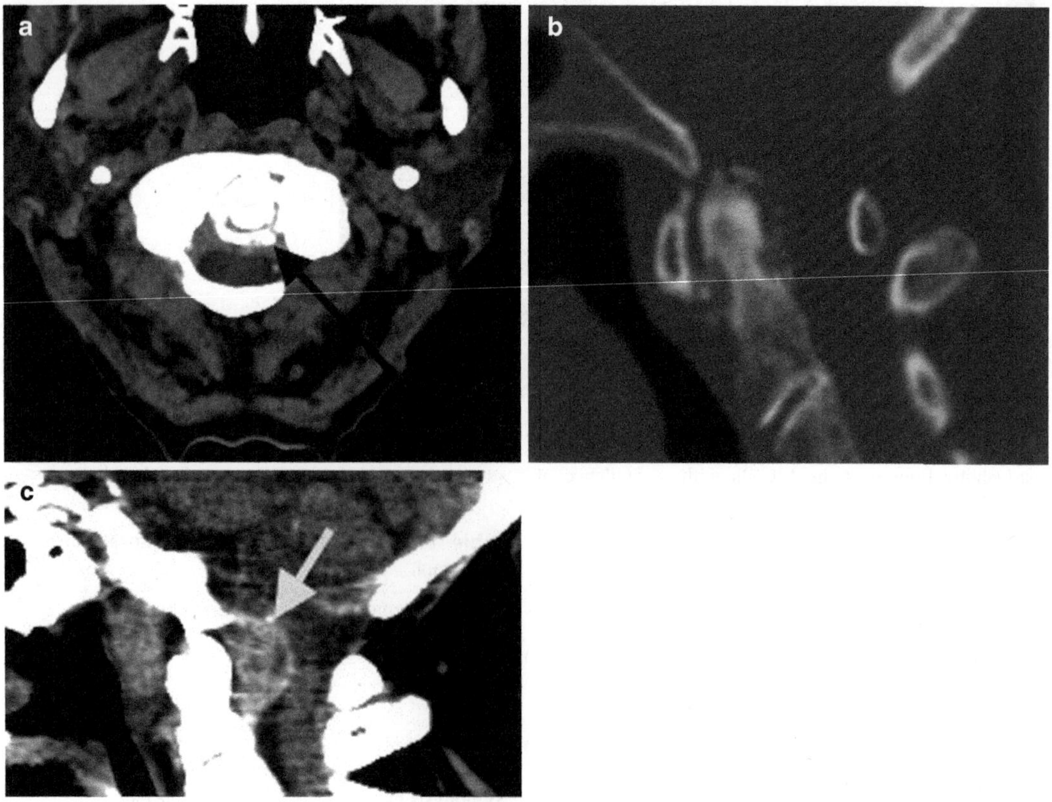

Fig. 8.11 Incidental finding of atlantoaxial CPPD arthropathy on CT head examinations. (**a**) Axial CT of an 81-year-old female demonstrating dense ligamentous calcification (*black arrow*, (**b**) the same patient, sagittal reformats on bone windows with ligament calcification, sclerosis odontoid and pressure-type "erosive" changes of the base of the odontoid, (**c**) sagittal reformat in a different patient with significant capsular distension of the calcified material (*white arrow*) with secondary spinal canal stenosis

Chondrocalcinosis of hyaline cartilage on MRI may cause a blooming artefact, focal low signal intensity, which appears larger than area involved by the crystal aggregates however may also cause no artefact and may not be visible on MRI. Fibrocartilage involvement may cause intermediate signal intensity of the menisci simulating tears on proton density. Calcification in tendons may also be missed as tendons are normally of low signal intensity, unless specific sequences such as gradient echo are performed where the calcification will cause a blooming artefact as described above. Acute arthritis will demonstrate typical acute nonspecific inflammatory changes on MRI including joint effusion, enhancing synovitis, bone marrow oedema and periarticular soft tissue oedema. It may help identify areas for synovial fluid aspiration for diagnosis if ultrasound is unavailable.

Hydroxyapatite Deposition Disease (HAAD)

Overview

Hydroxyapatite crystal depositional disease (HADD) is a systemic crystal depositional disease of unknown aetiology. Hydroxyapatite (HA) crystals are deposited into periarticular soft tissues, involving predominantly tendons but also ligaments, capsule and synovium. All ages are affected including children, but it is commonest in middle age with equal distribution between the sexes. The aetiology of the calcification is unknown, but it is thought to occur in areas of limited vascularity subjected to stress and microtrauma. It is less common than CPPD, but like CPPD is often asymptomatic and may only be discovered incidentally on radiographs. It is usually oligoarticular. HA crystals are needle-like and smaller than CPP. Electron microscopy, X-ray diffraction analysis or radioisotopic techniques can be used but are rarely required clinically. Alizarin red S stain can be useful as a rapid screening test using an ordinary light microscopy.

Presentation

HADD is often asymptomatic but may present acutely with symptoms of pain, stiffness, swelling and tenderness and may have a low-grade fever. ESR may be mildly elevated. The shoulder is the commonest joint involved but may involve any peripheral joint and/or the spine. Spinal disease can have a varied presentation depending on site involvement. Involvement of the longus colli is the most common with acute onset of neck pain and rigidity. Similar to CPPD it may present with the crowned dens syndrome.

Imaging Features

Radiographs (Figs. 8.12, 8.13, and 8.14)
Tendon calcification usually commences as periarticular amorphous cloudlike calcification and gradually becomes more defined and denser. Calcification may change in size and shape over time and may be reabsorbed and occasionally reappear. There are four recognised stages: *formative, calcific, resorptive and reparative*. Patients may or may not be symptomatic during these phases.

The periarticular soft tissues of the shoulder are commonly involved, particularly the supraspinatus. This can be identified on radiograph as focal calcification overlying the greater tuberosity on external rotation. The infraspinatus, subscapularis, long head biceps and teres minor may all be affected. Calcification may rupture through the tendon inciting a bursitis, e.g. subacromial subdeltoid bursitis when involving the supraspinatus. Bursitis is usually associated with an acute exacerbation of symptoms and can cause significant localised pain, tenderness and limited range of motion. There may be underlying cortical irregularity, early erosion and bone marrow oedema. The latter is apparent with MRI.

Rupture of calcification into the joint may incite enzyme release, including collagenase, with subsequent progressive degeneration of the cartilage and joint and rotator cuff rupture leading to a *Milwaukee shoulder* with joint space loss, bony destruction and loose

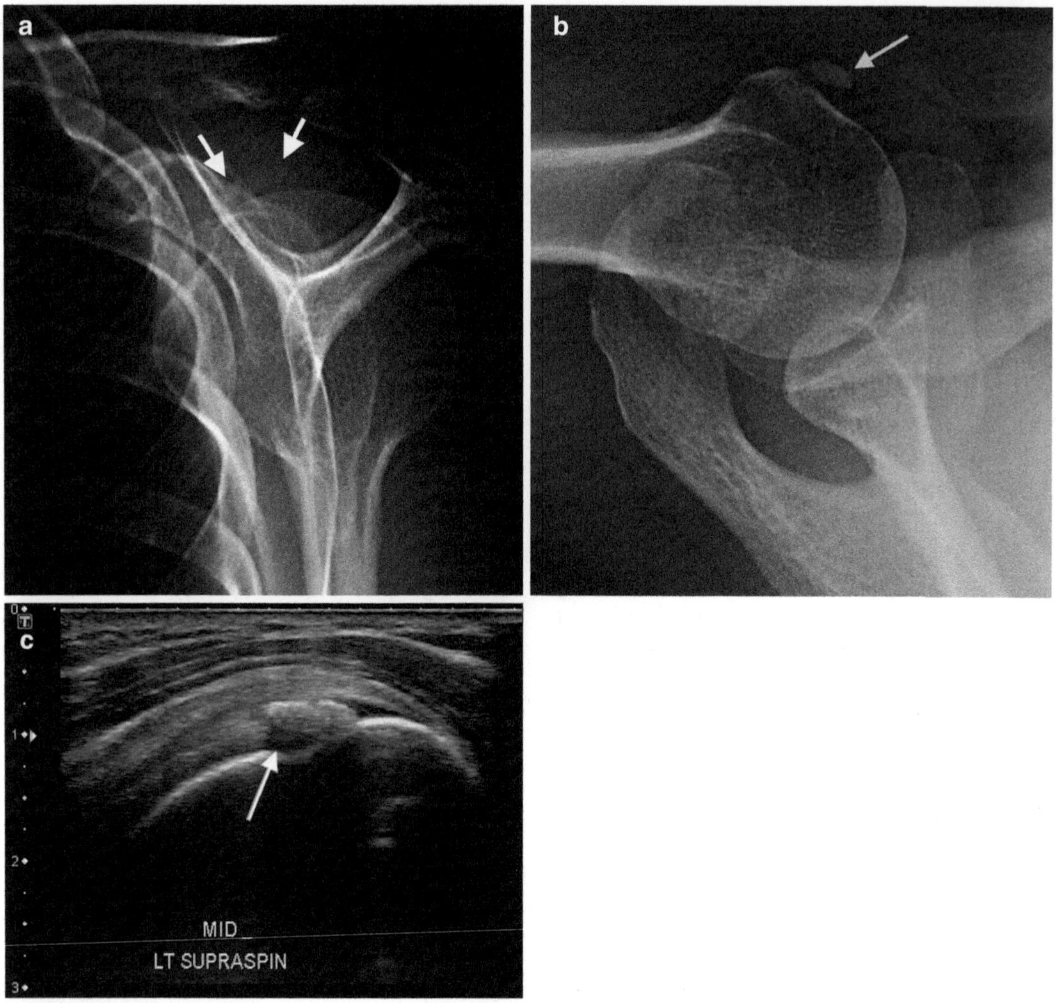

Fig. 8.12 Calcific tendinosis (*arrows*) in a 43-year-old female, (**a**) lateral radiograph of the shoulder demonstrating calcification in the expected location of the supraspinatus, also seen over the greater tuberosity on AP (not shown), (**b**) axial radiograph with calcification within the subscapularis and (**c**) longitudinal ultrasound of the supraspinatus demonstrating intra-tendinous hyperechoic focus with posterior shadowing in keeping with radiographic findings (**a**), no visible bursal distension. Note patient was not tender on compression over the areas of calcification during the ultrasound examination

intra-articular osseous bodies. Alternatively, the rotator cuff may rupture first with subsequent release of HA into the joint. Calcification around the greater trochanter of the hip is common, involving the glutei tendons. There may be related bursal calcification, bursitis or underlying osseous erosive changes. Periarticular soft tissue of any peripheral joint may be involved.

Spinal involvement may be occult or symptomatic. Radiographs may demonstrate ill-defined calcification anterior to the upper cervical spine with involvement of the longus colli muscles, usually occurring in adults. Calcification at the C1/2 level, best identified on a lateral radiograph, is typical. There is associated soft tissue inflammation which is poorly visualised on x-ray and is best appreciated on MRI. In the *crowned dens syndrome*, amorphous

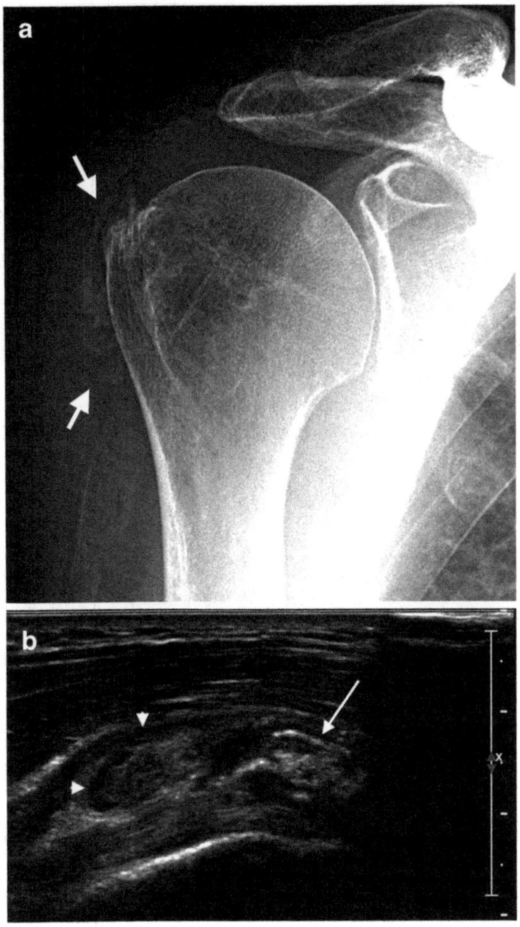

Fig. 8.13 A 52-year-old female drug abuser with severe shoulder pain, ultrasound and radiograph were requested to assess for septic arthritis. (**a**) AP radiograph demonstrating extensive calcification over the lateral margin of the greater tuberosity and focal calcification within the supraspinatus, (**b**) ultrasound confirming extensive calcification within the SASD bursa (*arrow*) with complex fluid and synovitis (*arrowheads*). No joint effusion present; the patient had severe tenderness over the bursa and supraspinatus tendon in keeping with acute calcific bursitis

calcification can be seen surrounding the dens. This is also seen in CPPD. Calcification and any associated erosions are best visualised with CT; MRI is less sensitive to calcifications but is excellent at assessing associated soft tissue inflammatory changes, synovitis and bone marrow oedema which may be associated. HADD may cause disc calcification, paraspinal ligamentous calcification and rarely apophyseal joint involvement.

Ultrasound (Figs. 8.12, 8.13, and 8.15)

Ultrasound demonstrates hyperechoic foci within a tendon, usually close to tendinous insertion. Depending on the formative stage of the calcification, it may be cloudlike without posterior shadowing, well-defined hyperechoic foci with posterior shadowing or a hyperechoic lesion without shadowing. Documenting whether the patient is symptomatic directly over the area of calcification during the ultrasound examination may be helpful in determining whether the calcific tendinosis is the cause of symptoms. Ultrasound can also identify the underlying cortical changes and any related bursitis as detailed above. Calcific tendinosis may be amenable to ultrasound-guided barbotage (see Chap. 4).

CT

CT is rarely required in the diagnosis of HADD and is more often identified as an incidental finding. Depending on the phase of development, calcification is identified within tendons but may also be seen within ligaments and intra-articularly as amorphous and heterogeneous or well-defined solid calcification. CT is excellent at identifying any underlying osseous changes but is relatively insensitive to soft tissue inflammatory changes and is unable to assess bone marrow oedema.

MRI (Fig. 8.16)

MRI is somewhat limited in the evaluation of tendinous calcification, as tendon and calcific deposits will both be of low SI on T1- and T2-weighted sequences albeit calcification is of lower SI. It is best appreciated on sequences that demonstrate susceptibility artefact, such as gradient echo sequence, whereby the calcification will become more obvious and will appear black. Related bursitis, high SI fluid on T2, low on T1 with thickened bursal wall, joint effusion which has a similar signal intensity, and intra-articular synovitis, intermediate to high SI on T2 with intermediate to low SI on T1 with post-gadolinium enhancement, may be present. MRI may also identify erosive-like changes with related bone marrow oedema. The oedema is of high SI on T2 sequences and may enhance post gadolinium.

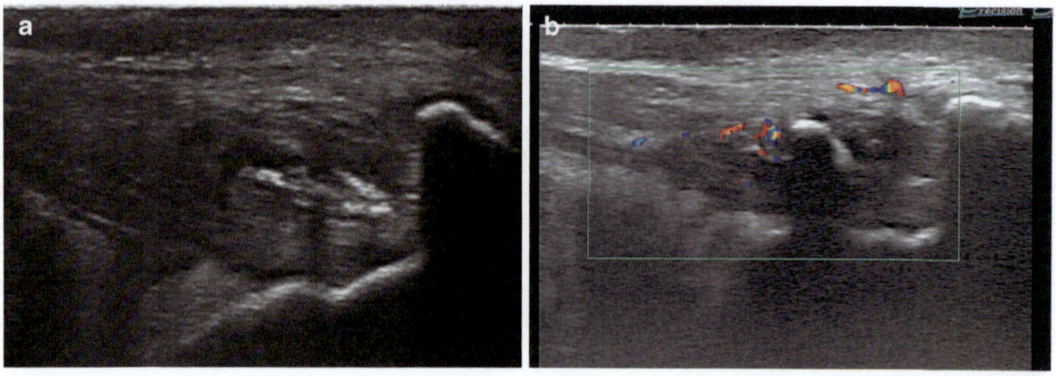

Fig. 8.14 Milwaukee shoulder in a 78-year-old female with progressive shoulder pain and limited range of motion. (**a**) AP and (**b**) oblique radiographs demonstrate marked joint distension with calcified soft tissue and subluxation and osseous destruction of the humeral head (*arrow*)

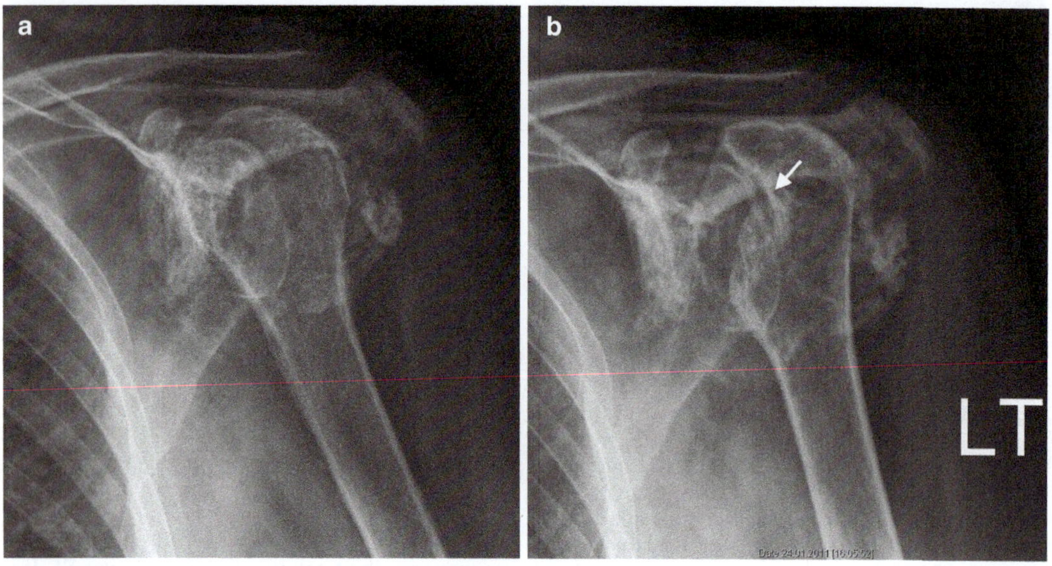

Fig. 8.15 A 54-year-old male with calcific tendinosis of the Achilles tendon (AT) on ultrasound. (**a**) Longitudinal ultrasound with hyperechoic foci within heterogeneous distal AT and (**b**) demonstrating increased internal flow on Doppler ultrasound

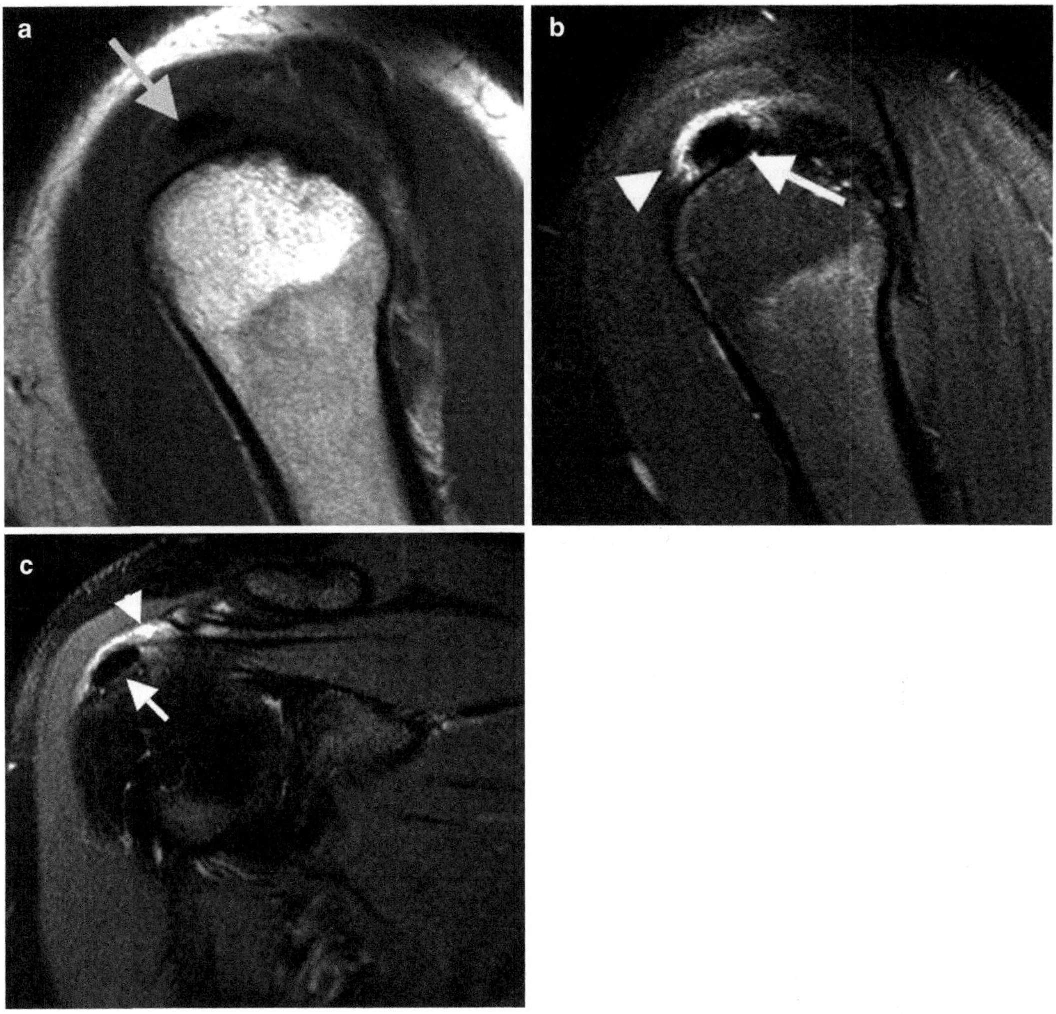

Fig. 8.16 MRI of the left shoulder with calcific tendinosis (low SI on imaging sequences, *arrow*) of the supraspinatus tendon extending to its bursal surface and overlying SASD bursal distension (*arrowhead*), due to leakage of crystals into the bursa and inciting an acute inflammatory response, in a 23-year-old female, (**a**) Sag T1, (**b**) Sag and (**c**) Cor T2FS

Further Reading

Gout

1. Carter JD, Kedar RP, Anderson SR, et al. An analysis of MRI and ultrasound imaging in patients with gout who have normal plain radiographs. Rheumatology (Oxford). 2009;48(11):1442–6.
2. Dalbeth N, Doyle A, McQueen FM. Imaging in gout: insights into the pathological features of disease. Curr Opin Rheumatol. 2012;24(2):132–8.
3. Dalbeth N, Schauer C, Macdonald P, et al. Methods of tophus assessment in clinical trials of chronic gout: a systematic literature review and pictorial reference guide. Ann Rheum Dis. 2011;70(4):597–604.
4. de Ávila Fernandes E, Kubota ES, Sandim GB, et al. Ultrasound features of tophi in chronic tophaceous gout. Skeletal Radiol. 2011;40(3):309–15.
5. Desai MA, Peterson JJ, Garner HW, Kransdorf MJ. Clinical utility of dual-energy CT for evaluation of tophaceous gout. Radiographics. 2011;31(5):1365–75; discussion 1376–7.
6. Glazebrook KN, Guimarães LS, Murthy NS, et al. Identification of intraarticular and periarticular uric acid crystals with dual-energy CT: initial evaluation. Radiology. 2011;261(2):516–24. Epub 2011, Sep 16.

7. Hamburger M, Baraf HS, Adamson TC, et al. Recommendations for the diagnosis and management of gout and hyperuricemia. Postgrad Med. 2011;123(6 Suppl 1):3–36.
8. Khoo JN, Tan SC. MR imaging of tophaceous gout revisited. Singap Med J. 2011;52(11):840–6.
9. Thiele RG. Role of ultrasound and other advanced imaging in the diagnosis and management of gout. Curr Rheumatol Rep. 2011;13(2):146–53.
10. Zhang W, Doherty M, Bardin T, et al. EULAR evidence based recommendations for gout. Part II: management. Report of a task force of the EULAR Standing Committee for International Clinical Studies Including Therapeutics (ESCISIT). Ann Rheum Dis. 2006;65(10):1312–24. Epub 2006 May 17.

CPPD

11. Doita M, Shimomura T, Maeno K. Calcium pyrophosphate dihydrate deposition in the transverse ligament of the atlas: an unusual cause of cervical myelopathy. Skelet Radiol. 2007;36(7):699–702.
12. Ellabban AS, Kamel SR, Omar HA. Ultrasonographic diagnosis of articular chondrocalcinosis. Rheumatol Int. 2012;32(12):3863–8. doi:10.1007/s00296-011-2320-1. Epub 2011 Dec 23.
13. Magarelli N, Amelia R, Melillo N. Imaging of chondrocalcinosis: calcium pyrophosphate dihydrate (CPPD) crystal deposition disease – imaging of common sites of involvement. Clin Exp Rheumatol. 2012;30(1):118–25.
14. Tsui FW. Genetics and mechanisms of crystal deposition in calcium pyrophosphate deposition disease. Curr Rheumatol Rep. 2012;14(2):155–60. doi:10.1007/s11926-011-0230-6.
15. Zhang W, Doherty M, Bardin T. European League Against Rheumatism recommendations for calcium pyrophosphate deposition. Part I: terminology and diagnosis. Ann Rheum Dis. 2011;70(4):563–70.

HADD

16. Choi MH, MacKenzie JD, Dalinka MK. Imaging features of crystal-induced arthropathy. Rheum Dis Clin N Am. 2006;32(2):427–46, viii.
17. Feydy A, Lioté F, Carlier R, et al. Cervical spine and crystal-associated diseases: imaging findings. Eur Radiol. 2006;16(2):459–68.
18. Hurt G, Baker Jr CL. Calcific tendinitis of the shoulder. Orthop Clin N Am. 2003;34(4):567–75.
19. Paparo F, Fabbro E, Ferrero G, et al. Imaging studies of crystalline arthritides. Reumatismo. 2012; 63(4):263–75.
20. Siegal DS, Wu JS, Newman JS, et al. Calcific tendinitis: a pictorial review. Can Assoc Radiol J. 2009; 60(5):263–72.

Endocrine and Miscellaneous Arthropathies

9

Viktoria Pavlova and John O'Neill

Amyloidosis

Overview

Amyloidosis is a rare disease that is caused by the extracellular deposition of a fibrous protein-polysaccharide complex called amyloid into different organs or tissues. Amyloid may be primary or secondary to a chronic inflammatory condition. Amyloid often deposits into the heart, kidney, gastrointestinal tract, and nervous system. Signs and symptoms of amyloidosis are various depending on organ involvement. Amyloid can deposit within the skeletal system, although rarely. Musculoskeletal manifestations due to amyloid deposition may be subtle, subclinical, and only apparent when a tissue biopsy is carried out. Chronic rheumatic disorders with poor inflammatory control may be either the cause or the result of amyloidosis.

Proteins that form amyloid fibrils differ in amino acid sequence, size, function, and native structure. Amyloidosis is now classified based on chemical structure. Twenty-three different fibril proteins are described in human amyloidosis, with variable clinical features. Amyloid A protein, β_2-microglobulin, immunoglobulin light chain, and transthyretin are a few of the well-known forms of fibril deposition.

V. Pavlova, MD, FRCPC (✉)
Assistant Clinical Professor,
Division of Rheumatology, Department of Medicine,
McMaster University, Ancaster,
ON L9G 3K9, Canada
e-mail: viktoria@viktoriapavlova.com

J. O'Neill, MB, BAO, BCh, MRCPI, MSc, FRCR
Associate Professor, Musculoskeletal Imaging,
Diagnostic Imaging, McMaster University/
St Joseph's Healthcare,
Hamilton, ON L8N 4A6, Canada
e-mail: joneill2@me.com

Musculoskeletal Presentation

Musculoskeletal manifestation of amyloidosis may involve either the axial skeleton, especially the cervical spine, or the peripheral skeleton. Amyloid arthropathy results from localized amyloid deposition in and around the joints. Pathogenesis is multifactorial. Amyloid arthropathy is often observed in long-term hemodialysis patients due to deposition of β_2-microglobulin since standard dialysis membranes do not filter this protein. Amyloid arthropathy is typically seen in the large joints, i.e., shoulders, knees, wrists, and elbows. Shoulder pain is the most common clinical manifestation. Joint involvement is symmetrical. Amyloid arthropathy usually lacks the intense distal synovitis. Synovial fluid is noninflammatory and contains amyloid fibrils.

Carpal tunnel syndrome is another common clinical manifestation of MSK amyloidosis due to β_2-microglobulin deposition. Patients can also develop osteolytic bone lesions (amyloidomas) that lead to pathologic fractures. Muscle

J. O'Neill (ed.), *Essential Imaging in Rheumatology*,
DOI 10.1007/978-1-4939-1673-3_9, © Springer Science+Business Media New York 2015

weakness due to amyloid infiltration (myopathy) has been described in some patients.

Imaging Features

Radiographs (Fig. 9.1)

Radiographic findings of large joint amyloid arthropathy resemble inflammatory arthritis including juxta-articular soft tissue swelling, mild periarticular osteoporosis, and subchondral cystic lesions, usually with well-defined sclerotic margins. The joint space is preserved until late in the course of the disease. Distribution is frequently bilateral. Osseous amyloidomas are well-defined lucent lesions of the medullary cavity or are subcortical with scalloping. Patients may present with a pathologic fracture.

MRI (Fig. 9.2)

MRI can identify amyloid deposition in the muscle and bone. The MR imaging appearance of amyloid infiltration within or around the joint consists of extensive deposition of an abnormal soft tissue that has low or intermediate signal intensity on both T1- and T2-weighted images. This abnormal material covers the synovial membrane, fills subchondral defects, and extends to the periarticular soft tissue. Joint effusion is usually present.

Ultrasound

Ultrasound is a simple and useful tool in confirming joint effusions and synovial proliferation. Inhomogeneous hypoechoic synovial thickening without increased flow on Doppler is typically seen within the joint or bursa. Similar ultrasound appearance can be found in the soft tissue, e.g., infiltrating around the median nerve with intratendinous and peritendinous involvement in carpal tunnel syndrome.

Nuclear Medicine

Nuclear medicine has a limited role in the assessment of MSK involvement in amyloidosis. Scintigraphy with radiolabeled serum amyloid P component is a specific investigation that can provide a map of amyloid deposition in tissues.

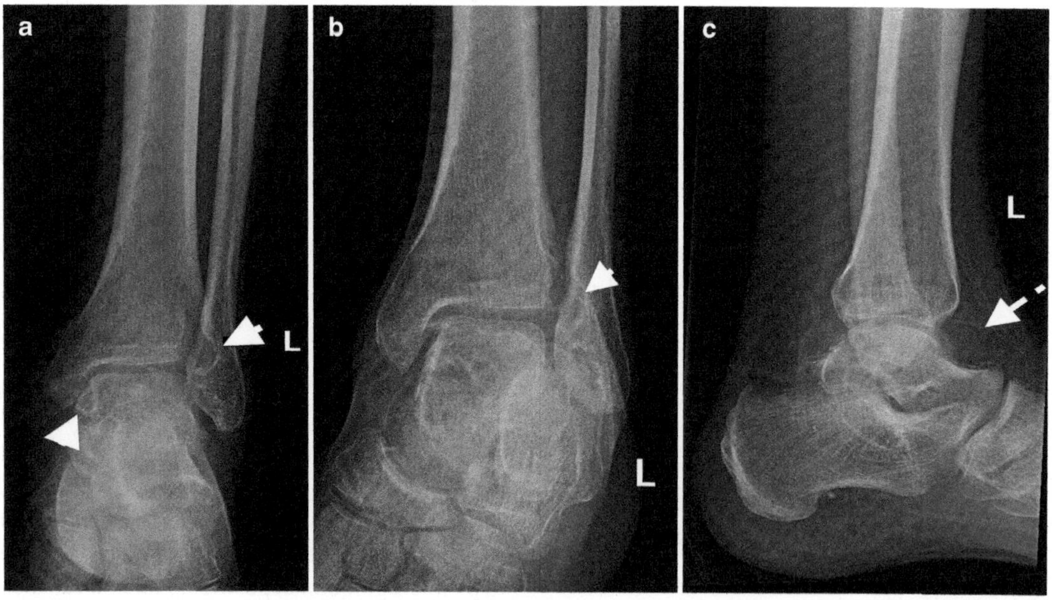

Fig. 9.1 A 50-year-old male with CRF on long-term hemodialysis with right ankle swelling secondary to amyloid arthropathy. (**a**) AP, (**b**) mortise view, and (**c**) lateral radiographs demonstrate well-defined erosions in the tibia, fibula, and talus with well-defined sclerotic margins (*arrowheads*) and joint distension (*arrow*)

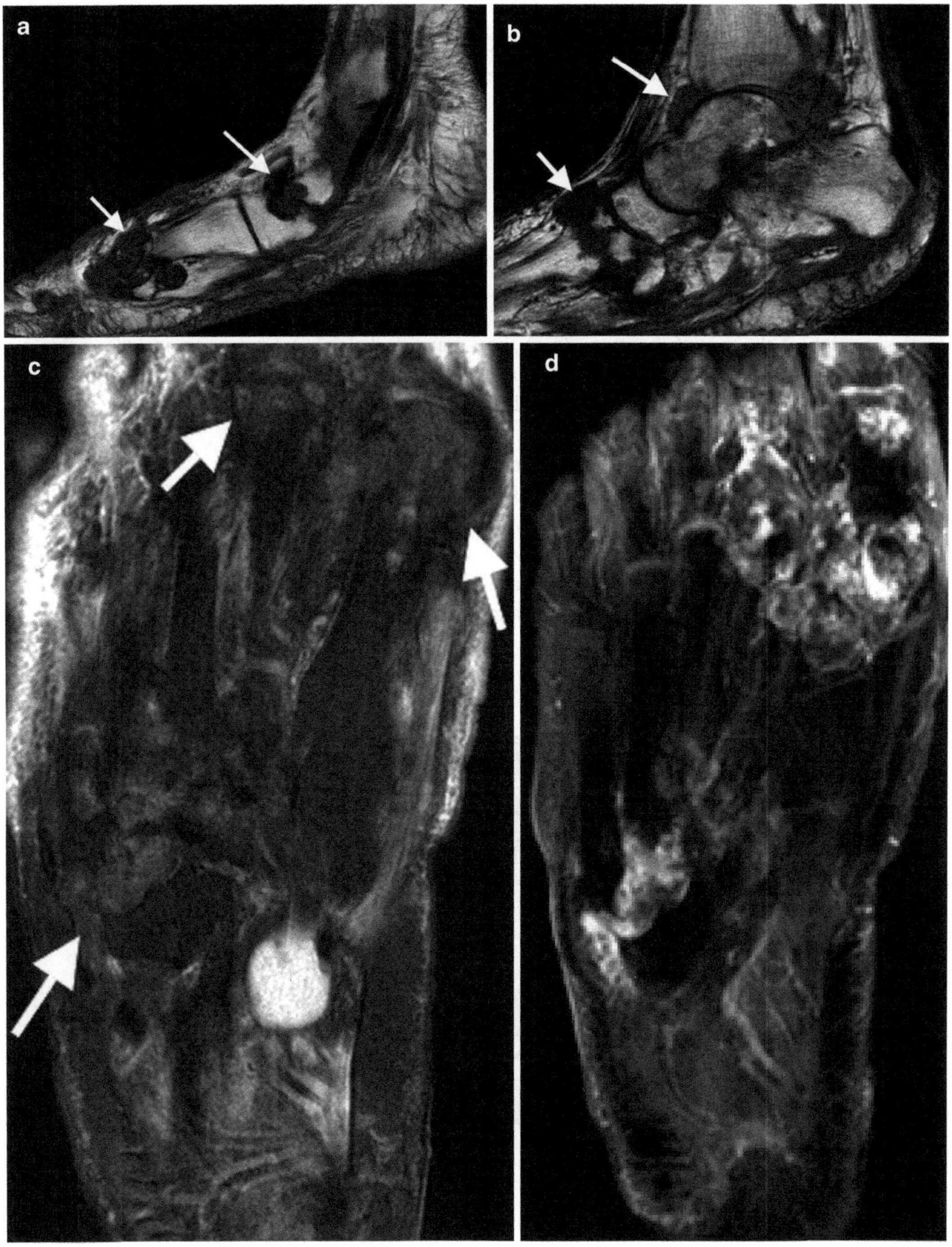

Fig. 9.2 A 60-year-old male on long-term hemodialysis with bilateral swelling in the feet and pain, MRI demonstrates features in keeping with amyloid arthropathy, (**a**, **b**) Sag TI foot with multifocal well-defined erosions (*arrows*) with sclerotic margins at intertarsal and tarsometatarsal joints and ankle joint distension, (**c**) axial T2FS with intermediate to low SI tissue (*arrows*) at involved joints, and (**d**) axial T1FS PG demonstrating heterogeneous enhancement of intra-articular soft tissue at sites of erosions

CT

CT has a limited role in the assessment of MSK involvement in amyloidosis particularly with the availability of MRI.

Acromegaly

Overview

Acromegaly is a rare disorder secondary to hypersecretion of the growth hormone from the pituitary gland, usually secondary to a pituitary adenoma. Presentation will differ between children with unfused growth plates and adults. In the former, there is excessive growth of bone leading to gigantism. In older children with fused growth plates and adults, there is also bone overgrowth but more so in width with related overgrowth of soft tissue and is termed acromegaly. Diagnosis is often delayed as symptoms and clinical features develop slowly.

Musculoskeletal Presentation

There is coarsening of the facial features with an enlarged protruding jaw (prognathism) and forehead (frontal bossing), poor dental occlusion, enlargement of the tongue, and coarse skin. The hands are enlarged and often described as spade-like with soft tissue enlargement of the tufts, increased number of sesamoid bones, and exostoses at tufts with similar changes occurring in the feet. In addition, there is increased heel fat pad thickness, >25 mm. Common musculoskeletal presentations include arthralgia, osteoarthritis, CPPD arthropathy, carpal tunnel syndrome, and back pain.

Imaging Features (Figs. 9.3 and 9.4)

There are characteristic features of the acromegaly. Radiographs of the hands demonstrate joint space widening due to cartilage overgrowth. The cartilage however is not as durable as normal car-

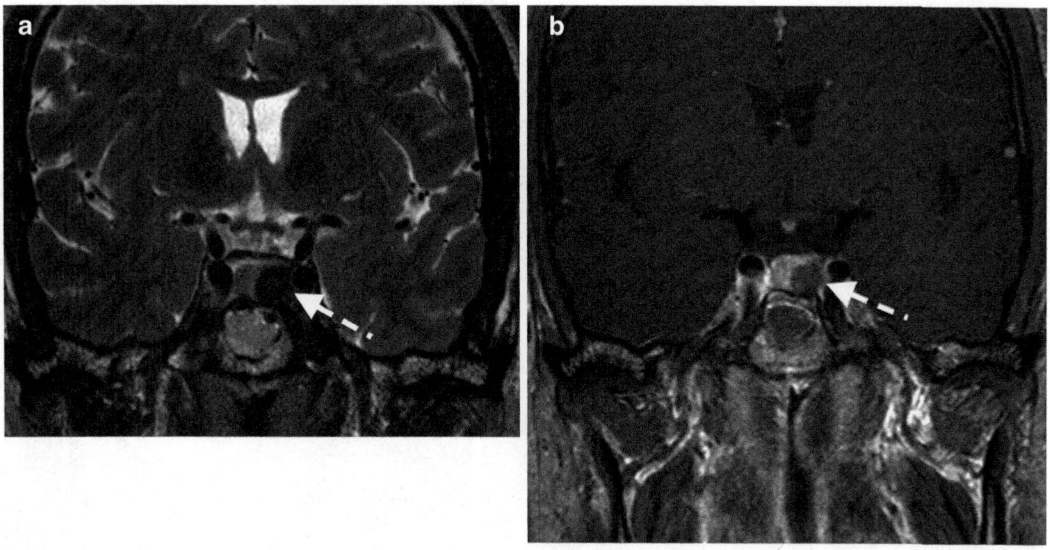

Fig. 9.3 MRI sella in patient with acromegaly demonstrating a left-sided pituitary adenoma (*dashed arrows*), (**a**) Cor T2 demonstrates low SI adenoma and (**b**) Cor T1 PG normal enhancing pituitary with limited enhancement of the adenoma

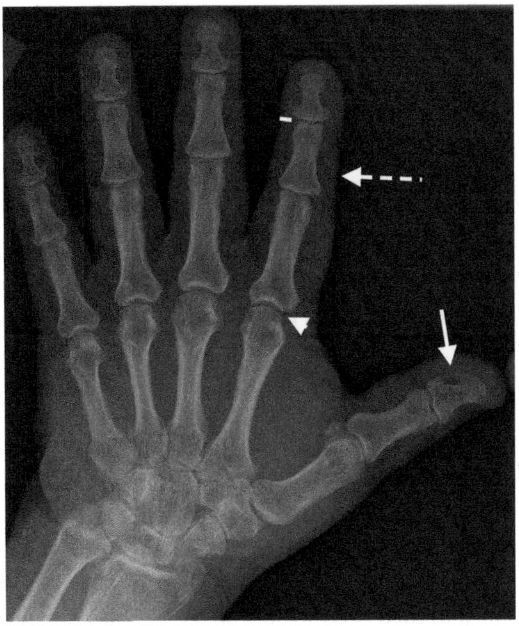

Fig. 9.4 PA radiograph in patient with acromegaly, note thickening of soft tissue (*dashed arrow*), widened joint spaces (*arrowhead*), and prominent ungual tufts (*arrow*). The metacarpals and phalanges are thickened with early osteophytes at the MCPJs (Kindly submitted by Dr. Gina Di Primio, University of Ottawa, Ontario, Canada)

tilage and predisposes to early degenerative osteoarthritis. The short bones of the hand are widened particularly the bases of the distal phalanges. There are small bone outgrowths at the site of ligament and tendon attachments. In addition, there is widening of the tufts with small exostoses and overlying soft tissue thickening. The sesamoid at the first Metacarpophalangeal joint (MCPJ) is enlarged and has been used as a radiographic feature of acromegaly via the sesamoid index. Changes on foot radiographs are similar to those described for the hands.

A lateral skull radiograph may demonstrate prognathism, overgrowth of the paranasal sinuses that, via the frontal sinuses, contributes to frontal bossing. The pituitary fossa may be enlarged and there may be thickening of the skull vault. Spinal radiographs demonstrate enlargement of vertebrae in AP and lateral dimensions, prominent end plate osteophytosis, and posterior vertebral scalloping. The intervertebral disk is enlarged. There is increased thoracic kyphosis and lumbar lordosis.

Alkaptonuria

This is a rare autosomal recessive metabolic disorder related to the absence of an enzyme, homogentisic acid oxidase, with subsequent accumulation of homogentisic acid (HA) in the body. HA is deposited in various organs and induces a bluish-black discoloration of tissues including the cartilage of the ear (ochronosis). HA is excreted in the urine, which turns dark if left to stand. Musculoskeletal presentation, secondary to HA deposition in cartilage and connective tissue, includes arthralgia and back pain from large joint and intervertebral disk involvement. The intervertebral disks demonstrate calcification, disk degeneration, and vacuum phenomenon. The outer fibers of the annulus fibrosus may ossify and simulate syndesmophytes. The vertebrae are osteoporotic. Degenerative changes are common at the sacroiliac joints, symphysis pubis, and large joints. Degenerative changes in large joints may be atypical, e.g., involving just one compartment of a multicompartmental joint or involve a joint not exposed to primary osteoarthritis such as the glenohumeral joint. Tendinous calcification may occur.

Wilson's Disease

Wilson's disease, also known as hepatolenticular degeneration, is a rare autosomal recessive metabolic disorder with excessive accumulation of copper in tissues and subsequent organ dysfunction. Features are most prevalent in the liver (cirrhosis), the brain and basal ganglia (movement disorders including ataxia and parkinsonism, psychiatric disorders), kidneys (renal tubular acidosis), and the cornea (Kayser-Fleischer rings). Ceruloplasmin is usually low. Musculoskeletal involvement includes a CPPD-like arthropathy, chondrocalcinosis, subchondral bone fragmentation, and degenerative changes particularly in large joints, osteopenia, and osteomalacia.

Hemochromatosis

Overview

Hemochromatosis, primary and secondary, is a disease of abnormal iron metabolism causing chronic iron overload and iron deposition in parenchymal organs. Primary hemochromatosis is a common autosomal recessive genetic disorder, which is caused by a defect in the HFE gene, the protein product of which regulates iron absorption from the gastrointestinal tract. Of two known important mutations in HFE, C282Y and H63D, C282Y is the most important and accounts for more than 95 % of symptomatic cases of hemochromatosis. Primary hemochromatosis affects 1:200 persons of Northern European decent with the highest prevalence being in people of Celtic origin. Although the genetic defect is distributed equally among men and women, the iron loss as a result of menstruation is protective, resulting in a clinical male predilection (M: F ~ 2–10:1). In men, the diagnosis usually becomes evident in middle age (30–40 years of age), whereas in women, clinical manifestation is delayed until the postmenopausal period.

Typical organs involved are the joints, liver, heart, pancreas, pituitary, nerves, and skin. The most common manifestation is hyperpigmented skin ("bronze" skin) and hepatomegaly. Arthralgia is present in up to 50 % of patients. Diabetes, heart failure, arrhythmia, hypothyroidism, hypogonadism, and hypopituitarism are other well-recognized clinical manifestations of hemochromatosis.

Secondary iron overload is rare but can be due to frequent blood transfusions, hemolytic anemia, myelodysplasia, juvenile hemochromatosis, and Friedreich's ataxia.

Musculoskeletal Presentation

Hemochromatosis can affect most joints in the body, but the primary articular manifestation of the disease is a characteristic symmetric, noninflammatory arthritis affecting the second and third MCPJs. Given this joint distribution, hemochromatosis may mimic rheumatoid arthritis. Absence of inflammatory features (increased warmth and erythema) helps to differentiate it from rheumatoid arthritis. Patients with hemochromatosis may also have recurrent attacks of pseudogout secondary to calcium pyrophosphate deposition (CPPD) (see chap. 8). Hemochromatosis arthropathy has an insidious onset and may occur at any stage during the course of the disease; in rare cases, it is the initial manifestation. Over time, large joints such as the hips, knees, and shoulders can be affected. The pathogenesis of hemochromatosis arthropathy has been associated with the presence of iron in joint tissue, a defect in cartilage metabolism, and immunological dysfunction. It is usually a slowly progressive non-deforming disease.

Imaging Features

Radiographs (Fig. 9.5)
Radiographs are the mainstay of musculoskeletal imaging in hemochromatosis and occasionally may provide the first suggestion of the disease. Hemochromatosis arthropathy presents with features of degenerative joint disease on plain radiograph. Hemochromatosis causes

destruction of joint cartilage due to defect in cartilage metabolism, and patients present with features of a secondary osteoarthritis. Radiographs demonstrate joint space narrowing, sclerosis, and osteophytosis with associated diffuse osteoporosis. However, in hemochromatosis, radiographs show degenerative changes with some unusual features. These include involvement at the joints that are not commonly involved in degenerative joint disease, such as the MCPJs, wrists, elbows, and glenohumeral articulations. Hooklike osteophytes on the radial aspect of the metacarpal heads of the second and third MCPJs are characteristic.

Furthermore it may be characterized by global joint space narrowing and chondrocalcinosis, an

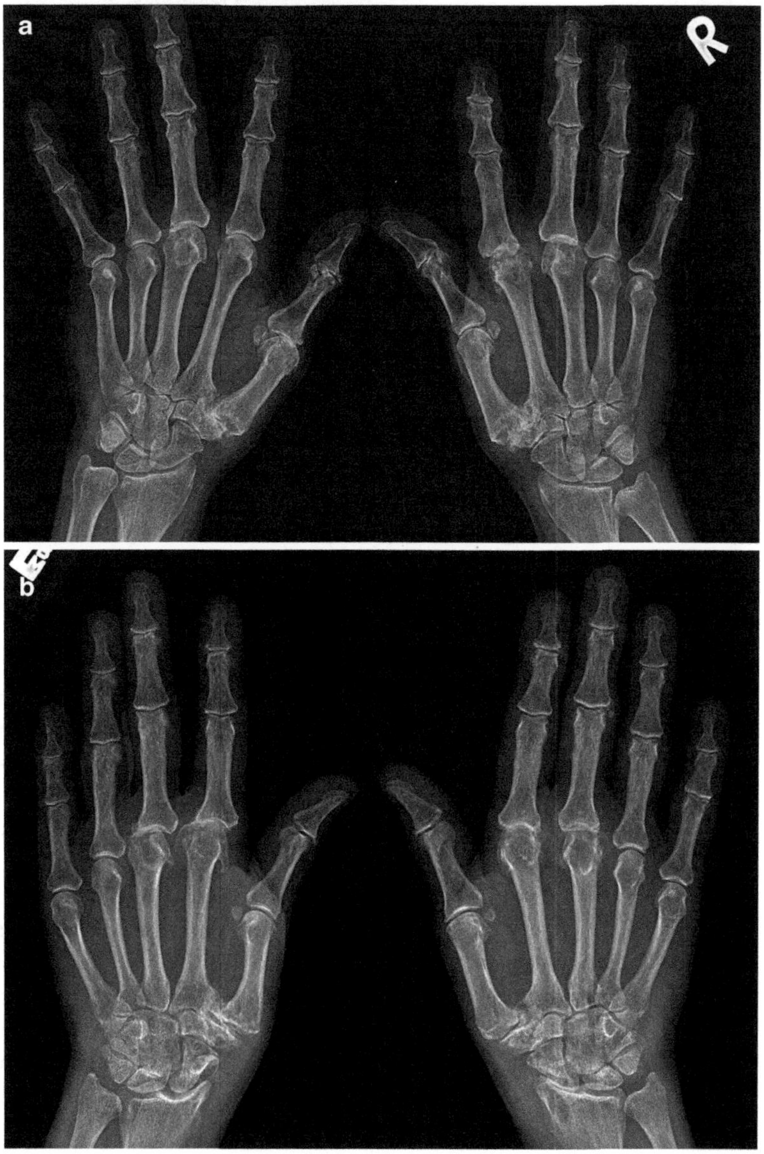

Fig. 9.5 (**a**) A 62-year-old female with hemochromatosis, AP radiography of the bilateral hands demonstrates degenerative changes at the MCPJs, most pronounced at the second and third and the first CMC joints, subtle chondrocalcinosis of the left TFC. (**b**) AP radiograph bilateral hands with more advanced degenerative changes and hooklike osteophytes of the MCPJs in a 48-year-old male with hemochromatosis, also radiocarpal degeneration with scalloping radius and subchondral cyst formation, typically seen in CPPD arthropathy. (**c**) The same patient, AP knee radiograph with chondrocalcinosis and large medial tibiofemoral osteophytosis. (**d**) CT abdomen with secondary cirrhosis, liver is atrophic with surface nodularity (*dashed arrow*)

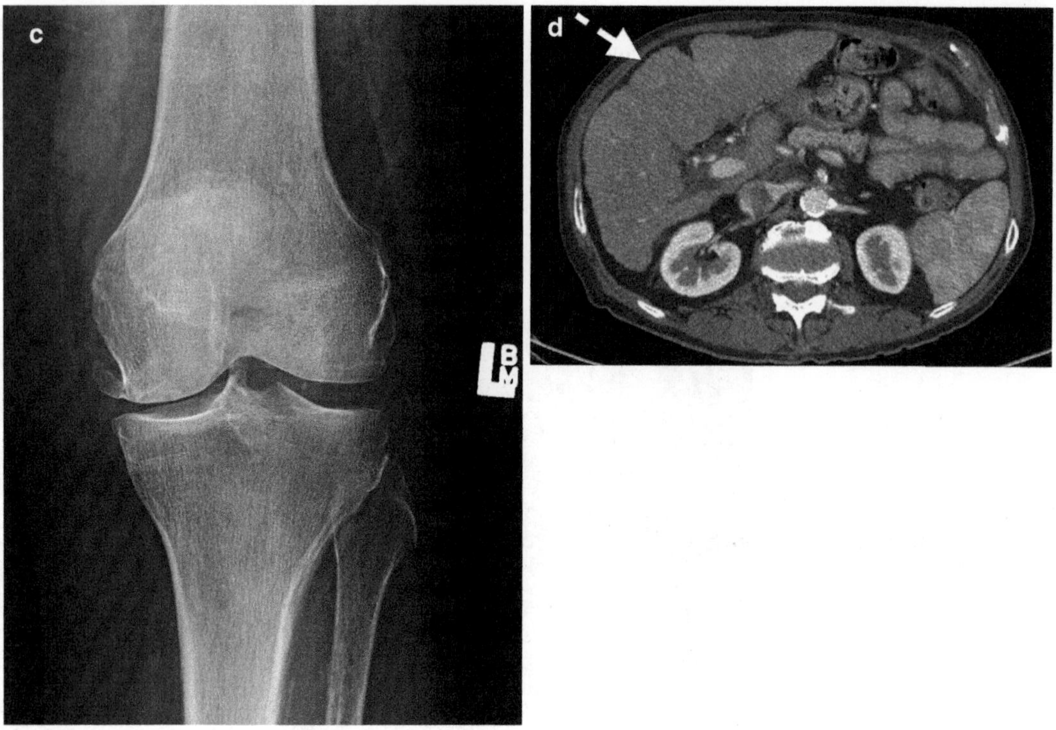

Fig. 9.5 (continued)

unusual finding in degenerative joint disease. Arthropathy may be associated with multiple cysts in the subchondral bone, which can occasionally reach a large size. The joint space loss is associated with subchondral bony eburnation and cyst formation. Periarticular erosions and deformities are not features of hemochromatosis. Subchondral radiolucency of the femoral head and atypical stripping of the cartilage from the subchondral bone are thought to be specific radiographic and histological changes of hemochromatosis arthritis.

MRI/CT/US/Nuclear Medicine

These modalities are usually not required in the assessment of hemochromatosis-related arthropathy. Occasionally MRI or ultrasound can be used for assessment of active synovitis.

Hemophilia

Overview

Hemophilia is a rare inherited bleeding disorder. Hemophilia A (factor VIII deficiency) affects less than 1 in 10,000 people. Hemophilia B (factor IX deficiency) is even less common, affecting approximately 1 in 50,000 people. The most severe forms of hemophilia almost always affect males due to X-linked inheritance pattern. Females can be seriously affected only if the father is a hemophiliac and the mother is a carrier or in the case of X-inactivation that occurs at an early stage of embryogenesis resulting in unusually low levels of factor VIII or IX. These cases are extremely rare. The degree of factor VIII deficiency correlates with the extent of bleeding, and hemophilia A can be classified as severe (<1 % activity), moderate (1–5 %), or mild (5–25 %). Common symptoms of hemophilia are surface bruising, hematuria, and peritoneal, retroperitoneal, and intracranial bleeding as well as MSK involvement.

Musculoskeletal Presentation

Musculoskeletal involvement includes soft tissue muscle hemorrhage, hemarthrosis, and intraosseous hemorrhage. The most commonly affected joints are the large joints, i.e., knees, elbows, ankles, hips, and shoulders. In patients with severe form of hemophilia, spontaneous bleeding occurs with minimal or no trauma. Joint involvement in severe forms of hemophiliac patients occurs in up to 90 % of patients by the age of 10 years. Recurrent intra-articular bleeding resulting in arthropathy is a leading cause of morbidity in hemophilia.

Hemophilic arthropathy is a joint-destroying disorder that is more prevalent before adulthood. Hemorrhage begins in the synovium before extending into the joint space. Blood causes an inflammatory response in the synovium, resulting in synovial hypertrophy and joint hyperemia. These responses make further bleeding more likely. Intra-articular bleeding is associated with joint effusion that can persist for days without treatment. Recurrent intra-articular hemorrhages cause hemosiderin deposition. Periarticular osteoporosis and regional soft tissue swelling are commonly seen with repeated bleeding. Initially the joint space is preserved. As arthropathy progresses, symmetric cartilage destruction and joint space narrowing are observed. Later manifestations of hemophilic arthropathy include osseous irregularity and erosions with secondary severe degenerative joint disease, including osteophytes, large subchondral cysts, and sclerosis. Subchondral cystic changes are thought to be due to both synovial intrusions through fissures in the joint surface and primary intraosseous hemorrhage. Eventually joint ankylosis may occur.

Imaging Features

Radiographs (Figs. 9.6 and 9.7)

Plain radiography is the primary imaging tool for evaluation of hemophilic joint disease. Radiographic features depend on the stage of the disorder. In the initial hemarthrosis, the radiographic finding is similar to a joint effusion. Increased density within the joint may reflect synovial hypertrophy and/or hemosiderin deposition following repeated hemorrhages. Later radiographic findings include extensive erosive and degenerative joint changes as described above with osteopenia.

MRI (Fig. 9.8)

MRI is the best imaging modality in order to assess and monitor hemophilic arthropathy. MRI can demonstrate synovial hypertrophy, intra-articular bleeding, hemosiderin deposition, cartilage damage/loss, and periarticular soft tissues changes. Destructive arthropathy with erosive disease and secondary degenerative changes are clearly visualized with MRI. Hemosiderin deposits can be seen on T1- and T2-weighted images as multiple, intra-articular low-signal-intensity irregular foci with blooming artifact on gradient echo sequences. Joint effusions are common findings at all stages of joint disease and blood products are commonly demonstrated. MRI is excellent in demonstrating soft tissue hemorrhages particularly in the deeper soft tissue where ultrasound may be limited. Signal intensity of soft tissue hematomas is variable. In the acute stage, hemorrhage is isointense to high signal intensity with respect to muscle on T1 and central low with peripheral high signal on T2 and changing to

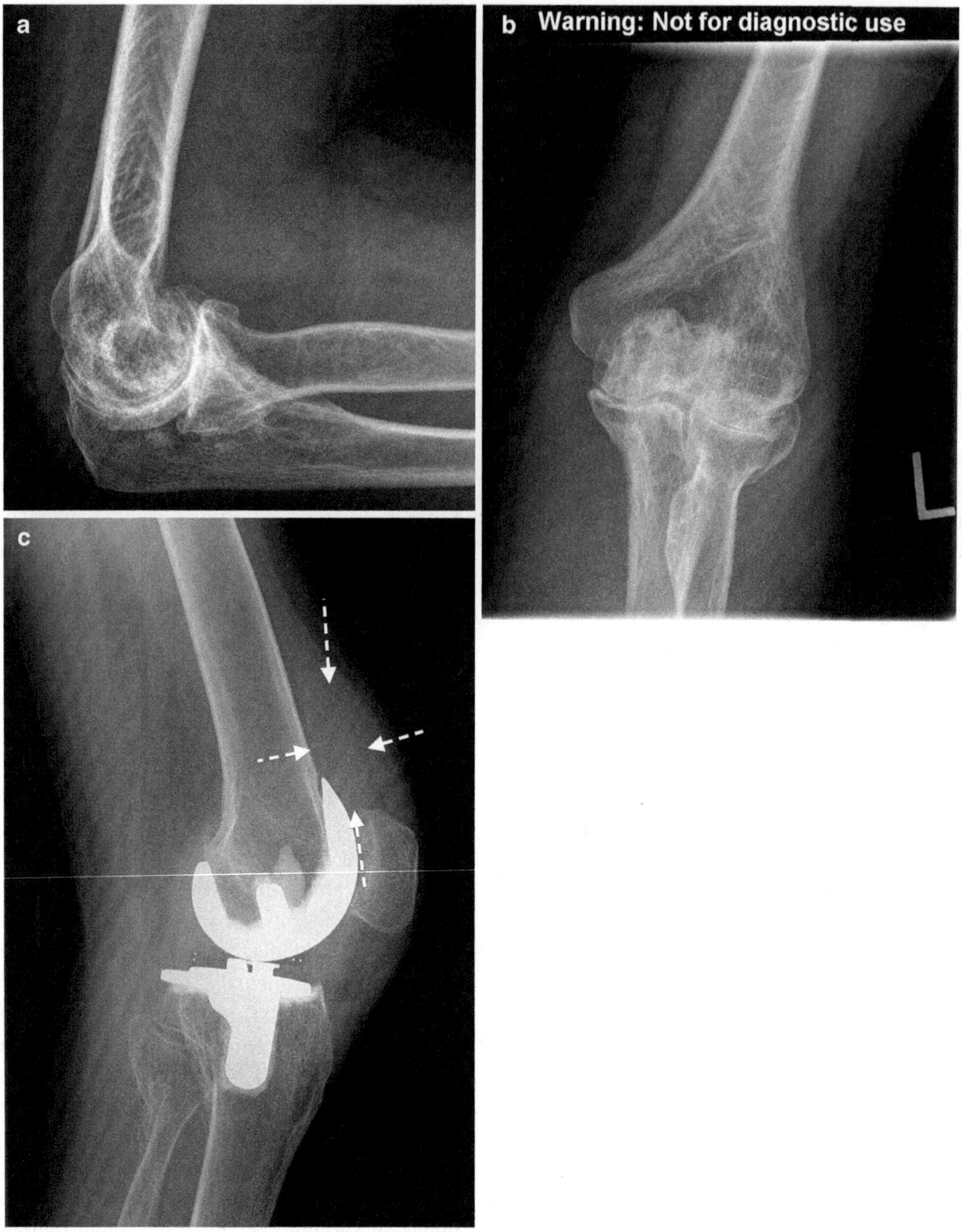

Fig. 9.6 (**a**) AP and (**b**) lateral radiographs of the elbow in a 25-year-old male with secondary degenerative changes secondary to recurrent hemarthrosis. (**c**) A 37-year-old-male hemophiliac with recurrent hemarthrosis (*dashed arrows*) at the knee joint with prior arthroplasty for secondary degenerative disease

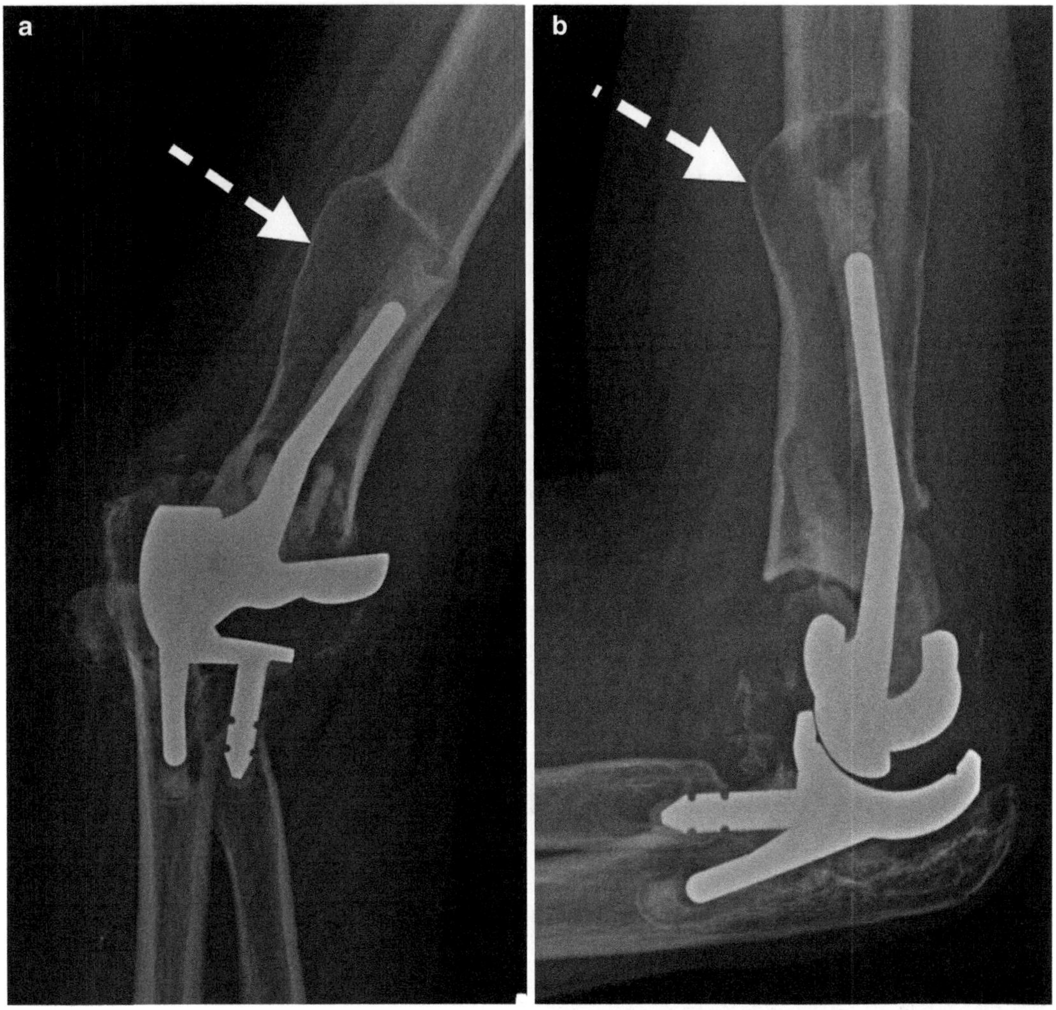

Fig. 9.7 (**a**) AP and (**b**) lateral radiographs of the left elbow in a hemophiliac with prior arthroplasty demonstrating pseudotumor appearance with secondary loosening prosthesis. Note intramedullary lucency and expansion with cortical thinning of the distal humerus (*dashed arrows*)

central high signal intensity on T2 after several days. Gradient echo sequences demonstrate low-signal-intensity foci with blooming artifact related to hemosiderin deposition.

US

Ultrasound can be useful for displaying joint and synovial fluid. Ultrasound is also useful in assessing intramuscular and soft tissue bleeds. The modality has a limited role in the assessment of chronically affected joints in hemophilia.

Radionuclide Scintigraphy

This is rarely required, although it can survey the whole skeleton, identifying target joints for further investigation where clinical findings are equivocal.

CT

CT has a limited role in the assessment of MSK involvement in hemophiliac patients. However, one can order CT to confirm deep tissue hemorrhage, i.e., retroperitoneum, iliopsoas muscle group, or intraosseous.

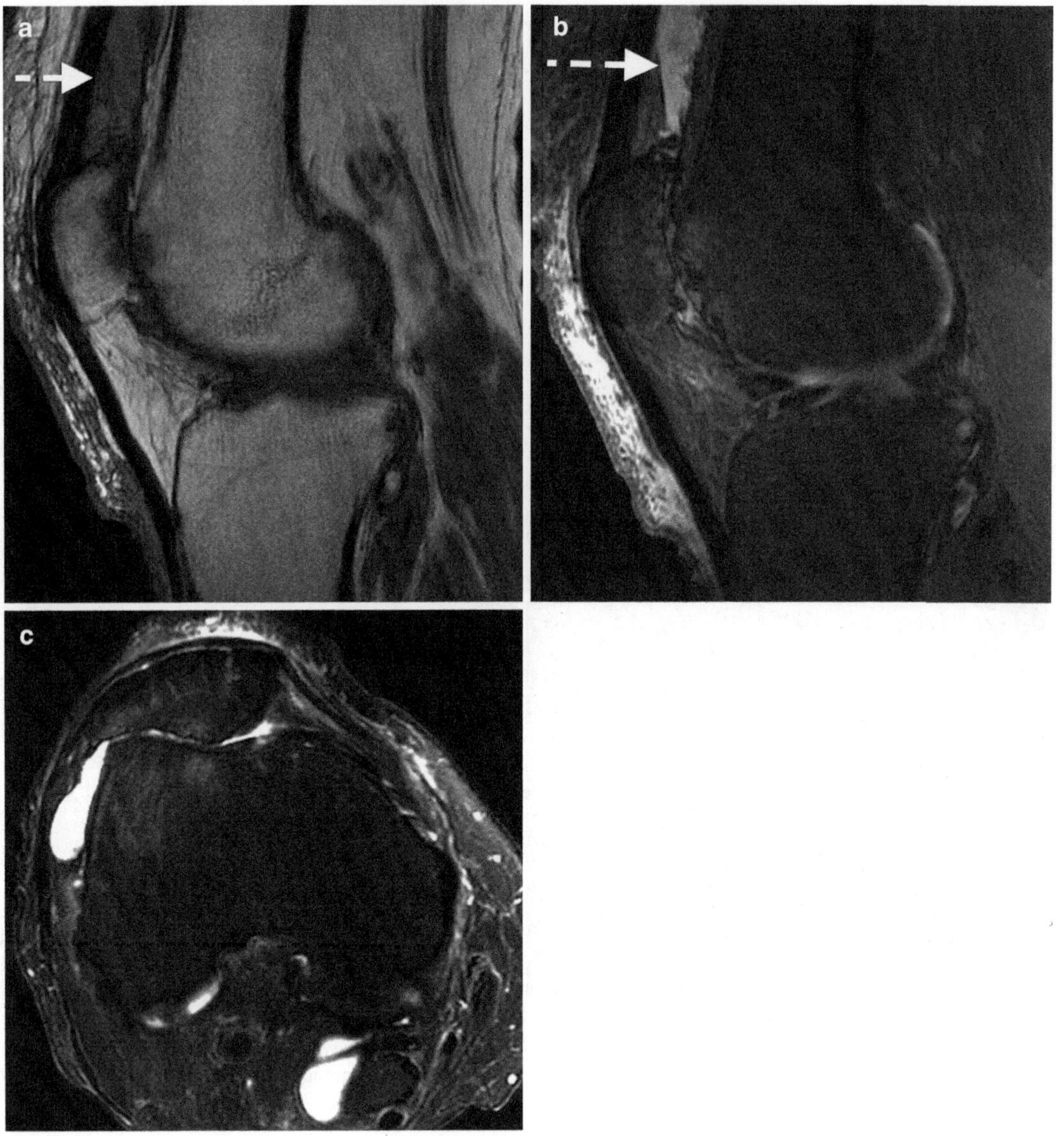

Fig. 9.8 Hemorrhagic suprapatellar recess effusion. (**a**) Sag T1 and (**b**) Sag T2FS demonstrate high SI effusion (*dashed arrows*) in keeping with hemorrhagic effusion and (**c**) axial T2 FS with significant patellofemoral degenerative change with denuded articular cartilage and subchondral bone marrow edema, cortical irregularity, and osteophytosis

Hypertrophic Osteoarthropathy

Overview

Hypertrophic osteoarthropathy (HOA) is a paraneoplastic syndrome that is characterized by digital clubbing, periostitis of the long bones, and symmetrical polyarthritis. It is associated with many illnesses, i.e., malignancy, chronic infectious and inflammatory processes, congenital heart disease, hepatic cirrhosis, inflammatory bowel disease, primary biliary cirrhosis, celiac disease, and Graves disease. Classically, it was described in patients with lung cancer and called hypertrophic pulmonary osteoarthropathy. Non-small cell lung cancer is the strongest malignant association. Thus, patients presenting with digital clubbing and joint and bone pain and/or found to have proliferative periostitis should be investigated for possible underlying malignancy and particularly intrathoracic cancer. HOA can present prior to any clinical signs or symptoms of malignancy. HOA predominantly affects adults with age and gender distributions corresponding with the underlying condition. Disease progression varies depending on the course of the primary disease. HOA can also occur in a primary form that is a rare hereditary autosomal dominant condition. It appears in childhood or at puberty and is not associated with other underlying diseases. Its course is usually self-limited.

Laboratory findings are nonspecific. Often patients may have elevated inflammatory markers due to underlying malignancy or inflammatory or infectious process. Connective tissue workup is typically negative. Synovial fluid is a noninflammatory type.

Musculoskeletal Presentation

Patients complain of pain and paresthesia in the affected extremities. They describe severe burning and deep aching pain in the long bones. Patients may also have swelling in extremities. Arthralgia in the small and large joints is common. Joint involvement is symmetrical with rheumatoid arthritis-type distribution. Small and large effusions may be present. Clubbing of the fingers and toes is a prominent clinical sign of this paraneoplastic syndrome; however, the presence of arthritis and periostitis symptoms is enough to make the diagnosis of an incomplete form of HOA.

Imaging Features (Fig. 9.9)

Radiographs

Plain radiography is a useful tool in diagnosing proliferative periostitis of the long bones. New bone formation is typically a bilateral and symmetrical process in HOA. The bone changes begin as a low-grade inflammatory process in the periosteum followed by new bone formation. Multiple layers of new bone are deposited which results in cortical thickening that can be seen on plain film. Periosteal changes are seen as a continuous thin line of sclerotic new bone separated from the cortex by a radiolucent space. Over time, the periosteal new bone thickens and fuses with the cortex.

Periosteal thickening initially appears in the distal diaphyseal regions of the long bones and later extends proximally to the diaphysis and metaphyses. The tibia, fibula, radius, ulna, and femur are usually involved. Other bony involvements include the scapula, clavicles, ribs, and pelvic bones. The abnormalities are more obvious in the lower than upper extremities and in the bones distal to the knees and elbows rather than in the femurs and humeri.

Another radiological pattern of hypertrophic osteoarthropathy is acro-osteolysis that is most frequently associated with cyanotic congenital heart disease. Acro-osteolysis affects the distal tufts of the phalanges causing their marked destruction and usually a sign of advanced stage of clubbing.

Chest radiograph should be done to investigate for potential pulmonary malignancy or infection in patients presenting with hypertrophic osteoarthropathy.

Nuclear Medicine

Bone scan demonstrates increased uptake in the periosteum. It may be positive prior to plain film changes. Bone scan shows solid continuous linear distribution of the tracer along the shafts of long bones. The clubbed digits may also show increased uptake. In case of synovitis, involved joints demonstrate increased uptake.

MRI

MRI can be ordered to investigate bone pain and may also show bilateral symmetrical periostitis.

CT

This modality has a limited role in the assessment of HOA itself but is helpful in diagnosis of intrathoracic pathology associated with HOA.

US

Ultrasound can be useful for confirming joint fluid and synovial thickening.

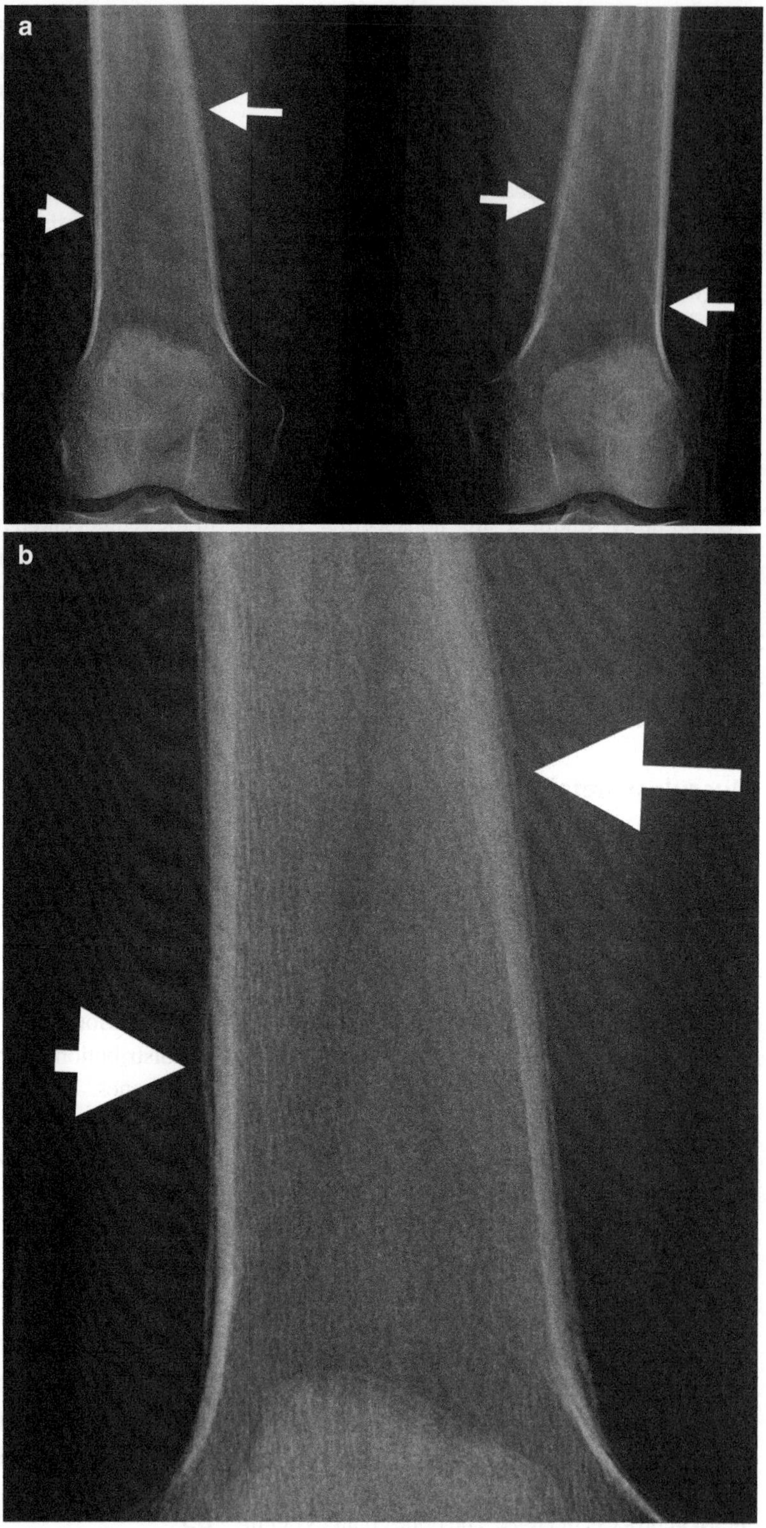

Fig. 9.9 Hypertrophic osteoarthropathy. (**a**) AP radiograph distal femurs with bilateral symmetrical periosteal reaction (*arrows*), (**b**) magnified view, (**c**) delayed bone scan, anterior and posterior views, with increased symmetrical uptake bilateral tibias and femurs in keeping with periostitis (*arrows*) and (**d**) chest radiograph with left perihilar lesion (bronchogenic carcinoma) (Kindly submitted by Dr. David Woods, St Joseph's Healthcare, Hamilton, Ontario, Canada)

Fig. 9.9 (continued)

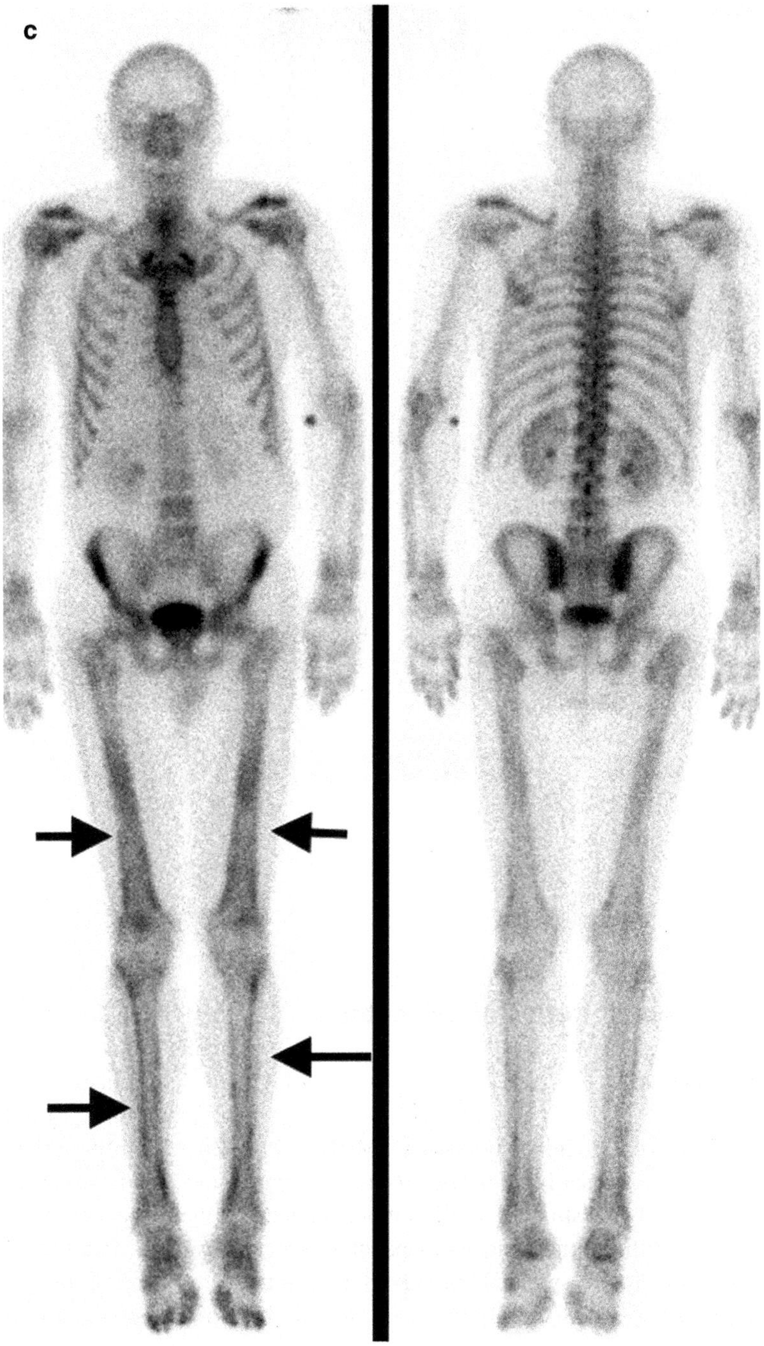

Fig. 9.9 (continued)

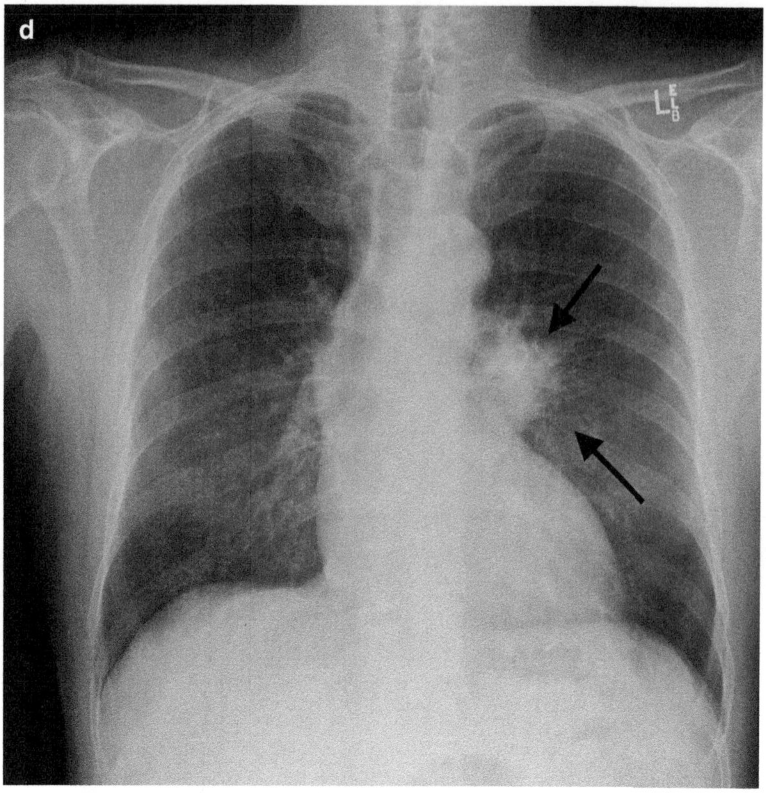

Multicentric Reticulohistiocytosis

Overview

Multicentric reticulohistiocytosis (MRH) is a rare systemic disorder of unknown etiology characterized by histiocyte proliferation. Patients present with multiple cutaneous papules associated with erosive symmetrical polyarthritis in up to 50 % of cases. The articular disease may be highly destructive. Involvement of the interphalangeal joints of the hands is typical and can lead to significant disability. MRH may affect any joint but most commonly the peripheral joints. Marked synovitis may be present, and synovial fluid cellularity is highly variable, ranging from bland to highly inflammatory. Most often synovial fluid analysis may demonstrate non-specific polymorphonuclear leukocytes or mononuclear cells.

The classic skin lesions are multiple firm flesh-colored to reddish-brown nontender nodules mainly on the dorsal aspects of the hands, face, and the periungual region but may occur on any part of the body, measuring up to 1–2 cm in size. Papules are classically described as "coral bead" in appearance. Cutaneous nodules demonstrate an infiltrate of histiocytic multinucleated giant cells with eosinophilic ground-glass cytoplasm. Histopathologic findings in combination with a clinical picture is the key to make a diagnosis. MRH has been reported primarily in Caucasians and more commonly in women with a female-to-male ratio of 2–3:1. MRH may occur at any age but usually in the fourth decade of life.

MRH is associated with malignancy in one third of patients. No specific site or type of malignancy has been identified, but the most frequently seen malignancies are in the lung, GI system, breast, ovary, and cervix. Malignancy may be preceded by or be present concomitantly with the cutaneous manifestations of MRH. MRH is also associated with other medical conditions such as diabetes mellitus, hypothyroidism, hyperlipidemia, rheumatoid arthritis, systemic lupus erythematosus, Sjögren syndrome, primary biliary cirrhosis, tuberculosis, and pregnancy. Pulmonary involvement by MRH is rare, but a few cases of nonspecific pulmonary findings, i.e., pleural effusions and infiltrates associated with MRH, have been described in the literature.

Imaging Features

Radiographs (Fig. 9.10)

Radiographs plays a very important diagnostic role. Radiologic findings include well-circumscribed marginal erosions that may be disproportionate to the cartilage loss. Lesions may resemble gouty erosions. Gout can be excluded given the symmetrical involvement. Severe progression of the disease can lead to arthritis mutilans (foreshortening of the fingers and telescoping of the digits). Widening of joint spaces due to cartilage loss and significant resorption of subchondral bone are also observed in MRH. Periarticular osteoporosis is usually absent or mild. Involvement of the distal interphalangeal

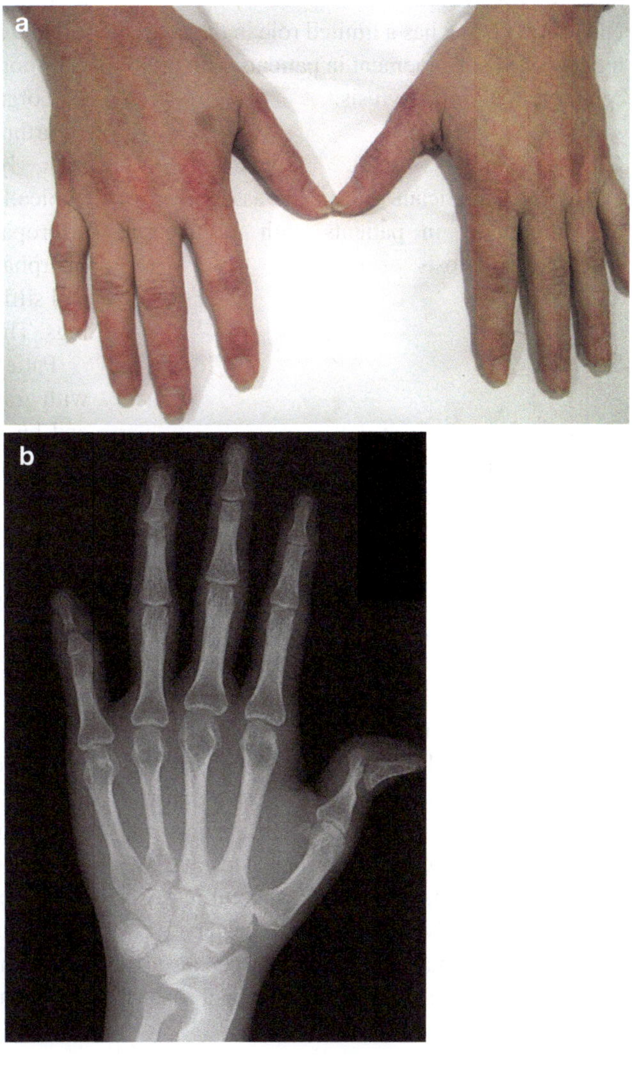

Fig. 9.10 Multicentric reticulohistiocytosis. (**a**) Photograph of the bilateral hands with classic reddish nodules on dorsal hands, (**b**) destructive, symmetric (right hand not shown) disease of the DIPJs, carpal involvement, and distal ulna erosive change, no new bone formation or periosteal reaction, minimal periarticular osteopenia present at the MCPJs (Kindly submitted by Dr. Larry Dixon, Associate Professor, University of Chicago)

joints presents in 75 % of patients and helps to differentiate from rheumatoid arthritis. Absence of new bone formation, e.g., periosteal reaction, helps to differentiate from psoriatic arthritis.

US

Ultrasound can be used to confirm joint effusion and demonstrate synovial proliferation and soft tissue changes.

MRI

MRI may be helpful in establishing the presence of synovitis in patients with normal radiographs and uncertainty regarding the presence of inflammatory changes.

Nuclear Medicine

Nuclear medicine has a limited role in the assessment of MSK involvement in patients with multicentric reticulohistiocytosis.

CT

CT has no significant role in the assessment of the arthropathy in patients with multicentric reticulohistiocytosis.

Sarcoidosis

Overview

Sarcoidosis is a multisystem noncaseating granulomatous disease of unknown etiology with variable presentation and prognosis. Sarcoidosis involves multiple organs, most commonly the lungs, lymph nodes, liver, skin, and eyes. Musculoskeletal involvement has been reported in 1–13 % of sarcoidosis patients, with an estimated average of 5 %. Patients are usually between 20 and 40 years and more common in females. African-Americans appear to be most commonly affected in North America. Clinical signs and symptoms include nonspecific constitutional symptoms (fatigue, weight loss, general malaise, and less commonly fever). Approximately 50 % of patients remain asymptomatic. Hypercalcemia may be present due to increased intestinal absorption of calcium, which results from activation of vitamin D by macrophages in sarcoid granulomas. Angiotensin-converting enzyme (ACE) level is usually elevated. The CD4:CD8 ratio in the blood serum is commonly decreased. These abnormalities are helpful in making the diagnosis of sarcoidosis; however, they are not specific and may be seen in other granulomatous diseases.

Musculoskeletal Presentation

Primary skeletal involvement without other organ involvements is extremely rare. Approximately 80–90 % of patients have concurrent pulmonary involvement. *Patients mostly complain of bone and joint pain. Arthropathy is usually symmetrical and transient.* The hands and feet are the most commonly affected bones.

Löfgren syndrome is a well-recognized triad of arthralgia, erythema nodosum, and bilateral hilar lymphadenopathy due to sarcoidosis. Typically patients present with bilateral ankle arthropathy but can involve the knees, proximal interphalangeal joints, wrists, and elbows. Pain and stiffness are often worse than objective findings. There is usually no joint effusion.

Patients with sarcoidosis may also present with granulomatous arthritis that causes synovitis and has a chronic transient or relapsing course. This form of sarcoidal arthritis is commonly associated with cutaneous sarcoidosis, but not with erythema nodosum. It is usually oligoarthritic process that involves two or three joints, including the knees, ankles, proximal interphalangeal joints, and occasionally the wrists or shoulders. Dactylitis of the fingers can be observed. Pain is usually not intense.

Muscular sarcoidosis is a rare condition but can present as two types: myopathic and nodular. The myopathic type presents as polymyositis with symmetric proximal weakness, elevated serum creatine kinase and aldolase levels, and myopathy at electromyographic evaluation. The nodular type affects extremities and causes solitary or multiple nodules. Those nodules are usually nontender.

Imaging Features

Radiographs (Fig. 9.11)

Classic sarcoidal lesions in the small bones of the hands and feet are well characterized and diagnosed with conventional radiographs and demonstrate a "lacelike" trabecular pattern, areas with cyst-like radiolucency of different sizes, and/or extensive bone erosions. Small, cortical, punched-out lytic lesions in the phalangeal heads are the most common manifestation. Middle and distal phalanges of hands and feet are most frequently involved. Adjacent soft tissue swelling is often present. Joint spaces are typically preserved. Other changes include subperiosteal bone resorption, acro-osteolysis, acro-osteosclerosis, and bone destruction with pathologic fractures.

Large bone and axial skeleton sarcoidosis is not common. They may present as lytic, sclerotic, or mixed lesions. Vertebral sarcoidosis is rare. Lesions tend to affect the lower thoracic and upper lumbar spine. Intervertebral disk spaces are preserved. Radiographic appearance may simulate osteomyelitis or tumor and biopsy helps to make a diagnosis.

MRI (Fig. 9.12)

MRI is a useful tool in identifying inflammatory changes in the joints that may not be appreciated on radiographs including synovitis and tenosynovitis. MR findings are nonspecific and may require biopsy for diagnosis of granulomatous involvement.

Although MR imaging is not necessary for the diagnosis of small bone sarcoidosis, it may reveal an early erosive process that is occult on plain radiography. Other MRI findings may include bone marrow lesions, extension of granulomas beyond the cortex, periosseous soft tissue involvement, or fine perpendicular lines extending from the ghost cortex and resembling periostitis.

Large bone sarcoid lesions may be indistinct or well marginated and of varying sizes on MRI. The signal intensity characteristics are variable depending on the activity of the disease process. Lesions typically have low intensity on T1 and increased intensity on STIR and T2. Lesions may enhance after contrast administration. In case of muscular sarcoidosis, nodular-type characteristic nodules may appear on

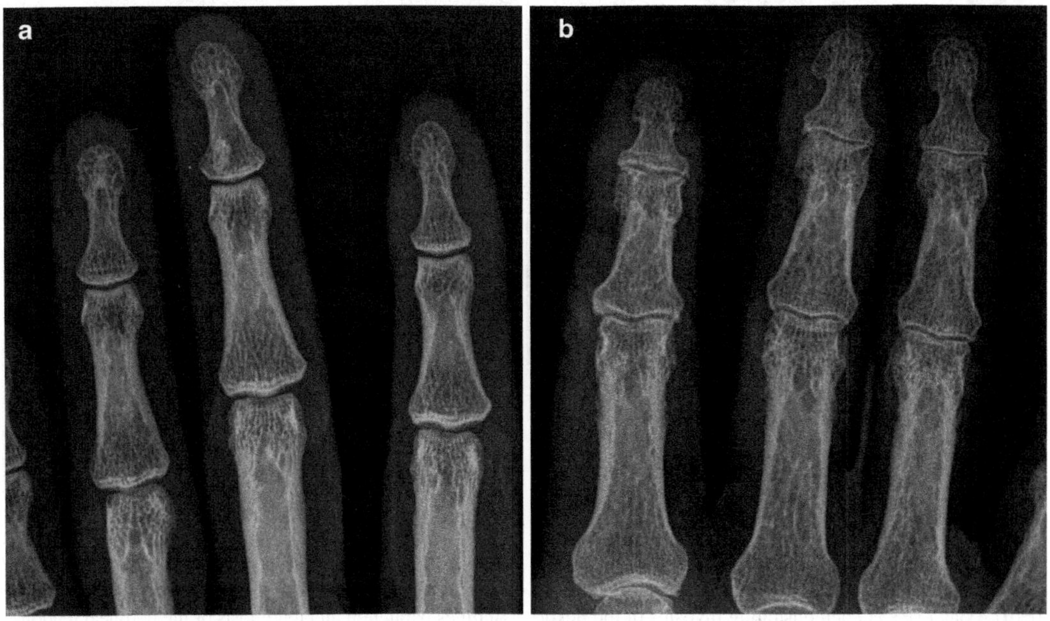

Fig. 9.11 Sarcoid changes in the hands. (**a**, **b**) Demonstrate lacelike trabecular pattern most pronounced in the metaphyseal regions and early cyst formation in (**b**)

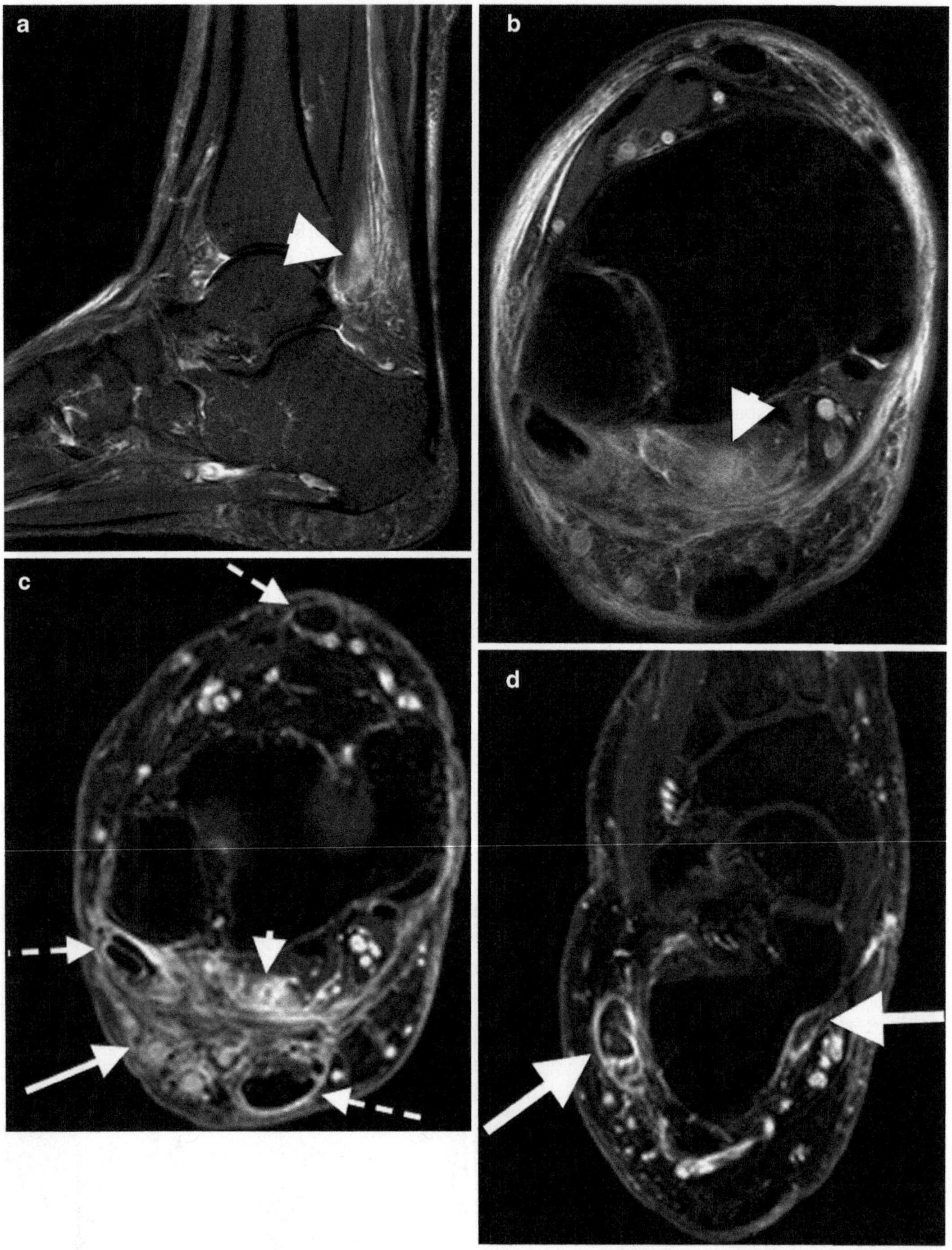

Fig. 9.12 MRI of the left ankle in a 55-year-old female with known sarcoid and persistent soft tissue pain and reduced range of motion. (**a**) Sag T2FS and (**b**) axial T2FS. (**c**, **d**) Axial T1FS PG demonstrating myositis of the flexor hallucis longus (*arrowhead*), edema of the adjacent Kager's fat pad (*arrow*), and multifocal tenosynovitis (*dashed arrows*). Note the postgadolinium enhancement of the Achilles paratenon and tendinosis of the peroneal tendons

MRI. The sarcoid nodules appear as focal intramuscular masses, usually at the musculotendinous junction. They are multiple and bilateral in distribution with a lower extremity predominance. Sarcoidal nodules are typically hyperintense on T2 with low signal intensity centrally, which is related to the fibrotic changes. Nodules enhance after administration of contrast. In myopathic sarcoid myopathy, MRI findings reveal symmetric proximal muscle atrophy with fatty replacement and increased signal intensity of involved muscle on T2WI.

Ultrasound

Ultrasound can be useful for displaying joint fluid, active synovitis, and tenosynovitis. Ultrasound is excellent for soft tissue image-guided biopsies if required.

CT

CT has a limited role in the assessment of MSK involvement in sarcoid.

Nuclear Medicine

Bone scintigraphy shows high sensitivity and somewhat lower specificity in assessing bone sarcoidosis. Scintigraphic findings become usually positive even before the lesions become manifest at radiography. Sarcoidal lesions show localized increased uptake that can be also seen in a variety of processes, such as bone metastasis, traumatisms, infections and inflammatory lesions, and degenerative disease. As a result, the diagnostic value of bone scanning in sarcoidosis is limited.

Paget's Disease

Overview

Paget's disease of the bone is an uncommon, chronic bone condition that occurs slightly more often in men than in women (3:2). It is usually seen after the fourth decade. The pelvis, sacrum, skull, spine, and extremities are favored locations. Distribution is usually asymmetric and polyostotic. Monostotic disease occurs in approximately 10–20 % of cases. The cause of Paget's is still unknown, although some have hypothesized an underlying viral trigger including exposure to measles and canine temper virus. Genetics also appears to play an important role after the identification of a mutation in the gene sequestosome 1 (SQSTM1), which is found in 46 % of patients with familial Paget's. Paget's is primarily a disease of increased osteoclast activity. The disease course of Paget's evolves through various stages of activity. There is initially an osteolytic phase which involves aggressive bone resorption characterized by significant increases in osteoclast activity. This is subsequently followed by a phase of excessive remodeling and new bone formation by osteoblasts. However, there are insufficient quantities of substrate to produce osteoid, given the rapid increase in osteoclastic activity. As a result, the osteoblasts lay down collagen instead, which ultimately leads to the production of woven bone with a mosaic pattern which is structurally inferior. After the osteoblastic activity slows down, this remodeling phase is then followed by an inactive phase, where the remaining bone becomes heavily calcified and there is a predominant osteosclerotic appearance associated with the inactive phase. Serum alkaline phosphatase (ALP) is often elevated.

Presentation

Patients are often asymptomatic, and a diagnosis is incidentally made on radiographs done for other reasons. Patients are also commonly diagnosed after an isolated elevation in alkaline phosphatase is identified. In patients with symptomatic disease, the clinical manifestations can vary depending on the distribution of involved skeletal sites. Paget's disease can involve any bone in the body but most commonly affects the skull, thoracolumbar spine, pelvis, and femur. Patients typically present with local pain at the involved sites. The degree of pain can be debilitating, is often worse at night, and does not seem to be associated with exertion activities.

Complications associated with skull lesions include headaches, hearing loss, visual disturbance, and alteration of the skull shape due to softening of the bone. Lesions of the thoracolumbar spine can result in compression fractures and bony proliferation. Vertebral involvement can be complicated by spinal stenosis, cauda equina syndrome, and focal radiculopathy. Femoral involvement can result in a bowing deformity of the femur with resultant limb shortening and complicated by early osteoarthritic changes. Patients with Paget's are at increased risk of fractures, since bowing of the weight-bearing bones may result in small fissure fractures of the cortical bone. There is a low but increased risk of osteosarcoma in areas involved with Paget's disease.

Imaging Features

Radiographs (Figs. 9.13, 9.14, and 9.15)

Radiographs are essential in establishing the diagnosis of Paget's disease. Early changes of Paget's disease are characterized by intense osteoclastic activity which cause osteolysis (lucent areas). The mixed (middle) phase of Paget's disease presents both the lytic and the blastic phases. Most patients present in the mixed phase. Osteolysis, coarsening and thickening of bone trabeculae, cortical thickening, and osseous widening characterize the mixed phase. The blastic, or late inactive, phase of Paget's disease manifests as osteosclerosis and presents predominantly sclerotic changes and bony enlargement.

Pelvis

Paget's disease of the pelvis usually presents with cortical thickening and sclerosis of the iliopectineal and ischiopubic lines and enlargement of the pubic rami and ischium. Para-acetabular changes can produce acetabular protrusion.

Skull

In the skull, osteolysis is seen as large and well-defined areas of radiolucency. They usually affect the frontal and occipital bones and are described as "osteoporosis circumscripta." Skull lesions are most prominent in the inner calvarial tables and usually cross the suture lines. Both inner and outer calvarial tables are involved, with the former usually more extensively affected.

Focal osteosclerosis in the skull presents as a cotton-wool appearance with globular to fluffy foci of variable density on plain x-ray.

Thickening of the inner calvarial table produces marked enlargement of the diploic space. It is referred as a "tam-o'-shanter" skull (a tam-o'-shanter is a Scottish cap that is broad and flattened). This new bone remodeling can cause nerve and brain compression resulting in neurologic symptoms.

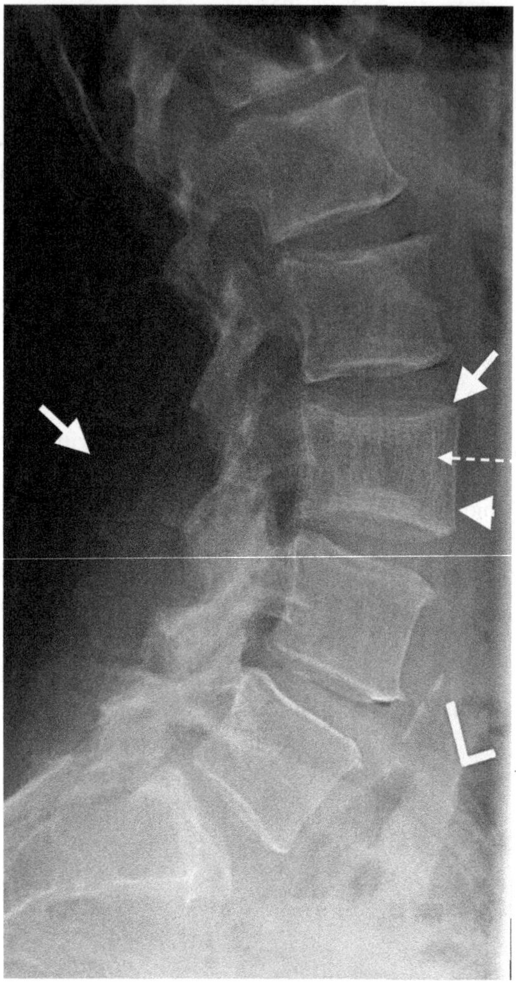

Fig. 9.13 A 42-year-old male with Paget's disease of the spine, asymptomatic. L3 vertebra (*arrow*) involvement, vertebra is enlarged, both anterior and posterior elements, when compared to adjacent vertebrae but without evidence of cortical destruction, there is thickening of the trabeculae (linear striations within the vertebra) (*dashed arrow*) and thickening of the cortex (*arrowhead*) giving a "picture-frame" appearance

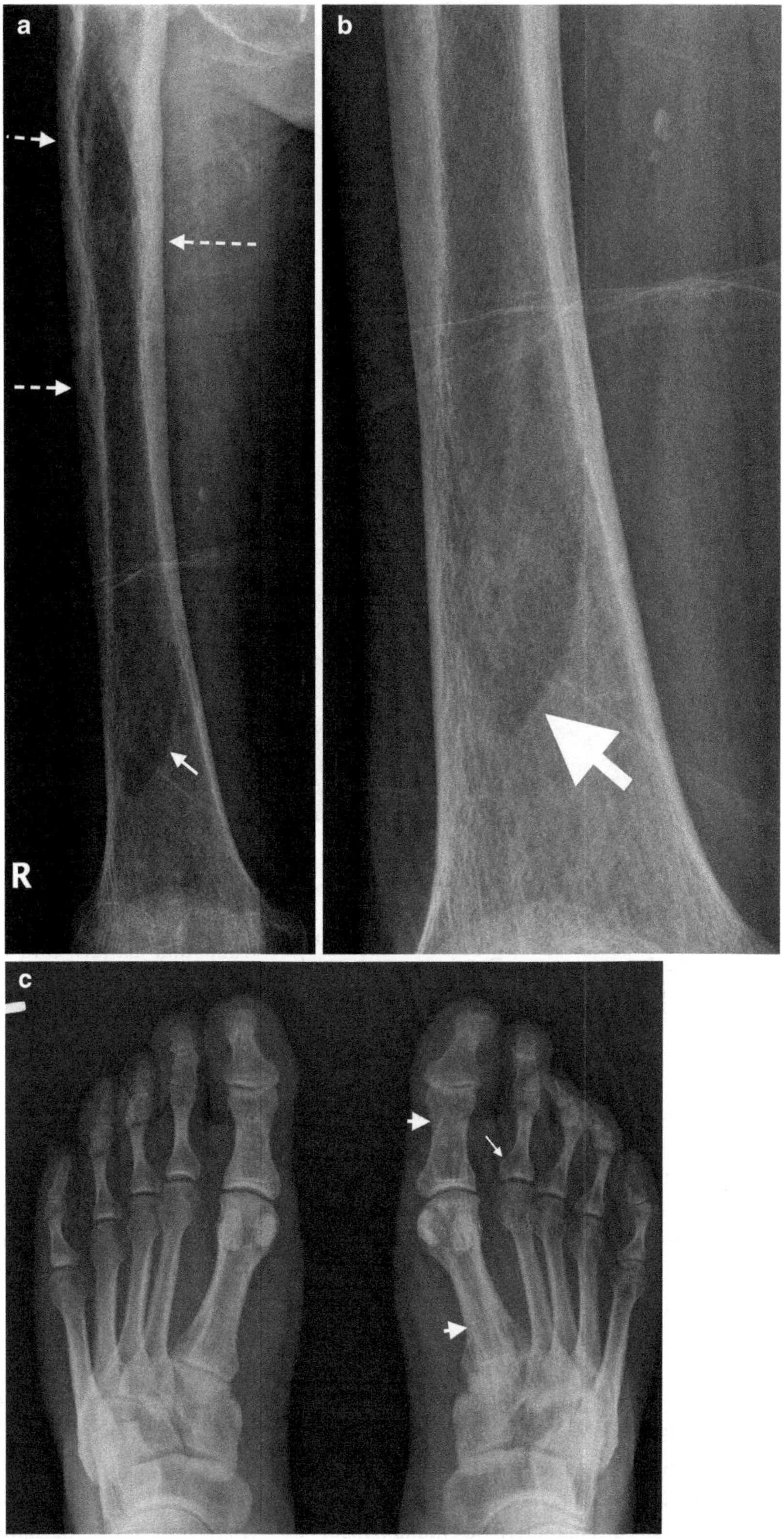

Fig. 9.14 A 71-year-old male with mixed osteolytic osteoblastic phase Paget's disease of the right femur on AP radiograph, (**a**, **b**) flame-shaped, also termed "blade of grass," appearance of the distal diaphysis with osteolysis (*arrow*) with more proximal cortical thickening (*dashed arrow*), (**c**) right foot involvement with enlargement of the right first metatarsal, thickened trabeculae (*arrowheads*), and subchondral osteopenia (*arrow*)

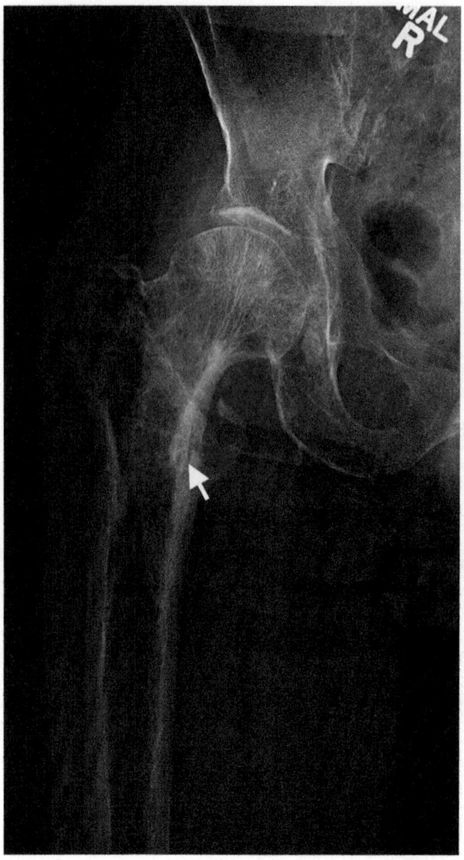

Fig. 9.15 A 72-year-old male with Paget's disease of the right femur with mixed phase disease demonstrates osteolysis of the medullary cavity with thickened cortex, and secondary intertrochanteric fracture (*arrow*). Note that fractures may be difficult to appreciate in Paget's disease due to the altered bone architecture and osteopenia as in this case

Spine

Paget's disease of the spine frequently manifests with cortical thickening along all four margins of the vertebral body, which creates the picture-frame appearance on radiographs. On lateral radiographs, flattening or squaring of the normal concavity of the anterior margin of the affected vertebral body also adds to the rectangular appearance. Additional changes may include coarsening of the trabecular pattern.

Long Bones

In the long bones, osteolysis begins as a subchondral area of lucency. As it progresses, it manifests as a characteristic metaphyseal to diaphyseal wedge-shaped area of radiolucency that assumes the configuration of a flame or blade of grass. Subperiosteal cortical thickening and accentuation and coarsening of the trabecular pattern with enlargement of bone contours can be seen in the later stages. Conversely, on occasion within the area of radiolucency, trabeculae can be obliterated and a hazy ground glass or "washed-out" pattern is observed. In rare cases, the disease is isolated to the diaphysis, most commonly in the tibia, rather than subchondral bone, which can cause diagnostic confusion.

Later in mixed phase, changes in the long bones manifest both as advancing osteolysis that extends toward the diaphysis and as focal bone sclerosis in the epiphysis and metaphysis.

In the long bones and pelvis, coarsening of the trabeculae and cortical thickening, with marked widening and enlargement of bones, are seen. Because of excessive deposition of abnormal bone, the bones are weak, and transverse fatigue fractures, which are referred to as "banana fractures," may occur. Multiple fractures and abnormal bone repair are associated with the development of progressive bowing deformities.

Hands and Feet

Although involvement of short tubular bones of the hands and feet is unusual, accentuated trabecular pattern and bone enlargement may be visualized in the mixed phase of the disease.

CT

CT scan is more demonstrative of the plain radiographic findings. CT demonstrates increased cortical thickness, accentuation of the trabecular pattern with coarseness, and enlarged bones (Fig. 9.16a–c). Additionally, should biopsy be indicated for the diagnosis of sarcoma, CT typically is the guidance modality of choice.

Bone Scintigraphy

Bone scan is a test that helps identify which bones have been affected by Paget's disease assessing the extent and activity of the disease. Bone scan is highly sensitive but not specific (Fig. 9.16d). Scintigraphy demonstrates marked increased uptake in all phases of disease with

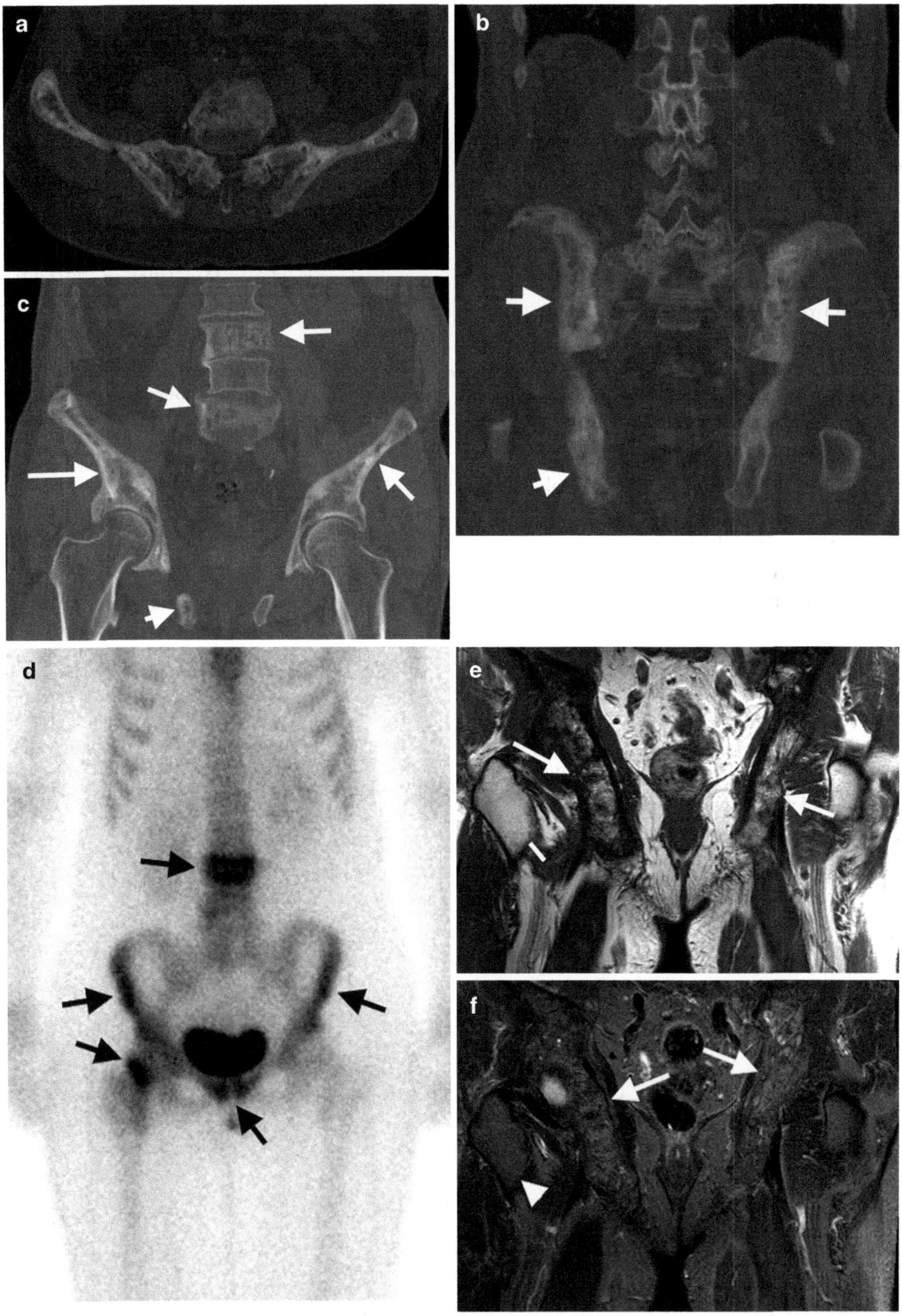

Fig. 9.16 A 67-year-old female with Paget's disease of the pelvis, (**a**) axial CT superior pelvis with diffuse mixed sclerotic and lucent bone, (**b**, **c**) coronal reformat with multiple areas involved (*arrows*), (**d**) bone scan of the same patient with increased uptake (*black arrows*) corresponding to CT, (**e**) Cor T1 and (**f**) Cor T2 FS of the same patient with thickened cortex and altered marrow signal intensity (*arrows*) when compared to normal marrow (*arrowhead*)

exception of burnt-out sclerotic phase, which may demonstrate normal uptake.

MRI

MR imaging is not generally used in diagnosis of Paget's disease. MRI is good for assessing sarcomatous transformation that may occur in up to 1 % of the cases. Preservation of normal marrow fat is a characteristic finding of the lytic phase of Paget's disease on MRI and allows it to be distinguished from most tumors.

MRI also helps to assess for other complications of Paget's disease—including basilar invagination, spinal stenosis, and nerve or spinal cord compression. The anatomy is well demonstrated by cross-sectional imaging in complex structures:

- Hypointense area or area of signal void on T1WI + T2WI (cortical thickening, coarse trabeculation) (Fig. 9.16e, f)
- Widening of bone
- Reduction in size and signal intensity of medullary cavity due to replacement of high-signal-intensity fatty marrow by medullary bone formation
- Focal areas of higher signal intensity than fatty marrow (from cyst-like fat-filled marrow spaces)
- Areas of decreased signal intensity within marrow on T1WI and increased intensity on T2WI (fibrovascular tissue resembling granulation tissue)

Further Reading

1. Armstrong DJ, et al. Hypertrophic pulmonary osteoarthropathy (HPOA) (Pierre Marie–Bamberger syndrome): two cases presenting as acute inflammatory arthritis. Description and review of the literature. Rheumatol Int. 2007;27:399–402.
2. Doria AS. State-of-the-art imaging techniques for the evaluation of hemophilic arthropathy: present and future. Haemophilia. 2010;16 Suppl 5:107–14.
3. Ioana F, et al. Ultrasound findings in AL musculoskeletal amyloidosis. Med Ultrason. 2011;13(1):76–9.
4. Jäger HJ, Mehring U, Götz GF, et al. Radiological features of the visceral and skeletal involvement of hemochromatosis. Eur Radiol. 1997;7(8):1199–206.
5. Resnick D, Kransdorf MJ. Bone and joint imaging. 3rd ed. 2004.
6. Roger K. Imaging of musculoskeletal complications of hemophilia. Semin Musculoskelet Radiol. 2003;7(N 2):127–36.
7. Santilli D, et al. Multicentric reticulohistiocytosis: a rare cause of erosive arthropathy of the distal interphalangeal finger joints. Ann Rheum Dis. 2002;61:485–7.
8. Sheldon PJ, et al. Imaging of amyloid arthropathy. Semin Musculoskelet Radiol. 2003;7(N 2):195–203.
9. Smith SE, Murphey MD, Motamedi K, et al. From the archives of the AFIP. Radiologic spectrum of Paget disease of bone and its complications with pathologic correlation. Radiographics. 2002;22(5):1191–216.
10. Vardhanabhuti V, Venkatanarasimha N, Bhatnagar G, et al. Extra-pulmonary manifestations of sarcoidosis. Clin Radiol. 2012;67(3):263–76.

Osteoarthritis

10

Alfred Cividino and John O'Neill

Overview

Osteoarthritis (OA), also termed degenerative joint disease, is the most common arthritis. There are two main forms, primary and secondary. *Primary OA* is an age-related disease with a genetic susceptibility in some individuals to earlier onset and more rapid progression. It occurs in joints without local predisposing factors. Primary OA may be localized or generalized. OA is a complex interaction of advancing age, genetic predisposition, mechanical stress, obesity, as well as metabolic and biochemical factors all of which may affect the degree, extent, and progression of disease. Obesity is the only modifiable risk factor. Primary OA increases significantly in prevalence after the age of 50 with the majority of individuals demonstrating some form of OA after the age of 70 years.

Secondary OA on the other hand occurs in abnormal joints. Predisposing conditions include but are not limited to traumatic joint injuries, inflammatory arthropathies, CPPD, prior septic arthritis, congenitally abnormal joints such as congenital hip dysplasia, metabolic- and endocrine-related arthropathies, and avascular necrosis.

Inflammatory markers are usually normal, and there is no increased prevalence of rheumatoid factor positivity above the general population. *Erosive OA* is a subset of primary OA and is also termed inflammatory OA. Middle-aged and elderly women are predominantly affected with a male:female ratio of 1:12. It usually presents with abrupt onset with pain and swelling of the hands and is discriminated by the development of central erosions. The pathological changes of OA include degradation and loss of articular cartilage, sclerosis and remodeling of subchondral bone, development of osteophytes, and synovial inflammation

Presentation

Clinical features include joint pain worse with use, mild stiffness often worse with immobility, pain on movement, restricted range of motion, periarticular tenderness, bony enlargement, soft tissue swelling, and joint crepitus. The joints

A. Cividino, MD, FRCPC (✉)
Director, Division of Rheumatology,
Department of Medicine, McMaster University,
Hamilton, ON L8N 2B6, Canada
e-mail: Cividino@mcmaster.ca

J. O'Neill, MB, BAO, BCh, MRCPI, MSc, FRCR
Associate Professor, Musculoskeletal Imaging,
Diagnostic Imaging, McMaster University/St Joseph's
Healthcare, Hamilton, ON L8N4A6, Canada

J. O'Neill (ed.), *Essential Imaging in Rheumatology*,
DOI 10.1007/978-1-4939-1673-3_10, © Springer Science+Business Media New York 2015

most frequently affected include the knees, hips, feet, hands, and cervical and lumbar spine. The diagnosis is usually clinical, and further investigations are usually not required. Radiographs can confirm the diagnosis and assess the degree and extent of the disease. The characteristic features of hand OA include the development of deformity with bony enlargement of the DIP and PIP joints with so-called Heberden's and Bouchard's nodes, respectively, and squaring of the first carpometacarpal phalangeal joint. Though uncommon the second and third MCP joint can be affected. Hemochromatosis may be suspected in these cases.

Erosive inflammatory OA often presents with joint swelling in a typical OA distribution however clinically resembles RA or PsA. Knee osteoarthritis is insidious and associated with pain on weight bearing. Joint swelling, flexion contracture, and varus or valgus deformities can develop. Hip osteoarthritis results in groin pain radiating down the anterior thigh to the knee, frequently insidious, and associated with weight bearing. Referred back pain may mimic these findings. OA of the foot typically affects the first metatarsophalangeal joint with accompanying hallux valgus and bony enlargement. Spinal disease is reviewed in detail in Chap. 15.

Imaging Features

Key radiographic features of osteoarthritis include joint space narrowing, osteophytosis, altered bone contour, bone sclerosis and cysts, periarticular calcification, and soft tissue swelling (Fig. 10.1). Additional imaging descriptions have been provided in Chap. 3.

The subchondral region bone plate is located deep to the articular surface, separated only by a thin layer of calcified articular cartilage (Fig. 10.2). When there is loss of the overlying cartilage, as in osteoarthritis, the subchondral bone is directly exposed to the stresses across the joint with subsequent trabecular collapse, flattening and *eburnation* (Fig. 10.3). Cartilage loss is discussed in greater detail in Chap. 3 and the Outerbridge classification of cartilage loss is outlined (see Table 3.5). The subchondral regions in areas of lower stress become increasingly vascularized. This stimulates endochondral ossification with new bone formation, *osteophytes* (Fig. 10.4). They are usually marginally growing as an extension of the joint margin. New bone formation may also occur centrally in areas of full cartilage loss and appear as new bone formation at the cortical surface, often with an irregular margin.

Subchondral cysts develop between the deformed trabeculae in areas of eburnation (Fig. 10.5). They are of variable size. The overlying cortex may be intact or may have a focal defect allowing communication of the cyst with the joint space. Prominent subchondral cyst formation raises possibility of underlying crystal disease. Joint space loss has long been attributed to cartilage thickness; however, in the knee, meniscal degenerative changes can also contribute to narrowing. Marked joint space narrowing is seen in advanced disease (Fig. 10.6).

On *radiographs* eburnation is noted as subchondral sclerosis and may demonstrate flattening and collapse of its surface. Osteophytes are noted as new bone forming at the periphery of the joint space. Subchondral cysts are variable in size, have a thin sclerotic margin, and may demonstrate communication with the joint space, e.g., intra-articular gas may extend into the cyst. The overlying cortex is usually intact or demonstrates a focal defect. Occasionally it may be difficult to differentiate a subchondral cyst from an erosion if there is collapse of the cyst overlying cortical margin. Subchondral cysts are however associated with joint space loss, subchondral sclerosis, and osteophytosis. Additional studies other than radiographs are rarely required, and the above changes however can be detailed on other imaging modalities when performed for alternative indications.

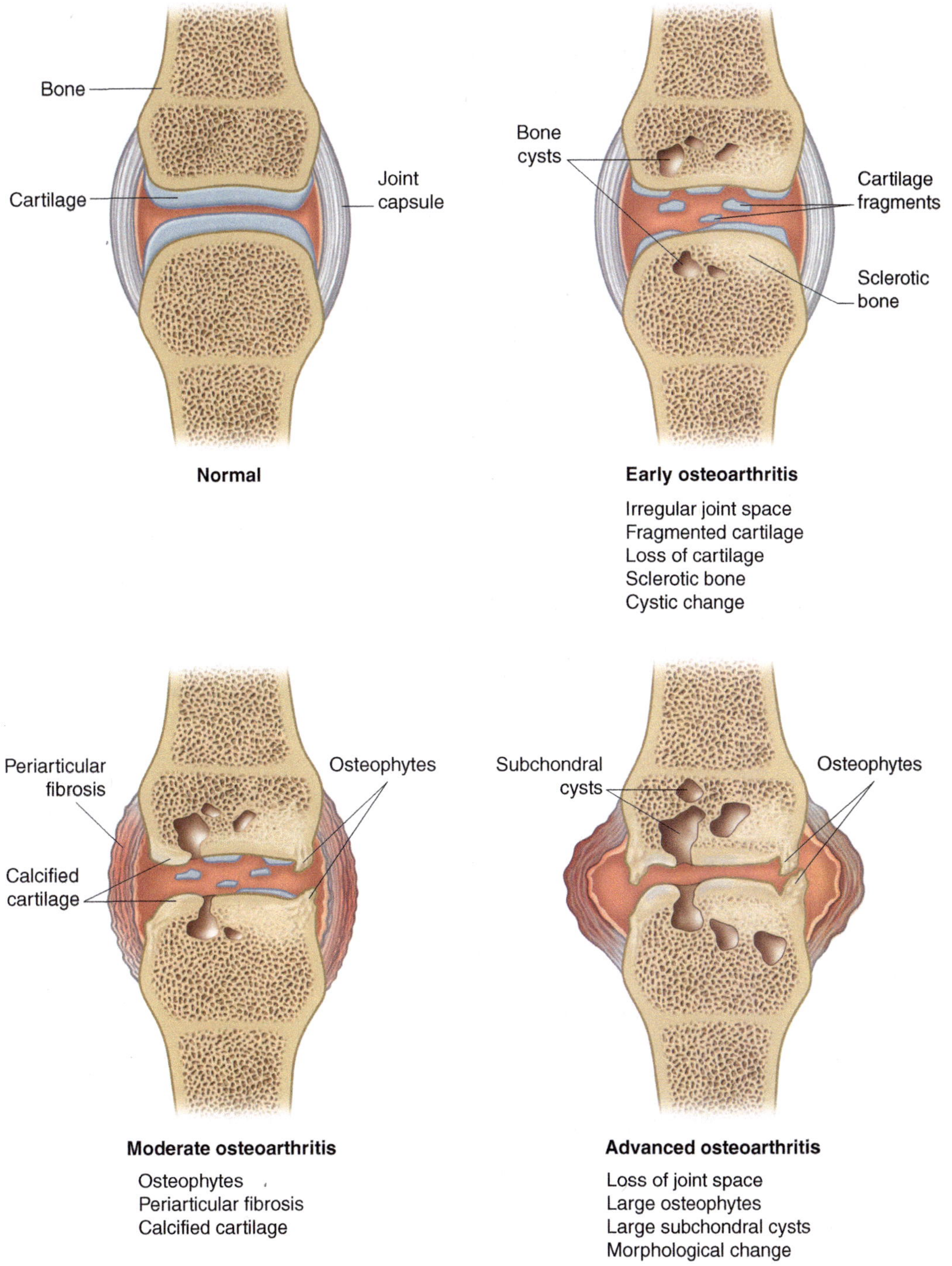

Fig. 10.1 Development and progression of osteoarthritis

Fig. 10.2 Cartilage layers and subchondral bone

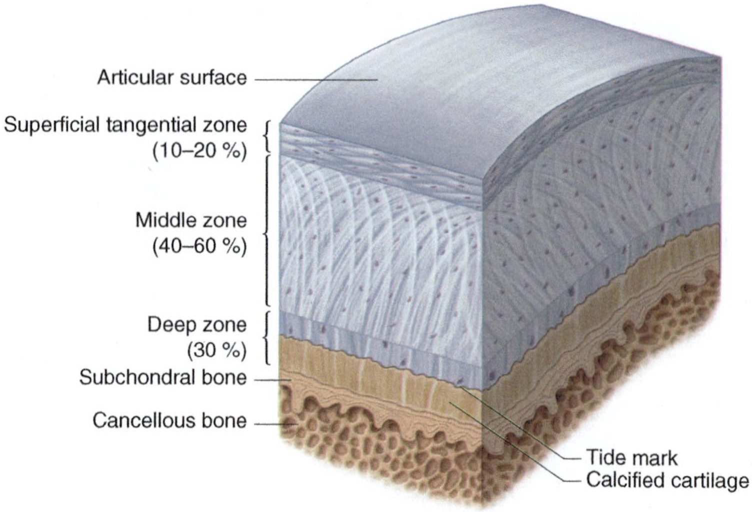

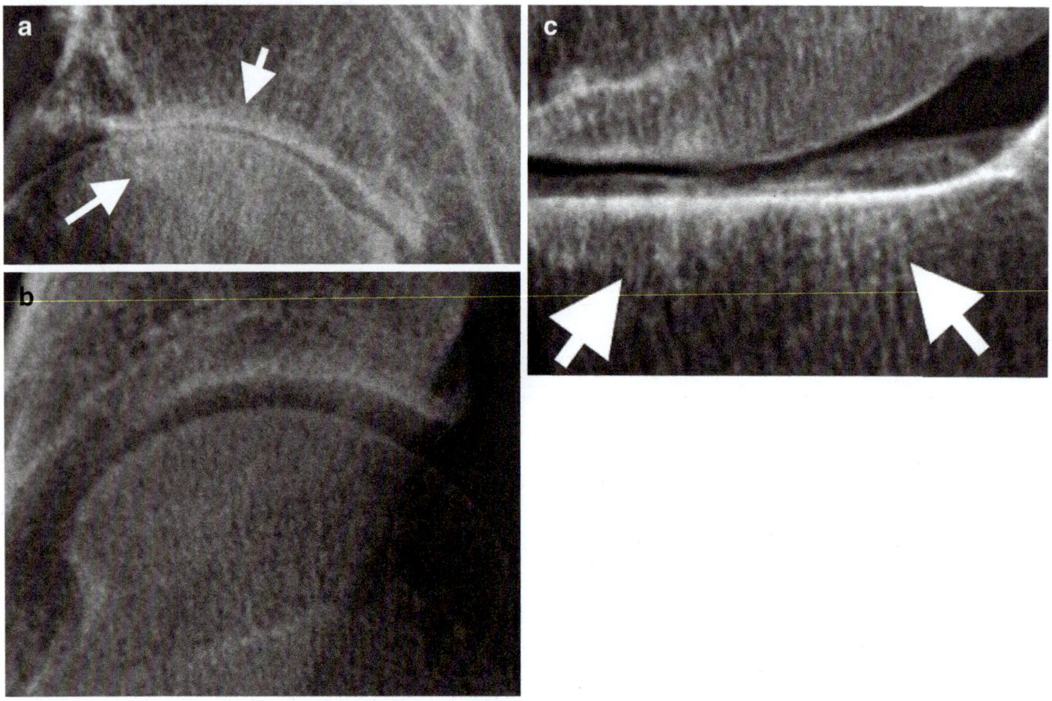

Fig. 10.3 Eburnation (*arrows*) on radiograph, (**a**) magnified AP subchondral region hip joint demonstrating increased subchondral sclerosis on both sides joint, (**b**) normal example for reference, (**c**) similar sclerosis secondary to degenerative disease medial tibiofemoral joint space

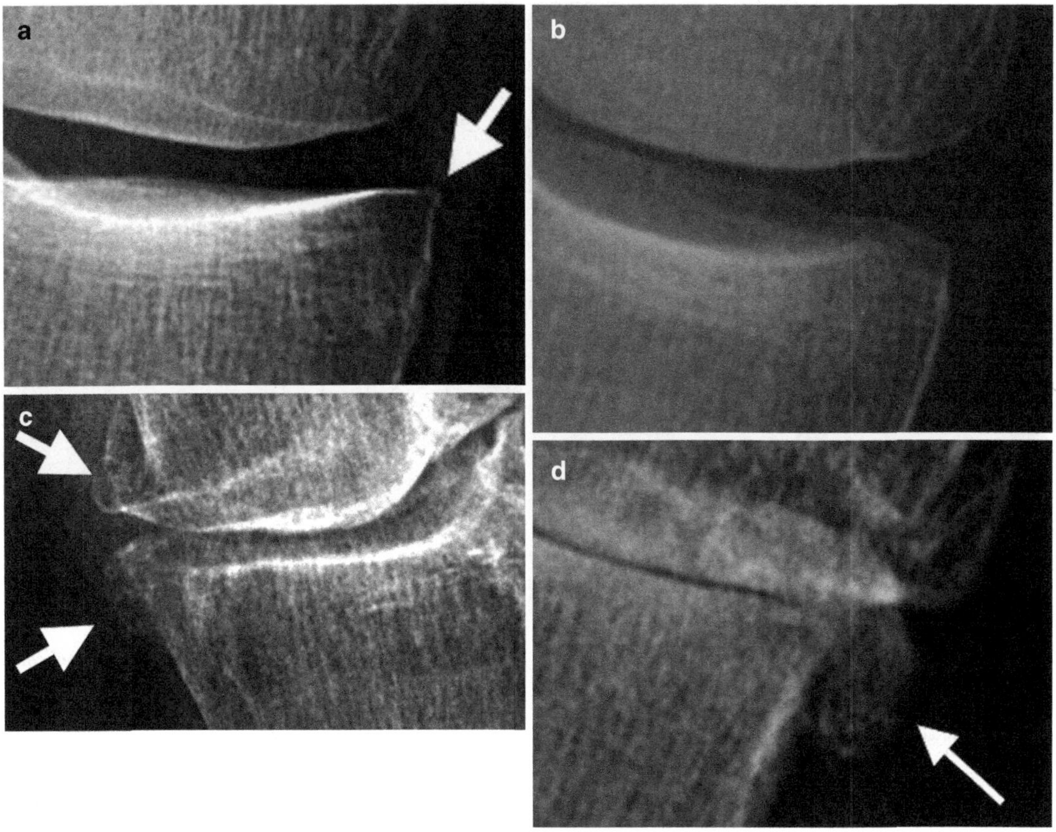

Fig. 10.4 Osteophyte on radiograph, (**a**) early osteophyte formation medial margin of the medial tibial plateau, (**b**) normal example for reference, (**c**) moderate and (**d**) large osteophytes (*arrows*)

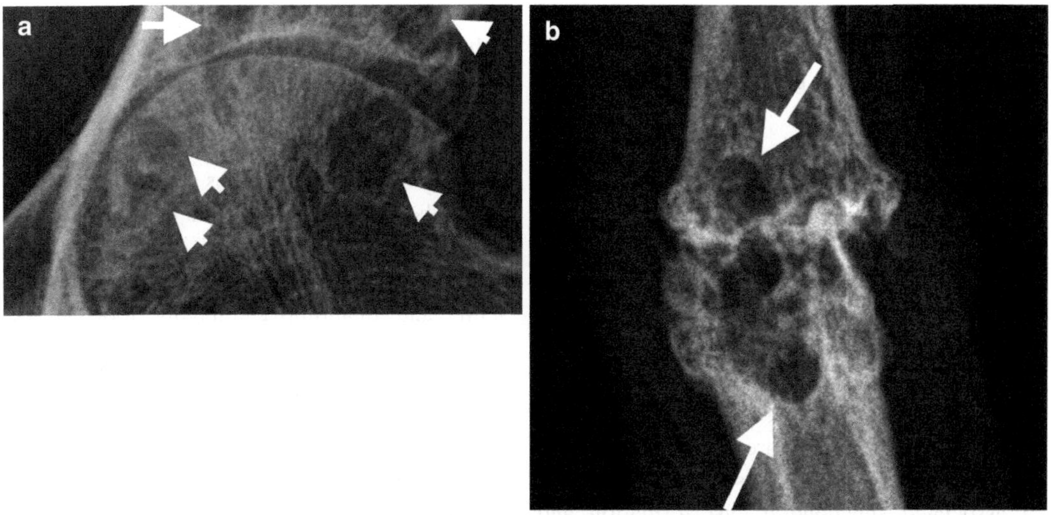

Fig. 10.5 Subchondral cysts (*arrows*) on radiographs, (**a**) well-defined subchondral lucencies with well-defined sclerotic margins in a degenerative hip joint (normal example for reference, see Fig. 10.3b), (**b**) large subchondral cysts in a degenerative PIPJ hand

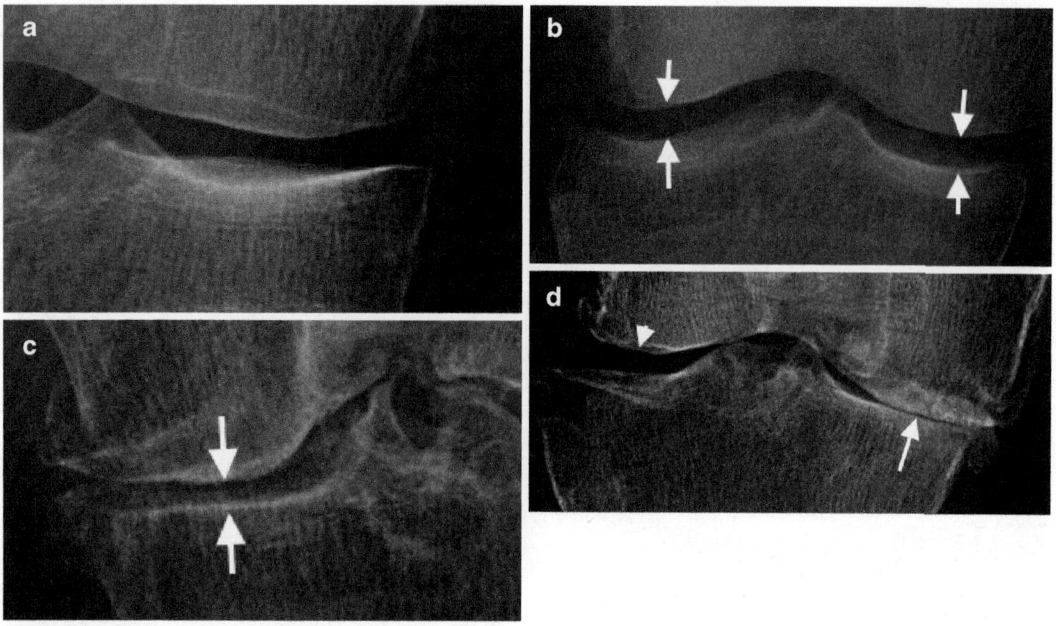

Fig. 10.6 Joint space (*arrows*) loss on radiographs. (**a**) Mild medial tibiofemoral joint space loss, (**b**) normal example for reference, (**c**) moderate to severe, and (**d**) severe, almost complete, joint space loss medially; note maintained lateral tibiofemoral joint space (*arrowhead*). True joint space loss is best assessed on standing for weight-bearing joints

CT demonstrates exquisite detail of subchondral changes as described in the above radiographic findings; however, it is rarely required in the assessment of OA. CT is occasionally used for assessment of intra-articular loose bodies and residual bone mass, e.g., glenoid, prior to joint replacement (Fig. 10.7).

Subchondral sclerosis on *MRI* is of low SI on both T1- and T2-weighted sequences. Subchondral cysts may contain proteinaceous material or joint fluid if they communicate with the joint and are of high SI on T2 and usually low SI on TI. MRI is the gold imaging standard in assessing cartilage. Cartilage abnormalities include changes in signal intensity, fibrillation cartilage surface, fissuring eventually extending full-depth cartilage, and areas of full-thickness cartilage loss (Fig. 10.8). These are often the sites of associated subchondral cyst formation and bone marrow edema. MRI of joints also allows visualization of the soft tissues including ligaments, capsule, synovium, and bone marrow changes. It should be stressed however that although MRI is useful in detecting lesions that are not possible with radiographs, they may not add to the clinical picture when plain radiographs demonstrate osteoarthritic changes. Further imaging beyond radiographs in clinical practice should be considered when the results will affect the management of the patient.

There is an array of studies using MRI as a semi- and quantitative imaging tools in the assessment of osteoarthritis. These studies are focused predominantly on the knee, hand, and hip. The required high-resolution imaging required for detailed cartilage review is mainly confined to research studies at this time due both to the extended time required to acquire and interpret

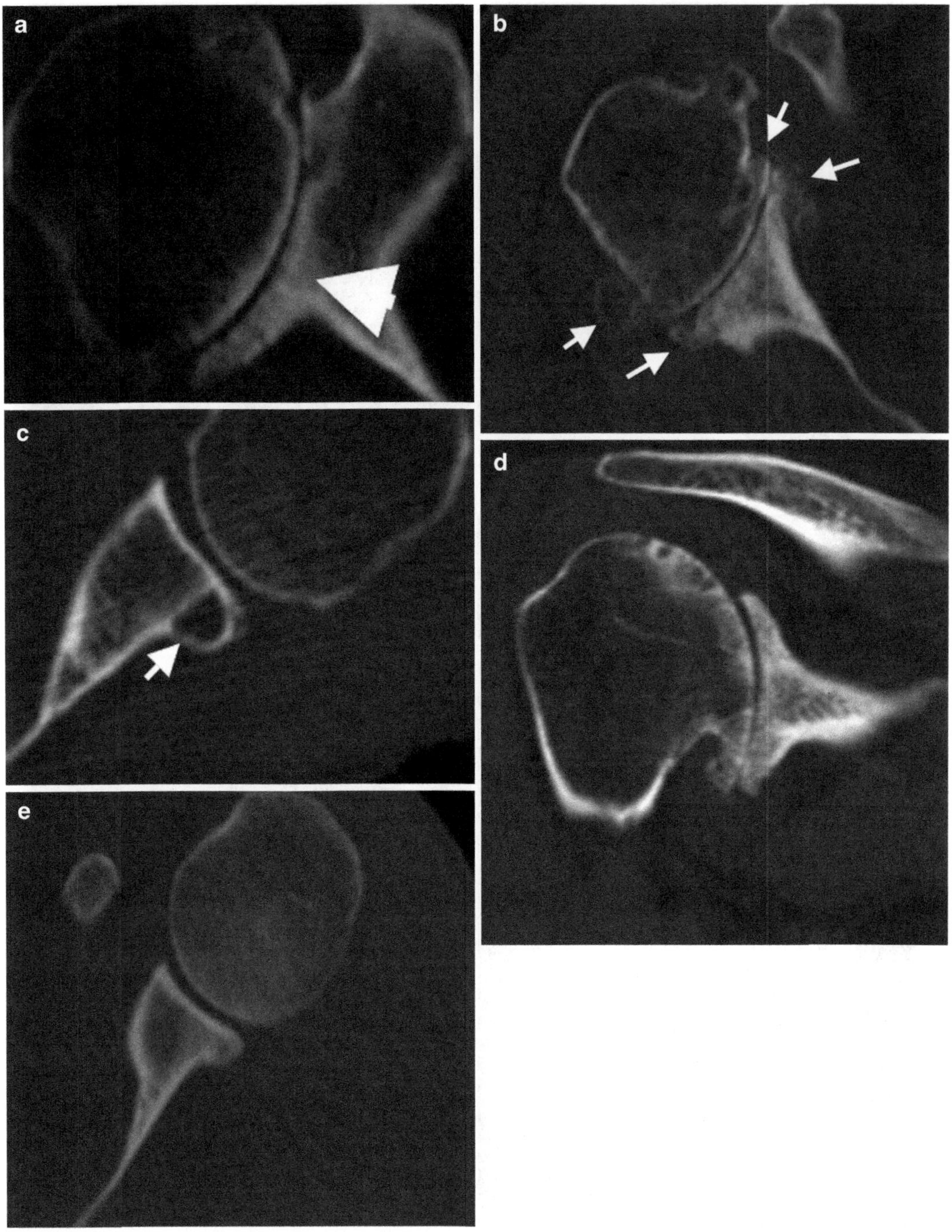

Fig. 10.7 CT secondary degenerative joint disease on the right shoulder. (**a**) Subchondral sclerosis/eburnation (*arrowhead*); (**b**) moderate osteophytosis (*arrows*); (**c**) subchondral cyst glenoid with well-defined sclerotic margins (*arrow*); (**d**) reformatted coronal image with joint space loss, subchondral sclerosis, osteophytes, and subchondral cysts; (**e**) normal axial CT for reference

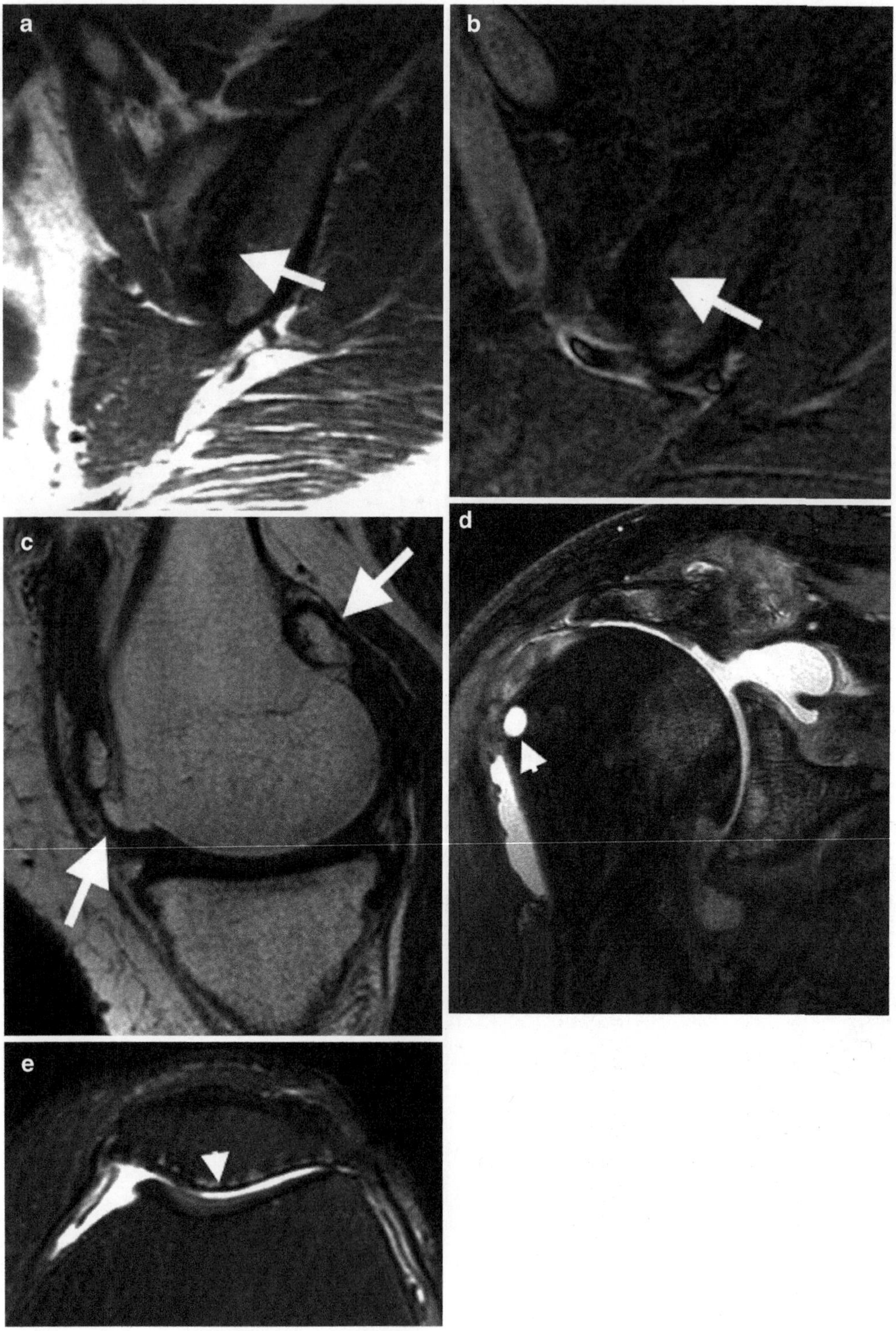

Fig. 10.8 MRI degenerative disease. (**a**) Subchondral sclerosis (low SI on all imaging sequences) left sacroiliac joint in patient with osteitis condensans ilii (OCI) with subchondral low signal (*arrows*) on Cor T1 and (**b**) Cor T2FS. (**c**) Moderate osteophytosis in medial femoral condyle on sagittal T1 (*arrowheads*), (**d**) rotator cuff arthropathy on the right shoulder with joint space loss, complete cartilage loss, subchondral bone marrow edema, and early subcortical cyst formation on Cor T2FS (*arrowhead*) low SI sclerotic rim on the greater tuberosity, (**e**) cartilage loss, full-thickness patellar aspect patellofemoral joint (*arrowhead*) with mild subchondral edema

these sequences and whether these sequences affect clinical management beyond currently performed sequences. *Ultrasound* is used predominantly for assessment of joint fluid and synovitis. Ultrasound can also demonstrate associated changes such as joint space loss, cartilage thinning and loss in the periphery of superficial joints, cortical irregularity, and osteophytosis. Nuclear medicine is generally not indicated.

The description of osteoarthritis will be subdivided into primary OA of large and small joints with typical examples provided.

Osteoarthritis: Small Joints

Osteoarthritis of the *hand* will be used to demonstrate the typical changes within small joints. The proximal and distal interphalangeal joints and the first carpometacarpal joint are the most commonly affected small joints. The PIP and DIP joints may demonstrate a symmetrical appearance in joints involved and the degree of osteoarthritis (Fig. 10.9). Localized bony outgrowths from the DIP and PIP joints are termed Heberden's and Bouchard's nodes, respectively. The joint

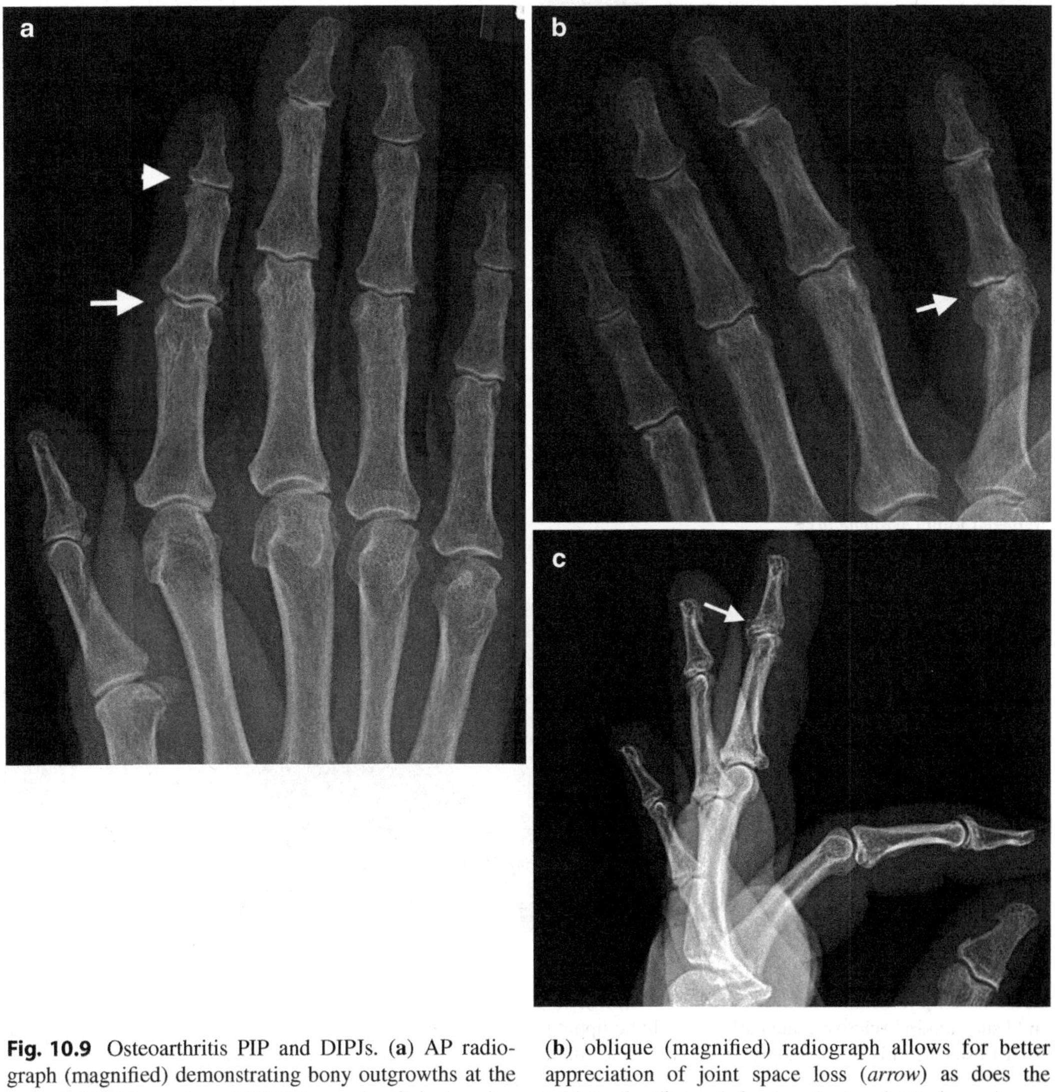

Fig. 10.9 Osteoarthritis PIP and DIPJs. (**a**) AP radiograph (magnified) demonstrating bony outgrowths at the second PIPJ (*arrow*) and DIPJ (*arrowhead*) in keeping with early Bouchard's and Heberden's nodes, respectively, (**b**) oblique (magnified) radiograph allows for better appreciation of joint space loss (*arrow*) as does the (**c**) lateral radiograph for dorsal osteophytes (*arrow*)

spaces are narrowed with subchondral sclerosis. There may be mild radial or ulnar subluxation. Metacarpophalangeal joint involvement occurs usually in the presence of more advanced disease

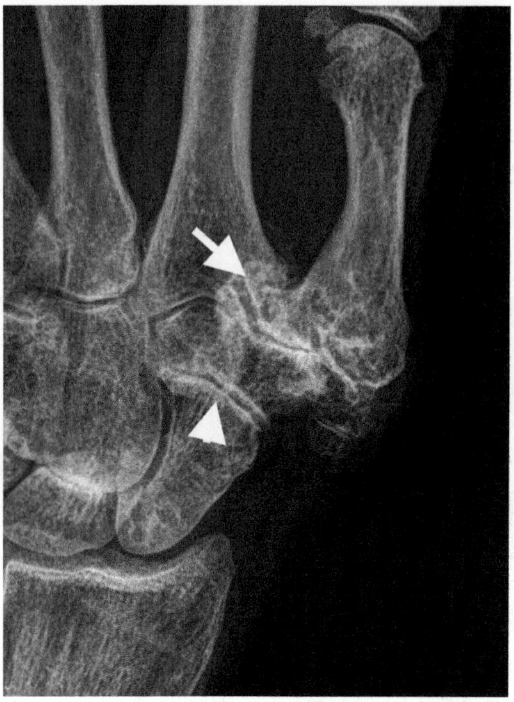

Fig. 10.10 AP radiograph (magnified) demonstrates advanced degenerative disease at the 1st CMC joint (*arrow*) and mild to moderate degeneration at the scapho-trapezial joint (*arrowhead*)

at the PIP and DIP joints. If disease is predominantly at the MCP joints, then one should consider alternative underlying pathology such as CPPD arthropathy and hemochromatosis.

The first carpometacarpal joint is predisposed to degeneration given its multidirectional capabilities and the various articulations involved (Fig. 10.10). Initially the joint space may be widened due to ligamentous laxity. Joint space loss, subchondral cysts, intra-articular (ossified and chondral) bodies, and subluxation may occur. Degeneration may progress to involve the scaphotrapezial joint. The first CMC is also commonly involved in CPPD arthropathy, and review for supporting changes for OA (PIPJ and DIPJ) or CPPD (chondrocalcinosis, radiocarpal degeneration) should be actively sought (Fig. 10.11).

Erosive Osteoarthritis

Erosive or inflammatory OA is a subset of primary OA and predominantly involves the hands. The PIP and DIP joints are more commonly involved although any of the above joints in primary OA may be involved. There are bony outgrowths at the joint margins, joint space loss, and central erosions. The latter produces the "sea gull" appearance (Fig. 10.12). Disease may progress with eventual ankylosis. Lack of marginal

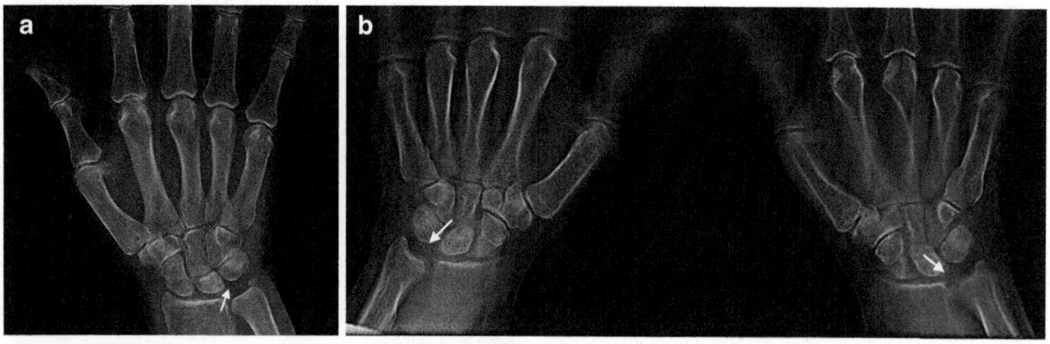

Fig. 10.11 CPPD arthropathy. (**a**) AP radiograph (magnified) of the right hand with joint space loss at the MCPJs, mild subchondral sclerosis, and early osteophytic lipping. MCPJ osteoarthritis is commonly secondary. Note subtle calcification (*arrows*) wrist, lunotriquetral ligament better appreciated on (**b**) single image from tomosynthesis series, also present contralateral hand. Incidental sclerosis and subchondral cyst lunate related to a prior injury

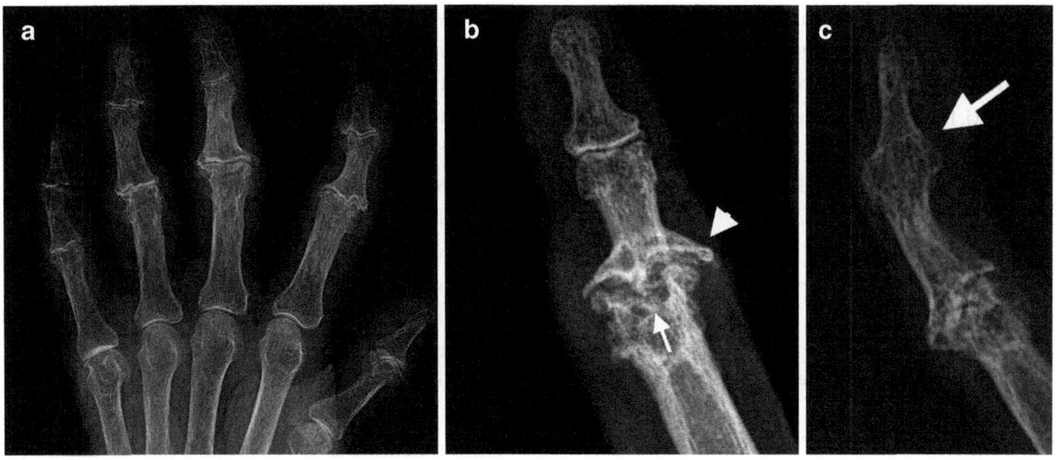

Fig. 10.12 Erosive osteoarthritis on radiographs, (**a**) magnified AP left hand central erosions, (**b**) soft tissue swelling and moderate degenerative changes at the PIPJs and DIPJs with joint space loss, osteophytosis, (**b**) magnified AP second digit different patient with central erosion (*arrow*) with gull wing appearance and moderate osteophytes (*arrowhead*), and (**c**) osseous fusion across fifth DIPJ secondary to erosive osteoarthritis (*arrow*)

erosions, periosteal reaction, and new bone formation, other than osteophytes, helps to separate the disease from psoriatic arthropathy.

Osteoarthritis: Large Joints

Knee

The knee joint is commonly involved with osteoarthritis, often with nonuniform involvement of the patellofemoral and medial and lateral tibiofemoral articulations. Standing radiographs allow for better assessment of joint space loss versus supine studies. Thus when comparing progression of disease, consistent patient positioning is important for an accurate assessment. The medial tibiofemoral joint is more commonly involved than the lateral space and may progress to cause a varum deformity (Fig. 10.13). Joint space in the tibiofemoral space is related both to articular cartilage and the menisci. Occasionally the dominate etiology is meniscal, prior meniscectomy or severely torn and displaced meniscal tissue, and there will be joint space loss without the characteristic additional changes of osteoarthritis.

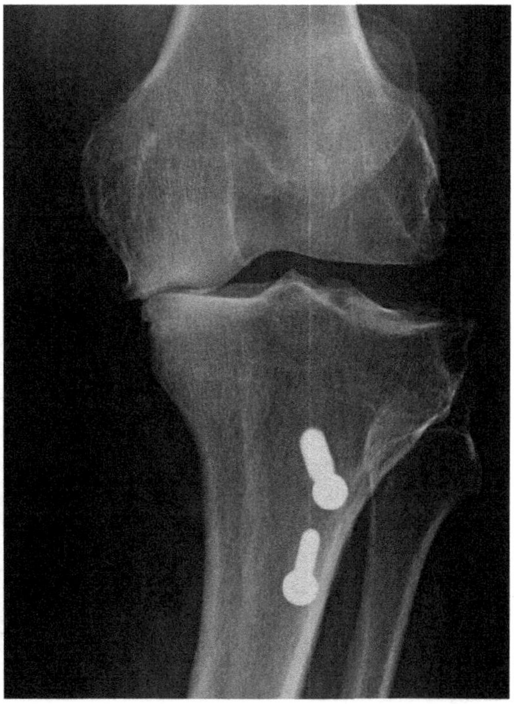

Fig. 10.13 AP radiograph of the left knee with severe medial tibiofemoral joint space loss, osteophytosis, subchondral sclerosis, and secondary genu varum. Orthopedic screws related to prior surgery and repositioning tibial tuberosity

There are several radiographic scoring systems available with the Kellgren and Lawrence classification being most commonly cited (Table 10.1, Fig. 10.14). This system grades conventional x-ray based on a scale of 0–4 by assessing the presence and severity of osteophytes, joint space narrowing, subchondral bony sclerosis, and deformity of the bony contour.

Table 10.1 Kellgren and Lawrence radiographic scoring of knee OA

Grade 0: Normal
Grade 1: Doubtful narrowing of joint space and possible osteophytic lipping
Grade 2: Definite osteophytes, possible narrowing of joint space
Grade 3: Moderate multiple osteophytes, definite narrowing of joint space, some sclerosis, and possible deformity of bone contour
Grade 4: Large osteophytes, marked narrowing of joint space, severe sclerosis, and definite deformity of bone

Knee joint effusion is often present with distension of the suprapatellar recess. This is best appreciated on a lateral radiograph with increased soft tissue attenuation between the post quadriceps and pre-femoral fat pads (Fig. 10.15). Intra-articular loose bodies, osseous and chondral, are also common. Occasionally soft tissue prominence may be identified in the popliteal fossa and represent a Baker's cyst, which often communicates with the joint (Fig. 10.15). Osseous bodies can be identified within the Baker's cyst when a communication exists. Rupture of a Baker's cyst can be confirmed on ultrasound. When dominant involvement of the patellofemoral joint is present, one should consider CPPD arthropathy, which may be present in the absence of radiographic chondrocalcinosis in the same joint.

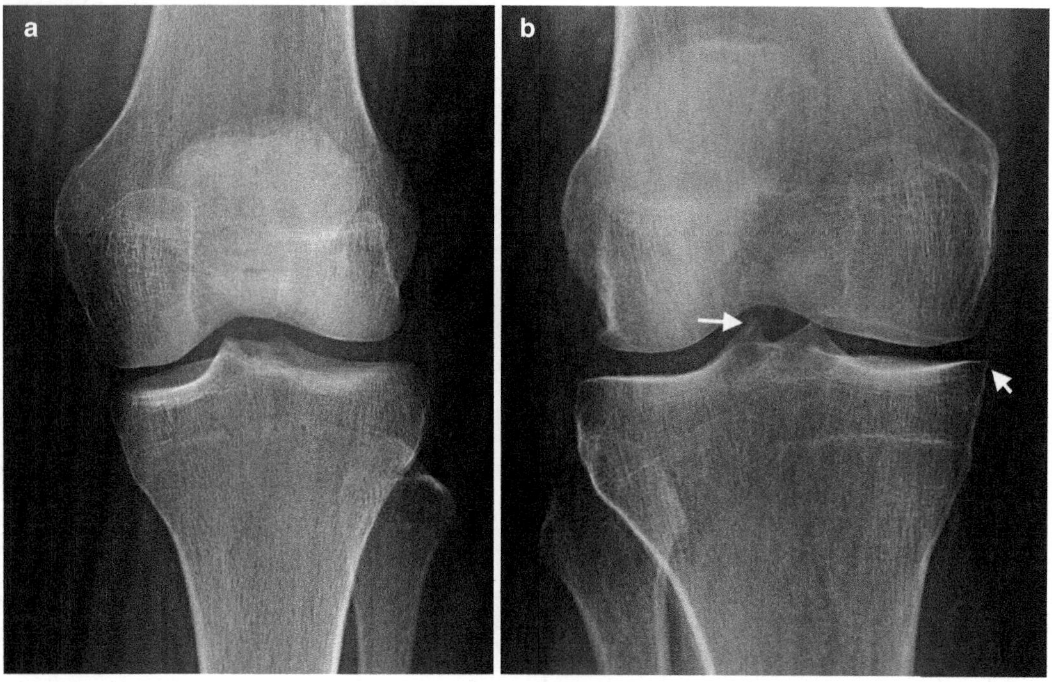

Fig. 10.14 Kellgren and Lawrence radiographic scoring of knee OA. (**a**) Normal AP radiograph of the left knee, grade 0. (**b**) Grade 1: doubtful narrowing of joint space and early osteophytic lipping (*arrow*). (**c**) Grade 2: definite osteophytes, possible narrowing of joint space. (**d**) Grade 3: moderate multiple osteophytes, definite narrowing of joint space, some sclerosis, and possible deformity of bone contour. (**e**) Grade 4: large osteophytes, marked narrowing of joint space, severe sclerosis, and definite deformity of bone

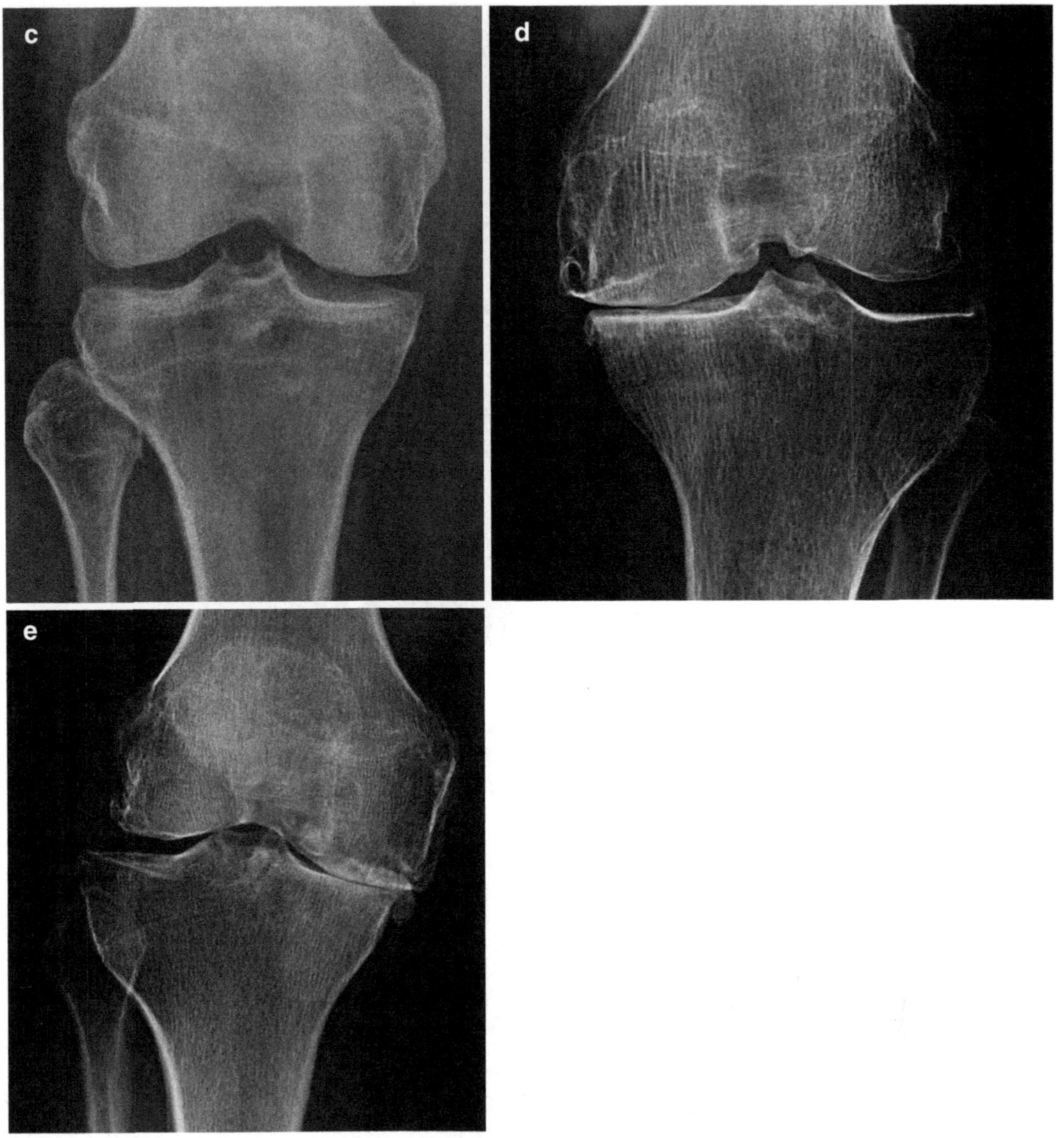

Fig. 10.14 (continued)

Hip

Joint space loss and subsequent migration of the femoral head may occur superolaterally, medially, or axially. Superolateral is the most common with joint space loss most pronounced on the upper and outer aspect of the hip joint, with subsequent migration of the femoral head (Fig. 10.16). The altered dynamics exaggerate secondary OA changes of subchondral sclerosis, cysts, and osteophyte formation. Medial migration may also occur and is more common in women and may relate to acetabular over coverage and subsequent pincer type femoroacetabular impingement. Axial migration occurs in line with the femoral neck and suggests secondary OA, usually related to inflam-

Fig. 10.15 A 58-year-old female lateral radiograph knee demonstrating patellofemoral advanced degeneration, with scalloping of the anterior margin distal femur (*arrowhead*). More pronounced degeneration at the patellofemoral joint should always raise the possibility of CPPD as in this case. Note suprapatellar recess moderate effusion (*small arrow*), soft tissue swelling within the popliteal fossa (*long arrow*) in keeping with a distended Baker's cyst (confirmed with ultrasound)

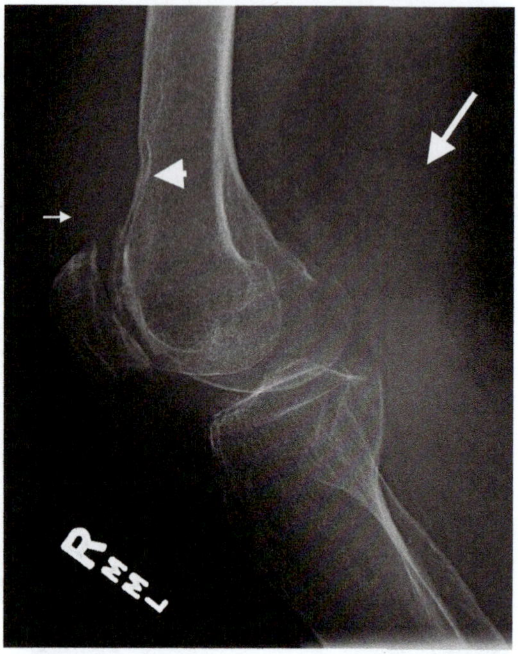

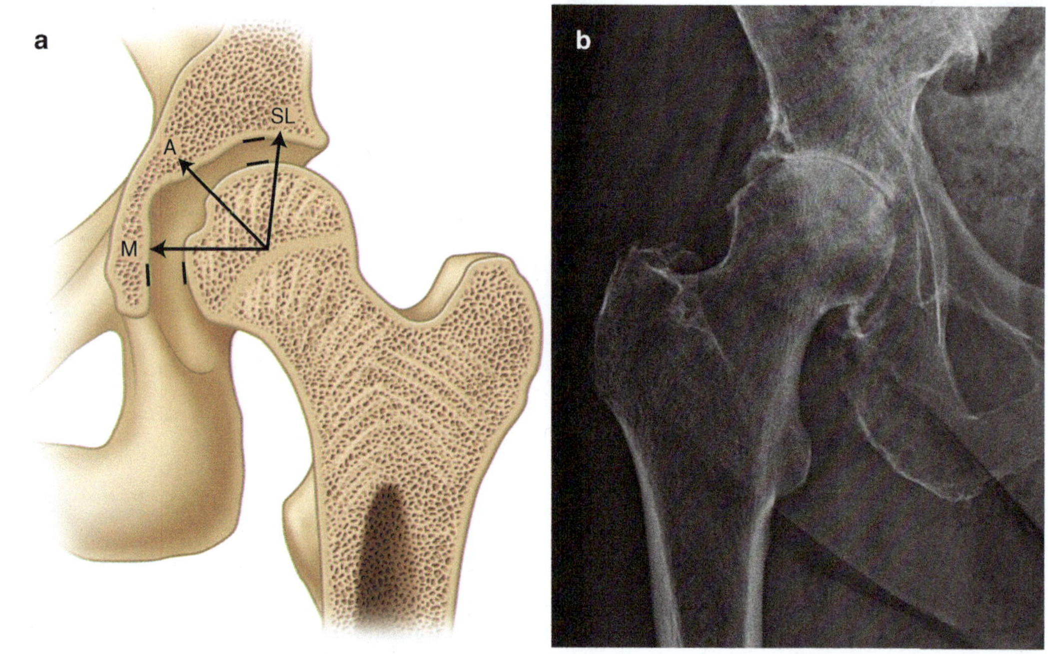

Fig. 10.16 (**a**) Femoral head migration patterns, *SL* superolateral, *A* axial, *M* medial. (**b**) AP radiograph hip with superolateral migration femoral head with joint space loss most pronounced on the upper and outer aspect of the hip joint. (**c**) Axial migration occurs in line with the femoral neck and suggests secondary OA, in this case secondary to CPPD arthritis which is suggested by the prominent subchondral cysts. (**d**) Axial migration with acetabular overcoverage. (**e**) Normal radiograph for comparison

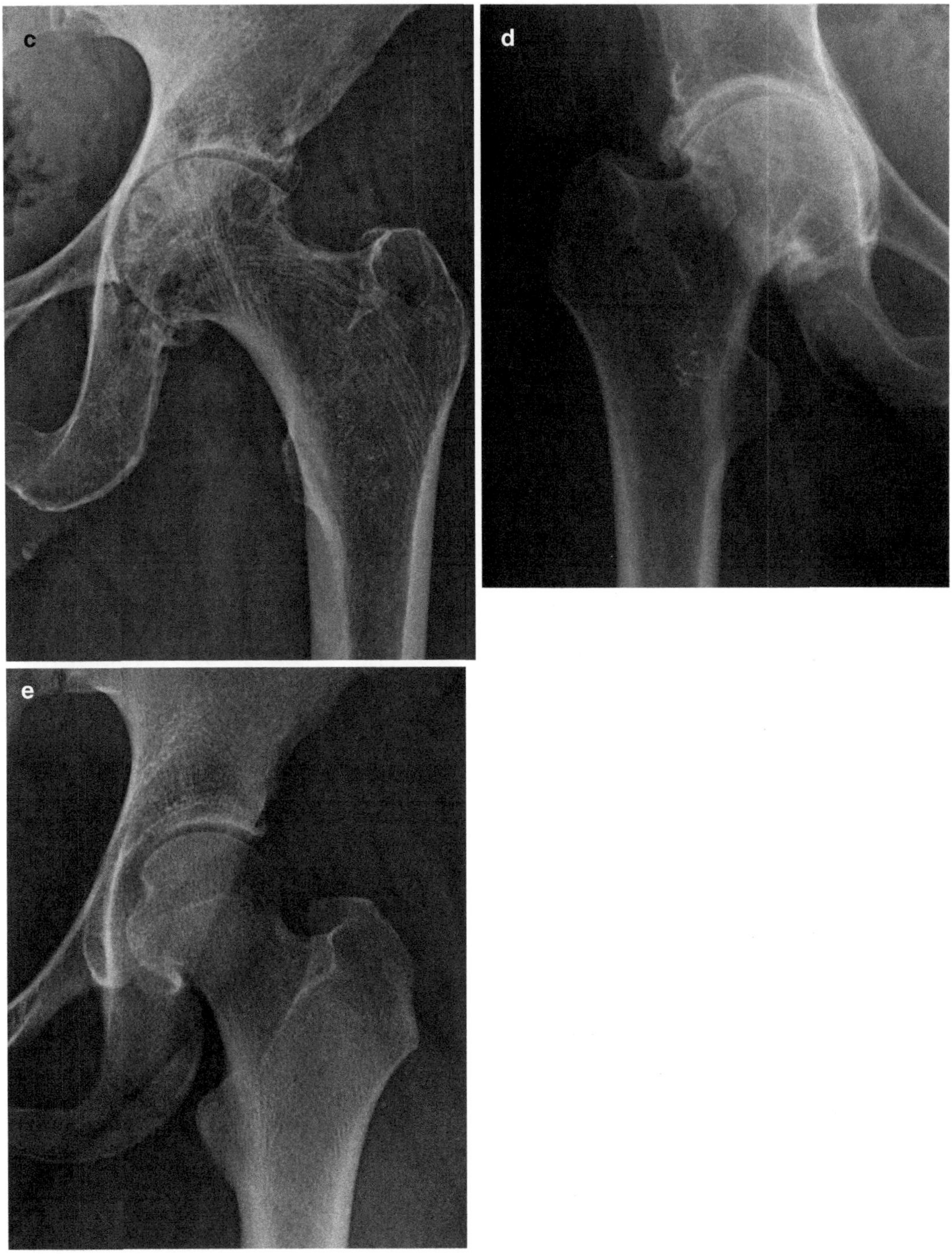

Fig. 10.16 (continued)

matory arthropathy such as rheumatoid arthritis. Buttressing, thickening of the medial cortex femoral neck with endosteal and periosteal new bone formation, is a stress response related to altered dynamics upon the hip joint due to OA.

Femoroacetabular impingement is an increasingly recognized cause of premature osteoarthritis. There are two main types, which often coexist to varying degrees in up to 80 % of patients, Cam and Pincer. Cam type, described after a cam mechanism, occurs in the presence of a femoral head neck dysplasia, i.e., abnormal bone formation at the femoral head neck junction, usually anterior or anterolaterally. This bony "bump" impacts upon the acetabulum on flexion and internal rotation of the hip with subsequent injury to the acetabular labrum and adjacent cartilage. It is more common in males. Pincer type is more common in middle-aged women and is related to acetabular overcoverage (Figs. 10.17 and 10.18). Note that these radiographic abnormalities may be present in joints that are asymptomatic and have no evidence of osteoarthritis.

Postel's coxarthropathy is an uncommon rapidly progressive destruction of the hip joint. It is thought to be secondary to insufficiency fracture with collapse and osteolysis of the femoral head. Degenerative changes are present; however, there is little osteophyte formation. The condition usually occurs unilaterally in elderly women (Fig. 10.19). Differential includes crystal arthropathy.

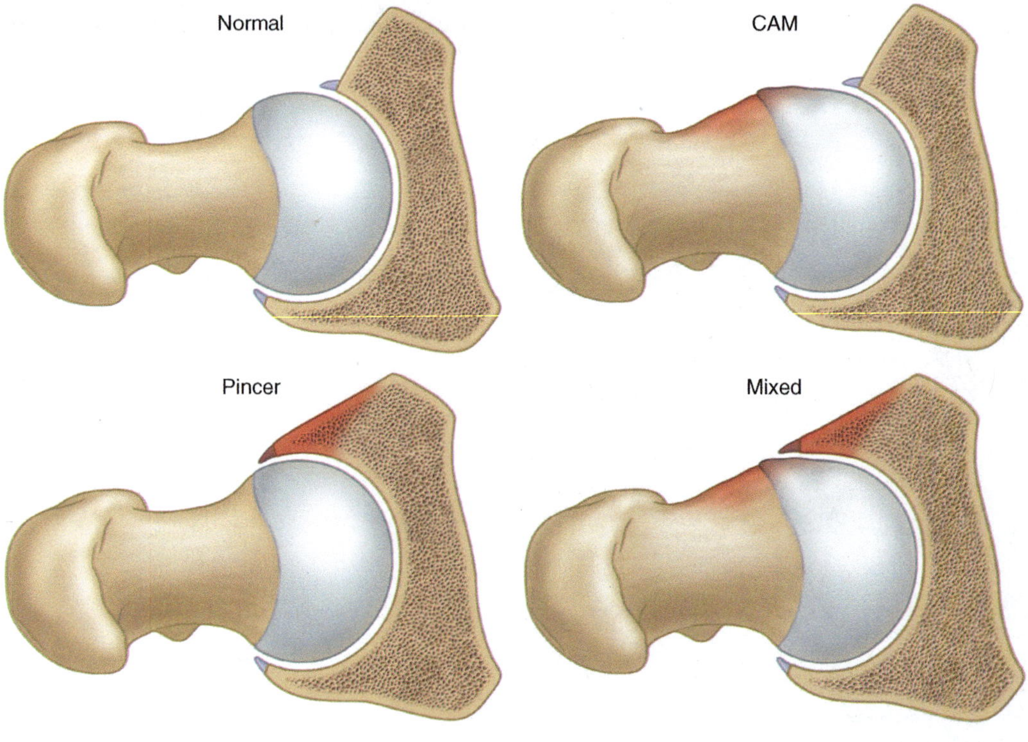

Fig. 10.17 Different types of femoroacetabular impingement

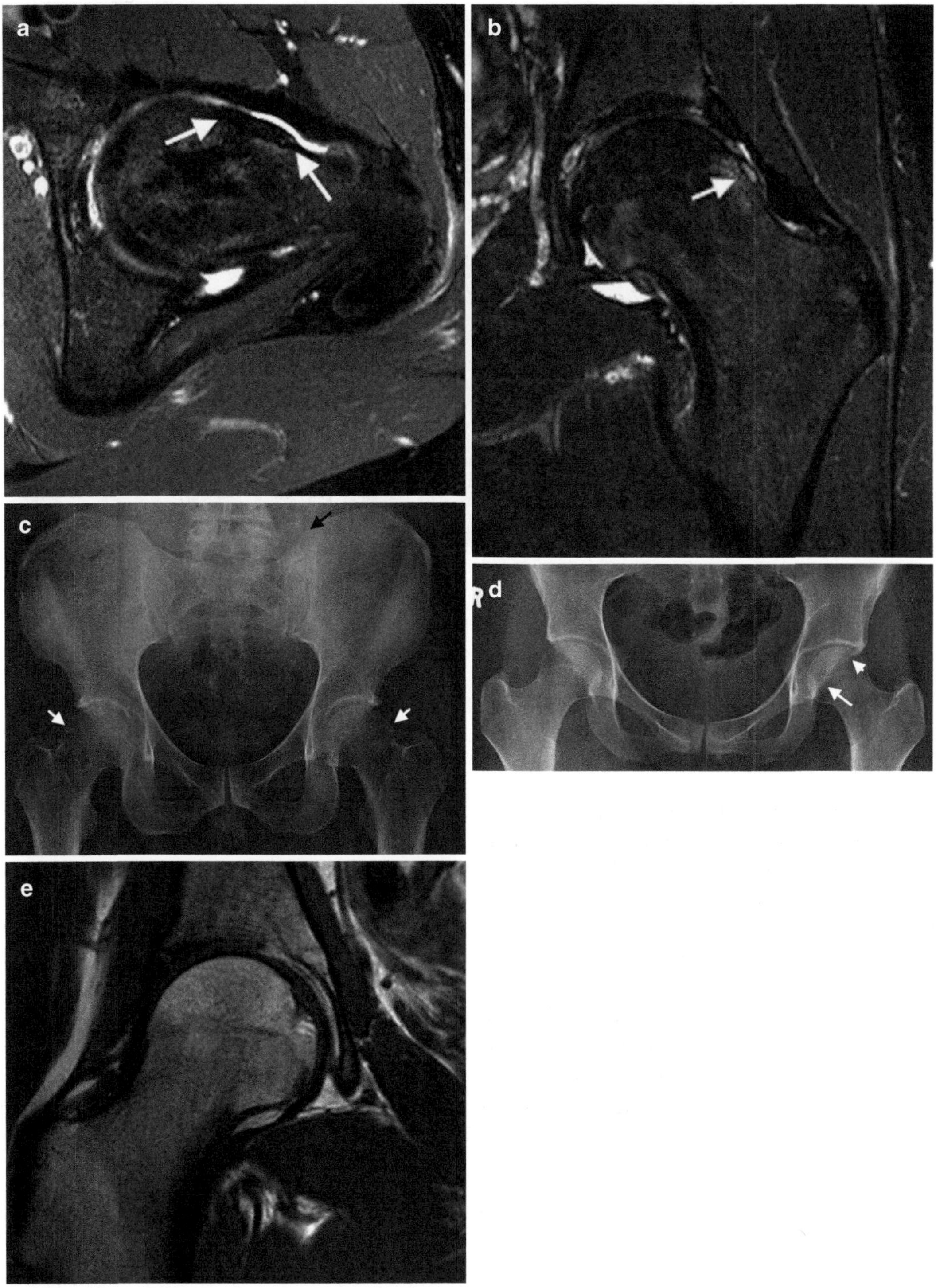

Fig. 10.18 (**a**) Axial oblique and (**b**) Coronal T2FS demonstrating femoral head-neck dysplasia (*arrows*) with associated mild bone marrow oedema; (**c**) AP pelvic radiograph demonstrating femoral head–neck dysplasia (*arrows*), incidental left transitional vertebra; (**d**) acetabular retroversion and (**e**) normal Cor T1 MRI right hip for reference

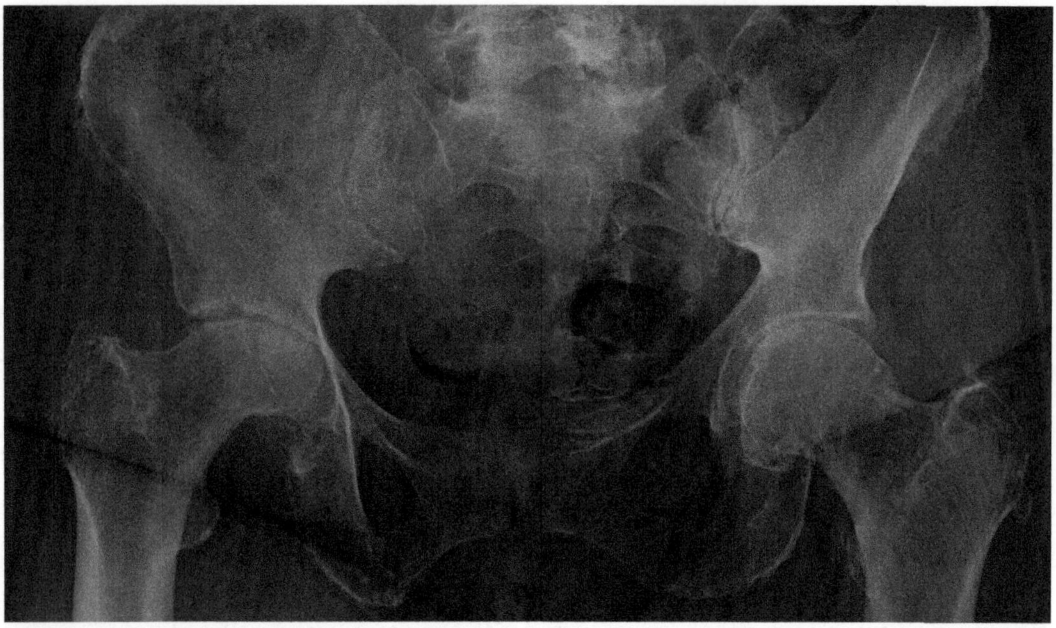

Fig. 10.19 AP radiograph of bilateral hips. Partial collapse right femoral head, likely related to previous undiagnosed insufficiency fracture on a background of degenerative disease. Note degenerative changes left hip and prominent enthesophyte formation; the later is related to known DISH in this patient

Glenohumeral OA

Glenohumeral osteoarthritis is almost always secondary in nature. Predisposing factors include prior trauma, instability, crystal disease, rotator cuff disease, and inflammatory, metabolic, and endocrine arthropathies. Rotator cuff arthropathy, common in the elderly patient, occurs in the presence of a complete tear of the supraspinatus tendon and often tears of the remaining rotator cuff and long head biceps (Fig. 10.20). There is secondary superior translation of the humeral head due to the unopposed upward pull of the deltoid muscle. The humeral head erodes the undersurface of the acromion with cortical loss, irregularity, and cyst formation, particularly within the superior humeral head and greater tuberosity. The inferior humeral head subsequently articulates abnormally with the glenoid with cartilage and joint space loss and inferior glenohumeral osteophytosis. This progresses to diffuse glenohumeral degeneration. In the absence of rotator cuff disease, trauma history, or evidence of an inflammatory arthritis, crystal disease should be considered and is reviewed in greater detail in Chap. 8.

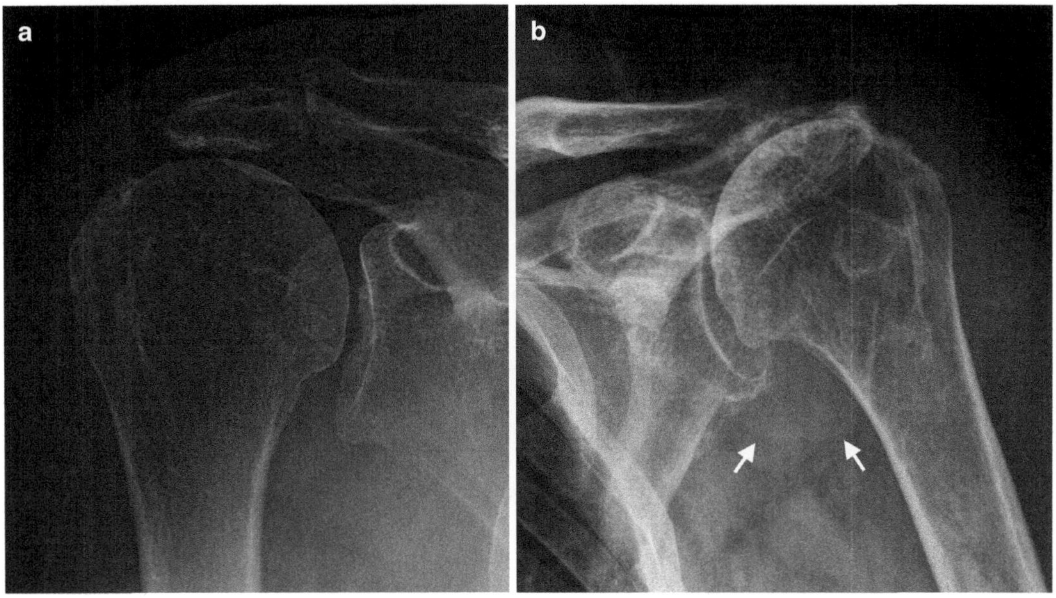

Fig. 10.20 Rotator cuff arthropathy in (**a**) 67-year-old female with massive rotator cuff tear, secondary superior translation humeral head and early cortical changes acromial undersurface to impaction from the humeral head, note cortical irregularity greater tuberosity secondary to rotator cuff disease (**b**) more advanced rotator cuff arthropathy in a 78-year-old male with osteophytosis inferior glenohumeral joint and extensive erosion acromion. Note joint effusion with soft tissue joint distension inferiorly (*arrows*)

Further Reading

1. Banks SE. Erosive osteoarthritis: a current review of a clinical challenge. Orthop Clin North Am. 2013;44(4): 575–89.
2. Guermazi A, Hayashi D, Eckstein F. Imaging of osteoarthritis. Rheum Dis Clin North Am. 2013;39(1):67–105.
3. Guermazi A, Hayashi D, Roemer FW. Osteoarthritis: a review of strengths and weaknesses of different imaging options. Rheum Dis Clin North Am. 2013;39(3):567.
4. Kellgren JH, Lawrence JS. Radiological assessment of osteo-arthrosis. Ann Rheum Dis. 1957;16:494–50.
5. Ornetti P, Brandt K, Hellio-Le Graverand MP. OARSI-OMERACT definition of relevant radiological progression in hip/knee osteoarthritis. Osteoarthritis Cartilage. 2009;17(7):856–63.
6. Resnick D, Kransdorf MJ. Bone and joint imaging. 3rd ed. Philadelphia, WB Saunders. 2004.
7. Rogers AD, Payne JE, Yu JS. Cartilage imaging: a review of current concepts and emerging technologies. Semin Roentgenol. 2013;48(2):148–57.
8. Sankar WN, Matheney TH, Zaltz I. Femoroacetabular impingement: current concepts and controversies. Clin Rheumatol. 2010;29(7):697–706.

11 Metabolic Bone Disease

Arthur N. Lau, John O'Neill, and Jonathan D. Adachi

Osteoporosis

Overview

Osteoporosis is a systemic disorder of bone metabolism. It is characterized by a decreased bone mineral density and deterioration in bone microarchitecture. This decline in both bone quantity and bone quality puts osteoporotic patients at a high risk of sustaining fractures. Osteoporotic fractures are very common and have a significant impact on patient's health-related quality of life and ability to function. Fractures of the hip, spine, wrist, humerus, ribs, pelvis, femur, and lower leg are considered osteoporotic fractures in the appropiate clinical presentation, while the skull, fingers, and toes are not. Osteoporotic or fragility fractures occur after minimal trauma defined as a force less than that sustained from a fall from a standing height. Hip fractures and vertebral fractures have also been shown to increase mortality rates. After a vertebral or hip fracture, the 5-year mortality rate is increased by about 20 %. The highest rate of mortality occurs within the first 6 months after a hip fracture. In addition, osteoporosis poses a significant economic impact on the health-care system.

A.N. Lau, MD, FRCPC (✉)
Clinical Scholar, Division of Rheumatology, McMaster University, Hamilton, ON L8N1Y2, Canada
e-mail: arthur.lau@medportal.ca

J. O'Neill, MB, BAO, BCh, MRCPI, MSc, FRCR
Associate Professor, Musculoskeletal Imaging Diagnostic Imaging, McMaster University/ St Joseph's Healthcare, Hamilton, ON L8N4A6, Canada
e-mail: joneill2@me.com

J.D. Adachi, MD, FRCPC
Professor, Department of Medicine, McMaster University/St. Joseph's Healthcare, Hamilton, ON L8N1Y2, Canada

Types of Osteoporosis

Osteoporosis can develop as a primary or a secondary disorder. Primary osteoporosis is by far the most common form of osteoporosis in both men and women, accounting for over 95 % of cases in women and over 70 % of the cases in men. Estrogen is protective against osteoclastic differentiation and thus has a protective effect. After menopause, the protective effect of estrogen is lost, leading to increase osteoclast survival and differentiation, leading to an overall net bone resorption. Secondary causes are much less common and include endocrine disorders, malabsorption syndromes, chronic renal insufficiency, immobilization, and drug-induced among other causes (Table 11.1).

Prevalence

An estimated ten million people in the United States over the age of 50 years have osteoporosis. Approximately 30 % of women over the age of 75 years have sustained at least one vertebral fracture. It is estimated that the incidence of vertebral fractures is 500,000 per patient-year in the United States each year. The number of hip fractures worldwide is estimated to increase to 6.3 million by 2050.

J. O'Neill (ed.), *Essential Imaging in Rheumatology*,
DOI 10.1007/978-1-4939-1673-3_11, © Springer Science+Business Media New York 2015

Table 11.1 Secondary causes of osteoporosis

Endocrine disease (hyperparathyroidism, Cushing's disease, hyperthyroidism, hypogonadism)
Chronic renal failure (secondary hyperparathyroidism, osteomalacia, adynamic bone disease)
Gastrointestinal disease (malabsorption syndrome, inflammatory bowel disease, post-gastric bypass)
Rheumatologic disease (rheumatoid arthritis, systemic lupus erythematosus)
Immobilization (prolonged bed rest or immobility, stroke, spinal cord injury)
Drug-induced (glucocorticoids, heparin, antidepressants, antiepileptics, aromatase inhibitors)
Other (anorexia nervosa, cystic fibrosis)

Clinical Presentation

Vertebral fractures commonly occur in patients with osteoporosis. These fractures are asymptomatic or are misinterpreted as mechanical back pain, so they are often underdiagnosed. Many of these fractures are not associated with a preceding traumatic event. Only about one-third of patients with a vertebral compression fracture evident on radiographs will have clinical manifestations, thus leading to underdiagnosis. Severe back pain and loss of height are the most common events which trigger further investigations. When symptomatic though, these fractures have a significant impact on health-related quality of life and functioning. Hip fractures are commonly symptomatic, and have a devastating effect on functioning and quality of life, and are associated with a significant risk of mortality.

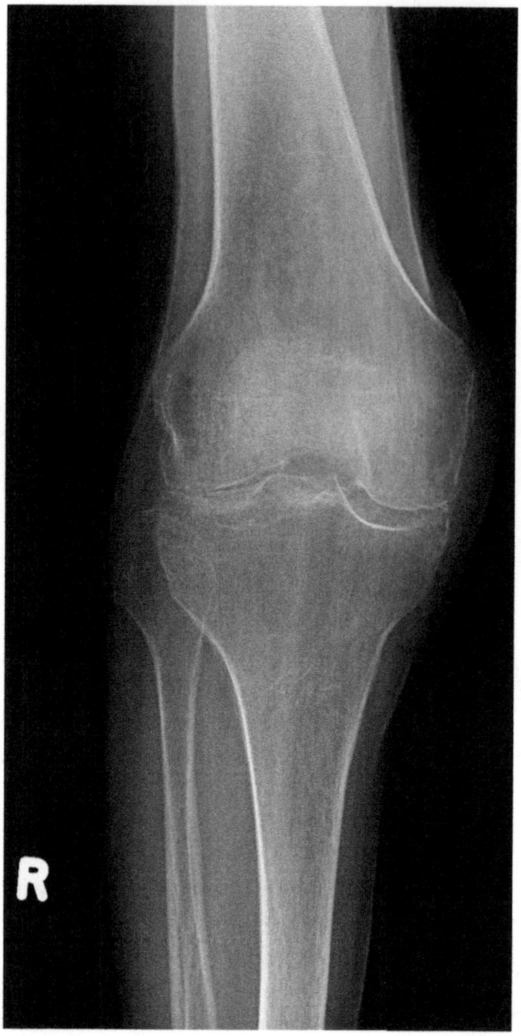

Fig. 11.1 AP radiograph of the right knee with marked osteoporosis with increased radiolucency, diminished cortical thinning, and loss of trabecular pattern

Imaging

Plain Radiographs

Plain radiographs are the most commonly utilized modality to assess for fractures in osteoporotic patients. Many of these fractures may be found incidentally, especially vertebral fractures given the asymptomatic symptoms in many cases. Radiographs in osteoporotic patients demonstrate a decrease in radiodensity of the bone with thinning of the bone cortex. Cortical thinning arises as a result of bone resorption in the endosteal, periosteal, and intracortical bone surfaces. On radiographs, these changes are most evident in both the axial skeleton and in the long bones (Fig. 11.1). The trabecular bone, especially is the most common area involved and most evident on radiographs. The earliest changes evident on radiograph are noted within the vertebrae and in the proximal long bones; both are usually not evident unless a significant amount of bone density is lost; thus radiographs are not very sensitive in early disease. As disease progresses there is increase in radiolucency of the vertebral bodies. In addition there is thinning or loss of the normal trabecular pattern of the vertebra bodies. This loss of transverse trabeculae leads to a vertical radiodense "bar" appearance, which is caused by a relative accentuation of remaining vertical trabeculae.

As stated earlier, the risk of fracture increases with progressive disease. Vertebrae are a very common site of fractures, and vertebral fractures are most commonly seen in the thoracic and thoracolumbar regions. Fractures result in a change of the shape of the involved vertebrae (Fig. 11.2). The most classical type of fracture seen in osteoporosis is a vertebral compression fracture, whereby the nature of mechanical forces involved causes a wedged or compressed appearance. This appearance is seen because the anterior portion of the vertebral body is unable to withstand the same degree of compressive force that the posterior portion is able to withstand, thus leading to the anterior wedging appearance. Normally, the posterior height of the thoracic and lumbar vertebrae should measure 1–3 mm more than the anterior height. A vertical height difference greater than 4 mm is considered a true vertebral compression. Vertebral fractures can be graded by their severity on radiographs, judged by the degree of deformity seen. A grade 1 (mild) vertebral fracture involves greater than 20 % but less than 25 % deformity. A grade 2 (moderate) vertebral fracture involves 25–40 % deformity, while a grade 3 (severe) vertebral fracture involves greater than 40 % deformity (Fig. 11.3). Higher-grade vertebral fracture correlates with significant clinical implications, as the risk for sustaining a future vertebral or hip fracture increases with a higher grade of vertebral fracture.

Aside from an anterior wedged appearance, other vertebral body shapes are seen as a result of fractures that arise from different mechanical forces. One appearance is a pancake vertebra where the vertebral body has lost both its anterior and posterior height; thus it has a flattened appearance reminiscent of a pancake. Another appearance is the codfish vertebra (also known as a fish vertebra), which describes a biconcave appearance of the vertebral body. A codfish vertebra appearance can also be seen in osteomalacia, Paget's disease, and hyperparathyroidism.

Radiographs of the hands in osteoporotic patients may also reveal characteristic findings. The thinning of cortical bone secondary to endosteal resorption is often seen in osteoporotic patients. The thinning of the cortex of the midportion of the non-dominant second metacarpal is involved, but this is often a late finding. The metacarpal index (MCI), the combined thickness of both cortices at the mid-metacarpal level divided by the with bone at the same level, can be measured for the index finger or as a combined measurement of the second to fourth digits (Fig. 11.4). It is a useful tool in the diagnosis of osteoporosis, can provide a computed BMD DXR measurement, and has been shown to correlate with risk of hip fracture. This is a useful tool that is readily available particularly for longitudinal assessment.

In the proximal femur, patterns of trabecular bone loss correlate well with the severity of underlying osteoporosis. Ward's triangle is an area of diminished trabecular bone seen in the femoral neck of hip radiographs. In osteopenia, when early trabecular resorption occurs, this results in an enlargement of the Ward's triangle, but it also becomes more indistinct due to loss of trabeculation. This is one of the methods that bone density can be assessed utilizing plain radiographs. With increasing severity of osteoporosis, there is further resorption of all trabecular groups, including the principal compressive group, which contains the most densely packed trabeculae and is seen only in the late stages of osteoporosis (Fig. 11.5).

Similar radiographic changes of cortical thinning and loss of trabeculae can also be seen in

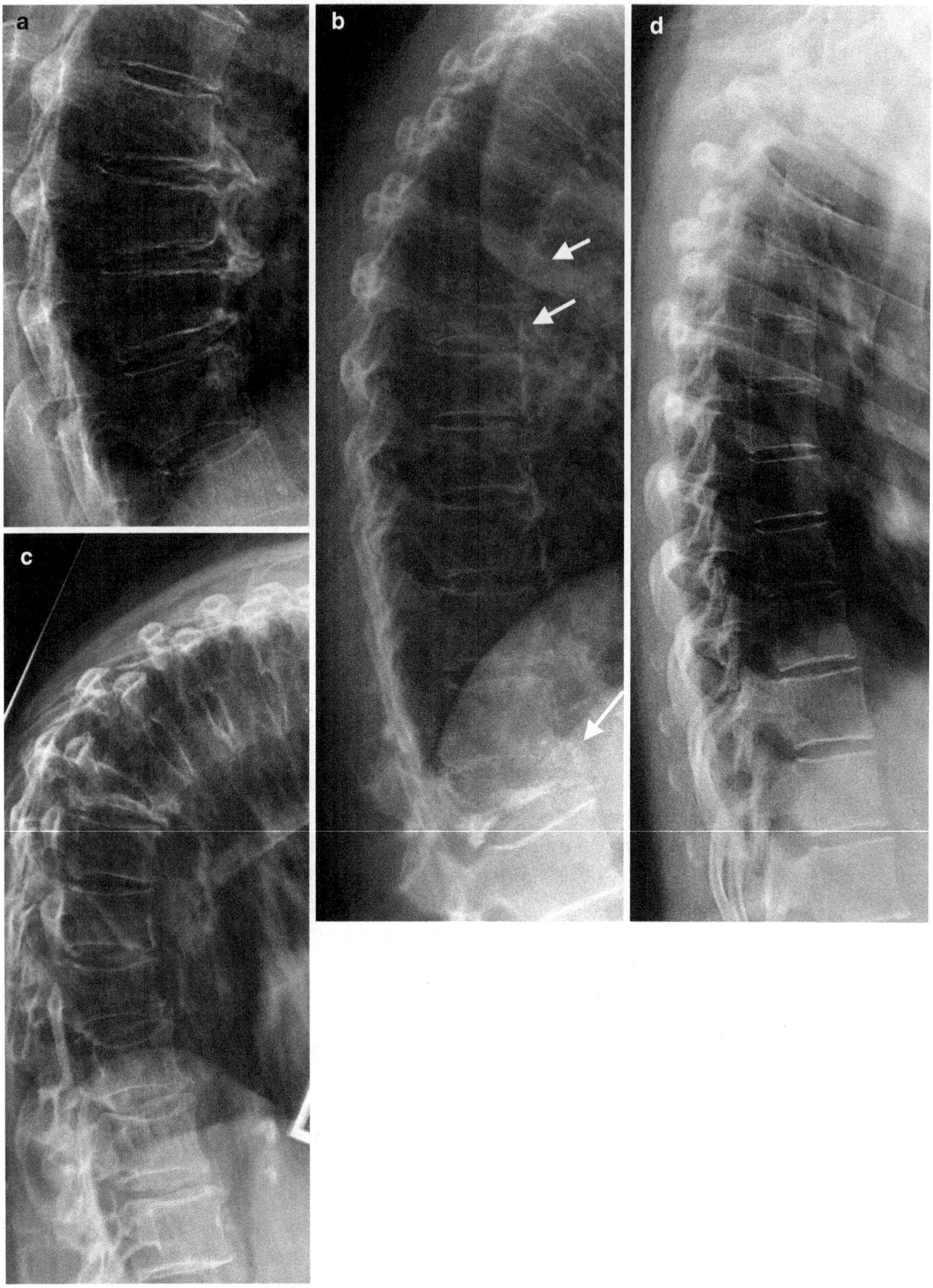

Fig. 11.2 (**a**) Osteoporotic lower thoracic vertebra on lateral radiography with anterior wedge compression fractures (**b**) Grade 2 and 3 anterior compression fractures (*arrows*) (**c**) Gibbus deformity secondary to compression fractures (**d**) normal lateral radiograph thoracic spine

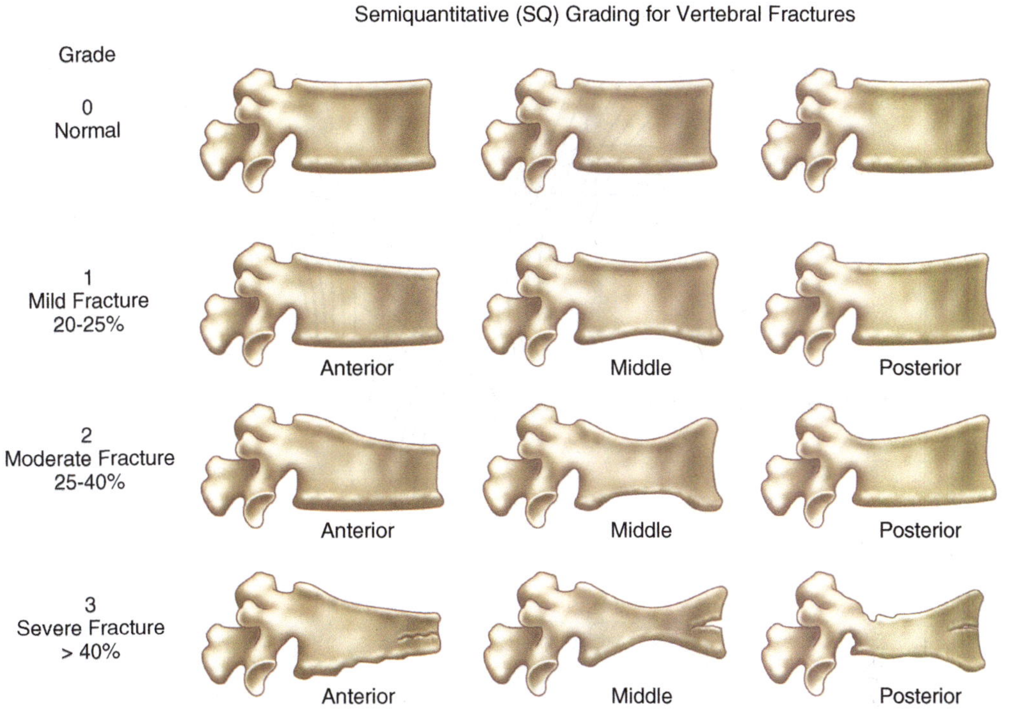

Fig. 11.3 Semiquantitative grading (*SQ*) for vertebral fractures

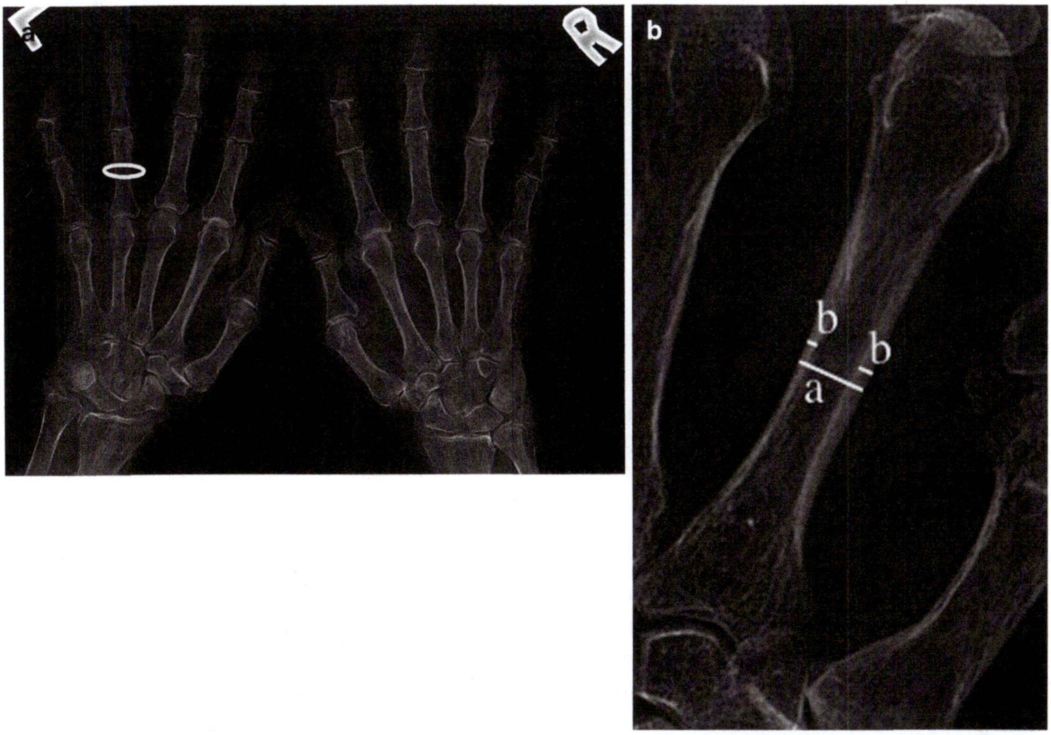

Fig. 11.4 Metacarpal index. (**a**) PA radiograph of hands with osteoporosis and (**b**) calculation of metacarpal index of the non-dominant second metacarpal, mid-diaphysis, measure width bone{a} and combined cortical thickness {b}, Index = a/b. References are available for different age groups and ethnicity

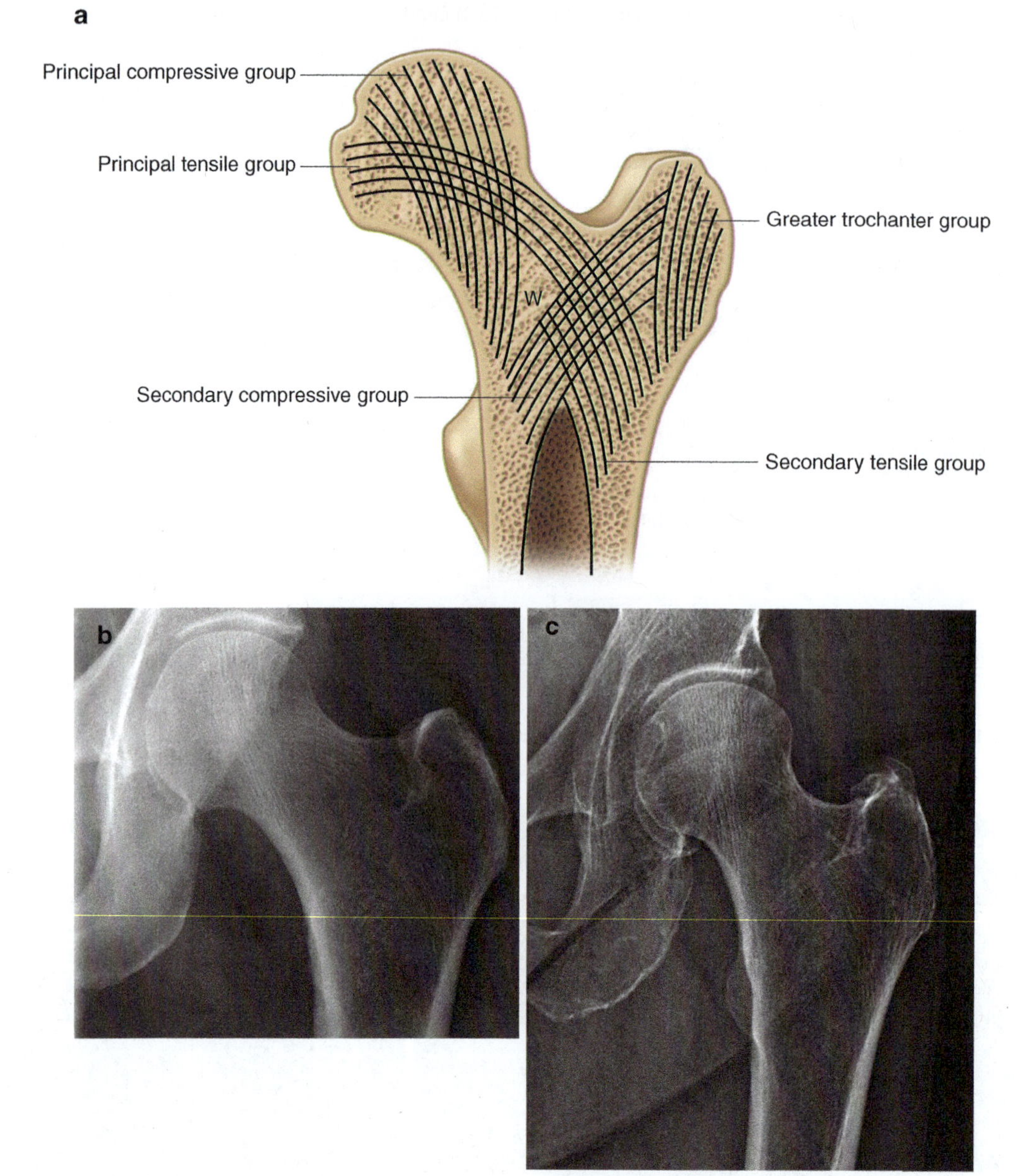

Fig. 11.5 Ward's triangle. (**a**) Illustration of trabecular pattern of left femoral head and neck, (**b**) corresponding normal radiograph, and (**c**) osteoporotic patient

other bones of the peripheral skeleton, especially in areas rich in trabecular bone. Insufficiency microfractures may also develop in osteoporotic patients. Common sites of these insufficiency fractures include the symphysis pubis, sacrum, supra-acetabular, pubic rami, calcaneus, pelvis, femoral neck, and sternum (Figs. 11.6 and 11.7). Areas of osteosclerosis may be seen if there are multiple underlying insufficiency fractures with subsequent development of callus in the reparative process.

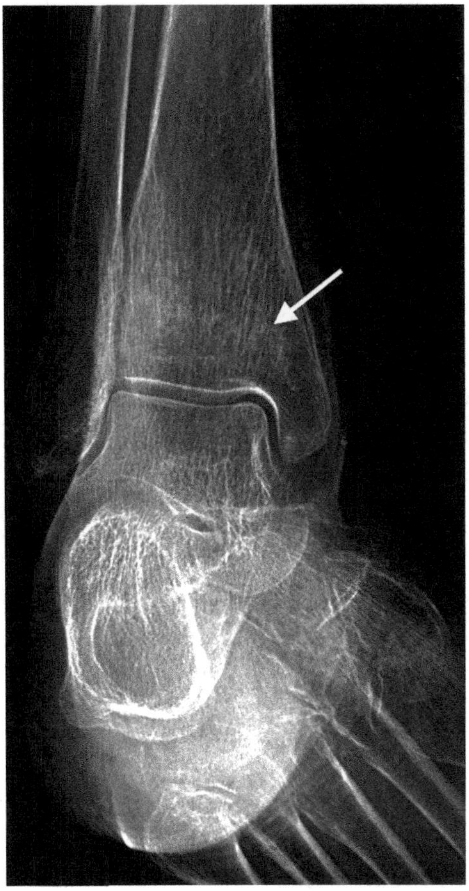

Fig. 11.6 An 80-year-old female with osteoporosis and severe ankle pain, AP ankle radiograph demonstrates diffuse osteoporosis and an ill-defined band of sclerosis (*arrow*) of the distal tibia in keeping with an insufficiency fracture

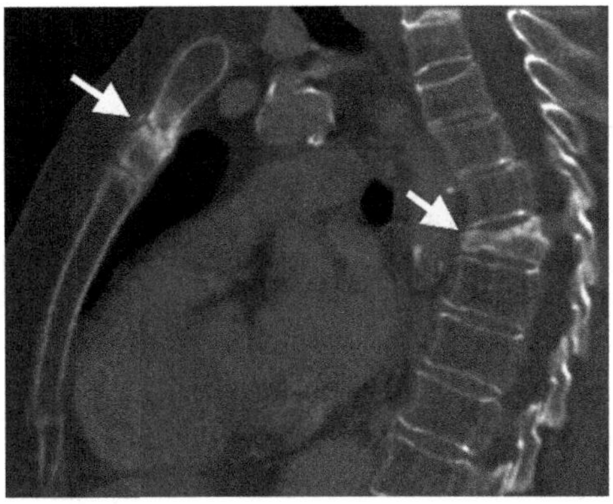

Fig. 11.7 Sag reformatted CT of the chest in a 68-year-old female with grade 3 osteoporotic fracture T6 (*short arrow*) and insufficiency fracture of the manubrium (*long arrow*)

Dual X-Ray Absorptiometry (Fig. 11.8)

Dual x-ray absorptiometry (DXA) is the gold standard tool for quantifying bone mass and to determine the bone mineral density (BMD). Measurements of BMD are reported as standard deviation units relative to the means of young, healthy reference population (*T*-score). Measurements are also reported as a standard deviation from age-matched BMDs (*z* score). The World Health Organization (WHO) uses specific BMD cutoffs for their definition of osteoporosis and osteopenia (Table 11.2). BMD measurements at the lumbar spine (L1 to L5), total hip, and femoral neck are the most common areas utilized. BMD assessment of the distal radius can be acquired if a BMD of the spine or hip cannot be obtained. Distal radius BMD assessments are particularly useful in certain patient populations, such as chronic renal failure patients on hemodialysis and those with severe obesity.

Epidemiological studies have demonstrated that BMD is a strong predictor of sustaining an osteoporotic fracture, and this relationship is independent of patient age. BMD measured by DXA accounts for about 70 % of the estimated bone strength. As the BMD declines, there is a corresponding increase in fracture risk. In general, each standard deviation decline in BMD increases the risk of fracture by 1.5- to 3-folds. A meta-analysis found that for each standard deviation decrease in femoral neck BMD, there is an associated 2.6-fold increase risk in sustaining a hip fracture. There is also an inverse relationship between BMD decline and the severity of fractures sustained, with an increased risk of sustaining malunion and early instability seen in patients with severely low BMDs. The majority of women under age of 50 years have a normal BMD unless there is a secondary cause of bone loss. However, with aging, BMD assessed by DXA gradually declines. By age 80, about 27 % of women will have a BMD in the osteopenic range, and 70 % will have a BMD in the osteoporotic range in at least one site.

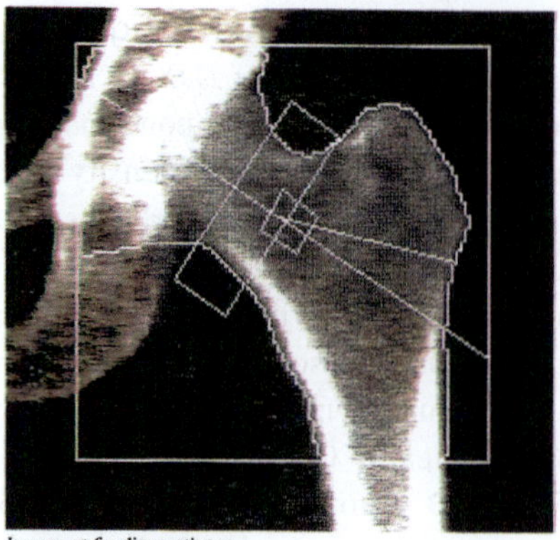

Image not for diagnostic use
k = 1.143, d0 = 49.0
96 x 94

Scan Information:

[redacted]

DXA Results Summary:

Region	Area (cm²)	BMC (g)	BMD (g/cm²)	T - Score	Z - Score
Neck	4.54	2.66	0.585	-2.4	-0.2
Troch	9.73	5.09	0.523	-1.8	-0.1
Inter	17.86	15.76	0.882	-1.4	0.3
Total	**32.13**	**23.51**	**0.732**	**-1.7**	**0.2**
Ward's	1.08	0.36	0.330	-3.5	-0.5

Total BMD CV 1.0%, ACF = 1.043, BCF = 1.032, TH = 6.026
WHO Classification: Osteopenia
Fracture Risk: Increased

Total

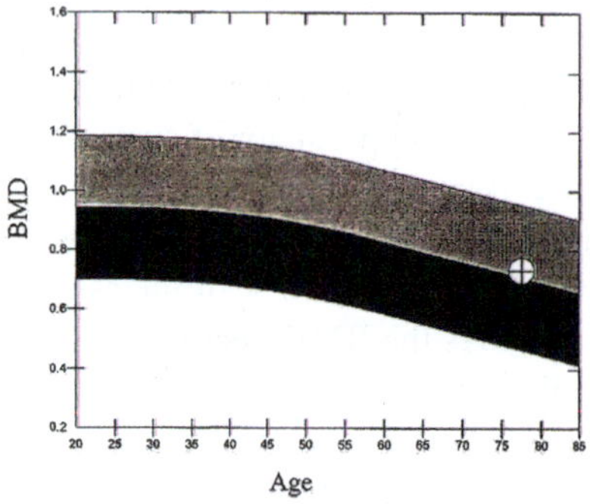

Reference curve and scores matched to White Female

Physician's Comment:

Fig. 11.8 Example of a DEXA scan report, femoral neck

Table 11.2 World Health Organization (WHO) diagnostic categories for osteoporosis based on bone mineral density (BMD)

Category	WHO definition
Normal	A BMD *T*-score of −1.0 or better
Osteopenia	A BMD *T*-score between −1.0 and −2.5
Osteoporosis	A BMD *T*-score of −2.5 or lower

BMD are recorded using DXA. *T*-scores are reported as standard deviations below the young adult mean

Quantitative Computed Tomography

Quantitative computed tomography (QCT) is another imaging modality to quantify bone density. QCT can reliably measure the BMD at the spine, proximal femur, and forearm. However, the benefit of QCT over standard DXA assessment is the ability to provide a true volumetric measurement of BMD rather than the areal measurement provided by DXA. This allows QCT to provide a more accurate measurement of bone density than what the DXA measurements allow. QCT can also differentiate between the densities of cortical and trabecular bone. QCT measurements are usually performed on the vertebrae, but there is a growing availability of peripheral QCT scanners (pQCT), which allows for the analysis of the forearm, tibia, and other sites. In addition, pQCT measurement of BMD at the tibia has been shown to provide highly reproducible measurements of total, cortical, and trabecular bone density. The pQCT scans have also been shown to provide accurate measurements of the muscle and fat cross-sectional area of the calf. In addition to having a low BMD as a risk factor for fracture, a newer concept is to assess for sarcopenia, which is the loss of skeletal muscle mass. Muscle density assessed by pQCT at the calf has been shown to be an independent risk factor for a history of fragility fractures in postmenopausal women.

MR Imaging

Magnetic resonance imaging (MRI) has become an increasingly useful tool in the management of patients with osteoporosis. The microstructure of bone can be assessed using micromagnetic resonance imaging (μMRI) and high-resolution magnetic resonance imaging (hrMRI). Therefore, it allows for the assessment of bone quality, in addition to just bone quantity, which is the bone density. These MRI imaging techniques have been established for peripheral imaging assessment of the distal radius, tibia, and calcaneus. The trabecular architecture derived on MR imaging correlates well with the underlying bone architecture seen on bone histology, thus providing an excellent assessment of underlying bone quality. In addition to providing a bone density measurement, MR imaging also provides additional information which can identify patients who sustained a fragility fracture. These MRI studies however are not widely available clinically.

Another clinically important utility of MR imaging in the setting of osteoporosis is its role in assessment of vertebral compression fracture (Fig. 11.9). MR imaging can help differentiate

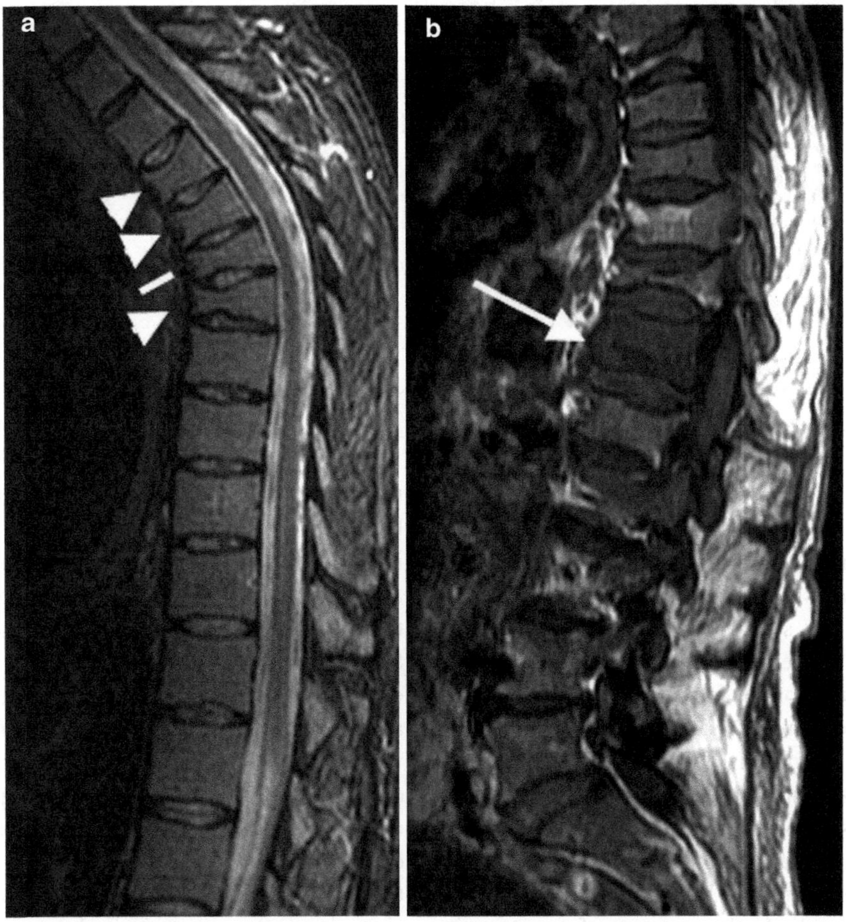

Fig. 11.9 (**a**) Benign compression thoracic fractures (*arrowheads* and line) of a 76-year-old female with history of osteoporosis. Low SI on Sag T2FS and normal marrow SI on T1 (not shown). (**b**) & (**c**) A 75-year-old female with history of OP vertebral fractures and acute lower thoracic pain demonstrates low-SI marrow diffusely at T12 on T1 and high SI on T2FS (*arrows*) and low T1 and high T2 SI fracture line paralleling the inferior endplate (*arrow*). (**d**) Cor T1 demonstrating a benign biconcave compression fracture

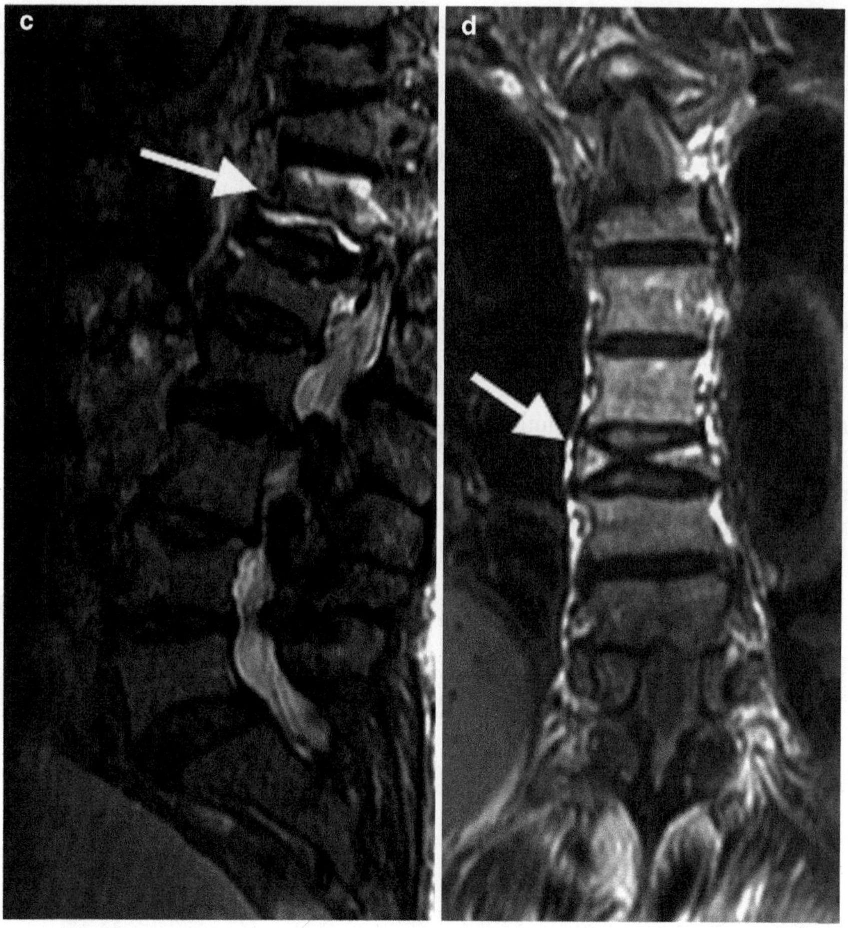

Fig. 11.9 (continued)

between a fracture related to osteoporosis versus a pathological fracture related to skeletal metastasis. In normal vertebrae, there is high signal intensity on T1-weighted images and an intermediate signal intensity on T2-weighted images in keeping with hemopoietic marrow mixed with normal fatty marrow SI. In the setting of bone metastasis, there is variable localized change in SI, dependent in turn on the mineralization of the metastatic deposit, e.g., osteoblastic metastatic deposit is low SI on T1 and T2, whereas an osteolytic metastatic deposit is high SI on T2 and intermediate to low on T1. Usually in the presence of a metastatic-related pathological fracture, the vertebral lesion is obscured by the acute edema related to vertebral collapse; however other deposits in the remaining vertebrae should be sought out to help arrive at a diagnosis (Fig. 11.10). Marrow infiltration with myeloma and lymphoma are also common etiologies of pathological fractures and demonstrate loss of normal marrow SI. In general 25 % of vertebral fractures in osteoporotic patients are pathological, and approximately 33 % of fractures in patients with known malignancy are benign. Helpful differentiating features suggesting a pathological fracture include the following: metastatic deposits or marrow infiltration within other vertebra, diffuse edema vertebral body with extension into the posterior elements, convex posterior cortex, paravertebral/epidural soft tissue mass, poorly formed fracture line, and persistent abnormal SI on follow-up imaging.

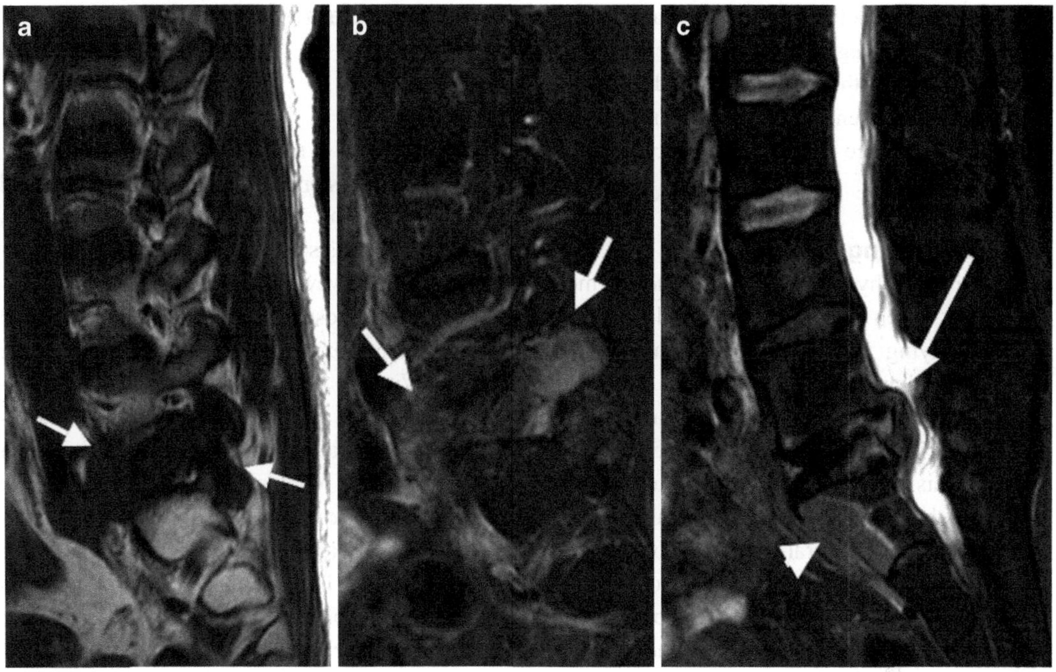

Fig. 11.10 A 49-year-old female with previous cervical carcinoma, presenting with metastatic disease with low-SI lesion at L5 on T1 (**a**) and high SI on T2 (**b**) (*arrows*), vertebral plana of L5 with posterior displacement of vertebral and soft tissue into spinal canal with secondary canal stenosis (**c**) (*long arrow*), on Sag T2FS paravertebral soft tissue thickening, and metastatic deposit at S1 (*arrowhead*)

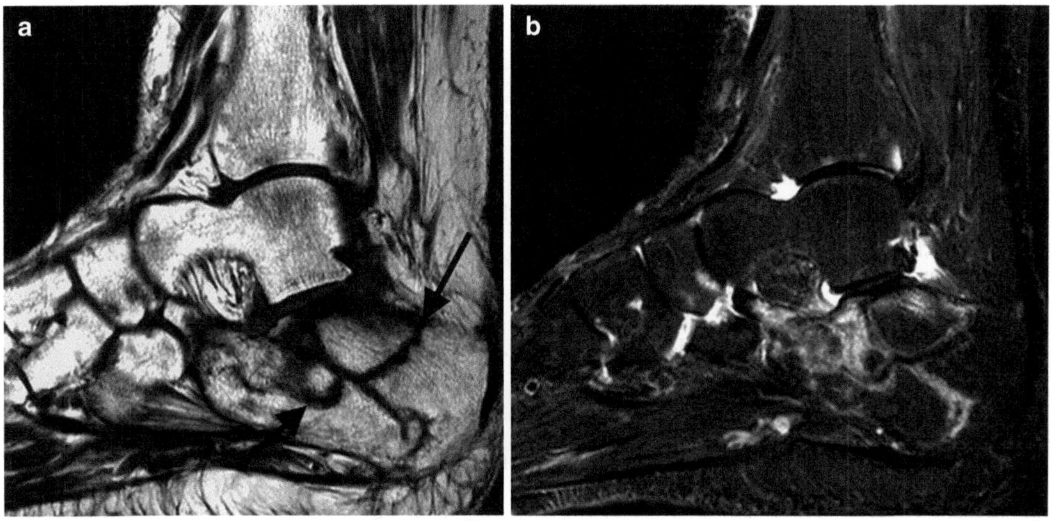

Fig. 11.11 Insufficiency fractures, acute and chronic, of the calcaneus. MRI of a 69-year-old female. (**a**) Sag T1 and (**b**) T2FS with low-SI fracture lines on T1 (*black arrows*) and surrounding bone marrow edema and high SI on T2

MR imaging is also a useful tool in detecting insufficiency fractures at extra-spinal sites. Bone marrow edema seen on MR is an early change associated with insufficiency fractures (Fig. 11.11). This edema has a low signal on T1-weighted images and a high signal on T2-weighted images. MR has a high sensitivity and specificity in detecting insufficiency fractures, especially in the pelvic bones, femoral neck, and intertrochanteric region. MR is a superior modality compared to either CT or plain radiographs in detecting insufficiency fractures and remains the modality of choice when an insufficiency fracture is in question.

Nuclear Imaging

Bone scintigraphy can be a useful nuclear medicine test which can assess bone lesions and the underlying bone metabolic status. These properties allow for it to be a useful tool in the assessment of metabolic bone diseases. It has little role in the diagnosis of uncomplicated osteoporosis. However, it is a useful tool to diagnose vertebral fractures and is useful in assessing the age of a vertebral fracture. However, MR imaging remains the modality of choice when the goal is to differentiate an acute vertebral fracture from a chronic one. In addition, bone scintigraphy can also be utilized to identify fractures at other sites, including the ribs, pelvis, and hips.

Summary

Osteoporosis is a common form of metabolic bone disease primarily seen in the elderly population, but can be seen in younger patients if a secondary cause is present. A decline in BMD subsequently increases the risk of sustaining a fracture. Osteoporotic fractures have been shown to increase patient morbidity and have a significant impact on patient health-related quality of life. Hip and vertebral fractures are also associated with increased mortality rates. Since many patients with osteoporosis are asymptomatic, even many with a prevalent vertebral fracture, screening strategies for the high-risk population are required. BMD assessment with DXA remains the gold standard. However, newer modalities including QCT and MR imaging provide insight into the underlying bone microarchitecture which provide important information into the underlying bone quality instead of just bone quantity. These modalities also provide insight into muscle and fat interactions, which may also play an important role in predicting those at high risk for fractures.

Osteomalacia and Rickets

Overview

Osteomalacia is a relatively common metabolic bone disease. It is primarily a disorder of impaired mineralization of the newly formed collagen matrix. Osteoblasts are still able to produce normal osteoid; however, there are no sufficient calcium and/or phosphate concentrations required for normal hydroxyapatite crystal formation in the osteoid. Vitamin D plays a pivotal role in regulating the serum calcium and phosphate concentration by regulating gastrointestinal absorption of calcium and renal secretion of calcium and phosphate. There are numerous causes of osteomalacia; some are acquired, while others are inherited (Table 11.3). Vitamin D deficiency is a common cause of osteomalacia, which may arise through decrease intake through the diet, lack of sun exposure, renal insufficiency, cirrhosis, and impaired gastrointestinal absorption. Phosphate deficiency is another common cause of osteomalacia, which may arise through decrease intake, vitamin D deficiency, antacid use, and secondary hyperparathyroidism. Compared to vitamin

Table 11.3 Causes of osteomalacia and rickets

Calcium deficiency
Decreased intake
Malabsorption
Phosphate deficiency
Decreased intake
X-linked hypophosphatemic rickets
Oncogenic osteomalacia
Vitamin D deficiency
Chronic kidney disease
Malabsorption
Lack of sun exposure
Fanconi syndrome
Acquired (multiple myeloma, lymphoma, amyloidosis, Sjogren syndrome)
Inherited (X-linked hypophosphatemic rickets, cystinosis, Lowe syndrome)
Drug-induced (6-mercaptopurine, gentamicin, valproic acid)
Aluminum antacid use
Drug-induced
Glucocorticoids, phenytoin, tenofovir, etidronate

D and phosphate deficiency, calcium deficiency is a rare cause of osteomalacia. Osteomalacia may also be in patients with Fanconi's syndrome, which is a disorder of the proximal convoluted tubules (PCT) of the kidneys which results in impaired renal reabsorption of phosphate, thus leading to an osteomalacia picture. Fanconi's syndrome can be due to an inherited cause or due to acquired causes, which includes myeloma, lymphoma, amyloidosis, Sjogren syndrome, and drug induced. Osteomalacia may also occur secondary to a variety of drugs. These drugs include antiseizure medications, glucocorticoids, and tenofovir and etidronate treatment in the setting of Paget's disease. As a result of the open growth plate, skeletal deformities, most famously the genu varum (bowed legged) deformity among others are seen in children with rickets, but not seen in adults with osteomalacia. Rickets shares the same pathogenesis as osteomalacia. However, the disease process occurs in children, where the growth plate is still open. Thus the bone formed by the growth plate is not mineralized due to insufficient substrate.

Clinical Presentation

Adults with osteomalacia do not present with any overt abnormalities to the skeleton like in rickets. These patients are often asymptomatic. Some adults with osteomalacia often present with nonspecific complaints, which include a diffuse throbbing bony discomfort, proximal muscle weakness, and myalgia. Patients with osteomalacia are also at an increased risk of sustaining a fragility fracture, which may occur in the ribs, vertebrae, and long bones.

Children with rickets often have multiple skeletal abnormalities. These abnormalities include bowing of the knees (genu varum), frontal bossing, and rachitic rosary overgrowths of the costochondral joints. Other clinical manifestations in children with rickets include severe muscle weakness, restlessness, delayed tooth eruption, and even seizures in severe cases.

Imaging

Plain Radiographs

There are a number of characteristic radiographic finding seen in patients with osteomalacia. However, these radiographic manifestations are not seen in all patients; thus these findings have a low sensitivity. Diffuse osteopenia is a common but nonspecific finding seen on radiographs. The trabeculae of the vertebral bodies also appear less clear, giving rise to a "fuzzy" appearance of the margins. Looser zone fractures (also known as pseudofractures) are a classical finding seen in osteomalacia. Looser zone fractures are radiolucent lines which often penetrate through the shaft of the long bones at right angles into the involved cortex. They typically have a sclerotic margin and are often asymmetrical (Fig. 11.12). These pseudofractures are often seen at the femoral neck, subtrochanteric region, pelvis (superior and inferior pelvic rami), scapula near the axillary

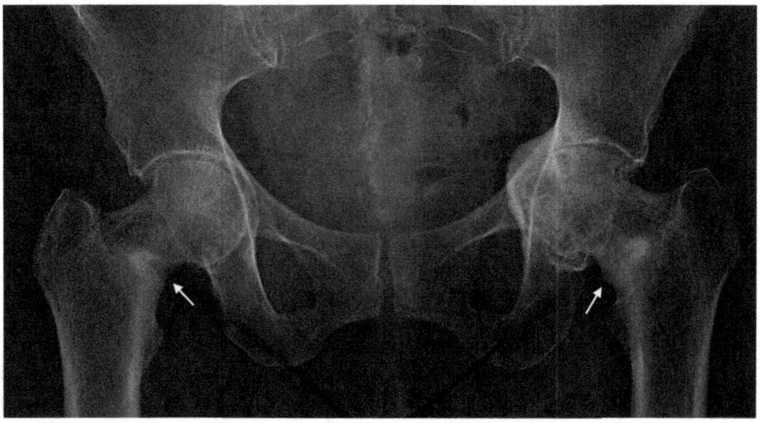

Fig. 11.12 AP radiograph bilateral hips demonstrating bilateral looser zone fractures (*arrows*) of the inner cortex of femoral neck (pseudofractures), radiolucent line extending up to 50 % diameter with surrounding fuzzy sclerosis and background osteopenia. Note significant left-sided protrusio acetabuli secondary to weakened bone related to osteomalacia

margins, and ribs. Looser zone fractures often occur on the concave edge of the involved bone. This differentiates looser zone fractures seen in osteomalacia from the pseudofractures seen in Paget's disease, which typically occur on the convex side of the affected bone.

Children with rickets have much more dramatic deformities compared to adults with osteomalacia since the growth plate has not yet closed. The earliest radiographic findings include widening of the growth plate and loss of the sclerotic zone of calcification on the metaphyseal side of the growth plate. These deformities are most noticeable in bones with the most active growth and most commonly involves the long bones. The most classical finding of rickets, as described earlier, is a genu varum deformity of the tibia and femur. This bowing deformity can also be seen in the upper extremities of toddlers who crawl. Greenstick fractures may also occur in long bones that have been weakened by the bowing deformities. Radiographs of the skull may reveal premature closure of the sutures. Radiographs of the long bones may reveal diffuse osteopenia and evidence of insufficiency fractures.

Dual X-Ray Absorptiometry

Since bone mineralization is impaired in osteomalacia and rickets, DXA can be utilized to assess abnormalities in bone mineral density. In osteomalacia and rickets, the BMD values are decreased, often in the osteoporotic range.

Nuclear Imaging

Bone scintigraphy may have a role in the diagnosis of osteomalacia and rickets. The typical finding seen is an uneven distribution of the radioactive tracer, with focal areas of increased tracer uptake. Bone scintigraphy can also identify focal lesions representative of pseudofractures or actual fractures, both of which can be seen in osteomalacia and in rickets and have a higher sensitivity in identifying these lesions compared to plain radiographs.

Computed Tomography Scan

CT scans are not routinely performed in the assessment of osteomalacia and rickets. They are more sensitive than plain radiographs in identifying the above-described findings and are more accurate in assessing the bone density.

Magnetic Resonance Imaging

MRI studies are not routinely performed for assessment of osteomalacia and Paget's. However, they are more sensitive than plain radiographs in identifying looser zone fractures.

Primary Hyperparathyroidism

Overview

Primary hyperparathyroidism is most commonly caused by a solitary parathyroid adenoma, followed by parathyroid hyperplasia. Parathyroid carcinomas are a very rare cause of primary hyperparathyroidism. Elevated serum level of parathyroid hormone (PTH) has a significant impact on bone metabolism. PTH is released from the parathyroid glands in response to a low serum calcium level. PTH acts on the renal tubules to increase calcium reabsorption and increases the hydroxylation of 25-OH vitamin D to form the active form, 1,25-OH vitamin D. In response to excess PTH, osteoclast activity is also increased, leading to increase bone resorption, especially loss of trabecular bone.

Clinical Presentation

Primary hyperparathyroidism is most commonly diagnosed in middle-aged and elderly women. Most patients with primary hyperparathyroidism are asymptomatic, but a small percentage of patients do present with a rheumatologic presentation. The incidence of gout and calcium pyrophosphate dehydrate crystal deposition (CPPD) is increased in patients with primary hyperparathyroidism. Due to an increase rate of bone resorption in the setting of elevated PTH, patients often have a decreased BMD detected by DXA, and some patients sustain fragility fractures. Hyperparathyroidism is not infrequently diagnosed in patients with osteoporosis after ordering an investigation to look for a secondary cause (Table 11.1). The pattern of bone loss is different from postmenopausal osteoporosis, as the lumbar spine BMD is often preserved in patients with primary hyperparathyroidism.

Imaging

Radiographs

Plain radiographs rarely reveal findings suggestive of primary hyperparathyroidism. One series of 52 patients with primary hyperparathyroidism found that less than 2 % of patients had any radiographic changes on plain radiographs. The earliest radiographic findings of hyperparathyroidism occur along the radial aspect of the middle phalanges of the hand, where subperiosteal resorption occurs (Fig. 11.13). Another finding is evidence of tuft resorption, leading to acro-osteolysis and the presence of Brown's tumors, which are lytic lesions made up of osteoclasts. Brown's tumors have the appearance of radiolucent lytic lesions on plain radiographs, and they tend to have a geographic appearance. They are most often seen in the phalanges of the hands, but they can also be seen in the proximal femur and in the hip girdle (Fig. 11.14).

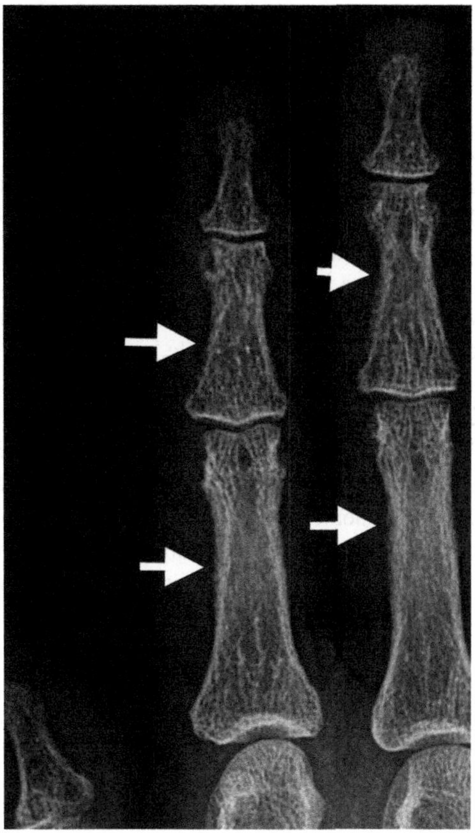

Fig. 11.13 AP radiograph of right hand, magnified, demonstrating changes of subperiosteal resorption (*arrows*)

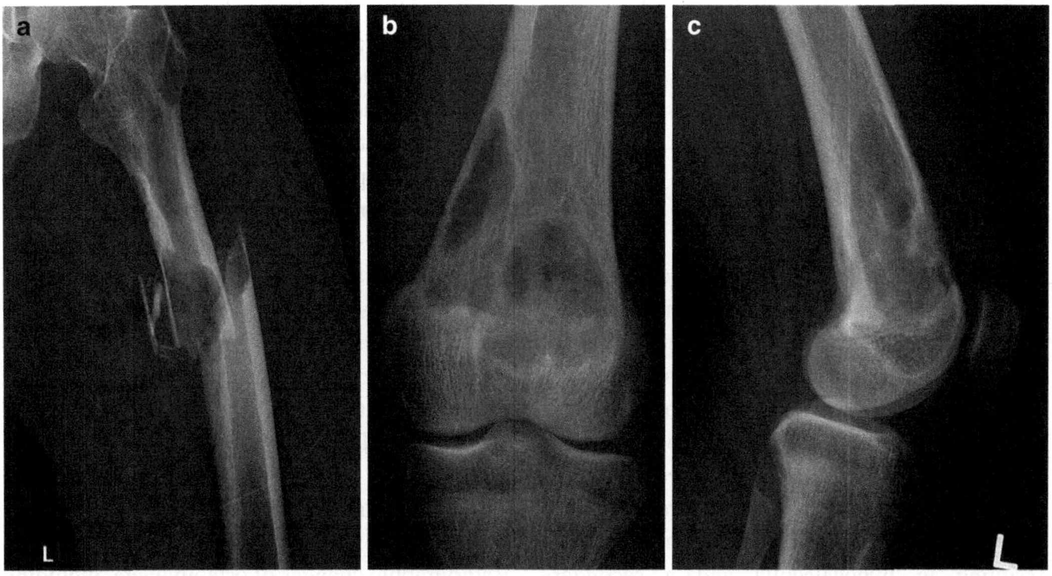

Fig. 11.14 (**a**) A 64-four-year-old male with a pathological fracture through a well-defined lytic lesion in the proximal diaphysis of the left femur. Lesion proved to be a brown tumor in a patient with a parathyroid adenoma (**b**) AP and (**c**) lateral radiograph of the knee in a different patient with well-defined lytic lesions with sclerotic margins in keeping with brown tumors

Patients with hyperparathyroidism also have evidence of diffuse osteopenia seen on radiographs and are susceptible to fractures. Fractures may be seen in the spine or at peripheral sites. Lesions may also occur in the skull, giving rise to a "salt-and-pepper" appearance of the skull. Other radiographic findings include the presence of chondrocalcinosis and soft tissue calcifications. Lesions may also be seen in the clavicles, which give rise to osteopenia, erosions, and resorption of the distal clavicle.

Computed Tomography Scan

CT scans are not routinely performed for the assessment of primary hyperparathyroidism. The CT studies demonstrate the same results seen on plain radiographs, such as subperiosteal resorption or Brown's tumors, but with better detail and higher sensitivity.

Magnetic Resonance Imaging

MRI studies are not routinely used to evaluate the osseous changes seen in hyperparathyroidism. However, MRI studies are more sensitive in detecting the osseous changes, which give an increased T2 signal intensity, although this is quite nonspecific. MRI studies are useful in identify Brown's tumors. Due to the high hemosiderin content inside Brown's tumors, the lesions have a hypo-intensity on both T1 and T2 images.

Renal Osteodystrophy

Overview

With progressive chronic kidney disease (CKD), bone metabolism is affected in a number of ways. Renal osteodystrophy is a heterogeneous group of metabolic bone disorders that may occur in patients with CKD. The earliest form of renal bone disease occurs as a result of secondary hyperparathyroidism due to impaired renal production of 1,25-hydroxy vitamin D from impaired hydroxylation of 25-hydroxy vitamin D, thus resulting in hypocalcemia and a secondary increase in PTH production. There is an exponential relationship between declining glomerular filtration rate and an increase in serum PTH levels. Bone histomorphometry remains the gold standard in differentiating the different types of renal osteodystrophy. Using double-tetracycline labeling, histomorphometric studies can differentiate between low, normal, and high states of bone turnover. Low bone turnover states include osteomalacia and adynamic bone disease. The histomorphometric studies in adynamic bone disease reveal a state of reduced bone formation rate, low or normal osteoid volume, and a reduced number of osteoblasts and osteoclasts. Adynamic bone disease is most commonly seen in CKD patients on dialysis therapy. High bone turnover states include osteitis fibrosa cystica, which is a state caused by secondary hyperparathyroidism. Mixed turnover states can be caused by mixed uremic osteodystrophy and in posttransplant bone disease. Differentiating between the types of renal osteodystrophy present is critical, since it will have implications on treatment strategy chosen.

Imaging

Plain Radiographs

Given that renal osteodystrophy is a heterogeneous group of metabolic bone diseases, there is also a heterogeneous set of radiographic changes that may be seen. The radiographic findings of both hyperparathyroidism and osteomalacia from 25-hydroxy vitamin D can be seen in renal osteodystrophy. The radiographic findings of secondary hyperparathyroidism are similar to those seen in primary hyperparathyroidism. A rugger jersey spine appearance can be seen due to cortical tunneling and osteosclerosis of the superior and inferior endplates. This gives the appearance of alternating sclerotic endplates with low-attenuating vertebral bodies, thus giving the appearance reminiscent of the stripes seen on a rugger jersey (Fig. 11.15). Renal osteodystrophy can also result in an erosive arthritis, involving primarily the MCPs and IP joints (Fig. 11.16). This form of arthropathy is often associated with subchondral erosions and cystic changes. Radiographic changes of osteomalacia, including looser zone fractures, can also be seen in renal osteodystrophy, and the findings are identical to those seen in osteomalacia from nonrenal causes.

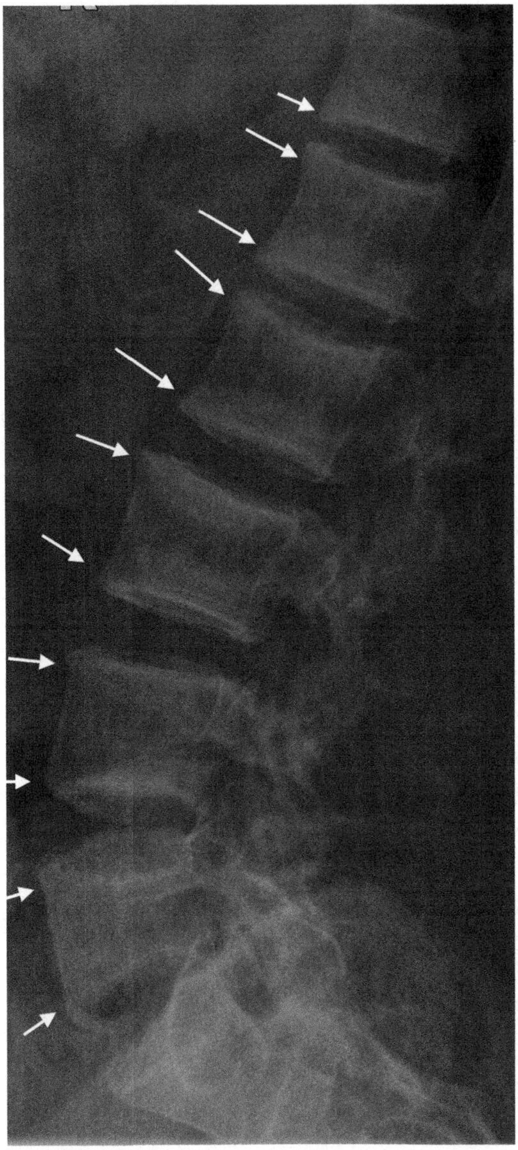

Fig. 11.15 Lateral radiograph of the lumbar spine demonstrating the typical feature of "rugger jersey" spine with endplate sclerosis (*arrows*) superimposed on osteopenic vertebrae

Soft tissue calcifications are commonly seen in patients with CKD which are due to calcium hydroxyapatite deposition in the subcutaneous fat. In addition, vascular calcifications of the vessel walls itself can also be seen in renal osteodystrophy, which is termed calciphylaxis (Fig. 11.17). Insufficiency fractures are also frequently seen in renal osteodystrophy and can be identified on plain radiographs

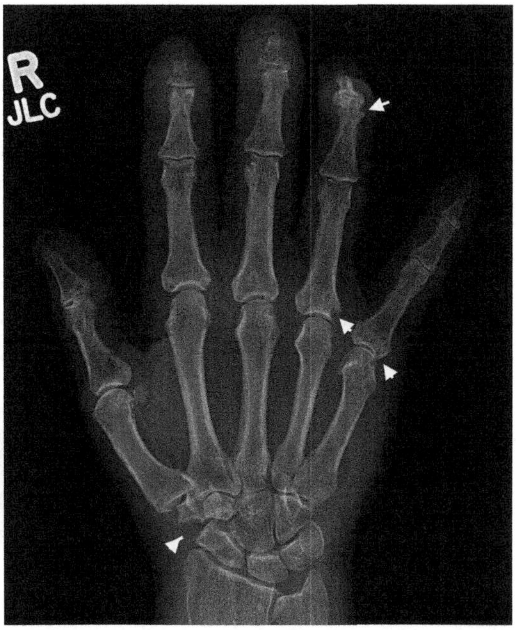

Fig. 11.16 PA radiograph of the right hand with osteopenia, periarticular erosions (*arrowheads*), tuft calcinosis cutis in a patient with CRF

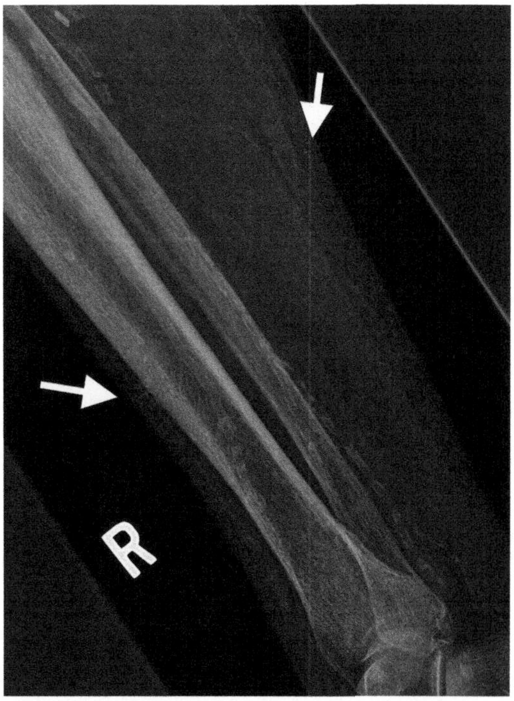

Fig. 11.17 Radiograph in a patient with chronic renal failure with heavy vascular calcification and calciphylaxis (*arrows*)

Dual X-Ray Absorptiometry

Bone mineralization abnormalities are seen in renal osteodystrophy, similar to the changes seen in osteomalacia and primary hyperparathyroidism. Serial BMD measurements using DXA is important to stratify patients into their degree of fracture risk.

Computed Tomography Scan (Fig. 11.18)

CT scans are not routinely performed in the workup of renal osteodystrophy. The findings described, including those of hyperparathyroidism, are more commonly seen on CT scans compared to plain radiographs. Compared to CT scans, MR studies are preferred if the goal is to assess for an insufficiency fracture.

Magnetic Resonance Imaging

Plain radiographs are still the first-line modality in the assessment of renal osteodystrophy. In patients with focal bone or soft tissue symptoms with normal plain radiographs, MRI studies are useful as it is more sensitive in identifying abnor-

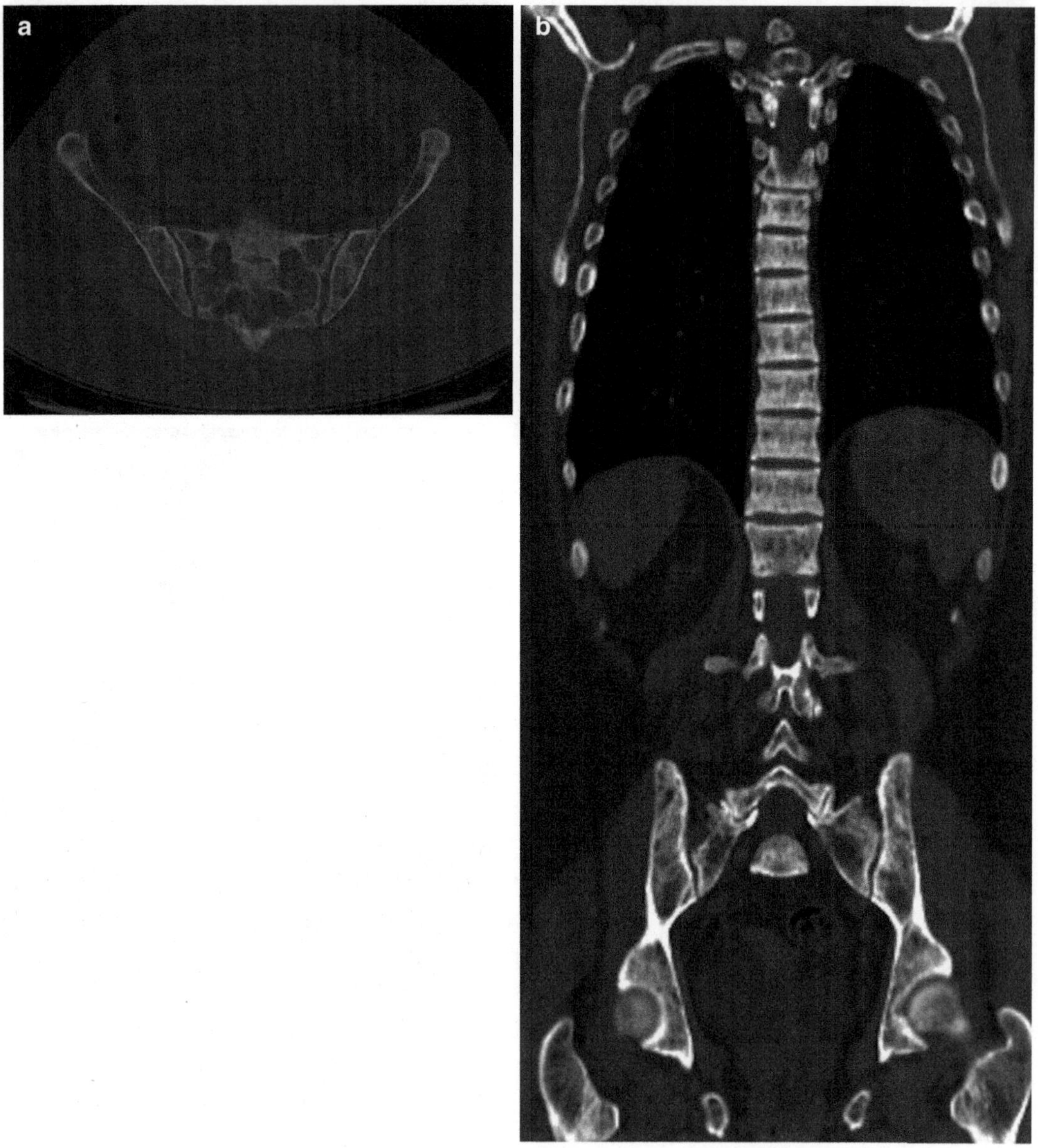

Fig. 11.18 A 47-year-old female with end-stage renal failure with changes of renal osteodystrophy, same patient as Fig. 11.15, (**a**) axial and (**b**) coronal reformatted CT with mixed sclerotic pattern on osteopenia and rugger jersey spine

malities such as insufficiency fractures, which are quite common and often missed on plain radiographs. MRI studies are also helpful in identify patients with carpal tunnel syndrome, which are a common complication of renal osteodystrophy.

Bisphosphonates and Atypical Fractures

In recent years, there has been an increasing concern about the development of "atypical" fractures that may occur in patients treated with bisphosphonates. These fractures typically occur in the subtrochanteric or diaphyseal region of the femur, a location which distinguishes them from the typical hip fractures seen in osteoporotic patients. Patients often present with a prodromal pain in the femur area, and pain is usually associated with prolonged treatment of bisphosphonates. They are extremely rare in patients treated with a bisphosphonate for 5 years or less. Overall, the incidence is about 1.46 per 1,000 patient-years on a bisphosphonate treatment. However, we would stress that although these fractures are seen in patients treated with a bisphosphonate, they do remain an effective therapy in the management of osteoporotic patients. It is estimated that for every atypical fracture caused by bisphosphonates, it prevents 99 osteoporotic hip fractures.

Plain Radiograph (Fig. 11.19)

Plain radiographs remain the modality of choice in the identification of these atypical femoral

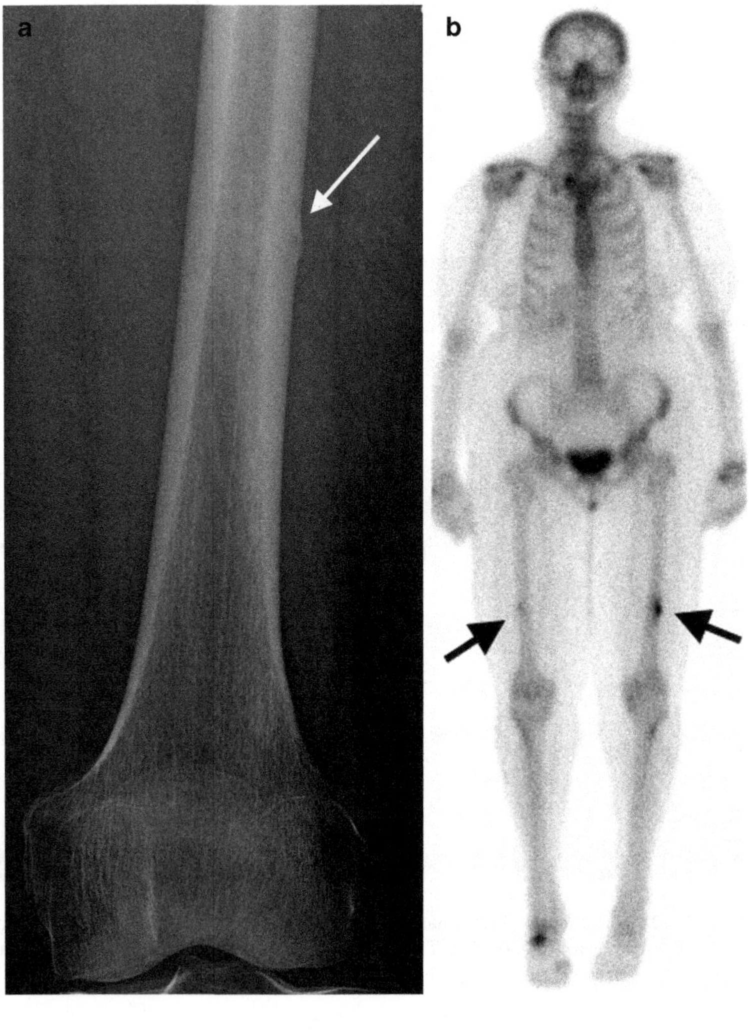

Fig. 11.19 Bisphosphonate-related fractures. (**a**) Incomplete fracture in the lateral cortical margin of the distal femur with associated periosteal reaction (*arrow*). (**b**) Bone scan in the same patient demonstrates an unsuspected fracture on the right (black *arrows*). (**c**) A 69-year-old female with right-sided fracture treated with internal fixation; note incomplete fracture on the left (*arrow*). (**d**) Acute left fracture when patient commenced limited weight bearing

Fig. 11.19 (continued)

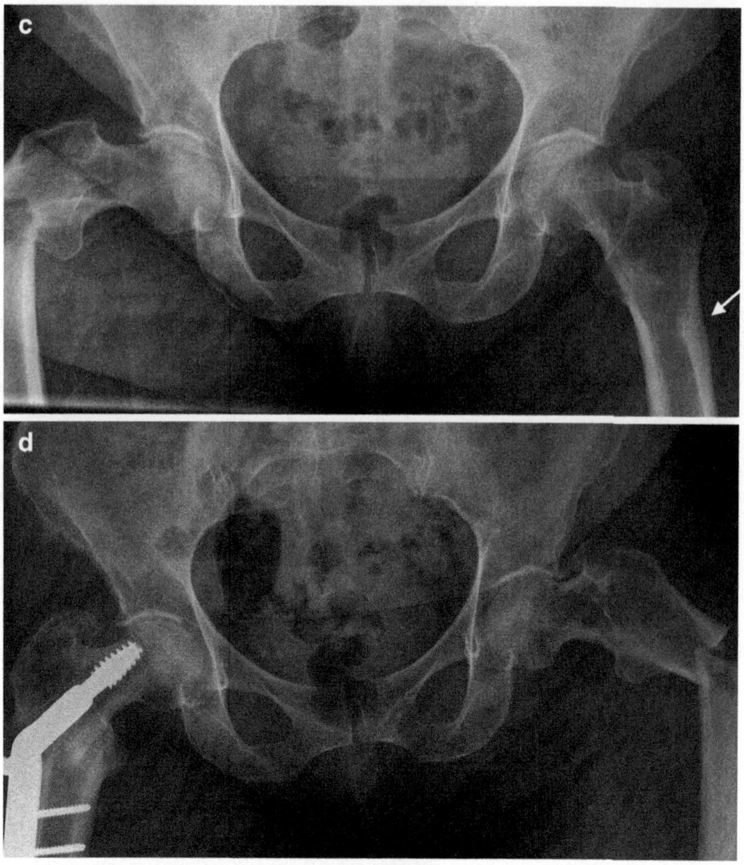

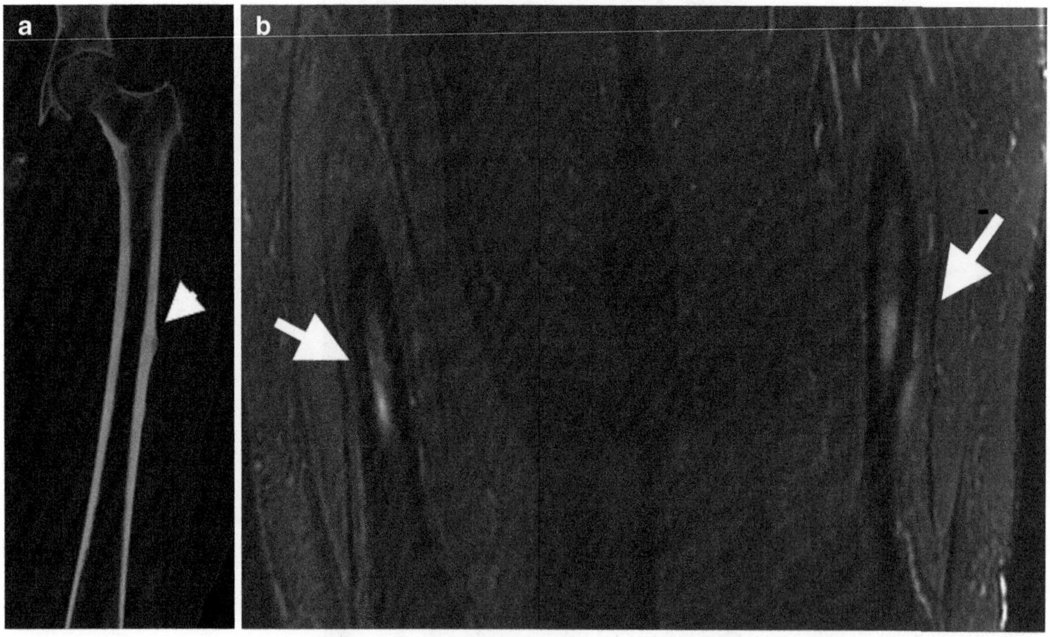

Fig. 11.20 (**a**) CT, coronal reformatted image, of left femur with incomplete fracture of the lateral cortex with periosteal reaction (*arrowhead*). (**b**) Cor T2FS MRI, same patient as in Fig. 11.19a, demonstrates bilateral fractures (*arrows*)

fractures. These fractures are usually seen in the subtrochanteric or diaphyseal region of the femur. There is often a cortical thickening of the femoral shaft or cortical breaking associated, although these features are not always seen. When a fracture does occur, they are usually simple transverse or oblique ($\leq 30°$) in nature and often on the lateral aspect of the femur. When a fracture is complete, a medial spike may be seen.

CT Scans (Fig. 11.20a)

CT scans are not typically used in the evaluation of patients with atypical fractures. The study may reveal a lateral cortical stress reaction which may be seen before the fracture becomes clinically evident.

MRI (Fig. 11.20b)

MRI scans are not typically used in the evaluation of patients with atypical fractures. Similar to the CT study, the MRI study may reveal a lateral cortical stress reaction, with a focally increased T2 signal seen and underlying bone marrow edema.

Oncogenic Osteomalacia

Overview

Oncogenic osteomalacia (also known as tumor-induced osteomalacia) is a rare paraneoplastic syndrome, which is caused by usually benign tumors. Phosphaturic mesenchymal tumors and hemangiopericytomas are the commonest tumors associated with this condition. However, oncogenic osteomalacia is also rarely associated with malignant tumors, such as osteosarcoma.

Oncogenic osteomalacia is characterized by hypophosphatemia due to impaired ability of the renal tubules to absorb phosphate. The tumor's secretion of fibroblast growth factor 23 inhibits this process at the renal tubules. The hypophosphatemic states subsequently results in the development of osteomalacia. Patients with this condition present clinically with symptoms suggestive of osteomalacia, including myalgia, boney pain, and recurrent fractures.

Imaging

Radiographs (Fig. 11.21)

There are few specific signs on radiographic examination to help diagnose oncogenic osteomalacia as the underlying process. Oncogenic osteomalacia may reveal the same radiographic findings as osteomalacia described earlier in this chapter. Findings include evidence of pseudofractures (looser zone fractures) and insufficiency fractures, both seen in osteomalacia. Once the diagnosis of oncogenic osteomalacia is made, the next step is to perform investigations to identify the causative tumor.

Computed Tomography Scan

CT scans can be useful modality to detect subtle changes of osteomalacia not detected on plain radiographs. However, it is not as sensitive as MRI in detecting insufficiency fractures or soft tissue masses associated with oncogenic osteomalacia.

Magnetic Resonance Imaging (Fig. 11.21b)

MRI is a very useful modality in oncogenic osteomalacia in identifying insufficiency fractures. It is superior to both CT and bone scans in identifying subtle fractures that may be seen in this condition. MRI is also useful in identifying soft tissue masses that are associated with osteogenic osteomalacia.

Hypophosphatasia

Overview

Hypophosphatasia is autosomal recessively inherited leading to a deficiency in tissue nonspecific alkaline phosphatase. This leads to severe hypomineralization and results in clinical finding similar to rickets and osteomalacia. There are multiple forms of hypophosphatasia which include a perinatal form, an infantile form, a childhood form, and an adult form. The perinatal form is characterized by profound hypomineralization, with

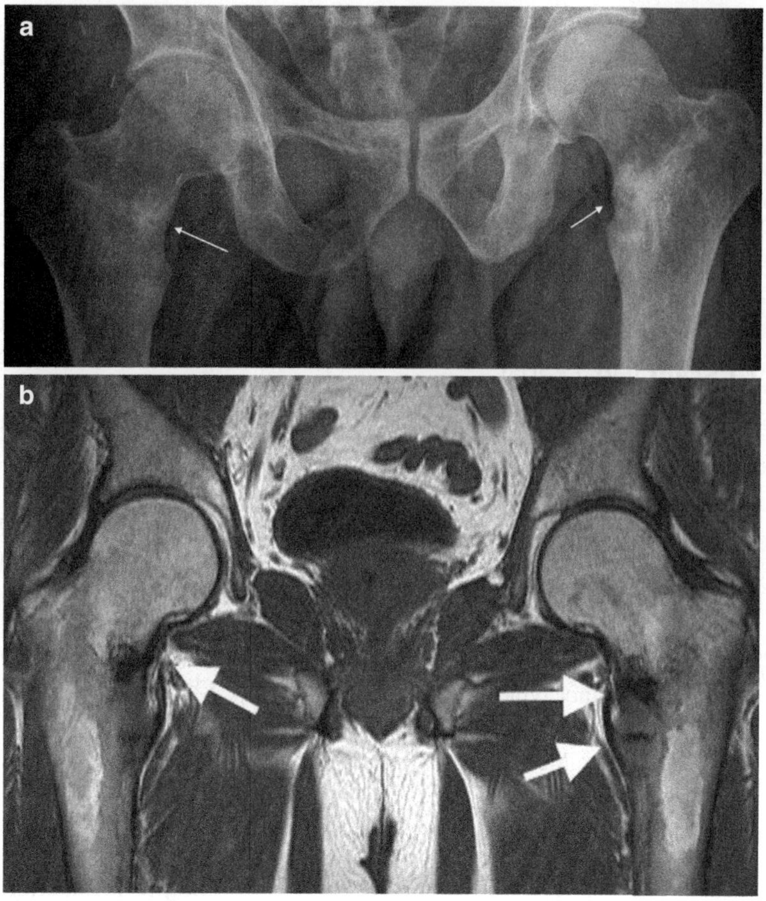

Fig. 11.21 Oncogenic osteomalacia. (**a**) AP radiographs of the hips with bilateral looser zone-type fractures (*arrows*) and (**b**) corresponding MRI, Cor T1 demonstrating fracture lines (*arrows*). Octreotide scan-positive primary lesion (not shown)

resultant extreme shortening of limbs and a soft calvarium (caput membranaceum). Many with in utero hypophosphatasia ultimately result in death shortly after birth due to respiratory failure. The adult form demonstrates many of the radiographic features of osteomalacia and rickets and is also characterized by early loss of dentition.

Imaging

Radiographs (Fig. 11.22)

The radiographic findings vary depending on the age of onset. In the adult form, pseudofractures are often found in the lateral subtrochanteric diaphysis, on the convex side. This contrasts with osteomalacia purely secondary to vitamin D deficiency, which often have pseudofractures along the medial subtrochanteric diaphysis (concave side). Fractures may also be seen in the ribs and in the metatarsals.

Hypophosphatasia presenting at younger ages have more characteristic radiographic findings. In newborns, radiographs feature marked under-mineralization of bone diffusely. The skull is also small in size and severely under-mineralized, often with calcification only at the frontal bones and at the base of the skull. There may also be lack of ossification, either partially or completely in one or more vertebrae. Bowdler spurs are commonly seen in the neonatal form, which are transverse bony spurs that may also be seen protruding from the radius, ulna, and fibula. These spurs can cause dimpling of the skin.

Computed Tomography Scan

CT scans are not routinely performed in the assessment of hypophosphatasia. They are more sensitive than plain radiographs in identifying the above-described findings and are more accurate in assessing the bone density.

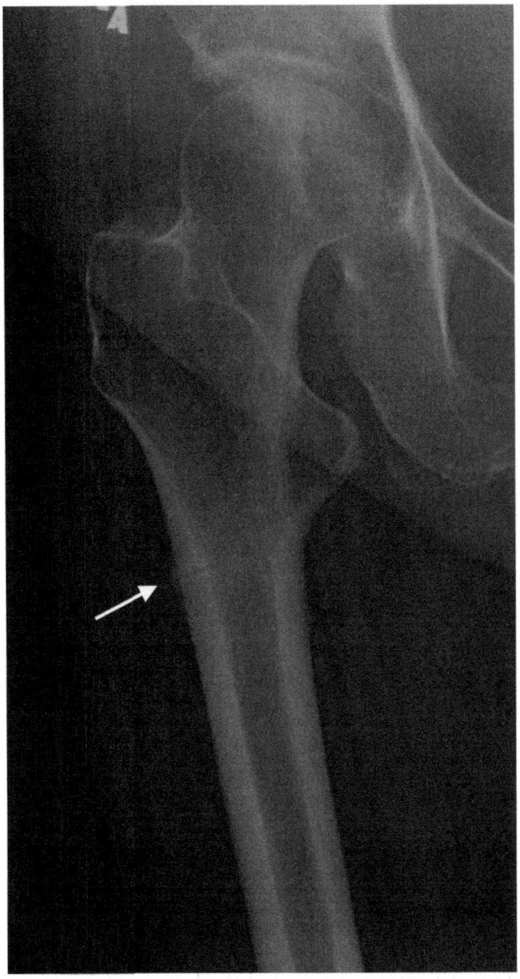

Fig. 11.22 AP radiograph of the right proximal femur with lateral cortical subtrochanteric fracture with periosteal reaction (*arrow*) in adult female with hypophosphatasia

Magnetic Resonance Imaging

MRI studies are not routinely performed for assessment of hypophosphatasia. However, they are more sensitive than plain radiographs in identifying pseudofractures.

Hypoparathyroidism

Overview

Hypoparathyroidism is a common cause of hypocalcemia. It can occur as a primary inherited disorder or as a secondary acquired disorder. The primary form is called DiGeorge syndrome, also known as type I polyglandular syndrome. This syndrome consists of hypoparathyroidism, mucocutaneous candidiasis, and adrenal insufficiency. Secondary causes of hypoparathyroidism include damage to the parathyroid glands, especially after head and neck surgeries. Other secondary causes include radiation to the head and neck area and infiltrative disorders, such as hemochromatosis and Wilson's disease.

Imaging

Radiographs

Plain radiographs are the most commonly used modality in the assessment of hypoparathyroidism. The most typical finding is the presence of diffuse osteosclerosis, although it can also be localized. This disorder is also characterized by calcifications at a number of sites. These calcifications may be seen in the subcutaneous tissue, ligaments of the spine (including the anterior longitudinal ligament), and entheseal insertion sites. Some of the changes of hypoparathyroidism may resemble those seen with a spondyloarthropathy, and care must be taken to differentiate between the two disorders. One key differentiating feature is that the sacroiliac joints are not involved in hypoparathyroidism and is usually a trademark seen in spondyloarthropathies.

Computed Tomography Scan

CT scans are not routinely performed in the assessment of hypoparathyroidism.

Magnetic Resonance Imaging

MRI scans are not routinely performed in the assessment of hypoparathyroidism.

Complex Regional Pain Syndrome

Overview

Complex regional pain syndrome (CRPS), formerly known as reflex sympathetic dystrophy, is a complex disorder that develops as a result of trauma to an affected limb. There are two types of CRPS. Type I develops after a noxious inciting event, but with no preceding nerve injury. Type II develops after an associated nerve injury. Common triggers for CRPS include peripheral trauma, fracture, lacerations, immobilization of a limb, or poststroke or myocardial infarction. CRPS may also develop after surgery, particularly for carpal tunnel release and resection of Morton's neuroma. Clinical manifestations, like the radiographic features, vary depending on the stage of disease.

In the acute stage (Stage I), CRPS is characterized by swelling and color change of the affected extremity. There is also significant pain, with the presence of allodynia and hyperalgesia which often extends beyond the area of the initial site of injury. There is also temperature changes noted between the affected limb and the contralateral limb. The acute stage usually lasts for 3–6 months. In the dystrophic stage (Stage II), the soft tissue swelling of the extremity become a hard edema, with associated atrophy of the adjacent soft tissue and muscles. The dystrophic stage typically lasts for 3–12 months. The atrophic stage (Stage III) is characterized by atrophic changes involving the skin, hair, and nails. Flexion contractures and limited joint range of motion develop during this stage. The development of trophic changes and muscle contractures indicate a poor prognosis.

Imaging

Radiographs (Fig. 11.23)

Conventional radiographs may be completely normal or may demonstrate osteopenia 2–3 weeks after the onset of the disease. Focal subchondral or subperiosteal osteoporosis is found in approximately 60 % of patients, but it is not specific and often represents changes of immobility secondary to the pain associated with CRPS.

There are five patterns of bone resorption on radiography:

1. Thinning of trabecular or cancellous bone of the metaphyseal regions, producing bandlike, patchy or periarticular osteoporosis
2. Subperiosteal cortical bone resorption resulting in a corrugated appearance of the outer margins of the diaphysis
3. Endosteal bone resorption resulting in irregularity of the endosteal surface and variation in the thickness of the cortices
4. Intracortical bone resorption resulting in excessive striation or tunneling within the cortex paralleling the longitudinal axis
5. Subchondral and juxta-articular erosions visible as small periarticular erosions and intra-articular gaps in the subchondral bone

Bone Scintigraphy

Three-phase bone scintigraphy has higher sensitivity and specificity compared to plain radiographs. The results of the bone scan using technetium-99m should be correlated with the stage of CRPS. The hallmark is diffuse increased perfusion (phase I) to the entire extremity and diffuse increased tracer accumulation on blood pool or tissue-phase images (phase II). Nuclear findings are abnormal in approximately 40 % of patients and blood pool findings in approximately 50 %. Delayed images demonstrate diffuse increased tracer throughout the extremity. Quantification may be helpful but is not used routinely. A normal bone scan does not exclude the diagnosis of CRPS.

Computed Tomography Scan

CT scans are not routinely performed in the assessment of CRPS.

Magnetic Resonance Imaging (Fig. 11.23b)

The findings of CRPS on MRI tend to be nonspecific. These nonspecific findings include bone marrow edema, muscle atrophy, and soft tissue edema of the affected limb. Given the nonspecific nature of the findings on MRI, it is not a modality commonly used in the assessment of CRPS.

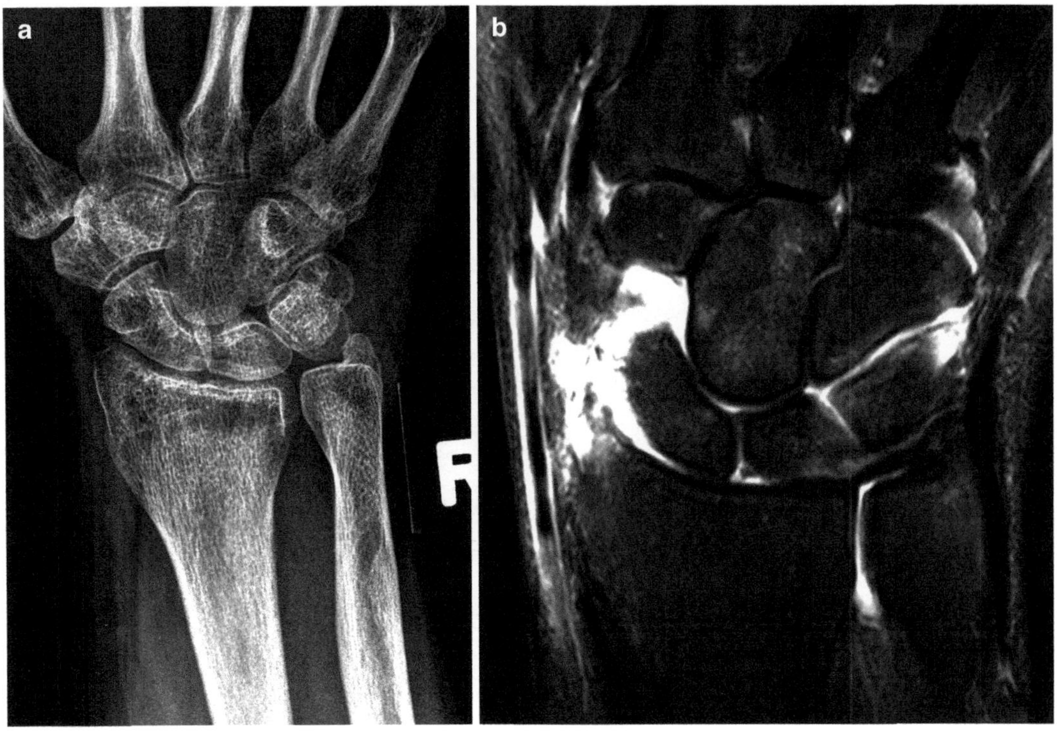

Fig. 11.23 CRPS in a 25-year-old male with post-right elbow fracture who developed swelling and hyperalgesia of the right wrist. (**a**) PA radiograph demonstrates patchy osteopenia and (**b**) Cor T2FS of the wrist demonstrates ill-defined foci of carpal bone marrow edema and joint effusions

Further Reading

1. Ashebu SD, Dahniya MH, Muhtaseb SA, Aduh P. Unusual florid skeletal manifestations of primary hyperparathyroidism. Skelet Radiol. 2002;31:720–3.
2. Assessment of fracture risk and its application to screening for postmenopausal osteoporosis. Report of a WHO Study Group. World Health Organ Tech Rep Ser 1994;843:1–129
3. Berry JL, Davies M, Mee AP, et al. Vitamin D metabolism, rickets, and osteomalacia. Semin Musculoskelet Radiol. 2002;6:173–82.
4. Cheung AM, Adachi JD, Hanley DA, Kendler DL, Davison S, Josse R, Brown JP, Ste-Marie LG, Kremer R, Erlandson MC, Dian L, Burghardt AJ, Boyd SK. High-resolution peripheral quantitative computed tomography for the assessment of bone strength and structure: a review by the Canadian Bone Strength Working Group. Curr Osteoporos Rep. 2013;11(2):136–46.
5. Genant HK, Wu CY, van Kuijk C, Nevitt MC. Vertebral fracture assessment using a semiquantitative technique. J Bone Miner Res. 1993;8:1137–48.
6. Harden RN, Oaklander AL, Burton AW, Perez RS, Richardson K, Swan M, Barthel J, Costa B, Graciosa JR, Bruehl S, et al. Complex regional pain syndrome: practical diagnostic and treatment guidelines, 4th edition. Pain Med. 2013;14:180–229.
7. Hruska KA, Teitelbaum SL. Renal osteodystrophy. N Engl J Med. 1995;333:166–74.
8. Hyldstrup L, Nielsen SP. Metacarpal index by digital x-ray radiogrammetry: normative reference values and comparison with dual x-ray absorptiometry. J Clin Densitom. 2001;4:299–306.
9. Melton 3rd LJ, Lane AW, Cooper C, Eastell R, O'Fallon WM, Riggs BL. Prevalence and incidence of vertebral deformities. Osteoporos Int. 1993;3:113–9.
10. Miller PD. Diagnosis and treatment of osteoporosis in chronic renal disease. Semin Nephrol. 2009;29:144–55.
11. Moe S, Drueke T, Cunningham J, et al. Definition, evaluation, and classification of renal osteodystrophy: a position statement from Kidney Disease: Improving Global Outcomes (KDIGO). Kidney Int. 2006; 69:1945–53.
12. Quek ST, Peh WC. Radiology of osteoporosis. Semin Musculoskelet Radiol. 2002;6:197–206.

13. Ross PD. Risk factors for osteoporotic fracture. Endocrinol Metab Clin N Am. 1998;27:289–301.
14. Schilcher J, Michaelsson K, Aspenberg P. Bisphosphonate use and atypical fractures of the femoral shaft. N Engl J Med. 2011;364(18):1728–37.
15. Silverberg SJ. Natural history of primary hyperparathyroidism. Endocrinol Metab Clin N Am. 2000;29:451–64.
16. Thawait SK, Marcus MA, Morrison WB, Klufas RA, Eng J, Carrino JA, et al. Research synthesis: what is the diagnostic performance of magnetic resonance imaging to discriminate benign from malignant vertebral compression fractures? Systematic review and meta-analysis. Spine. 2012;37:736–44.

Osteonecrosis

12

John O'Neill

Overview

Avascular necrosis (osteonecrosis, aseptic necrosis) of the femoral head is the occurrence of bone necrosis secondary to anoxia in a subchondral region. There are various pathophysiological mechanisms including traumatic vascular occlusion, altered coagulation, mechanical stress, and increased intraosseous pressure as may be seen in venous obstruction. A bone infarct differs from AVN only in that the bone necrosis occurs in the metaphyseal or diaphyseal regions. The femoral head is the most common site involved in AVN and will be described here in detail; these imaging findings can be reflected at other sites. Patients are usually middle aged, excluding SLE, men are more commonly affected.

AVN is a relatively common condition with an incidence of 20,000/year in the USA and is responsible for up to 10 % of hip replacements. There are multiple underlying etiological factors, with steroid and alcohol chief among the nontraumatic causes (Table 12.1). Traumatic AVN usually takes place in the setting of a femoral neck fracture or hip dislocation. There is a high incidence of bilateral involvement in atraumatic cases, up to 80 %, and is dependent on the underlying etiology. Multiple other sites may be involved and may remain asymptomatic. Common non-femoral head sites include medullary cavity long bones, humeral head, and femoral condyles. Common traumatic sites include the femoral and humeral heads, capitate, scaphoid, and talus.

Table 12.1 Etiologies of femoral head AVN

Trauma
Femoral neck fracture
Hip dislocation
Atraumatic
Alcoholism
Corticosteroids
SLE
Caisson disease
Coagulopathies
Sickle cell disease
Cushing disease
Gaucher disease
Pancreatitis
Chronic renal failure
Pregnancy
Smoking
Oral contraceptives
Hemoglobinopathies

Clinical Presentation

Atraumatic cases may be asymptomatic and may only be diagnosed when incidentally imaged, e.g., AVN femoral head/s identified during MRI examination for assessment of a pelvic renal transplant. Patients may complain of nonspecific groin pain, worse on weight bearing with

J. O'Neill, MB, BAO, BCh, MRCPI, MSc, FRCR
Associate Professor, Musculoskeletal Imaging, Diagnostic Imaging, McMaster University/St Joseph's Healthcare, Hamilton, ON L8N4A6, Canada
e-mail: joneill2@me.com

J. O'Neill (ed.), *Essential Imaging in Rheumatology*,
DOI 10.1007/978-1-4939-1673-3_12, © Springer Science+Business Media New York 2015

progression over time. Larger infarcts may present with more severe pain. Clinical examination demonstrates a decreased range of motion. There is progressive disability with femoral head collapse and secondary degeneration.

Staging

There are multiple staging systems available. The most commonly used are detailed in Tables 12.2 and 12.3.

Table 12.2 Classification of AVN of the femoral head

Stage	Radiograph	Diagnosis	Clinical
Stage 0 preclinical	Normal	Biopsy positive	Osteonecrosis suspected when definite disease in contralateral hip
Stage 1 preradiographic	Normal or subtle loss of clarity trabecular pattern, patchy osteopenia	Biopsy, bone scan, MRI[a] positive	50 % sudden pain in groin, limited range of motion
Stage 2a precollapse	Changes in trabecular pattern, sclerosis may be localized or diffuse, cysts may develop, mixed pattern	Radiograph, bone scan, MRI[a] positive	Clinical signs persist or worsen over several months
Stage 2b transition	Flattening, crescent sign (subchondral fracture)	Radiograph, bone scan, MRI[a] positive	
Stage 3 collapse	Sequestrum, break articular margin on both sides of the affected bone followed by collapse, normal joint space	Radiograph, bone scan, MRI[a] positive	Progressive increase and more constant pain, functional incapacity
Stage 4 osteoarthritis	Osteoarthritis superimposed on a deformed femoral head	Radiograph, bone scan, MRI[a] positive	Progressive decrease in range motion

From *Ischemia and Necroses of Bone*, by R. Paul Ficat, Jacques Arlet; edited and adapted by David S. Hungerford, Williams & Wilkins, 1980

[a]MRI was not included in original staging

Table 12.3 ARCO classification system 1992

Stage	Imaging	Subdivisions
Stage 0	Positive biopsy, negative imaging	
Stage 1	Positive MRI +/– bone scan, negative radiograph, CT	Lesion location: medial, central, or lateral
Stage 2	Radiograph positive: sclerotic/cystic/osteopenia	% femoral involvement
Stage 3	Radiograph: crescent sign (subchondral fracture)	Head
Stage 4	Radiograph: flattening of the femoral head	a <15 % b 15–30 c >30 %
Stage 5	Radiograph positive: flattening of the femoral head and osteoarthritis	Depression femoral head when fracture present (stages 4 and 5) a <2 mm b 2–4 mm c >4 mm
Stage 6	Complete joint destruction	

Reprinted with permission from ARCO (Association Research Circulation Osseous): Committee on terminology and classification. *ARCO News*. 1992;4:41–46

Imaging

Radiographs (Fig. 12.1)

Radiographs may be normal or demonstrate only subtle changes. Radiographs have a low sensitivity in early disease. In patients with suspected AVN, MRI is advised.

Early changes include patchy osteopenia and loss of clarity of the trabecular pattern. This progresses to areas of ill-defined sclerosis. The subchondral region should be closely evaluated for development of a lucent line, the "crescent sign," a subchondral fracture that heralds impending collapse. The convex outline of the femoral head should be maintained; any

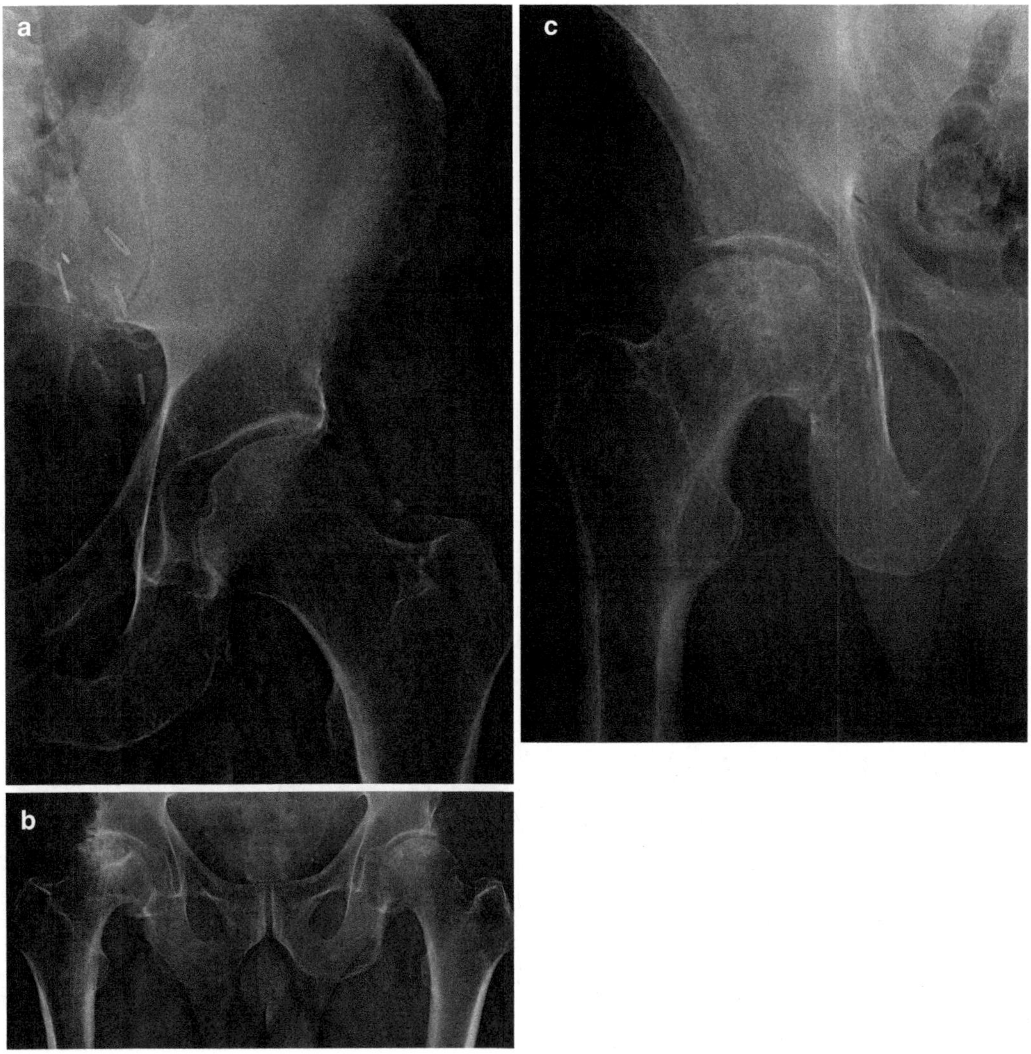

Fig. 12.1 (**a**) Modified AP radiograph of the left hemi-pelvis, surgical clips related to renal transplant, left hip pain, generalized osteopenia, no radiographic changes AVN, stage 1 AVN. (**b**) AVN of bilateral hips on AP radiograph, stage 4. The right hip demonstrates partial collapse of the femoral head and secondary degenerative changes, stage 2a; the left femoral head demonstrates localized sclerosis in a patient on long-term steroids. (**c**) AP radiograph of the right hip with stage 3 AVN, with collapse of the femoral head with maintenance of joint space. See Table 12.2 for detailed description of the staging of AVN

loss of convexity or flattening indicates early collapse. Collapse progresses with deformity of the femoral head and development of secondary degenerative changes such as joint space loss, osteophytes, subchondral sclerosis, and cyst formation. These latter changes may be more evident on the acetabular aspect of the joint as the femoral head collapses. Radiographic findings are detailed in Table 12.2.

MRI (Figs. 12.2, 12.3, 12.4, and 12.5)

MRI is the imaging gold standard for AVN with a sensitivity approaching 100 %. MRI clearly demonstrates early features of AVN not visible on radiographs, the preradiographic stage. Initial features include localized subchondral bone marrow edema, which becomes more defined with a peripheral serpentine rim of low signal intensity

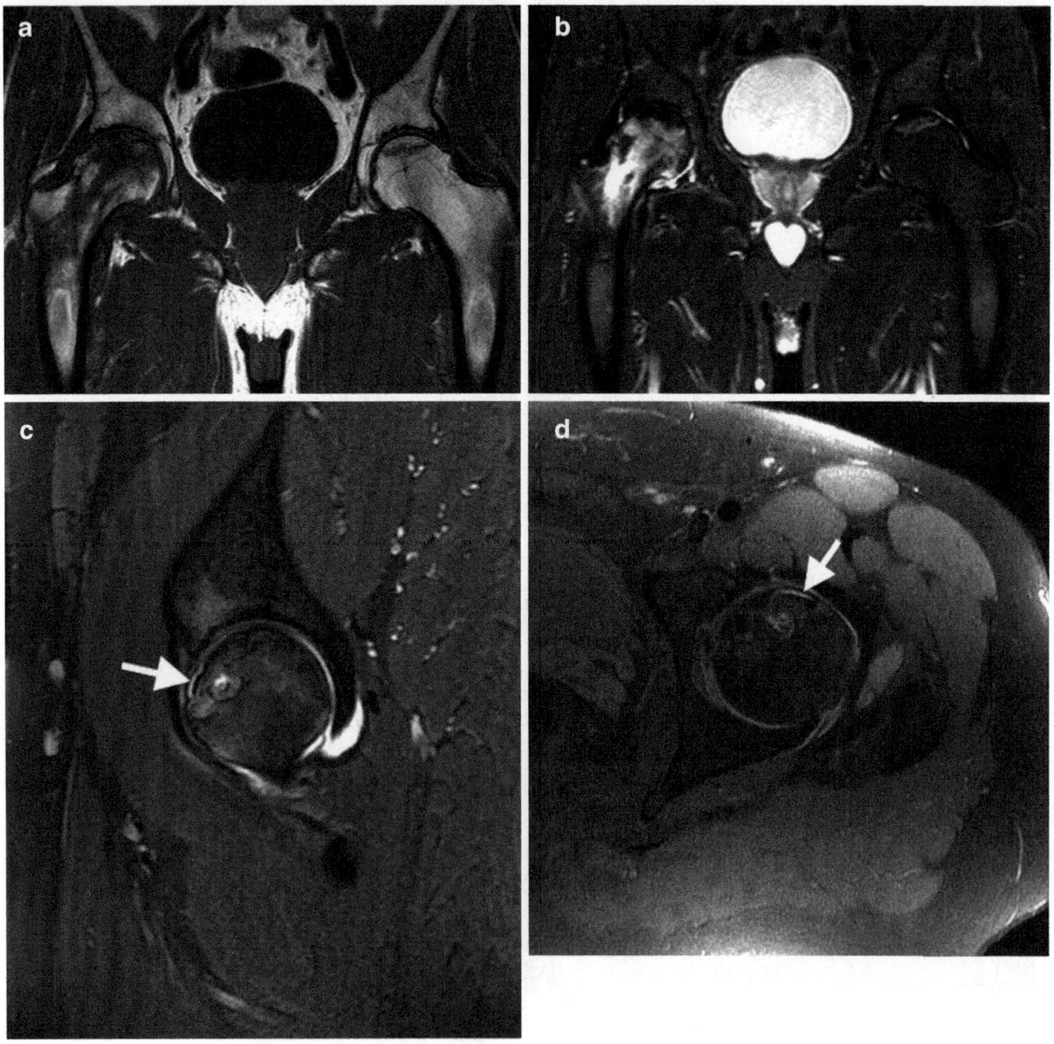

Fig. 12.2 (**a**, **b**) Cor T1 and T2FS, respectively, demonstrate bilateral AVN and chronic AVN of the left femoral head (note the double-line sign and acute AVN of the right femoral head with extensive bone marrow edema and small joint effusion). (**c**, **d**) Sag and axial T2FS, respectively, in a different patient, with subchondral fracture line (*arrow*), linear high signal intensity, and early cortical collapse

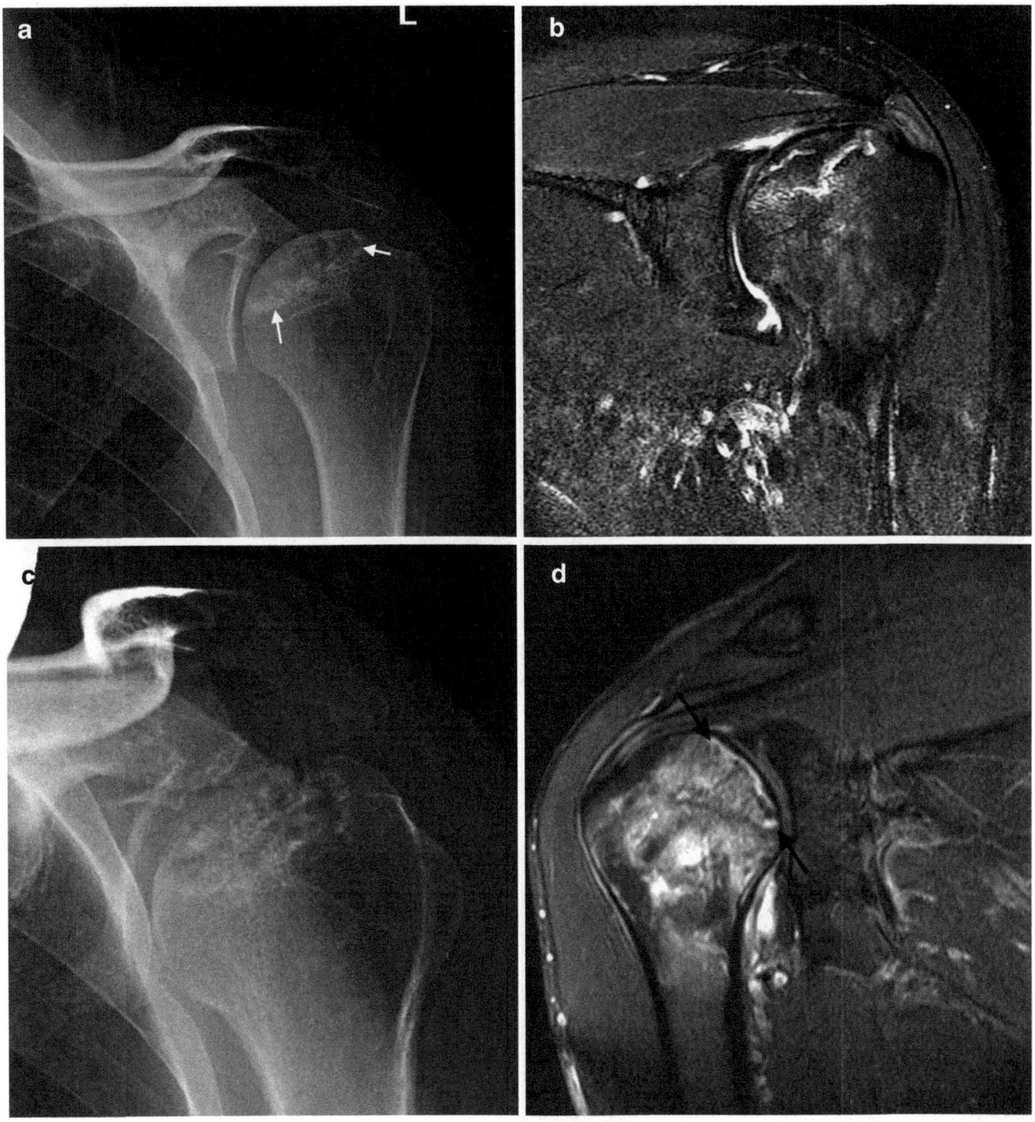

Fig. 12.3 (**a**) AP radiograph of the left shoulder demonstrating AVN of the humeral head, stage 2b, in a patient with Crohn's disease. (**b**) Corresponding Cor T2FS MRI. (**c**) 6 years later, AP radiograph, stage 3 AVN. (**d**) AVN of the right humeral head in a different patient with subchondral fracture (*black arrows*) and early collapse with flattening cortical margin

(SI) on T1 and T2. The lesion itself may demonstrate normal marrow SI, commonest appearance, edema, high T2 and low T1 SI, or fibrosis/sclerosis as low T1 and T2 SI. This peripheral ring is the interface between living and necrotic marrow. On T2-weighted sequences, the "double-line sign," which is pathognomonic for AVN, may be apparent in up to 80 % cases and consists of a low SI outer ring and inner high SI ring. It is likely related to chemical shift artifact, a misregistration of fat protons relative to water protons.

Bone marrow edema and joint effusion both correlate with patient's symptoms. As disease progresses, a subchondral fracture line may develop, with high SI T2 and low T1 with surrounding edema. Cortical contour should be

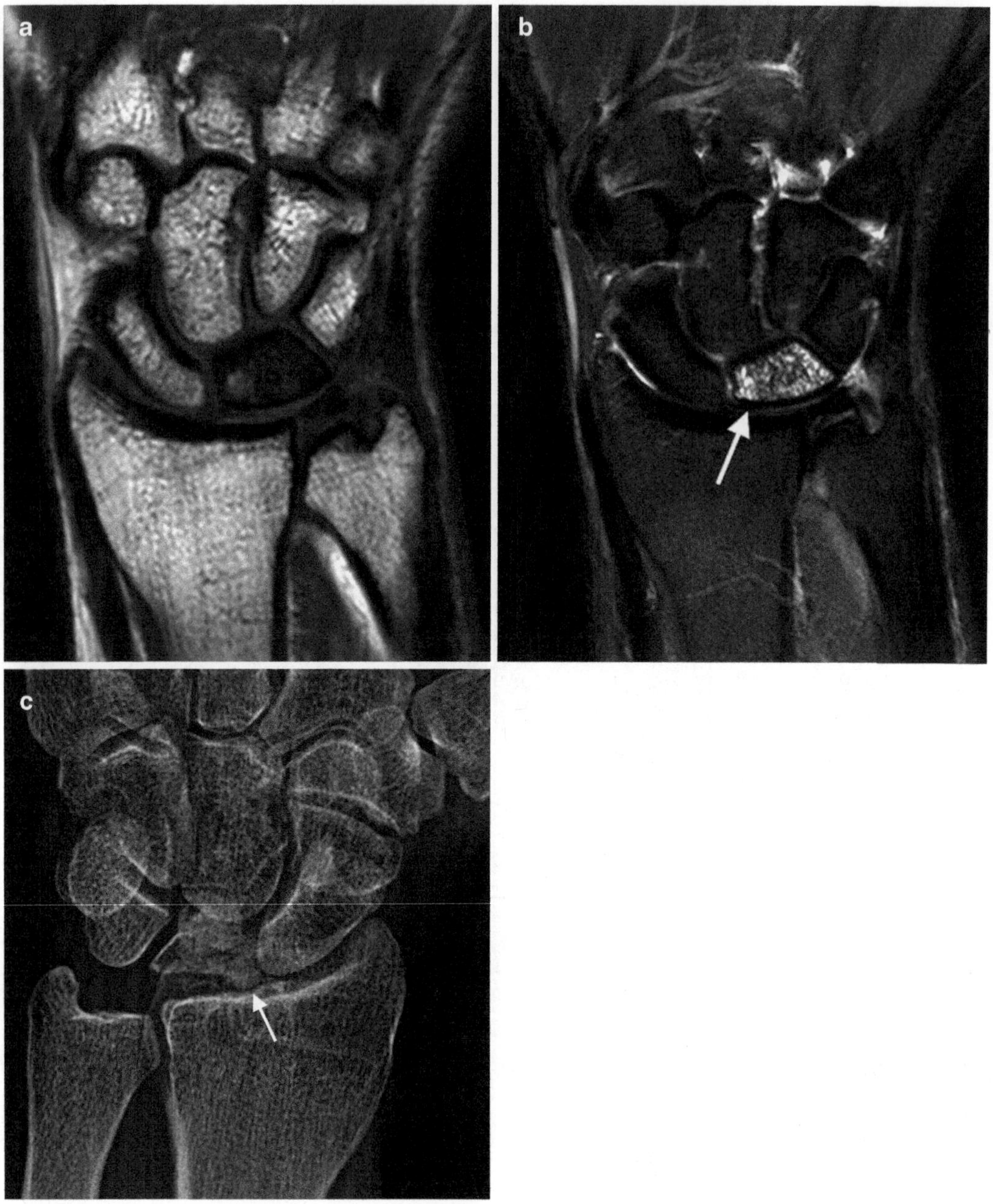

Fig. 12.4 42-year-old female patient, with a history of scleroderma and who is currently on steroid treatment presenting with wrist pain. (**a**, **b**) Cor T1 and T2FS, respectively, demonstrate Kienböck's disease with heterogeneous low SI on T1 and high SI on T2 in keeping with bone marrow edema (*arrow*) without evidence of collapse. (**c**) AP radiograph of the wrist 6 months later demonstrates progression of the disease, stage 3, with collapse and fragmentation of the lunate (*arrow*)

closely assessed on all planes to assess for early collapse. Once collapse occurs, there is unavoidable progression to degenerative joint disease.

Treatment at some centers in early disease may involve core decompressions of the femoral head and can be seen on radiographs, CT, and MRI as linear bands transversing the femoral head exiting laterally at the level of the greater trochanter. Core decompressions are thought to decrease intraosseous pressure and venous congestion.

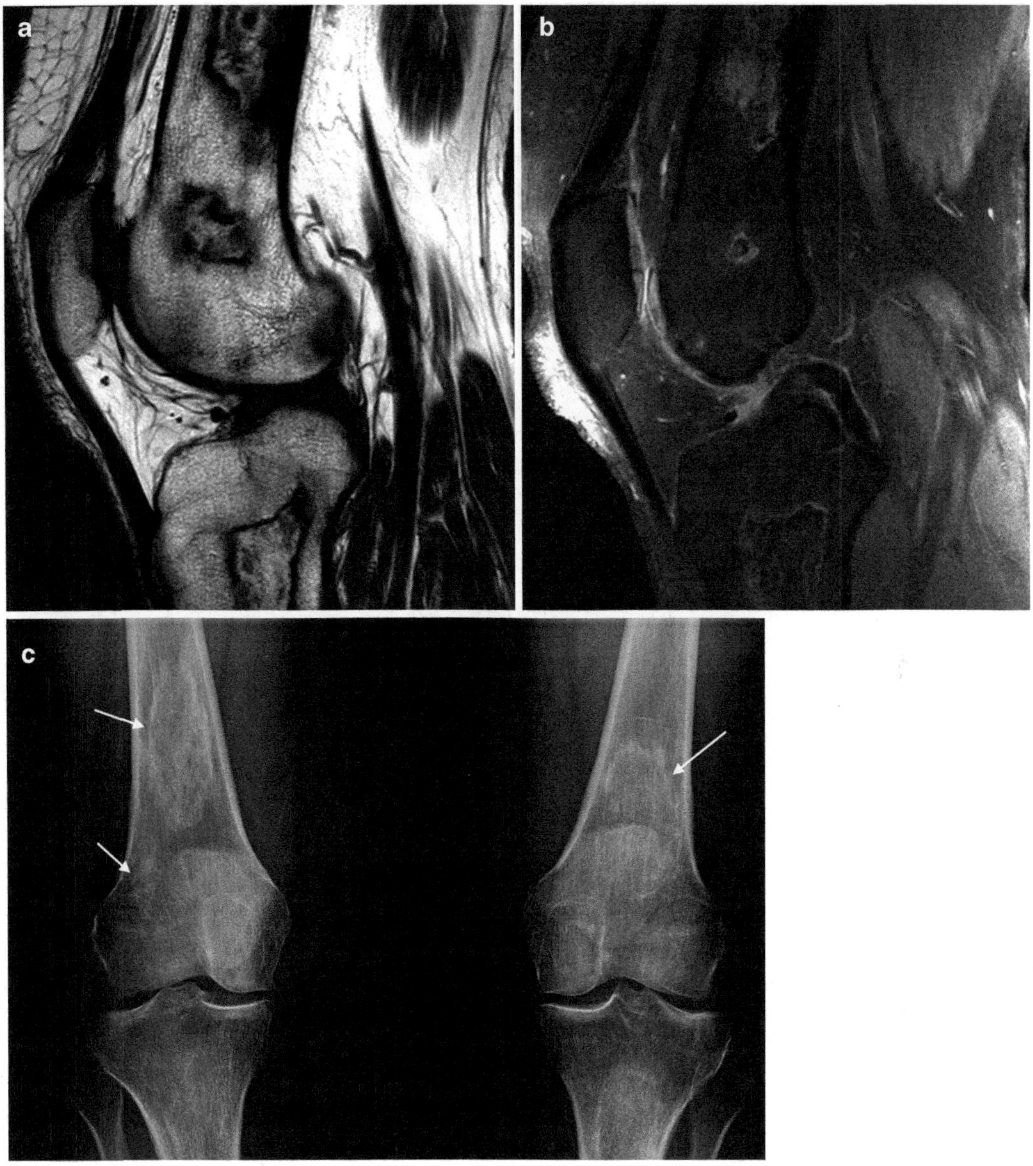

Fig. 12.5 A 46-year-old female with SLE with mild bilateral knee pain secondary to medullary infarcts. (**a**, **b**) Sag T1 and T2FS, respectively, demonstrate multiple intramedullary lesions within the diametaphysis with serpiginous margins of low SI on TI and high SI on T2 with some lesions demonstrating the double-line sign, and normal central marrow SI. (**c**) AP radiograph of the right knee and distal femur with classic radiographic features of medullary lesions with well-defined sclerotic margins (*arrows*) and central lucency

CT (Fig. 12.6)

CT is significantly less sensitive than MRI or bone scan in the early stages of the disease. There may be evidence of central sclerosis, the asterisk sign, within the femoral head. As disease progresses, CT becomes more sensitive. Subchondral fracture, cortical collapse, the volume of the femoral head involved, and early and advanced secondary degenerative changes can be assessed with similar sensitivities to MRI. CT does not demonstrate bone marrow edema and does, however, incur a radiation exposure and hence is usually employed only in specific cases, e.g., MRI unavailable and

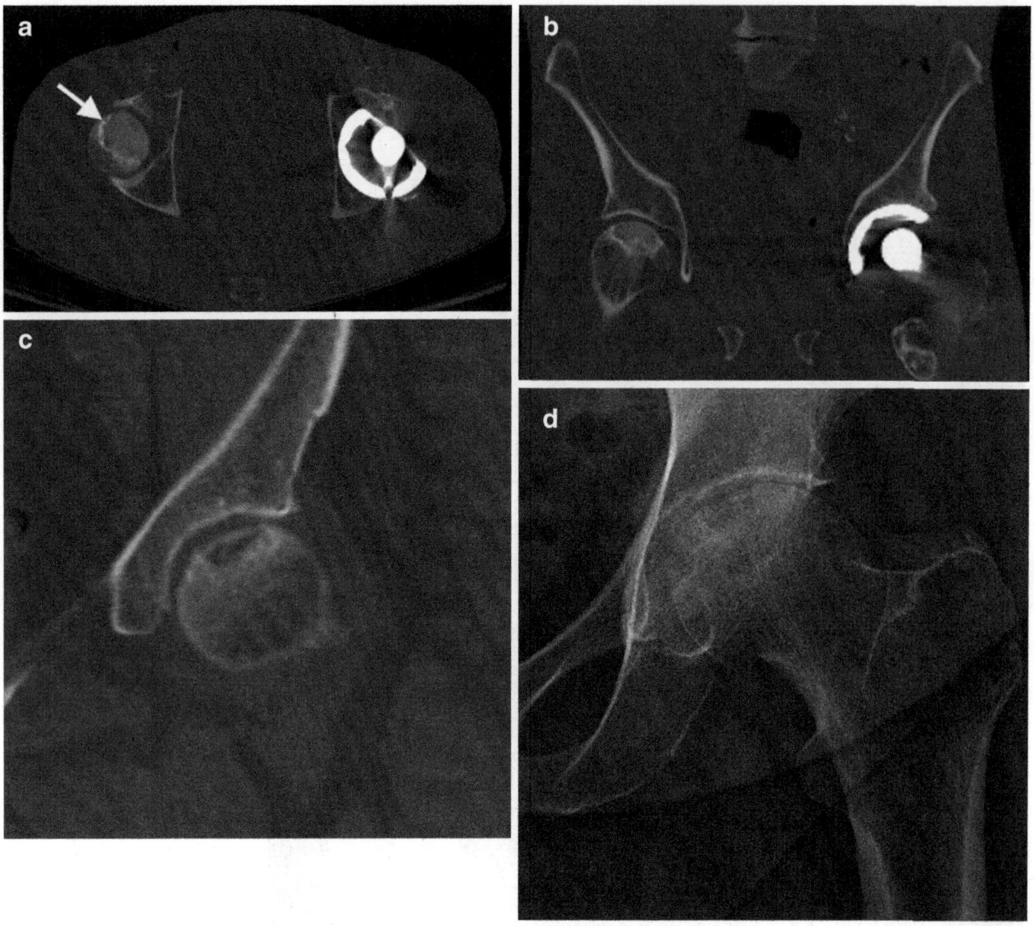

Fig. 12.6 CT AVN in a 63-year-old male COPD patient with a history of steroid use, prior left THR secondary to advanced AVN. (**a**) Axial and (**b**) Cor reformatted CT of bilateral hips demonstrate increased sclerosis of the right femoral head with well-defined sclerotic rim (*arrow*), stage 2a disease. (**c**) Cor CT and (**d**) AP radiograph of the left femoral head in a different patient with stage 3 disease, subchondral fracture with collapse

there is a questionable subchondral fracture, which may influence patient's management.

Bone Scan

Bone scan is used less frequently for investigating AVN as MRI has become more widely available. Bone scan is less sensitive and specific than MRI and incurs a significant radiation dose. In early AVN, there is absent uptake, a cold lesion, at the site of AVN. A peripheral ring of increased uptake develops representing a reparative rim with increased osteoblastic activity in conjunction with absent central uptake that is known as the "doughnut sign." Progression of degenerative changes can be seen as diffuse increased uptake on both sides of the joint. Bone scans should always be interrogated in conjunction with other imaging such as radiographs.

Ultrasound (Fig. 12.7)

Ultrasound has essentially no role in the evaluation of AVN. It may be helpful in excluding alternate periarticular soft tissue pathologies and for joint effusion/active synovitis.

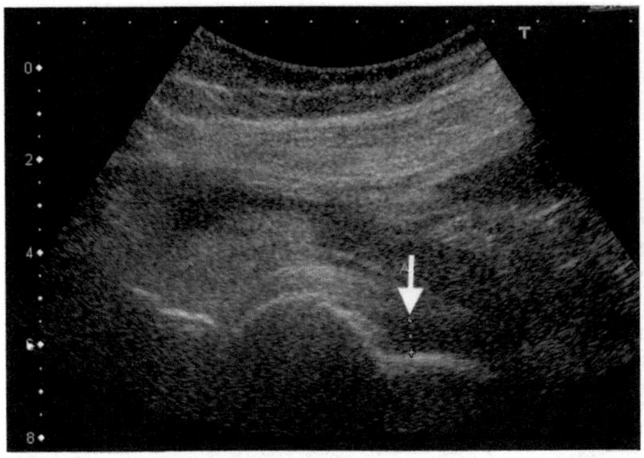

Fig. 12.7 Longitudinal ultrasound in a patient with AVN demonstrates joint effusion (*arrow*) but cannot demonstrate AVN (confirmed on follow-up MRI)

Differential Diagnosis

Differntial diagnosis includes transient bone marrow edema syndrome, insufficiency fracture, inflammatory arthropathies (Chaps. 5 and 7), and septic arthritis (Chap. 14).

Insufficiency Fractures of the Femoral Head

Subchondral insufficiency fractures of the femoral head have a similar imaging and clinical characteristics with avascular necrosis. Patients with insufficiency fractures are classically elderly osteoporotic female patients and present with progressive hip pain. The predisposing factors for AVN are usually not present. AVN is commonly bilateral, whereas insufficiency fracture is unilateral. Both can progress to femoral head collapse.

Clinical Presentation

Acute onset unilateral hip pain in elderly obese osteoporotic female patients that gradually worsens is the classical presentation. Femoral head insufficiency fractures have been documented in younger patients with no obvious predisposing factors but have been found to be osteopenic on bone mineral density testing. Subchondral fatigue fractures should be considered in the differential diagnosis. These are most commonly reported in young male military recruits undergoing heavy training.

Imaging

Radiographs (Fig. 12.8)
Radiographs may be normal or demonstrate subtle abnormalities. Predisposing osteopenia should be noted. In early fractures, increased resorption around the subchondral fracture can be make the fracture line difficult to appreciate. The convex contour of the femoral head should be closely inspected for localized flattening in keeping with early collapse. A subchondral linear lucency, crescent sign, also seen in AVN, may occasionally be seen. In subchondral fractures that progress, follow-up radiographs demonstrate ongoing collapse of the femoral head. Insufficiency fractures have been implicated in rapidly destructive arthrosis of the hip.

MRI (Figs. 12.8 and 12.9)
Extensive bone marrow edema is present, demonstrated by low signal intensity on T1 and high signal intensity on T2. It is best appreciated on STIR sequences or T2 with fat saturation. On T1 a subchondral low signal intensity line, the fracture line, is identified just deep to the low signal intensity of the cortex. The line is convex to the cortex and is irregular and discontinuous. On T2 the band is of high signal intensity corresponding to reparative tissue. In AVN T1, the line is also of low signal intensity; however, it is continuous, smooth, and concave to the articular surface and outlines the area of infarct. It may be difficult if not impossible to separate these two entities on imaging once the femoral head has collapsed. Assessment of different predisposing risk factors and other potential sites of involvement, including the contralateral hip in AVN, may help differentiate the underlying etiology.

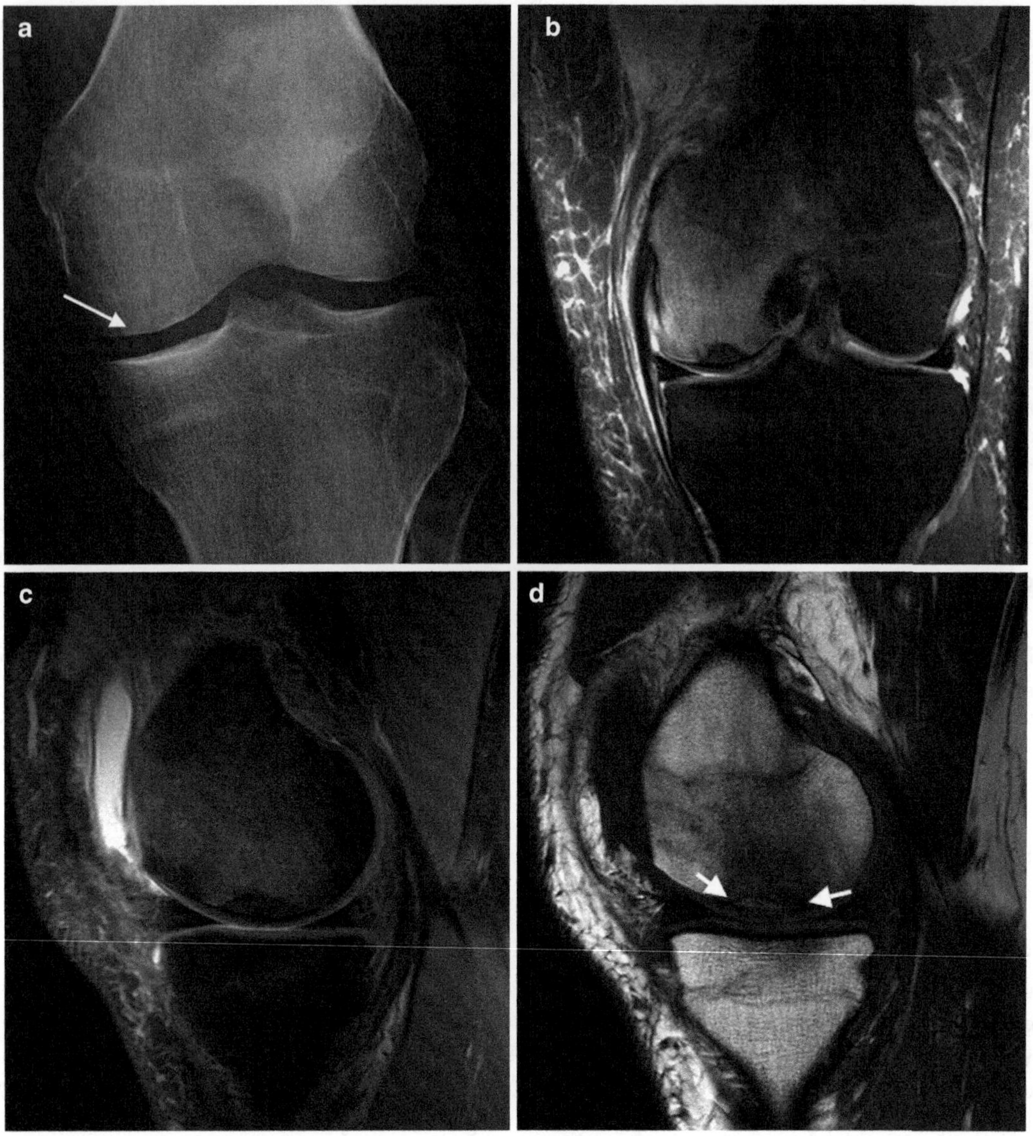

Fig. 12.8 A 52-year-old female with subchondral insufficiency fracture of the weight-bearing surface right medial femoral condyle (previously these lesions were termed "SONK," spontaneous osteonecrosis of the knee, until subchondral fracture lines were identified on MRI). (**a**) AP radiograph demonstrates subchondral sclerosis of the medial femoral condyle (MFC), without cortical collapse, and a subtle subchondral lucent line (*arrow*). (**b**) Cor and (**c**) Sag T2FS well-defined subchondral low SI with extensive edema MFC and (**d**) low SI fracture line (*arrows*) on Sag T1

CT

CT is less sensitive than MRI in diagnosing insufficiency fractures; this is related in part to underlying osteopenia, which can limit detection of fracture lines. In addition fracture lines are usually parallel to axial acquisition plane and may not be clearly visualized even on coronal and sagittal reconstructions. Fractures are usually anterosuperior at the site of major weight bearing. CT does not have the ability to detect marrow edema as detected on MRI. Reactive sclerosis can be seen in subacute cases but may be delayed in those that are severely osteoporotic. Early collapse with flattening of the femoral

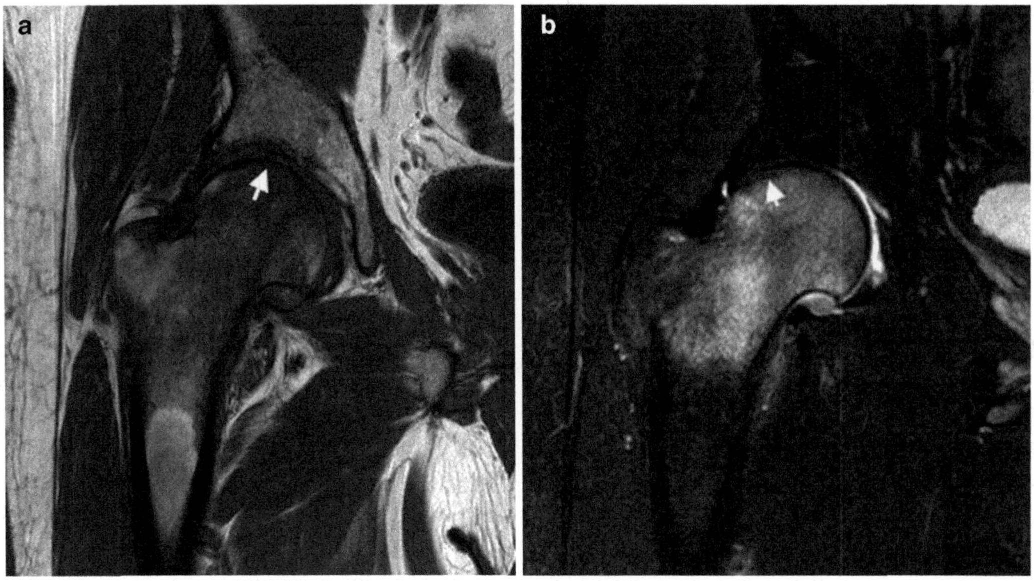

Fig. 12.9 A 62-year-old osteoporotic female with sudden onset of right hip pain; radiographs demonstrated osteopenia. (**a**) Cor T1 and (**b**) Cor T2FS demonstrate a low SI line (*arrows*) of the femoral head convex to cortex with extensive edema extending inferiorly to the intertrochanteric region

head, progression of collapse, and volume femoral head involved can be assessed.

Nuclear Medicine

Tc99m-MDP bone scan demonstrates increased uptake at fracture site due to increased osteoblastic activity. Patients may demonstrate decreased uptake as fracture heals. Progressive increased uptake is in keeping with progression fracture and collapse. Bone scans should be interpreted with radiographs. In osteoporotic patients, early bone scan may be normal or demonstrate minimal increased uptake. AVN findings are described above. A bone mineral density test should be performed in assessing osteoporosis.

Ultrasound

Ultrasound has essentially no role in the evaluation of subchondral fracture. It may be requested in patients with nonspecific hip pain where a nonspecific effusion is present. This should prompt close reevaluation of radiographs.

Transient Osteoporosis/Transient Bone Marrow Edema Syndrome

Overview

Transient osteoporosis of the hip was first described in 1959 in three pregnant patients, in their last trimester with hip pain and evidence of spotty demineralization on radiographs with resolution of radiographic findings after several months. It was initially termed transitory demineralization of the hip. The condition, however, is most common in middle-aged male patients. It is self-limiting and is of unknown etiology and symptoms, and imaging features resolve after several months.

Clinical Presentation

There is acute onset of unilateral hip or groin pain, exacerbated by weight bearing. The patient may have a limp and demonstrate decreased range of motion. Symptoms plateau after 3 months and then gradually improve with symptom resolution in less than 10 months. Previous reports have suggested progression to AVN or femoral head collapse, but it is unknown whether these patients had early evidence of AVN or possible insufficiency fractures that were not initially evident.

Imaging

Radiographs

Radiographs may initially be normal at the onset of symptoms. Progressive osteopenia develops, which may be spotty, in the femoral head. Bony trabeculae become indistinct with increased bone resorption, particularly of the subchondral bone plate. The joint space is preserved. There are no degenerative changes, evidence of periosteal reaction or cortical destruction. Radiographs gradually return to normal with resolution of clinical symptoms.

MRI (Fig. 12.10)

Transient bone marrow edema syndrome is the MRI equivalent of transient osteoporosis of the hip. MRI demonstrates changes before radiographs. There is diffuse bone marrow edema involving the subchondral femoral head extending inferiorly as far as the intertrochanteric region. The edema is homogenous with no high or low signal intensity foci within. It is low signal intensity on T1 and high on T2 fat-saturated or STIR sequences. There may be sparing of areas of red marrow such as the greater trochanter. Bone marrow enhances with contrast although contrast is usually not required. Careful search of the subchondral region is required to exclude a subchondral insufficiency fracture. A fracture may occur later in the course of the disease due to profound

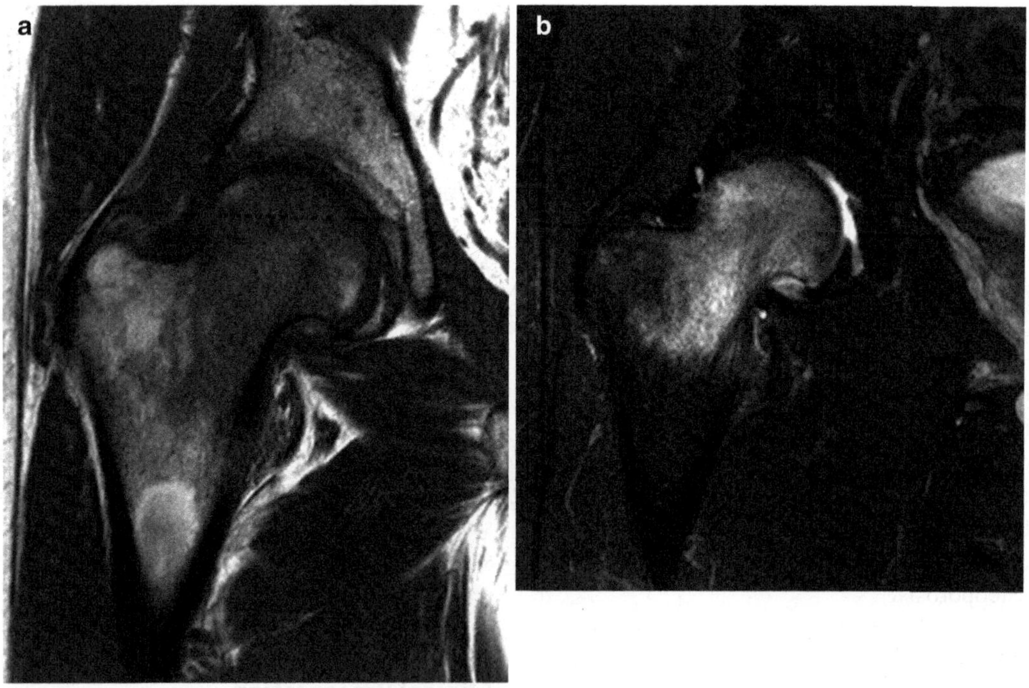

Fig. 12.10 A 38-year-old male with acute onset of severe right hip pain. (**a**) Cor T1 and (**b**) Cor T2FS demonstrate extensive subchondral bone marrow edema extending inferiorly to the intertrochanteric region. No insufficiency fracture lines identified, otherwise very similar in appearance to Fig. 12.8. Patient's age and risk factors are important in helping to arrive at final diagnosis. Many cases of TBMES are likely insufficiency fractures

osteopenia. A joint effusion is often present. MRI findings resolve completely with symptoms.

CT

CT is not routinely used in the diagnosis of transient osteoporosis of the hip but may be performed in cases of suspected insufficiency fracture, which have a similar clinical presentation. CT demonstrates significant osteopenia of the femoral head with thinning trabeculae but without evidence of fracture. Note that CT is not as sensitive as MRI in diagnosing fractures due to osteopenia as detailed in the discussion on insufficiency fractures above.

Nuclear Medicine

Bone scan demonstrates diffuse increased uptake within the femoral head and neck and is positive before radiographic changes develop. Findings are nonspecific on bone scan. MRI remains the gold imaging standard.

Ultrasound

Ultrasound may demonstrate a hip joint effusion but does not have a primary imaging role.

Regional migratory osteoporosis presents with similar clinical and imaging features as transient osteoporosis of the hip, but is not limited to the hip. Multiple sequential weight-bearing joints are involved, usually of the lower extremity, such as the hip, knee, and ankle. It is more common in middle age and in men.

Further Reading

1. Emad Y, Ragab Y, El-Shaarawy N, Rasker JJ. Transient osteoporosis of the hip, complete resolution after treatment with alendronate as observed by MRI description of eight cases and review of the literature. Clin Rheumatol. 2012;31(11):1641–7.
2. Ficat RP. Idiopathic bone necrosis of the femoral head. Early diagnosis and treatment. J Bone Joint Surg Br. 1985;67(1):3–9.
3. Gil HC, Levine SM, Zoga AC. MRI findings in the subchondral bone marrow: a discussion of conditions including transient osteoporosis, transient bone marrow edema syndrome, SONK, and shifting bone marrow edema of the knee. Semin Musculoskelet Radiol. 2006;10(3):177–86.
4. Ikemura S, Yamamoto T, Motomura G, et al. MRI evaluation of collapsed femoral heads in patients 60 years old or older: differentiation of subchondral insufficiency fracture from osteonecrosis of the femoral head. AJR Am J Roentgenol. 2010;195(1): W63–8.
5. Jackson SM, Major NM. Pathologic conditions mimicking osteonecrosis. Orthop Clin North Am. 2004;35(3):315–20.
6. Karantanas AH, Drakonaki EE. The role of MR imaging in avascular necrosis of the femoral head. Semin Musculoskelet Radiol. 2011;15(3): 281–300.
7. Karantanas AH, Nikolakopoulos I, Korompilias AV, Apostolaki E, Skoulikaris N, Eracleous E. Regional migratory osteoporosis in the knee: MRI findings in 22 patients and review of the literature. Eur J Radiol. 2008;67(1):34–41.
8. Starr AM, Wessely MA, Albastaki U, Pierre-Jerome C, Kettner NW. Bone marrow edema: pathophysiology, differential diagnosis, and imaging. Acta Radiol. 2008;49(7):771–86.

Imaging in Musculoskeletal Infection

13

Kimberly J. Legault and John O'Neill

Infectious agents can affect the musculoskeletal system by infecting the joint (septic arthritis), bone (osteomyelitis), or muscle (pyogenic myositis) or by causing soft tissue infections such as cellulitis, necrotizing fasciitis, or abscess formation. This chapter will review the various presentations of infection-related arthritis and their radiological characteristics.

Septic Arthritis

Overview

Septic arthritis is usually caused by bacterial infection but can occasionally be fungal. When considering bacterial infections, gonococcal and mycobacterial infections are typically considered separately from other bacteria due to the differences in clinical presentations. Bacterial septic arthritis typically arises from hematogenous spread but can also occur through direct inoculation of the joint space or via transfer from adjacent osteomyelitis. Risk factors for the development of septic arthritis are outlined in Table 13.1. Bacteria initially infect the synovial membrane with rapid dispersal into the synovial fluid, leading to purulent joint fluid. The ensuing inflammatory cells release cytokines and activate proteolytic enzymes that lead to rapid destruction of the joint cartilage, and superantigens, such as staphylococcal toxic shock syndrome toxin, contribute further to joint damage. The bacteria most commonly implicated in causing nongonococcal septic arthritis are presented in Table 13.2.

Table 13.1 Risk factors for septic arthritis

Age >80 years
Diabetes mellitus
Rheumatoid arthritis
Prosthetic joint
Recent joint intervention, including surgery and intra-articular steroid injection
Soft tissue infection
IV drug use
Alcoholism

Table 13.2 Bacteria causing nongonococcal septic arthritis

Staphylococcus aureus
Streptococcal species
Gram negatives
Mycobacterial species
Borrelia burgdorferi
Mycoplasma hominis

K.J. Legault, MD, FRCPC (✉)
Division of Rheumatology, Department of Medicine, McMaster University, Hamilton, ON, Canada
e-mail: kimberly.legault@medportal.ca

J. O'Neill, MB, BAO, BCh, MRCPI, MSc, FRCR
Associate Professor, Musculoskeletal Imaging, Diagnostic Imaging, McMaster University/St Joseph's Healthcare, Hamilton, ON L8N4A6, Canada
e-mail: joneill2@me.com

J. O'Neill (ed.), *Essential Imaging in Rheumatology*,
DOI 10.1007/978-1-4939-1673-3_13,

Clinical Presentation

The presentation is typically monoarticular, with >1 joint involved in only 20 % of cases. The joint most commonly infected is the knee. Patients typically present acutely with a hot, red, swollen joint with severe pain on active and passive range of motion. Fever is usually, though not always, present. Given the associated rapid joint destruction, joint aspiration should be performed as soon as possible. Arthrocentesis typically exhibits high numbers of white blood cells: the likelihood ratio associated with septic arthritis increases with increasing number of leukocytes. For example, a WBC count of >100,000 × 10*6 cells has an associated positive likelihood ratio of 47 for septic arthritis. There are typically >80 % neutrophils. Erythrocyte sedimentation rate (ESR) and C-reactive protein (CRP) are usually elevated, sometimes dramatically so. Treatment is typically intravenous antibiotics initially for 2–3 weeks based on the gram stain and culture results, followed by several weeks of oral antibiotics. Joint drainage is indicated, preferably through arthroscopic or open surgical techniques.

Gonococcal arthritis often presents as an oligo- or polyarthritis in the setting of a gonococcal rash. It should be suspected in younger individuals with risk factors for sexually transmitted infections. *Neisseria gonorrhoeae* is not reliably isolated from gram stain or culture of the joint aspirate, and diagnosis requires culturing all potentially infected sites (urethra, cervix, pharynx, and blood), in addition to synovial fluid culture. Tuberculous arthritis is typically more indolent in presentation, with pain progressing over weeks to months, and fewer inflammatory joint symptoms with less erythema, swelling, and heat. The diagnosis is often delayed as the indolent nature of the symptoms leads to consideration of noninfectious arthropathies such as osteoarthritis or rheumatoid arthritis. Phemister's triad seen in TB arthritis includes periarticular osteopenia, marginal erosions, and progressive joint space loss. Acute viral arthritis, usually occurring in children, is self-limiting and benign. It may be mono- or polyarticular and may present like septic arthritis as described above or like an inflammatory arthropathy. Complications of septic arthritis include joint destruction, joint deformity, osteonecrosis of intra-articular bodies, premature osteoarthritis, and ankylosis.

Differential diagnosis of a septic arthritis includes crystalline arthropathies, seronegative spondyloarthropathies, and less commonly monoarthritic presentations of rheumatoid arthritis or other varieties of inflammatory arthritis. It is typically the crystalline arthropathies that mimic the septic joint most closely, with rapid onset of symptoms, erythema and swelling of the joint, and significant pain and disability. It must not be forgotten that infection and a crystalline arthropathy can coexist in the same joint. For these reasons, no modality aside from aspiration and analysis of synovial fluid can reliably and safely distinguish these entities.

Imaging Features

Radiographs (Fig. 13.1)

Radiographs in septic arthritis are often normal at presentation. Joint effusion, possibly leading to initial joint space widening, and/or soft tissue swelling may be detectable. Later findings include subchondral bony erosion/destruction that is present on both sides of the joint, uniform joint space narrowing secondary to cartilage damage, reactive bony sclerosis, and juxta-articular osteopenia.

Fig. 13.1 A 28-year-old male with soft tissue laceration of the radial aspect of the index finger overlying the DIPJ, (**a**) initial AP and (**b**) lateral radiograph demonstrating soft tissue swelling with no acute bone injury or retained metallic foreign body, metallic pin denotes site of injury and mild flexion deformity at DIPJ, (**c**) follow-up radiographic series 2 weeks later after minor trauma with fracture of the proximal diaphysis of the distal phalanx; however, there is now progressive joint space loss at the DIPJ and periarticular osteopenia with osteolysis at the ulnar margin of the distal phalanx in keeping with septic arthritis and osteomyelitis, (**d**) progression osteolysis and subluxation at the DIPJ

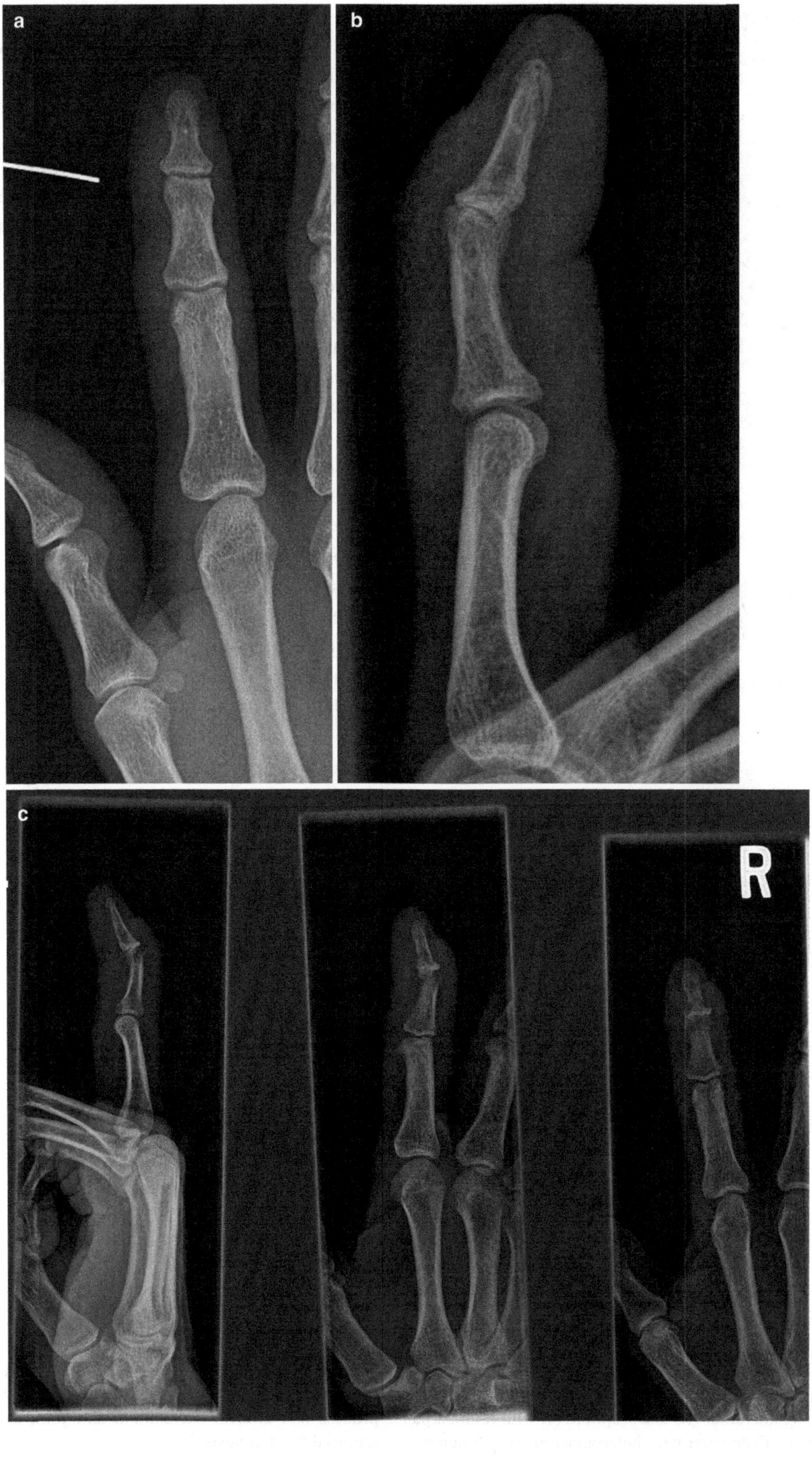
a
b
c
R

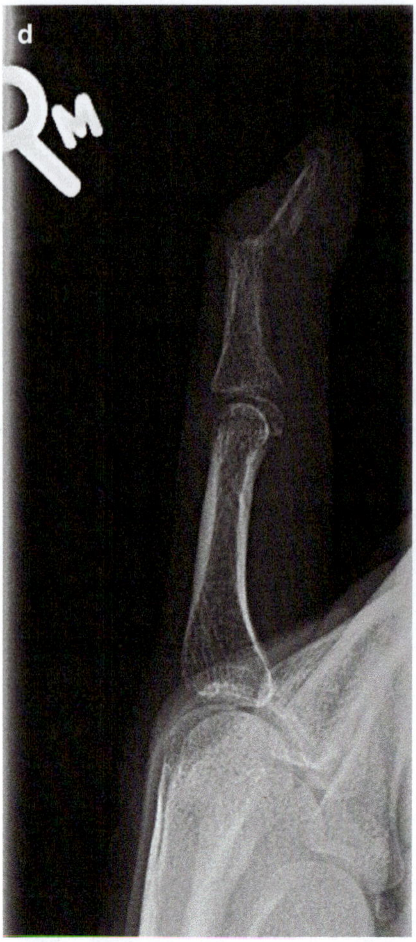

Fig. 13.1 (continued)

The regional osteopenia that develops in septic arthritis occurs as a result of the regional exuberant immune response with high levels of inflammatory cytokines and prostaglandins that act to inhibit regional bone formation and promote absorption. Coincident osteomyelitis is often present, leading to cortical destruction and reactive new bone formation of the periosteum termed "periosteal reaction" (see section entitled "Osteomyelitis"). There can be severe bony disorganization and destruction at this stage with secondary osteoarthritic change. Bony ankylosis can occur. Abscesses can form adjacent to the site of infection (see section "Abscess" below).

Ultrasound (Fig. 13.2)

Ultrasound can demonstrate a joint effusion, which may not always be present, before it becomes visible on a radiograph. Septic joint effusion is usually complex in appearance with hyperechoic appearance secondary to pus, internal septations, and debris. Occasionally effusions are anechoic. The joint capsule is diffusely thickened. Hyperemia with increased flow on Doppler may be seen within the synovium and capsule. Depending on the joint and accessibility to detailed ultrasound evaluation, other changes may be visible including cartilage destruction demonstrated as loss of the normal convex

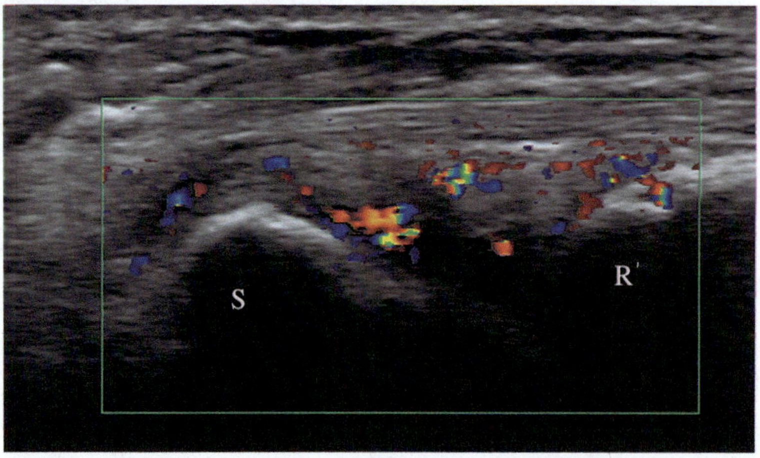

Fig. 13.2 Ultrasound in a 37-year-old female patient with septic arthritis of the wrist, longitudinal image demonstrating the radius (*R*) and scaphoid (*s*) with radiocarpal joint space distension with heterogeneous tissue demonstrating marked flow within on color Doppler. Note that ultrasound can only demonstrate an active inflammatory process and clinical correlation, and joint aspiration is required for diagnosis

hypoechoic cartilage contour which may be filled with hyperechoic synovium and complex fluid. Erosions, as focal cortical defects, and periosteal reaction with subperiosteal collection may also be visible. The adjacent soft tissues are also evaluated for associated collections. Assessment of osteomyelitis is limited and is best performed with MRI. Ultrasound can also confirm joint effusion and guide needle placement for joint aspiration.

MRI (Fig. 13.3)

While the diagnosis of septic arthritis should always be made based on appropriate synovial

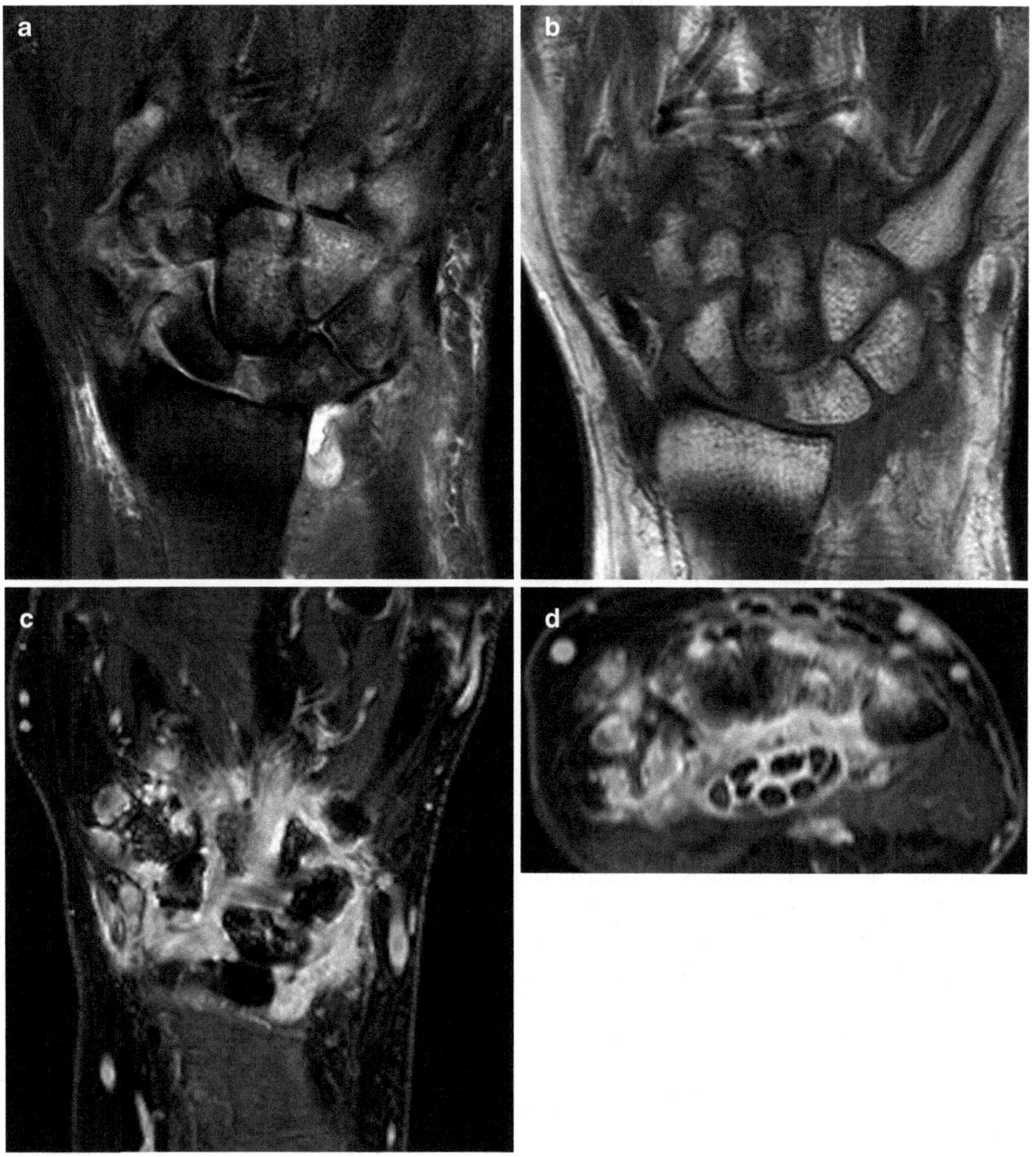

Fig. 13.3 MRI in a patient presenting with acute inflamed right wrist without prior history of inflammatory arthropathy, with septic arthritis of the radiocarpal joint with extension to the midcarpal and distal radioulnar joint with secondary multifocal osteomyelitis. (**a**) Cor T2FS and (**b**) Cor T1 demonstrating joint effusions and extensive osteitis. (**c**, **d**) Cor and reformatted axial T1FS, respectively, with diffuse enhancing synovitis, erosions, and osteitis with marked enhancement of flexor tendon sheaths (infective tenosynovitis) within the carpal tunnel. Imaging finding suggests the diagnosis, but aspiration is required for confirmation

fluid sampling and culturing techniques, MRI can be a helpful adjunct to diagnosis. Multiple suggestive findings occurring in concert should raise suspicion. The adjacent bone can demonstrate erosions. Erosion is defined as a loss of the normal cortical contour of the bone, seen in two adjacent slices on MRI. The erosion shows loss of the normal cortical hypointensity and the normal trabecular hyperintensity on T1W images. Erosions are caused due to proliferative synovitis leading to pannus formation that invades into the adjacent bone, and thus post-gadolinium images show contrast enhancement within the pannus within the erosion. This pannus can also be seen as abnormal hyperintense signal within the erosion on T2W images due to the high water content in the inflamed tissue. Erosions typically occur first in the "bare area" – the marginal area of the joint near the area of attachment of the capsule that is minimally covered by cartilage and thus relatively unprotected. With continuing inflammation, however, erosions can involve any area of the articular surfaces, and severe bony destruction can occur. Adjacent bone marrow edema is also characteristic, which manifests as hypointensity on T1 and hyperintensity on T2. Synovial thickening and edema can be present, as well as a joint effusion. IV gadolinium can be used as a contrast agent and can differentiate synovium from joint effusion – in early post-gadolinium administration, synovium enhances, while joint effusion will not enhance. Soft tissue edema is present and occasionally soft tissue collections develop.

There are some unique features of tuberculous septic arthritis that can be seen on MRI. Forty percent develop synovial granulomas, which manifest as hypointense lesions on T2-weighted images. Areas of synovial proliferation (termed "pannus") can be seen, and characteristically in tuberculous arthritis, there are both active (enhancing) and chronic (non-enhancing) pannus, which coexist. Intra-articular bodies, termed "rice bodies," are related to ischemia of the synovium with subsequent shedding synovium and encasement by fibrin. They are classically seen in tuberculous arthritis but may also be present in entities such as rheumatoid arthritis and SLE. There can also be findings of microabscesses and evidence of osteomyelitis. Synovitis, effusions, and erosive changes are also seen as in other types of septic arthritis. Both central and peripheral erosions are seen.

Bone Scan

Bone scan is not commonly used to aid in the diagnosis of septic arthritis as the findings are indistinguishable from other types of arthritis. Classically, there is joint hyperperfusion and hyperemia on early imaging, with increased activity at articular surfaces on delayed imaging. Occasionally a WBC scan is performed in cases where there is a differential diagnosis such as Charcot joint.

CT

CT scanning is not commonly used in the setting of acute septic arthritis. Like plain radiographs, it can be normal in early stages or show only evidence of joint effusion or soft tissue swelling. It may be more sensitive to early findings of joint space widening due to effusion and later changes of erosions or periosteal reaction than radiographs, however. It could be considered when MRI is contraindicated but is generally considered inferior to MRI in septic arthritis.

Osteomyelitis

Overview

Like septic arthritis, osteomyelitis can arise due to hematologic spread of infection, direct inoculation from trauma or surgery, or contiguous spread from adjacent structures, such as an infected joint. The vertebral body is the most commonly affected area in adults and the long bones in children. Risk factors for osteomyelitis include diabetes mellitus, particularly with vascular insufficiency, peripheral neuropathy, the presence of decubitus or other chronic ulcers, prosthetic joint material, and a history of trauma. The organisms typically involved depend on the site and mode of transmission. Osteomyelitis secondary to hematogenous seeding is most commonly due to a single bacterium. Staphylococcal species, particularly *Staphylococcus aureus*, and aerobic gram-negative bacteria are the most common causes, with streptococci and enterococci occurring less frequently. Osteomyelitis secondary to direct inoculation, such as in patients with chronic nonhealing ulcers, is more likely to be polymicrobial.

Osteomyelitis can present either acutely or chronically, and presentation can vary by chronicity and site. Hematogenous osteomyelitis affects the medullary area of bone initially, and the subsequent inflammatory reaction causes increased intramedullary pressure that can rupture through the bony cortex. This can compromise blood flow to the periosteal region, which can lead to necrotic areas that then become separated from the rest of the bone. These sequestrated necrotic areas are characteristic of chronic osteomyelitis and are referred to as "sequestra." These can be helpful in the identification of osteomyelitis radiologically. Typically a layer of granulation tissue separates the sequestrum from the living bone, and the sequestrum can then become encased in reactive bone (termed "involucrum"). Sinus tracts through the cortical bone to the medulla can also be seen. Abscesses can form, in the subacute to chronic phase of osteomyelitis, particularly within the ends of tubular bones, and may be single or multiple, "Brodie's abscess." Due to developmental changes in blood supply and end vessels, the epiphysis is a common location of osteomyelitis in the infant and the metaphysis in the child. Spondylodiscitis is reviewed in detail in Chap. 15

Clinical Presentation

Patients with acute osteomyelitis typically present with pain, warmth, and erythema of the affected site. Some sites, such as vertebral, hip, and sacroiliac, usually present with pain. Constitutional symptoms and signs such as fever and malaise may be present. In patients with ulcers, lack of improvement with appropriate wound care should raise the suspicion for underlying osteomyelitis. If an ulcer is larger than 2×2 cm in diameter or if bone is exposed, there is a high likelihood of underlying osteomyelitis. In these cases, treatment with antibiotics is often initiated empirically. A draining sinus tract and overlying tissue necrosis are also strong indicators.

Inflammatory markers such as erythrocyte sedimentation rate and C-reactive protein are usually elevated in osteomyelitis but are nonspecific. Blood cultures are only positive in approximately 50 % of patients with acute hematogenous osteomyelitis but should still be performed in all patients. The gold standard for diagnosis of osteomyelitis is bone biopsy, and a positive result for osteomyelitis on bone biopsy has both histopathologic and microbial components. The biopsy should show inflammatory infiltrate within the bone leading to bony resorption and subsequent necrosis on histopathology, and an offending organism should be isolated on microbial cultures. However, bone biopsy may not be feasible in the setting of inaccessible anatomic areas or if there is concern regarding lack of healing in patients with compromised vascularity, and in this case empiric treatment is typically undertaken. Superficial wound cultures are only consistent with bone biopsy results in about 30 % of cases and thus should not be used for diagnosis routinely.

Treatment of osteomyelitis is dependent on several factors, including culture and sensitivity results, chronicity, and amount of devitalized bone and necrotic tissue present, and involves a combination of antibiotic therapy and surgical debridement. Initial antibiotic therapy is typically administered intravenously. Chronic osteomyelitis and/or osteomyelitis associated with cutaneous ulcers in patients with compromised regional vascularity can require more prolonged courses of antibiotics. There is little randomized controlled data in this area to guide therapy. Uncomplicated hematogenous osteomyelitis in children can be treated for as few as 4 days with IV therapy, with transition to oral antibiotics for a period of 4 weeks. Chronic osteomyelitis in adults is typically treated with 2–6 weeks of IV antibiotics initially, then oral antibiotics subsequently to complete a course of 4–8 weeks. More prolonged courses can be required in more complicated infections. Recurrence rates in adults are quoted as being around 30 % at 1 year and even higher (~50 %) for infections with *Pseudomonas aeruginosa*. Bony debridement is indicated when there is necrotic tissue, and prosthetic material at the site of infection may need to be removed. Adjunctive modalities for treatment of osteomyelitis include hyperbaric oxygen therapy and negative pressure wound therapy with vacuum-assisted devices.

Imaging

Radiographs (Fig. 13.4)

Radiographs are always the first-line examination when assessing for the presence of osteomyelitis, though notably sensitivity is low, and a normal x-ray result does not rule out the presence of osteomyelitis, particularly in the early stages (i.e., the first 1–2 weeks). There may be soft tissue abnormalities such as swelling if there is an overlying penetrating wound or cellulitis.

Radiographs can reveal soft tissue swelling, regional osteopenia progressing to mixed lucencies with areas of osteopenia and bony sclerosis,

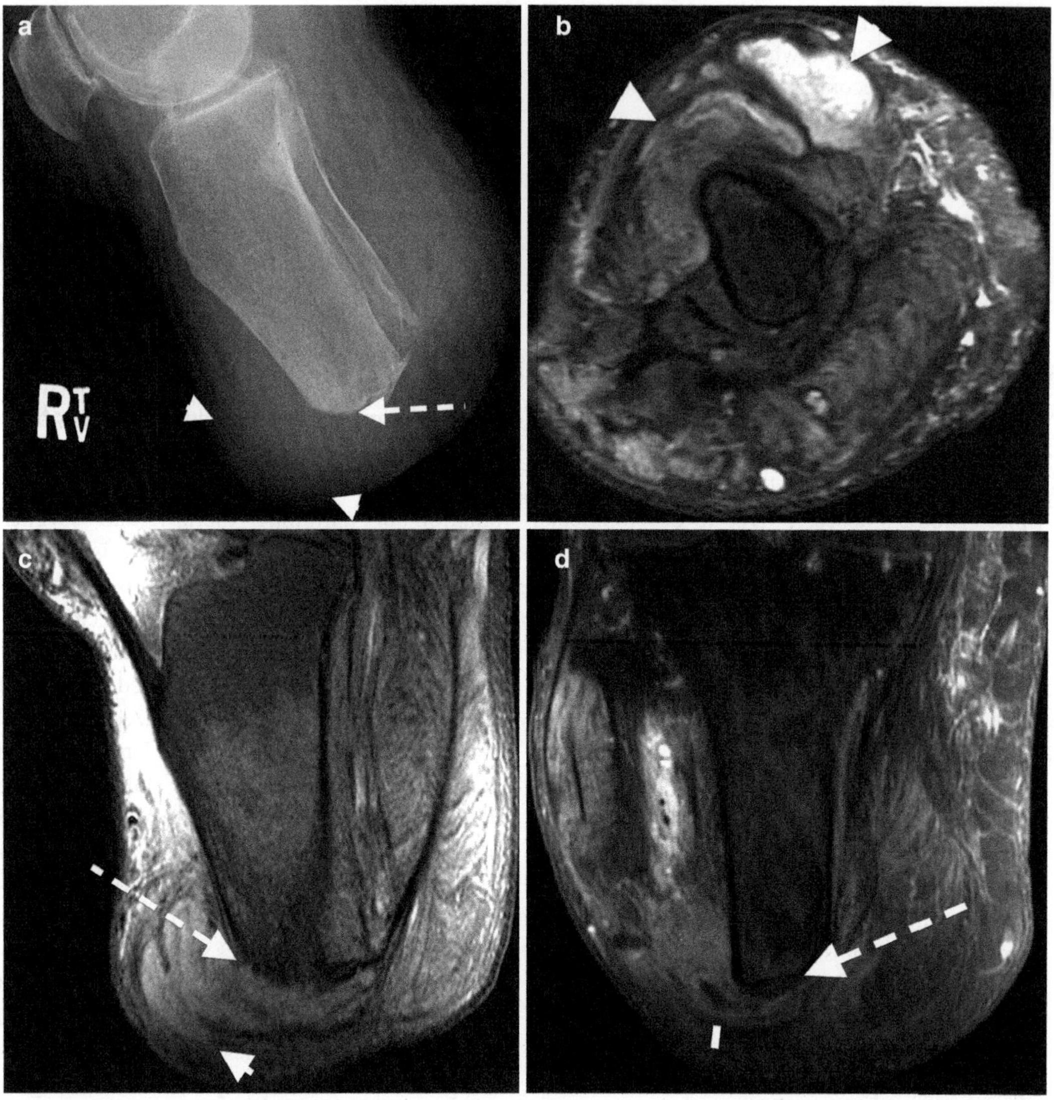

Fig. 13.4 A diabetic patient with right below-the-knee amputation presenting with soft tissue swelling, erythema, and fever. (**a**) Lateral radiograph stump demonstrates distal soft tissue swelling of increased density (*arrowheads*) when compared to adjacent soft tissue suggesting collection and underlying cortical irregularity, subtle periosteal reaction (*dashed arrow*), and adjacent mixed sclerosis and lucency in keeping with osteomyelitis. MRI of the same patient on the same day. (**b**) Axial T2FS with heterogeneous soft tissue collection (*arrowheads*), mild muscular edema (myositis), and subcutaneous edema (cellulitis) which enhance on T1FS PG. (**c–e**) The collection (line) demonstrates low central SI on (**e**) with rim enhancement (*arrowhead*) in keeping with a subcutaneous abscess (dashed arrow demonstrates adjacent osteomyelitis)

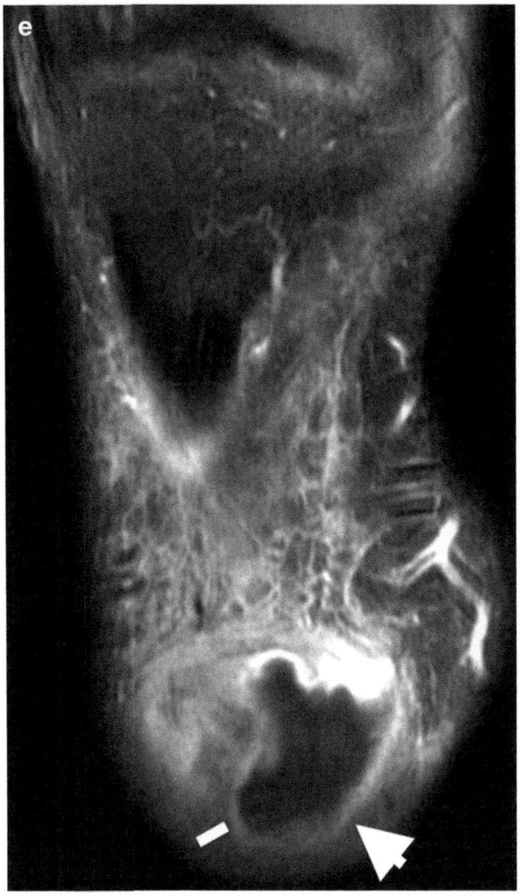

Fig. 13.4 (continued)

and later cortical destruction/erosions. Periosteal reaction is a very important finding and is very suggestive of osteomyelitis in the correct clinical setting. Brodie's abscess in subacute to chronic osteomyelitis appears as single or multiple radiolucencies surrounded by ill-defined sclerosis. Sequestra, necrotic bone, can be visualized by 6–8 weeks as isolated radiodense fragments surrounded by the involucrum, periosteal new bone. A sinus tract may develop at this time. In TB osteomyelitis and fungal infections, osteopenia is usually present, but there is limited sclerosis or periosteal reaction.

MRI (Fig. 13.4)

The earliest sign of osteomyelitis is alteration of the normal marrow signal. These changes are consistent with those typical for inflammatory changes, where the increased water content causing edema leads to hypointensity on T1W sequences and hyperintensity on T2W images. Low SI on T1 is more sensitive for osteomyelitis as high SI on T2 may represent early reactive changes. These changes can begin early, within the first few days of infection. However, the finding of bone marrow edema is nonspecific and can be seen in several other conditions affecting bone, such as osteonecrosis, post-traumatic changes, Charcot arthropathy, etc. Clinical correlation and the presence of additional imaging finding including ulceration adjacent to the area, bone marrow edema, cellulitis, or soft tissue collection will suggest osteomyelitis. Osteomyelitis may demonstrate restricted diffusion on diffusion-weighted imaging (DWI).

In subacute or chronic osteomyelitis, periostitis can be seen as an area of low signal intensity periosteal bone separated from the remainder of the bone by a higher signal intensity band of fluid or pus. Brodie's abscess characteristically appears as a target sign on enhanced T1-weighted images with four layers with alternating low to high SI from the center outward. In chronic osteomyelitis, sequestra demonstrate low signal intensity on T1W and STIR imaging and are non-enhancing with gadolinium. Surrounding granulation tissue can be seen as high signal intensity on T2W images, while the devitalized bony shell is low signal intensity. Gadolinium enhancement identifies areas of sinus tract formation and abscess. Areas of sclerosis and osteonecrosis can be seen as hypointense areas on both T1W and T2W sequences. Notably, the resolution of MRI changes related to osteomyelitis lags behind the clinical improvement, and thus MRI should not be used as the sole indicator of improvement with therapy.

CT (Fig. 13.5)

CT scan can show some changes of osteomyelitis, in particular cortical thickening and sclerosis, as well as detection of sequestra and sinus tracks that may not be distinguishable from adjacent bone on plain radiographs. Notably these findings occur relatively late in the infectious process; thus, CT is not a sensitive modality for early diagnosis. Both sequestra and involucra are more readily diagnosed on CT compared to MRI; however, CT is inferior to MRI for soft tissue

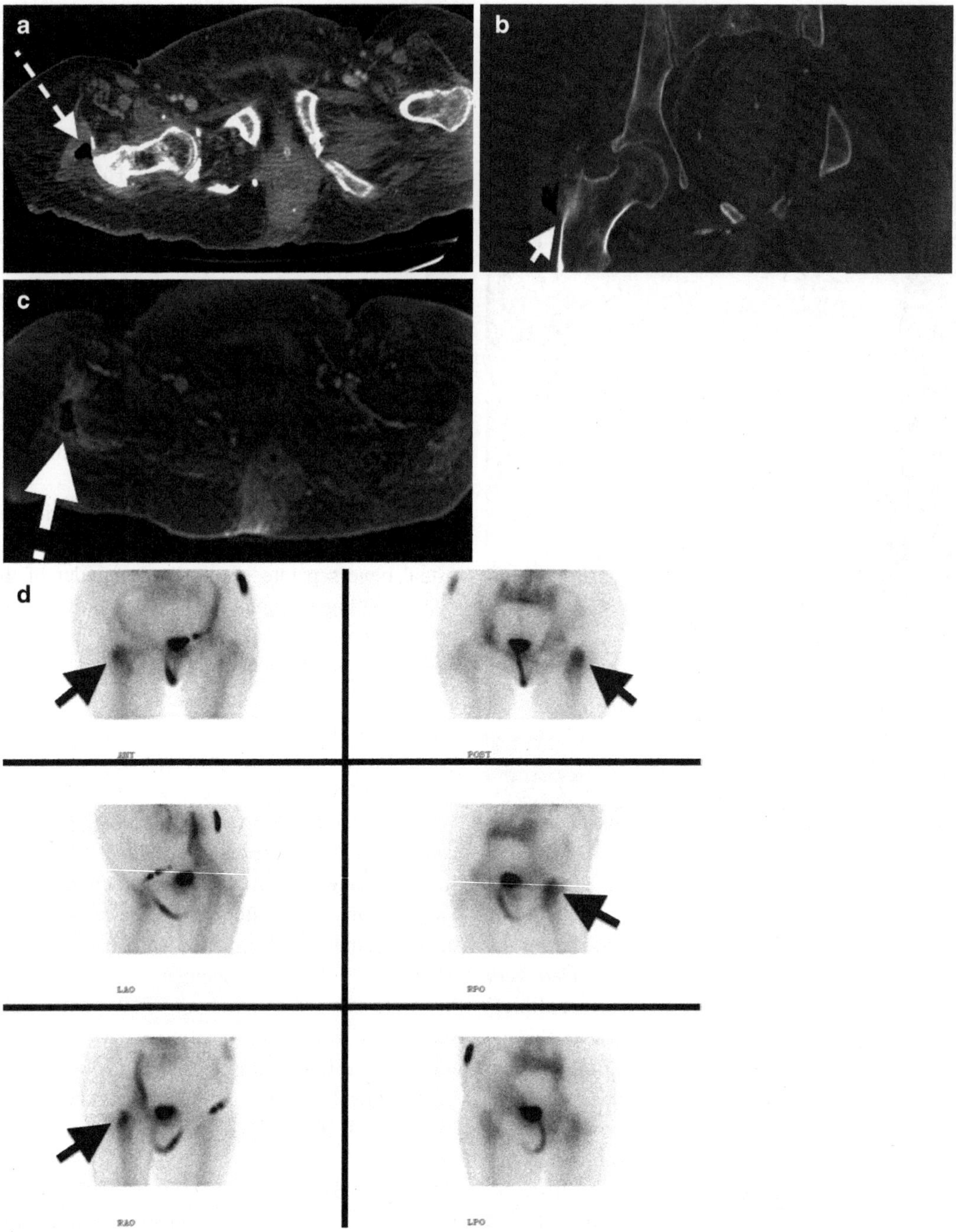

Fig. 13.5 Decubitus ulcer of the right greater trochanter with secondary osteomyelitis. (**a**) Axial CT, soft tissue windows, and (**b**) coronal reformatted image, bone windows, demonstrating ulceration extending to cortical surface with adjacent cortical sclerosis (*arrows*). (**c**) MRI, axial TIFS, corresponding to CT image (**a**) with air noted as black focus overlying the greater trochanter which has subtle osteitis and cortical erosions in keeping with osteomyelitis and surrounding soft tissue phlegmon (*dashed arrow*), (**d**) bone scan with localizer uptake at the right greater trochanter (*arrows*)

changes consistent with infection, and MRI is considered the diagnostic modality of choice, particularly in early infection. CT can be useful for guiding biopsy for diagnosis.

Bone Scan (Figs. 13.5 and 13.6)

Bone scanning reveals changes of osteomyelitis very early. On delayed imaging, increased uptake in the affected bony area is seen. Bone scan is very sensitive in detection of osteomyelitis; however, its specificity is low. In areas with suspected dual pathology, e.g., fracture or recent joint replacement with superimposed osteomyelitis, a bone scan will demonstrate increased uptake in both entities due to increased osteoblastic activity. Indium-labeled leukocytes may be helpful in this instance, localizing to area of infection and demonstrating increased uptake.

Ultrasound

Ultrasound is unable to penetrate cortical bone and thus has no direct role in evaluating osteomyelitis. For comprehensiveness, however, we will review the ultrasound findings that are suggestive

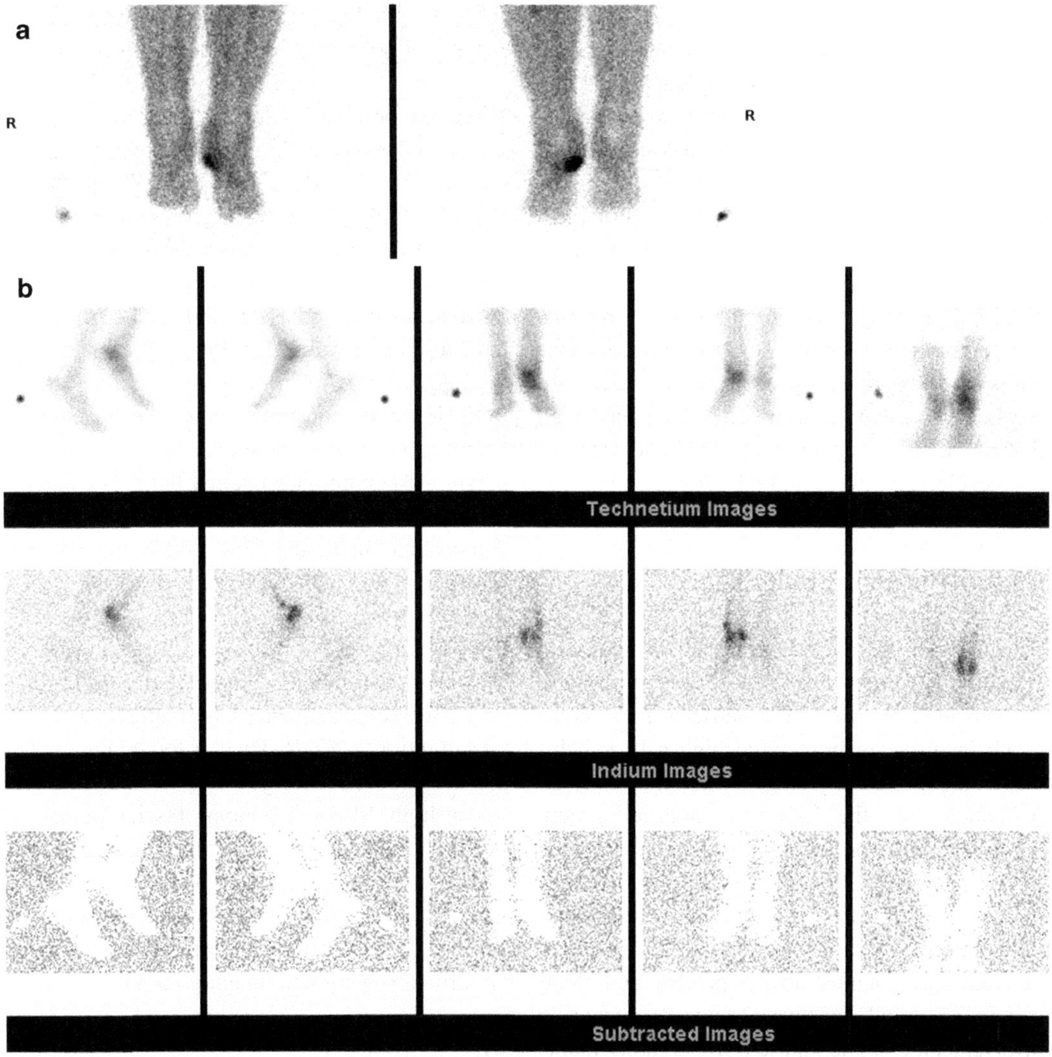

Fig. 13.6 (**a**) WCC scan (indium-labeled leukocyte) in a patient with positive bone scan, (**b**) for comparison, a patient with positive bone scan (*first row images*) and negative WCC on subtracted images (*last row images*)

of osteomyelitis. Early on, elevation of the periosteum by a hypoechoic layer of purulent material is characteristic. Cortical erosions can be seen later in the disease process. Abscesses can be identified as hypoechoic or anechoic fluid collections adjacent to bone. Power Doppler can show increased signal adjacent to the bone or within abscesses. Adjacent joints can be evaluated for features of septic arthritis.

Pyomyositis

Overview

Pyomyositis is an infection of skeletal muscle that typically occurs via hematogenous seeding of the muscle. It is most commonly seen in children in tropical countries but is becoming more commonly seen in temperate climates. Some of the risk factors include immunosuppression, particularly secondary to HIV, trauma, intravenous drug abuse, and malnutrition. The most common microbial pathogen is *Staphylococcus aureus*. Less commonly, group A streptococcus or other strep species or gram-negative enterics are implicated. Tuberculous pyomyositis has been described but is uncommon. Diabetic patients can develop polymicrobial infections.

Clinical Presentation

Patients with pyomyositis present with pain and cramping affecting one muscle group, usually accompanied by fever. The muscles most commonly involved are those of the thigh, calf, and gluteal areas. In the early stages, there may only be induration of the affected muscle group. As the infection progresses, the patient develops increasing pain and more signs of systemic toxicity. Edema of the affected area, often with a palpable fluctuant mass, can be appreciated on exam. Leukocytosis is almost always present, and blood cultures are usually positive. Despite severe muscle involvement, creatine kinase (CK) is rarely markedly elevated and can be normal or only exhibit mild elevations. ESR and CRP are typically elevated. Intravenous antibiotics based on either results from blood cultures or from sampling and culture of abscess from the affected muscle are the mainstay of treatment, though in the setting of abscess, drainage is indicated if possible. With extensive muscle involvement, surgical intervention for debridement may be required. Hyperbaric oxygen has recently been used with some success.

Imaging

Radiographs

Radiographs demonstrate no specific findings and may be normal. Soft tissue swelling may be present with loss of fat planes. It is useful for assessment of superficial or deep soft tissue air.

Ultrasound (Fig. 13.7a-d)

Findings depend on the stage of presentation and whether an abscess has formed. Initially the muscle is tender on probe placement and is swollen with a hyperechoic echotexture. Later, as areas of necrosis and abscesses develop, hypoechoic foci become evident. An abscess has developed when these foci have a defined wall. They demonstrate increased through transmission, i.e., tissues directly posterior to the lesion demonstrate increased echotexture in comparison to adjacent similar tissue at the same depth, in keeping with internal fluid. The latter is usually of heterogeneous echotexture. Doppler will demonstrate increased flow within the adjacent muscle and within the wall of the abscess.

MRI (Fig. 13.7e)

MRI demonstrates ill-defined edema as high SI on T2-weighted sequences, best appreciated with fat saturation or STIR. There is low SI on T1. The muscle may be enlarged and fluid appears as linear high SI on T2 along fascial planes. If abscess formation occurs, this appears as a heterogeneous encapsulated lesion of low SI on T1 and high SI on T2 with rim enhancement with contrast. It may demonstrate restricted diffusion on diffusion-weighted imaging (DWI).

CT

CT is limited in assessment and may demonstrate an enlarged muscle with low attenuation cystic lesion with rim enhancement.

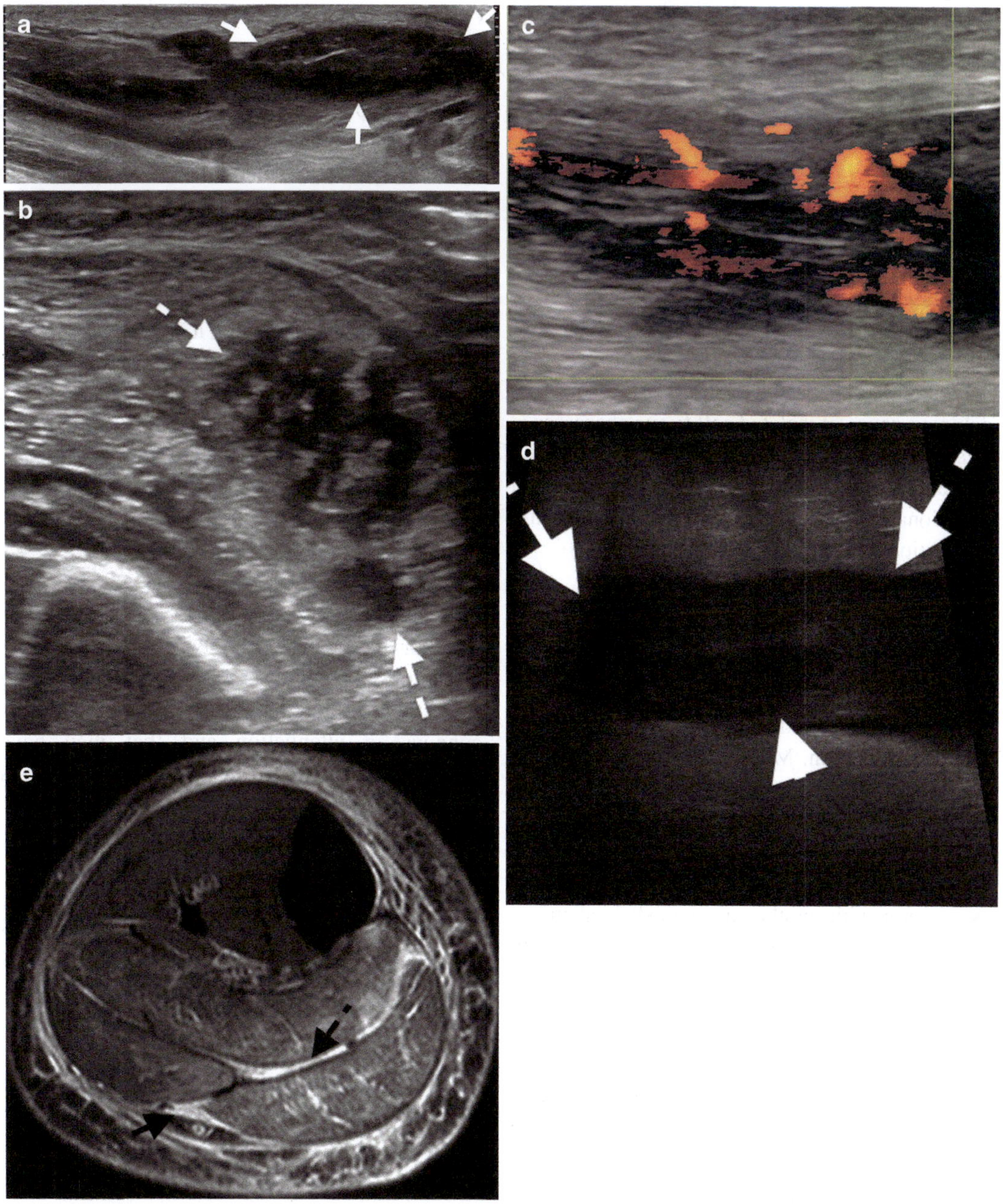

Fig. 13.7 (**a**–**c**) A 30-year-old female drug abuser with intramuscular abscess (*arrows*) and surrounding myositis of the right biceps with increased peripheral flow on power Doppler (**c**), (**d**) superficially infected intramuscular collection and abscess in a 68-year-old female post hip transplant on the longitudinal ultrasound image with central cystic component (*arrowhead*) and surrounding ill-defined muscle (*myositis/arrows*), (**e**) a 28-year-old female with group A streptococcus septicemia and calf pain, axial T2FS MRI image of the mid-calf demonstrates extensive muscular edema and fascial fluid (*black arrow*), extensive subcutaneous edema in keeping with cellulitis

Nuclear Medicine

Use of indium-labeled white cells can localize sites of infection but incurs a significant radiation dose and is not commonly used if nonionizing modalities are available.

Differential diagnosis in diabetic patients includes muscle infarction, usually occurring in poorly controlled diabetics.

Abscess

Overview

Abscesses can occur in conjunction with any of the musculoskeletal soft tissue infections. It is a collection of purulent material that becomes walled off from adjacent healthy tissue. The most common cause of isolated soft tissue abscesses is *Staphylococcus aureus*, though abscesses can be caused by many different pyogenic bacteria, and occasionally other organisms such as fungi, and in addition can be polymicrobial.

Clinical Presentation

The presentation of an abscess is dependent on site of infection and extent of associated surrounding infection. Most present with pain, and if the abscess is superficial, it may be palpated as a fluctuant mass. There can be surface erythema and warmth. Spontaneous drainage from the abscess can occur. If the abscess is occurring in association with another musculoskeletal infection, e.g., osteomyelitis and pyomyositis, then the features of the associated infection may dominate the clinical picture. The important issue arising with abscesses is that treatment almost always requires drainage of the abscess, either percutaneously, with the aid of imaging techniques such as ultrasound or CT, or surgically. Treatment of an abscess is dependent on the extent of associated soft tissue infection.

Imaging

Ultrasound (Fig. 13.7a–d)

Abscesses are seen on ultrasound as a well-demarcated walled-off collection that can demonstrate either increased or decreased echogenicity with respect to the surrounding tissue. There can be internal echoes seen due to necrotic debris. Septa or loculations may be seen as thin or thick bands of tissue transversing the abscess. Compression of the abscess with the probe can cause visible "swirling" of the purulent material. Power Doppler usually shows hyperemia of the walls and surrounding inflamed tissue. The real-time feature of ultrasound makes it well suited to guide abscess drainage.

MRI (Figs. 13.4e and 13.7e)

An abscess is seen on MRI with low signal intensity on T1W images, though it can have a hyperintense rim. Fluid-sensitive sequences such as T2 will reveal a core of high signal intensity with a hypointense rim. The rim enhances post-gadolinium administration. Gas within the abscess can be best appreciated on gradient echo sequences as low SI foci. It may demonstrate restricted diffusion on diffusion-weighted imaging (DWI).

CT

MRI or ultrasound are the preferred imaging modalities. Abscesses are seen as rim-enhancing collections of fluid that may be somewhat heterogeneous in attenuation and that may have admixed air within the purulent material that is visible on CT scan.

Nuclear Medicine

Use of indium-labeled white cells can localize sites of infection but incurs a significant radiation dose and is not commonly used if nonionizing modalities are available.

Necrotizing Fasciitis

Overview

Necrotizing fasciitis is an infection of the subcutaneous tissue and fascia that spares the underlying muscle. It can be a rapidly progressive disorder that can be limb- or life-threatening unless rapidly recognized and treated. Patients may have a history of minor trauma or skin abrasion. It is polymicrobial in more than 60 % of cases, and of the monomicrobial cases, *Streptococcus* species are the most common, particularly group A streptococcus; toxic shock syndrome commonly coexists.

Clinical Presentation

The extremities, the perineum, and truncal areas are all common sites for necrotizing fasciitis. The classic presentation is regional pain out of proportion to local findings on clinical examination, and a high index of suspicion is required for diagnosis. If diagnosis and treatment are delayed, the skin can progress from normal appearance to ill-defined erythema and edema, then to dusky blue discoloration, and finally to tissue necrosis. Bullous formation, with subsequent hemorrhage, can follow. During this period the patient will inevitably be exhibiting signs of severe sepsis and likely progress to septic shock. Most patients are very ill with evidence of multiple organ toxicity on laboratory investigations. Leukocytosis is invariably present, with elevation of inflammatory markers and often elevation of creatine kinase (CK) and lactate. Necrotizing fasciitis is a medical and surgical emergency requiring prompt surgical debridement, decompressive fasciotomy, and IV antibiotics.

Imaging

Radiographs (Fig. 13.8)

Radiographs in necrotizing fasciitis can show obliteration of the deep fat planes and soft tissue swelling. Most important, however, is the finding

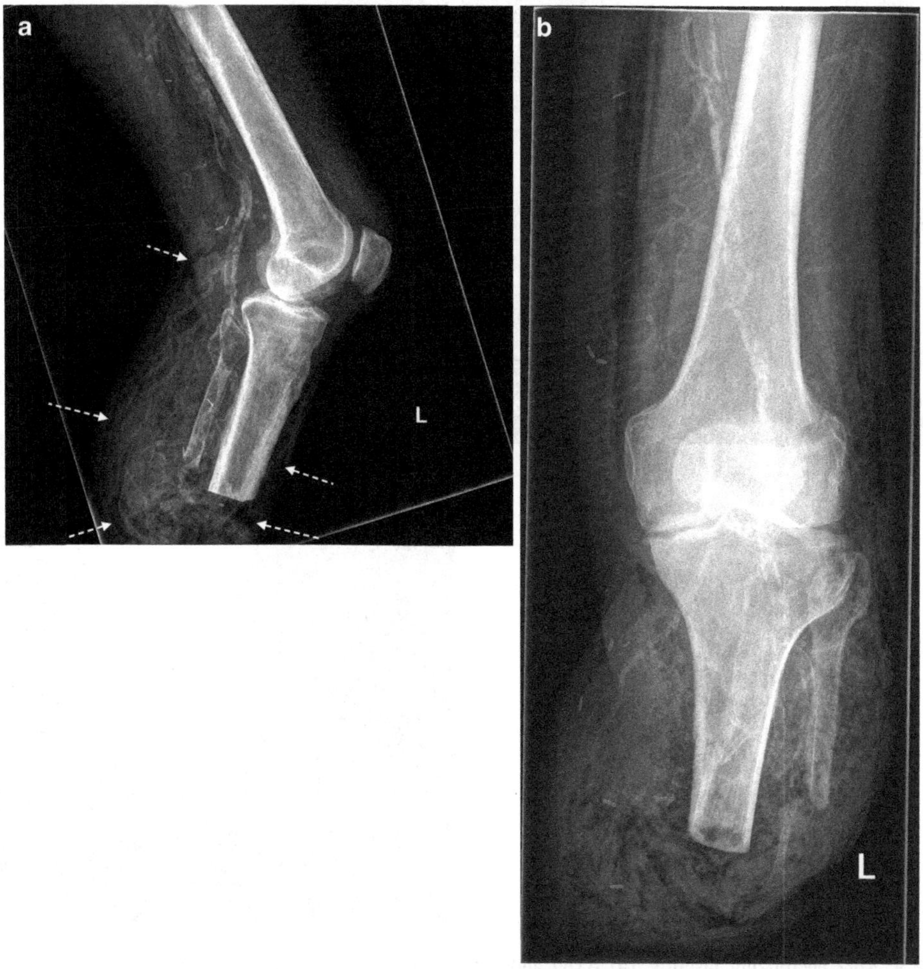

Fig. 13.8 A 78-year-old male diabetic with below-the-knee amputation. (**a**) Lateral and (**b**) AP radiographs demonstrate extensive soft tissue air with proximal extension along expected fascial planes (*dashed arrows*) in keeping with clinical diagnosis of necrotizing fasciitis

of gas in the tissues, which should make the viewer very suspicious of an infectious process. This finding demands immediate attention.

MRI (Fig. 13.9)

On MRI, there is abnormal T2W hyperintensity in the deep subcutaneous tissue adjacent to the fascial planes, with fluid collections. Fluid can be seen tracking within the intermuscular fascial planes, hyperintense on T2W, hypointense on T1W, and non-enhancing with gadolinium, consistent with necrotic tissue. Gas within the deep tissues can be best visualized on gradient echo sequences.

CT

CT is the most sensitive modality for the presence of gas in the tissues. Gas appears as very low attenuation in the deep subcutaneous region adjacent to the fascia. The fascia itself can also be seen as thickened. In addition there is involvement of the deeper fascia and muscles, not seen with cellulitis. When IV contrast is used, the fascia is non-enhancing due to necrosis. Assessment of deep soft tissue necrosis is limited in comparison to MRI. Overlying cellulitis is seen as edema in the soft tissues, which on CT has the appearance of fat stranding with increased attenuation.

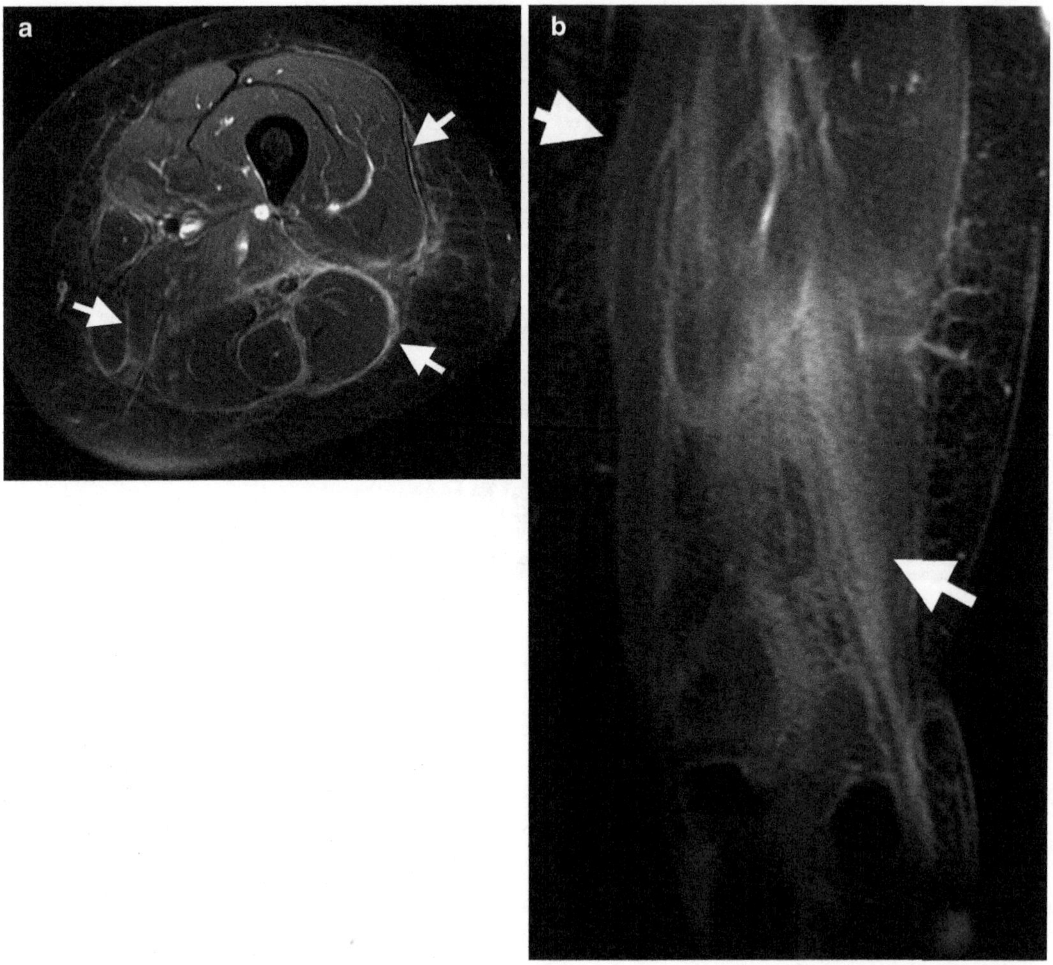

Fig. 13.9 MRI necrotizing fasciitis. (**a**) Axial and (**b**) Cor T2FS demonstrating extensive deep and interfascial thickening of high signal of the left thigh (*arrows*). No further sequences were acquired as the patient proceeded to emergency surgery

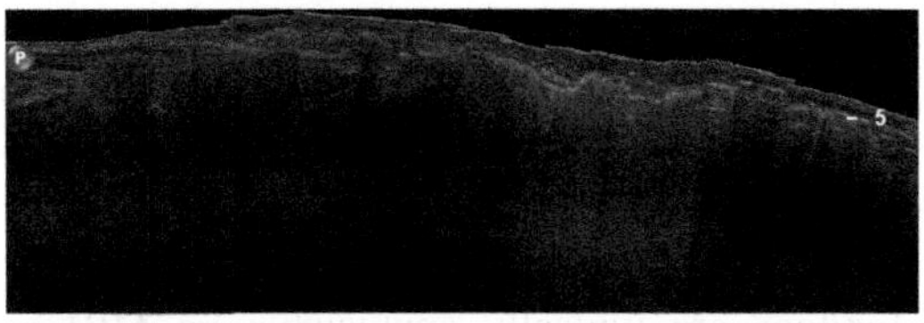

Fig. 13.10 Ultrasound of the calf in a patient with soft tissue swelling demonstrates extensive fascial hyperechogenicity with posterior dirty shadowing in keeping with fascial air and necrotizing fasciitis. Ultrasound is not routinely performed for NF. Findings were confirmed on radiograph prior to surgery

Ultrasound (Fig. 13.10)

Ultrasound does not have a primary role in the detection of necrotizing fasciitis. If performed in this setting, air within the soft tissues can be seen as echogenic foci with posterior ill-defined shadowing, known as "dirty shadowing." Subcutaneous and fascial edemas may be seen. MRI, CT, and radiography are preferred to ultrasound for this condition.

Nuclear Medicine

Bone scanning is not indicated in necrotizing fasciitis.

Infectious Tenosynovitis

Overview

Infectious tenosynovitis refers to infection of the synovial sheath surrounding the tendon with buildup of purulent material in the potential space between the visceral and parietal layers of tendons. Infection of a tendon sheath can spread between sheaths as well as to adjacent bursae. Tenosynovitis can result from direct inoculation from a puncture wound, contiguous spread from adjacent infections, or hematogenous spread. The organisms involved thus depend on the mode of infection. Infections resulting from direct inoculation are most commonly infected with gram-positive skin flora such as staphylococcal or streptococcal species; however, depending on the source of the inoculum, other organisms may be implicated, and infections may be polymicrobial. Infections such as these typically present acutely, with swelling along the tendon sheath; pain, particularly with stretching of the tendon sheath; and often erythema.

Subacute infections present similarly, though are more indolent. Mycobacterial infections or fungi such as *Sporothrix* are examples of implicated pathogens. Hematogenous spread can present either acutely or indolently. One common cause of hematogenous infectious tenosynovitis is *Neisseria gonorrhoeae*, though other neisserial species or mycobacteria have been implicated. Aspiration of fluid from the tenosynovial sheath is key to determining the offending organism and guiding antibiotic choice. Surgical intervention, comprising tendon sheath irrigation +/– debridement, is a main component of therapy and is necessary to gain source control.

Imaging

The imaging findings of tenosynovitis have already been reviewed in Chap. 3 Imaging cannot clearly differentiate between infectious and non-infectious tenosynovitis, but associated findings including clinical history, skin laceration, retained foreign body, and adjacent soft tissue or joint infection make infectious tenosynovitis more likely. Aspiration is required for confirmation and culture.

Radiographs

Plain radiographs typically reveal overlying soft tissue swelling and can see surface lacerations. It is minimally helpful in the evaluation of infectious tenosynovitis except in the circumstance of a necrotizing infection when gas in the tissues can be appreciated.

Ultrasound (Fig. 13.11)

In infected tenosynovitis it is predominantly the tendon sheath that is involved early in the course of the infection. The enclosed tendon, when involved, may appear enlarged but otherwise normal and can lose its normal fibrillar pattern and appear hyperechoic. The tendon sheath distends with fluid, typically heterogeneous with mixed hyperechoic and hypoechoic foci. There

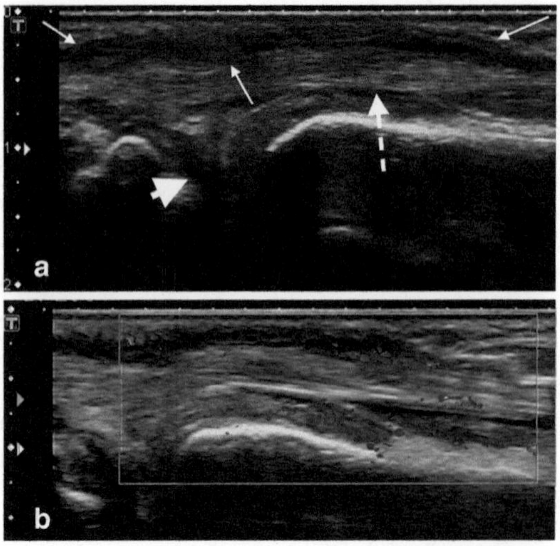

Fig. 13.11 Longitudinal ultrasound of infected tenosynovitis (*arrows*) and tendinosis of the extensor carpi ulnaris (*dashed arrow*) and small joint effusion (*arrowhead*), the same patient as in Fig. 13.2, without (**a**) and with (**b**) color Doppler. Note the heterogeneous tendon sheath distension and increased internal flow on Doppler. Note that ultrasound can only demonstrate an active inflammatory process and clinical correlation, and joint aspiration is required for diagnosis

is thickening of the sheath itself. On Doppler there is increased vascular flow within the sheath at sites of synovitis though not within the fluid. In general, the amount of fluid within the tendon sheath correlates with severity of infection. The ultrasound findings do not differentiate infectious from inflammatory tenosynovitis; thus, aspiration and culture of fluid are required in the appropriate clinical circumstances. Aspiration could be performed using ultrasound guidance.

Ultrasound is very sensitive in the assessment of retained foreign bodies including those not visible on radiographs such as glass and wood. Foreign bodies are hyperechoic with surrounding hypoechoic rim of granulation and fibrotic tissue. There is posterior shadowing (wood) and reverberation artifact.

CT

CT is usually not indicated for imaging infectious tenosynovitis. In infectious tenosynovitis, tendons can appear thickened and indistinct. Fluid distending the tendon sheath can be appreciable, with variable enhancement. Gas in the tissues is best seen on CT.

MRI (Fig. 13.12)

Tendons are typically appreciable on MRI as well-demarcated areas of low signal intensity, with no or minimal fluid within the tendon sheath. In infectious tenosynovitis, fluid distending the tendon sheath can be readily identified as hypointense signal on T1W images and hyperintense signal on T2W images. The synovial lining of the tendon can be thickened. The tendon loses its low intensity signal and becomes ill defined. The tendon sheath frequently shows enhancement with gadolinium, though the purulent fluid within the sheath does not.

Cellulitis

Overview

Infection of the dermis and superficial subcutaneous tissues is termed cellulitis. It typically occurs after a break in the skin allows bacteria to bypass the natural barrier that skin provides. The most commonly associated organisms are beta-hemolytic streptococcal species and *Staphylococcus aureus*; however, many other bacteria such as gram-negative enterics, anaerobic bacteria, and other organisms can cause cellulitis.

Clinical Presentation

Patients typically present with pain, erythema, and warmth at the site of cellulitis. The lower limb is the most common site of involvement. Lymphangitis and lymphadenopathy of regional lymph nodes are common. The patient may be febrile but only very rarely exhibits signs of systemic toxicity. In patients with systemic toxicity, a thorough search should be undertaken to look for deeper sites or alternative sources for infection. Laboratory investigations typically show leukocytosis. Blood cultures are infrequently positive (<5 % of cases), and treatment is typically

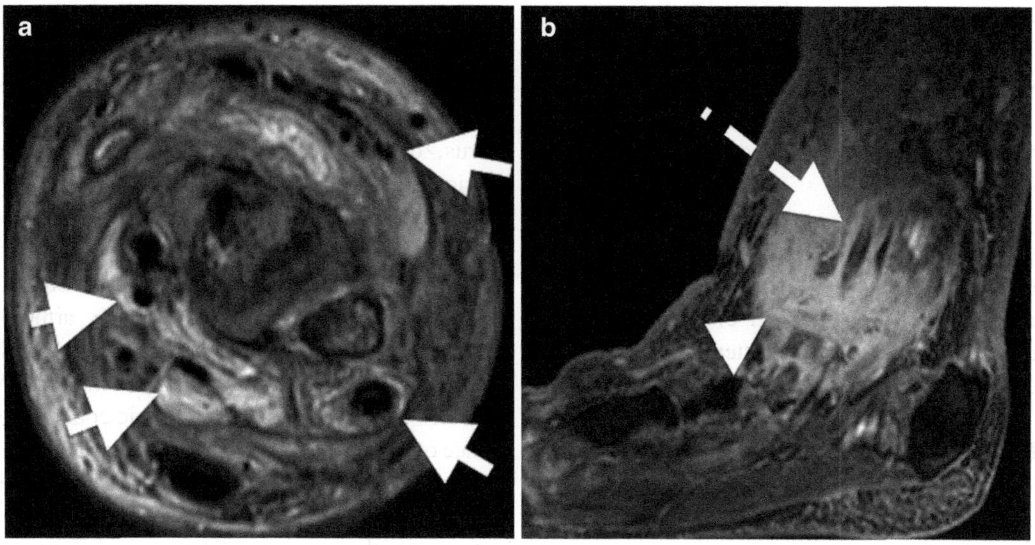

Fig. 13.12 MRI of the infected tenosynovitis, (**a**) axial T2FS and (**b**) Sag T1FS PG demonstrate extensive fluid SI distension of the tendon sheaths proximal to the ankle (*arrows*) in (**a**) and post-gadolinium enhancement (*dashed arrow*) in (**b**) with surrounding soft tissue enhancement (*arrowhead*). Patient also had septic arthritis of the ankle and osteomyelitis of the tibia

initiated empirically with antibiotics that cover the common offending organisms. Most patients can be treated with oral antibiotics; however, if there are signs of systemic toxicity or rapid progression, then IV antibiotics should be considered. Elevation of the affected limb and maintenance of skin hydration to avoid cracking of the skin are also important.

Cellulitis is a clinical diagnosis, but occasionally radiological methods are employed to rule out potential complications of the infection, such as abscess formation, or extension to deeper structures. In addition, cellulitis can be caused by foreign bodies that may be retained, and imaging can be helpful to identify these objects.

Imaging

Radiographs

Plain radiographs in cellulitis will show nonspecific soft tissue swelling.

Ultrasound (Fig. 13.13)

Cellulitis can be seen on ultrasound as edema of the subcutaneous tissues, which can manifest in

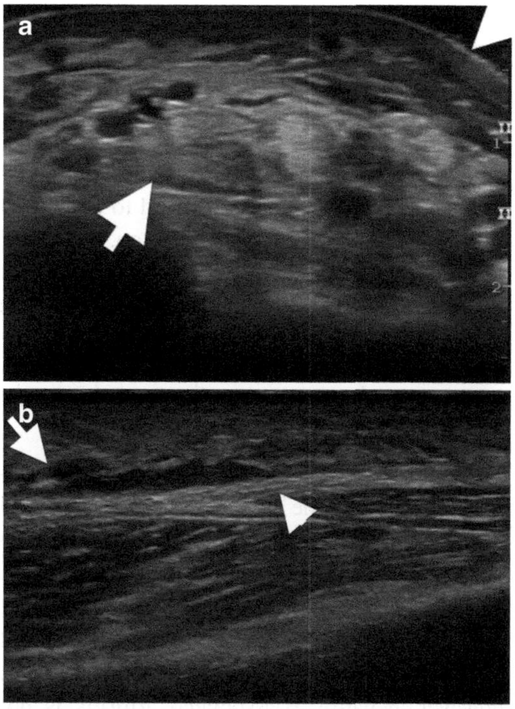

Fig. 13.13 (**a**) Ultrasound in a patient with lower-limb cellulitis with subcutaneous thickening of heterogeneous echotexture. Doppler, not shown, would demonstrate increased flow. (**b**) A 73-year-old female presenting with superficial peroneal nerve (SPN) symptoms and panniculitis (*arrow*) on ultrasound with irritation underlying SPN (*arrowhead*)

several ways: by diffuse thickening and increased echogenicity of the subcutaneous tissue or by the visualization of hypoechoic strands in between areas of hyperechoic fat – this can appear as a "cobblestone" pattern. Power Doppler can show hyperemia.

CT

CT reveals changes of skin thickening, septation of the underlying fat, and evidence of fascial thickening, with increased attenuation of the subcutaneous tissues in cellulitis.

MRI (Figs. 13.4, 13.5, 13.6, and 13.7)

Cellulitis is characterized by the findings of hypointensity on T1W images in the affected superficial subcutaneous tissue, enhancement on post-gadolinium T1W images, and hyperintensity on T2W images. No deep fascial or soft tissue involvement is present in isolated cellulitis.

Infection-Related Arthropathy

Some infections are associated with inflammatory arthritis without evidence of direct inoculation of the joints and are presumed to be caused by an immune-mediated phenomenon. Examples of such infections are those caused by hepatitis B and C virus, human immunodeficiency virus (HIV), as well as many other common viruses or those that may be seen as sequelae of particular bacterial infections such as in rheumatic fever and subacute bacterial endocarditis.

Hepatitis B and C are thought to cause inflammatory arthritis due to the deposition of viral products and immune complexes and the development of cryoglobulins within the synovium. Hepatitis B virus typically results in a small joint polyarthritis. Evidence of synovitis with joint effusion can be seen on ultrasound, CT, and MRI; however, hepatitis B-associated arthritis is not associated with erosive change or joint destruction. Hepatitis C virus can result in either a small joint polyarthritis or an oligoarthritis.

Many other viruses can result in arthralgia, arthritis, or tenosynovitis. Typically they are self-limiting and do not lead to erosive change or permanent joint sequelae. There are many examples of these viruses, such as parvovirus B19, alphaviruses, rubella virus, coxsackievirus, echovirus, mumps virus, dengue virus, and the herpes viruses varicella virus, cytomegalovirus, herpes simplex virus, and Epstein-Barr virus.

HIV infection can lead to a variety of different articular syndromes. Patients can demonstrate a self-limited oligoarticular lower-limb arthritis, though they can also develop a reactive arthritis that is similar to reactive arthritis seen in non-HIV infected patients with a more chronic course, presence of enthesopathy and tenosynovitis, and HLA B27 positivity. The self-limited oligoarthritis typically is managed with NSAIDs and supportive care, while the reactive arthritis typically requires more chronic management, with DMARDs or other therapy as in non-HIV infected patients. Patients with HIV also suffer from arthritic conditions such as psoriatic arthritis, rheumatoid arthritis, and systemic lupus erythematosus, often to a greater severity than seen in patients without HIV infection. Radiological manifestations of these conditions are similar to those in the non-HIV infected populations. Due to immunosuppression in HIV, patients are more prone to developing the wide range of musculoskeletal infections as outlined in this chapter including septic arthritis, osteomyelitis, and soft tissue abscesses.

Rheumatic fever is an immune-mediated syndrome occurring post streptococcal infection, with cardinal manifestations including inflammatory arthritis, chorea, subcutaneous nodules, erythema marginatum rash, and carditis that can lead to chronic valvular damage. The arthritis of rheumatic fever is typically a migratory oligoarthritis with severely painful joint swelling and loss of range of motion lasting 24–48 h and responding to aspirin. It is an acute arthritis with resolution without joint damage.

Subacute bacterial endocarditis can lead to an immune-mediated oligo- or polyarthritis as an immune-mediated phenomenon, possibly due to immune complex deposition in the synovium. This type of arthritis is nonerosive and nondeforming. Importantly, however, one must always have a high index of suspicion for septic arthritis in the setting of bacterial endocarditis, and joints should be aspirated for culture of organisms. Bacterial endocarditis is also associated with vertebral osteomyelitis. Radiological findings in these conditions are similar to those outlined in the sections entitled "Septic arthritis" and "Osteomyelitis."

Further Reading

1. Adhikari S, Blaivas M. Sonography first for subcutaneous abscess and cellulitis evaluation. J Ultrasound Med. 2012;31:1509–12.
2. Bancroft L. MR imaging of infectious processes of the knee. Radio Clin North Am. 2007;45:931–41.
3. Chou H, Teo H, Dubey N, Peh W. Tropical pyomyositis and necrotizing fasciitis. Semin Musculoskelet Radiol. 2011;15:489–505.
4. Delport A, Long S. Ultrasound of musculoskeletal infection. Semin Musculoskelet Radiol. 2011;26: 290–4.
5. Fayad L, Carrino J, Fishman E. Musculoskeletal infection: role of CT in the emergency department. Radiographics. 2007;27:1723–36. Hatzenbuehler J, Pulling T. Diagnosis and management of osteomyelitis. Am Fam Physician. 2011;84:1027–33.
6. Palestro C, Love C, Miller T. Imaging of musculoskeletal infections. Best Pract Res Clin Rheumatol. 2006;20:1197–218.
7. Pineda C, Espinosa R, Pena A. Radiographic imaging in osteomyelitis: the role of plain radiography, computed tomography, ultrasonography, magnetic resonance imaging, and scintigraphy. Semin Plast Surg. 2009;23:80–9.
8. Pineda C, Vargas A, Rodriguez A. Imaging of osteomyelitis: current concepts. Infect Dis Clin North Am. 2006;20:789–825.
9. Sanverdi S, Ergen F, Oznur A. Current challenges in imaging of the diabetic foot. Diabet Foot Ankle. 2012;3. doi:10.3402/dfa.v3i0.18754.
10. Sawlani V, Chandra T, Mishra R, Aggarwal A, Jain U, Gujral R. MRI features of tuberculosis of peripheral joints. Clin Radiol. 2003;58:755–62.
11. Toledano T, Fatone E, Weis A, Cotten A, Beltran J. MRI evaluation of bone marrow changes in the diabetic foot: a practical approach. Semin Musculoskelet Radiol. 2011;15:257–68.
12. Turecki M, Taljanovic M, Stubbs A, Graham A, Holden D, Hunter T, Rogers L. Imaging of musculoskeletal soft tissue infections. Skeletal Radiol. 2010;39:957–71.
13. Yu J, Habib P. MR imaging of urgent inflammatory and infectious conditions affecting the soft tissues of the musculoskeletal system. Emerg Radiol. 2009;16: 267–76.
14. Goldenberg, DL, Sexton DJ. Septic Arthritis. In: UpToDate, Sexton, DJ. (Ed), UpToDate, Waltham, MA. (Accessed April 2014).
15. Lalani T, Overview of Osteomyelitis in Adults. In: UpToDate, Sexton, DJ. (Ed), UpToDate, Waltham, MA. (Accessed April 2014).
16. Baddour, LM, Keerasuntornpong, A. Pyomyositis. In: UpToDate, Sexton, DJ. (Ed), UpToDate, Waltham, MA. (Accessed April 2014).

14 The Diabetic Foot

Kimberly J. Legault and John O'Neill

Diabetes mellitus can adversely affect the musculoskeletal system in a variety of ways. One of the more common complications that arise as a result of long-standing or poorly controlled diabetes is the "diabetic foot". The diabetic foot is an umbrella term for a spectrum of different pathologies affecting the foot in diabetes patients, including neuropathic arthropathy and infection, with each process either existing in isolation or in conjunction with others at any given time.

Pathogenesis of neuropathic arthropathy includes the neurotraumatic and neurovascular theories. Diabetes, particularly in long-standing disease, can have a significant impact upon the vasculature, with blockage and/or obliteration of both small and large peripheral vessels, leading to chronic tissue ischemia of the periphery, especially the feet. The vasa nervorum of the peripheral nerves also becomes ischemic, leading to small-fibre, predominantly sensory, peripheral neuropathy. The patient loses proprioception and the ability to sense and respond to trauma (neurotraumatic). Recurrent episodes of microtrauma to the desensitized joint play a major role in the development of the neuropathic joint (neurotraumatic). Bone, cartilage, ligamentous and tendon injuries occur. Motor fibres are involved with subsequent loss of muscle tone and function and can lead to joint instability and deformity. Altered vascular control may lead to hyperaemia, secondary bone resorption and weakening of subchondral bone (neurovascular). Autonomic involvement often presents as areas of dry skin and areas of fissures that predispose to ulceration.

Diabetic patients also have impaired immunity and are more susceptible to infections and thus can more readily develop secondary infections of the ulcers. Infection in the non-healing ulcers can penetrate into the deep tissues of the foot, and/or sinus tracts can develop. The sinus tracts tunnel between the skin and the underlying bone or joints, which can lead to osteomyelitis, septic arthritis and deep soft tissue infections. Ulcers occur at typical sites of bony prominences. In weight-bearing patients these include plantar aspects of the 4th and 5th metatarsal heads, tuft of great toe and at heel. Patients with rocker-bottom foot deformity develop ulceration under the fallen cuboid bone in the midfoot. Although the neuropathic joint is most commonly seen in chronic diabetic patients, it may also be seen in many conditions including the following pathologies: tabes dorsalis, congenital insensitivity to pain, spinal cord trauma, syringomyelia, meningomyelocele, alcoholism and amyloidosis.

The difficulty that both clinicians and radiologists face in managing these patients is in the identification of infections and distinguishing these from a neuropathic arthropathy. Both of

K.J. Legault, MD, FRCPC
Division of Rheumatology, Department of Medicine, McMaster University, Hamilton, ON, Canada
e-mail: kimberly.legault@medportal.ca

J. O'Neill, MB, BAO, BCh, MRCPI, MSc, FRCR (✉)
Associate Professor, Musculoskeletal Imaging, Diagnostic Imaging, McMaster University/St Joseph's Healthcare, Hamilton, ON L8N4A6, Canada
e-mail: joneill2@me.com

J. O'Neill (ed.), *Essential Imaging in Rheumatology*,
DOI 10.1007/978-1-4939-1673-3_14, © Springer Science+Business Media New York 2015

these phenomena can exist concurrently, which further complicates the picture and makes distinguishing between them difficult.

Neuropathic Arthropathy (Charcot Joint)

Isolated neuropathic arthropathy appears to occur due to repeated trauma and posttraumatic skeletal inflammation. It can present as an indolent process or as an acutely swollen, red, hot joint, thus mimicking a septic joint. Given the pain insensitivity due to peripheral neuropathy, the patient typically continues to weight-bear on the acutely inflamed joint, which then leads to trabecular microfractures and subsequent bone and joint damage with loss of the normal architecture and deformity. The management of an acute Charcot joint requires an attempt at early diagnosis through education and screening of patients by healthcare professionals and immediate total offloading of the affected joint to prevent further damage and to promote healing. This can be accomplished through the use of modified or specialty footwear.

Imaging can be helpful both in confirming a Charcot joint and in differentiating it from an infectious arthropathy. This section will focus on the findings of a Charcot joint. The following session discusses the imaging of infectious arthropathies in diabetes and will offer strategies on differentiating these from neuropathic arthropathies.

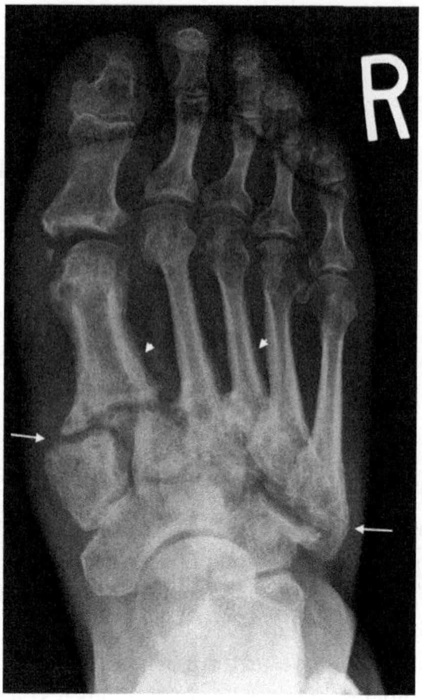

Fig. 14.1 AP foot radiograph in a 67-year-old female diabetic with long-standing foot problems. There is a homolateral Lisfranc fracture dislocation (*arrows*, the first to fifth metatarsals are dislocated laterally at the TMT joints with associated fractures), there is increased sclerosis, and there is periosteal reaction along the lateral proximal and mid-diaphysis of the first and third metatarsals (*arrowheads*). The first MTPJ is widened, bony destruction with periarticular erosions and intra-articular debris

Imaging

Several patterns of neuropathic arthropathy can occur and include atrophic, hypertrophic and mixed. In the atrophic form there is a dominance of bone resorption, whereas in the hypertrophic form, there is a dominance of new bone formation with large osteophytes, sclerosis and joint destruction. The atrophic form is most commonly seen in non-weight-bearing joints and upper motor neuron pathology.

Initially joints may appear normal. Diffuse periarticular soft tissue swelling and joint effusions are present early in the disease. Subtle subluxation may be present. There is progressive joint deformity and destruction. In mid- and late-stage disease, the *6 D's* are present in variable degrees: *d*eformity, *d*estruction (of bone and joint), *d*ebris (intra-articular bone and cartilaginous bodies), *d*ensity (increased subchondral sclerosis), *d*islocation and *d*egeneration (changes of osteoarthritis/attempted repair).

For the purpose of interpreting radiographic findings, the progression of neuropathic arthropathy has been classified into three stages by Eichenholtz and later a preradiographic stage was added: Stage 0 represents the earliest symptoms where reactive osseous oedema can be seen on MRI, while plain radiographs remain normal. In Stage 1 there is acute arthropathy with bone dissolution, Stage 2 represents the early repair phase (coalescence), and Stage 3 represents the chronic healing phase (remodelling). This staging is not commonly used in clinical practice but is useful in understanding the progression of a Charcot joint.

Radiographs (Figs. 14.1 and 14.2)

In Stage 0, radiographs are typically normal; however it may demonstrate joint space widening.

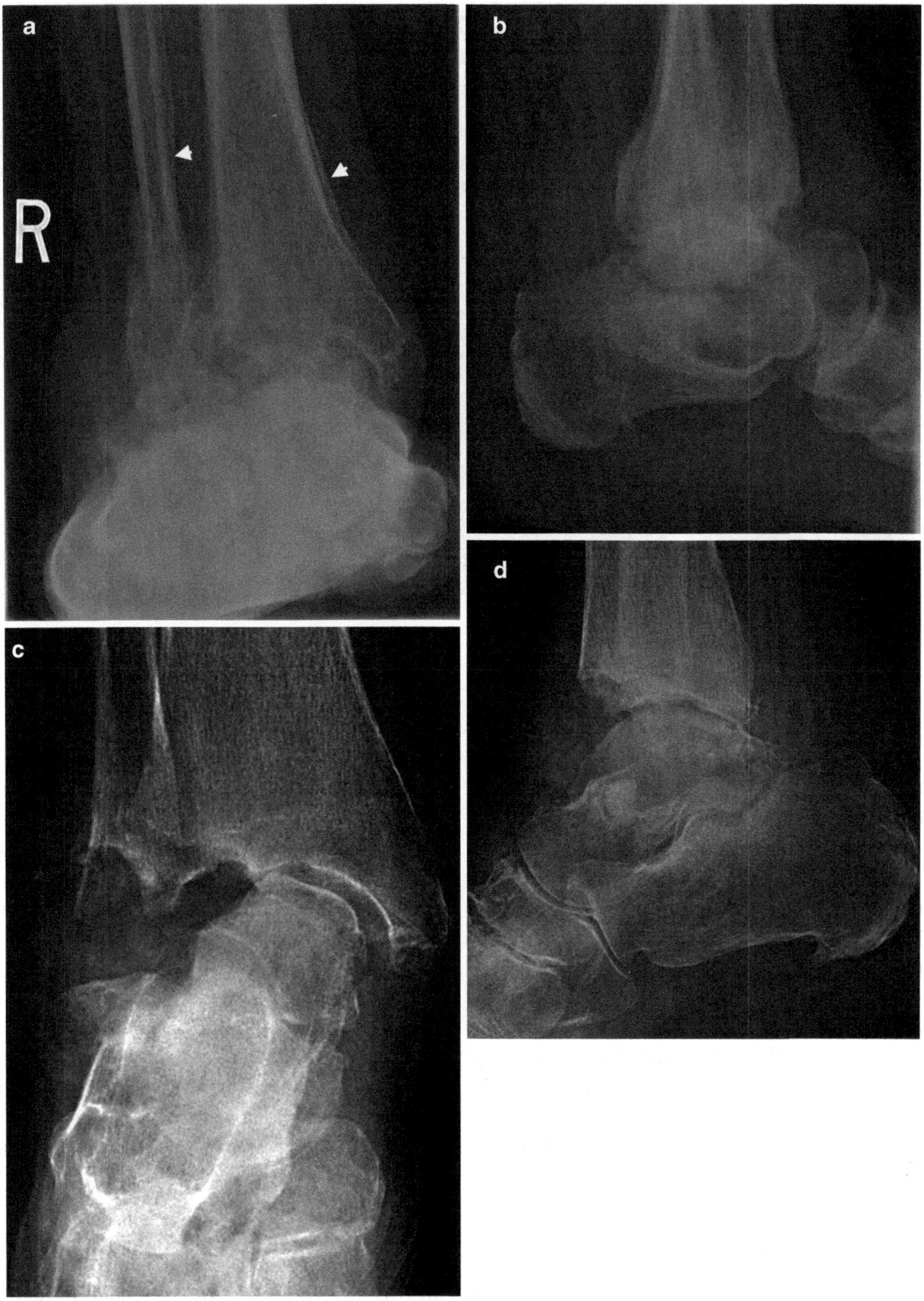

Fig. 14.2 A 55-year-old male diabetic with neuropathic arthropathy of the ankle joint. (**a**) AP and (**b**) lat radiographs demonstrate complete joint space loss, large joint effusion, destruction with partial collapse talar dome, extensive erosions tibia, sclerosis, internal debris, osteophytosis and chronic periosteal reaction (*arrowheads*) of the tibia and fibula. No soft tissue ulceration identifiable (**c**, **d**) in different patients with less advanced secondary degenerative change. (**e**, **f**) Sag reformatted CT on bone windows in a different patient demonstrates exuberant new bone formation post-ankle joint fusion which is seen in hypertrophic neuropathic joints

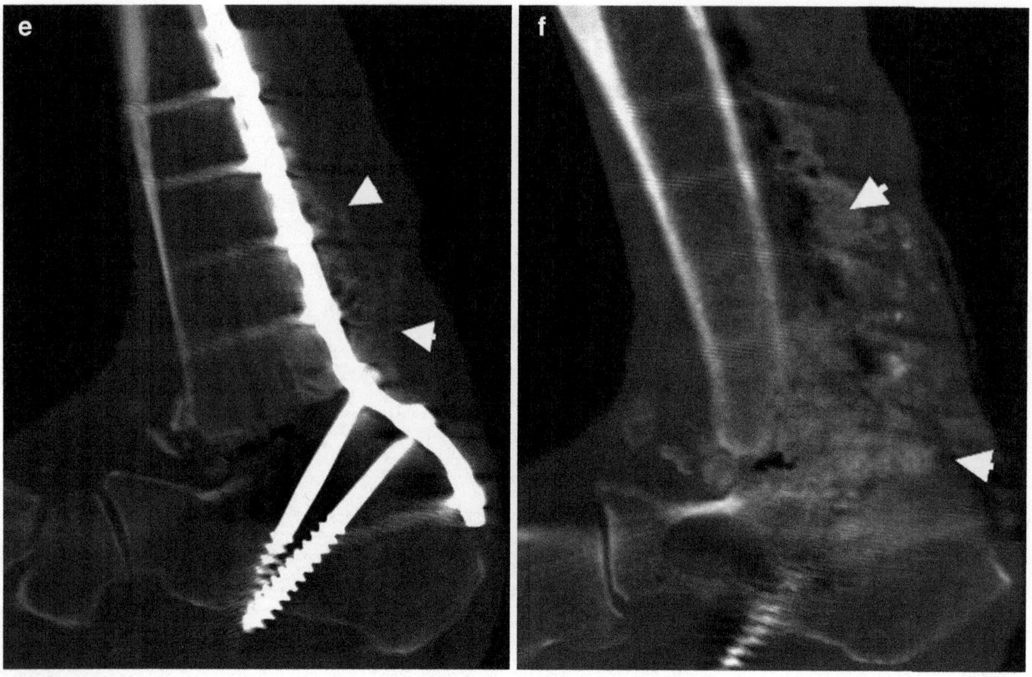

Fig. 14.2 (continued)

Radiographs of Stage 1 can show demineralization of the bone and findings of bone damage including fragmentation, disorganization, subluxations or osteoarthrosis with subchondral cystic changes. In Stage 2 there is evidence of healing with callus formation, reabsorption of bony fragments and debris and bony remineralization. Persistent changes of subluxations and bone deformity are often present. These changes also carry into Stage 3, though further rounding and smoothing of bony deformities are seen in this chronic healing stage, and bones can develop subsequent ankylosis and/or superimposed degenerative changes.

Magnetic Resonance Imaging (MRI) (Fig. 14.3)

The earliest finding in a neuropathic arthropathy on MRI is bone oedema, with hyperintensity on T2W imaging, often with visible trabecular stress fractures without cortical disruption, seen as hypointensities on T1W imaging. Joint effusion and cartilaginous damage or thinning can be seen. Soft tissue oedema is frequently visible as high signal intensity on T2W imaging of the soft tissues. There are periodically early deforming joint changes with subluxations, even prior to abnormalities on radiograph, though this is more prominent in the subsequent stages. Stage 1 changes encapsulate all of those seen in Stage 0 with progression of bony deformities and damage. In Stage 2, there tends to be improvement in the degree of bony and soft tissue oedema, with development of callus. In Stage 3, the acute oedematous changes have resolved, and persistent bony deformities and changes of osteoarthrosis are seen.

CT (Fig. 14.4)

CT will demonstrate similar bony and joint findings as described in MRI although it cannot assess bone marrow oedema and is limited in assessing the soft tissues. Occasionally CT will be acquired for a detailed bone assessment prior to surgery.

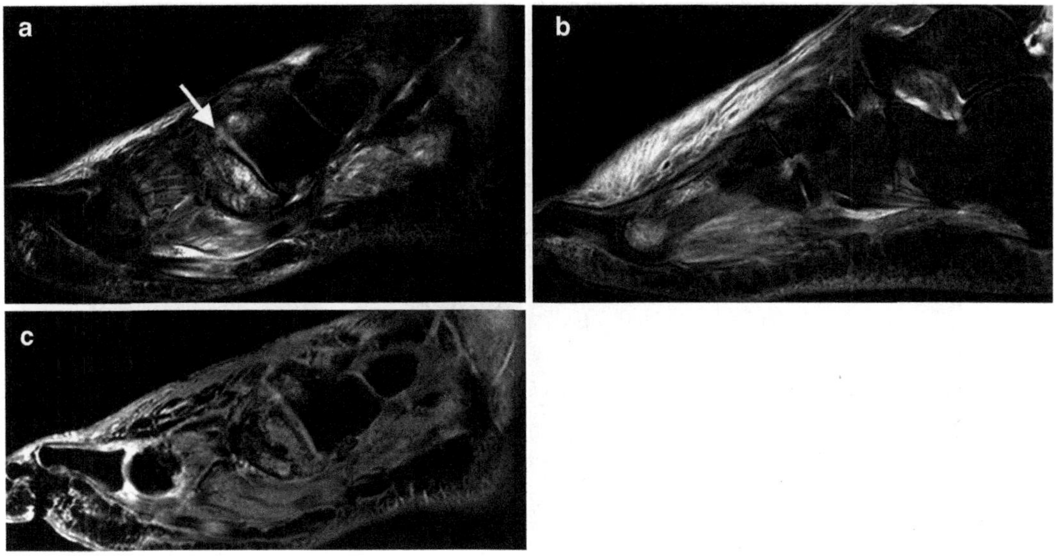

Fig. 14.3 A 44-year-old male diabetic with 6-month history of foot pain diagnosed with Charcot joint with fractures and diffuse soft tissue oedema and tenosynovitis. (**a**, **b**) Sag T2 FS of navicular-medial cuneiform (*arrow*) and 2nd MTPJ, respectively, with extensive bone marrow oedema, tenosynovitis, soft tissue and extensive dorsal subcutaneous oedema without soft tissue ulceration and (**c**) Sag T1FS PG demonstrate diffuse enhancement areas of oedema without evidence of soft tissue collections

Ultrasound (Fig. 14.5)
Ultrasound has a limited role. It is excellent in assessing related soft tissue pathology, excluding soft tissue collection and assessing joint effusions.

Nuclear Medicine
This has a limited role. The involved joint will demonstrate increased osteoblastic activity and increased uptake on bone scan, but this can be inferred from radiographic findings.

If successful treatment is initiated early, prior to the development of bony changes, the progression to later stages and subsequent permanent arthropathy and deformity can be avoided.

Diabetic Foot Infections

Given that the vast majority of diabetic foot infections occur as a result of direct inoculation of the affected site from skin barrier breakdown, the absence of an ulcer makes osteomyelitis or septic arthritis and a presentation of foot swelling and erythema in a patient with peripheral neuropathy and supportive radiographic findings is likely due to a neuropathic joint without superimposed infection. Clinically, infected ulcers appear as purulence of the ulcer with surrounding erythema. Those ulcers that are greater than 2 × 2 cm have a high likelihood of being complicated by underlying osteomyelitis. When the underlying bone is visible at the base of the ulcer or can be probed with a sterile instrument, osteomyelitis is almost certainly present.

Identification of an organism in a diabetic ulcer is best accomplished by culturing the tissue removed by curettage rather than merely swabbing the ulcer surface. The infections are most commonly due to gram-positive cocci; however they can be polymicrobial, and concurrent infection with gram-negative bacilli or anaerobic organisms is common. Treatment of diabetic foot infections is beyond the scope of this text; however some basic principles are outlined: All ulcers should receive appropriate wound care including mechanical offloading if possible. Antibiotics covering the cultured organisms, tailored to sensitivities, are the mainstay. Combination

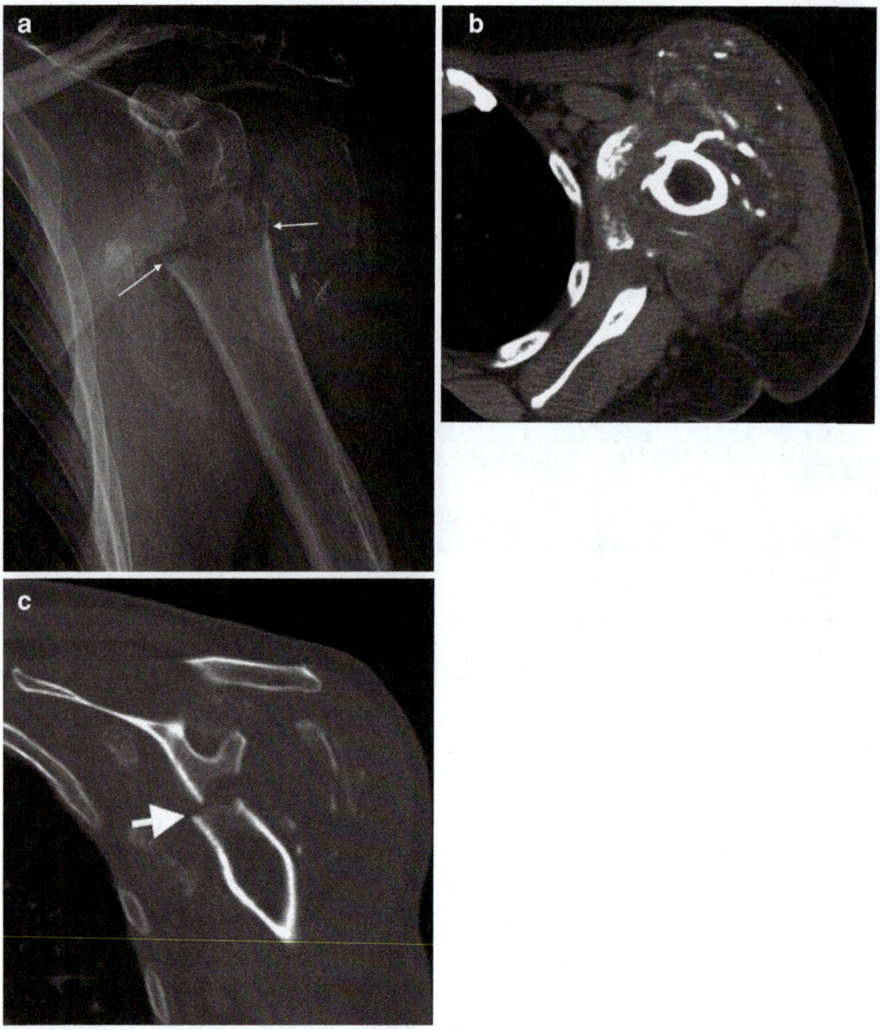

Fig. 14.4 Neuropathic arthropathy of the shoulder on (**a**) AP radiograph demonstrating diffuse soft tissue and joint swelling, multiple fractures with variable degree of osteolysis of bone fragments, bony debris, disorganization and dislocation without increased density in keeping with an atrophic neuropathic type joint. Note the straight transverse margin surgical neck humerus fracture (*arrows*); this is surgical like and should always raise possibility of a neuropathic joint when seen. (**b**) Axial soft tissue and (**c**) Cor reformatted on bone windows CT of the same joint demonstrating similar changes as described above

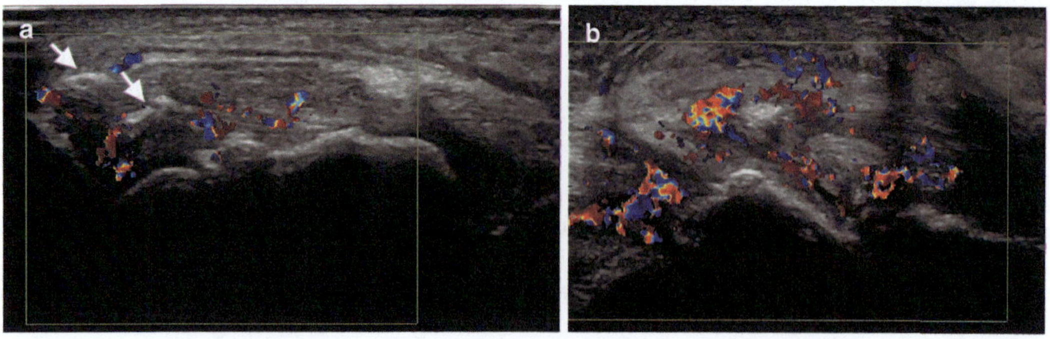

Fig. 14.5 Ultrasound of Charcot ankle joint demonstrating (**a**) increased internal flow on colour Doppler in keeping with active synovitis surrounding echogenic internal loose bodies (*arrows*) confirmed as avulsed bony fragments on radiographs (not shown) and (**b**) extensive periarticular tendinosis and tenosynovitis

antibiotic therapy may be required. Development of soft tissue infections and underlying osteomyelitis typically requires several weeks of intravenous antibiotics, with duration based on severity and patient response. Hyperbaric oxygen therapy has shown some benefit in non-healing ulcers. Surgery may be required in patients with severe infections, particularly those with significant vascular compromise, for removal of infected tissue or limb amputation if necessary.

Imaging can be helpful to assess for diabetic foot complications and in identification of osteomyelitis or septic arthritis and differentiating from an isolated neuropathic joint. MRI is particularly helpful in this regard; however other modalities can play a role as well. Osteomyelitis and septic arthritis are reviewed here. Cellulitis, abscesses and retained foreign bodies are reviewed in the chapter.

Imaging

Radiographs (Figs. 14.6 and 14.7)

Radiographs reveal predominantly major structural abnormalities of the bones of the foot. Both septic arthritis and neuropathic arthropathies can appear similar in this modality: Bony demineralization, disorganization, erosive change, bony fragmentation and joint narrowing and destruction can be present in both. Identification of superficial soft tissue deformity on radiograph

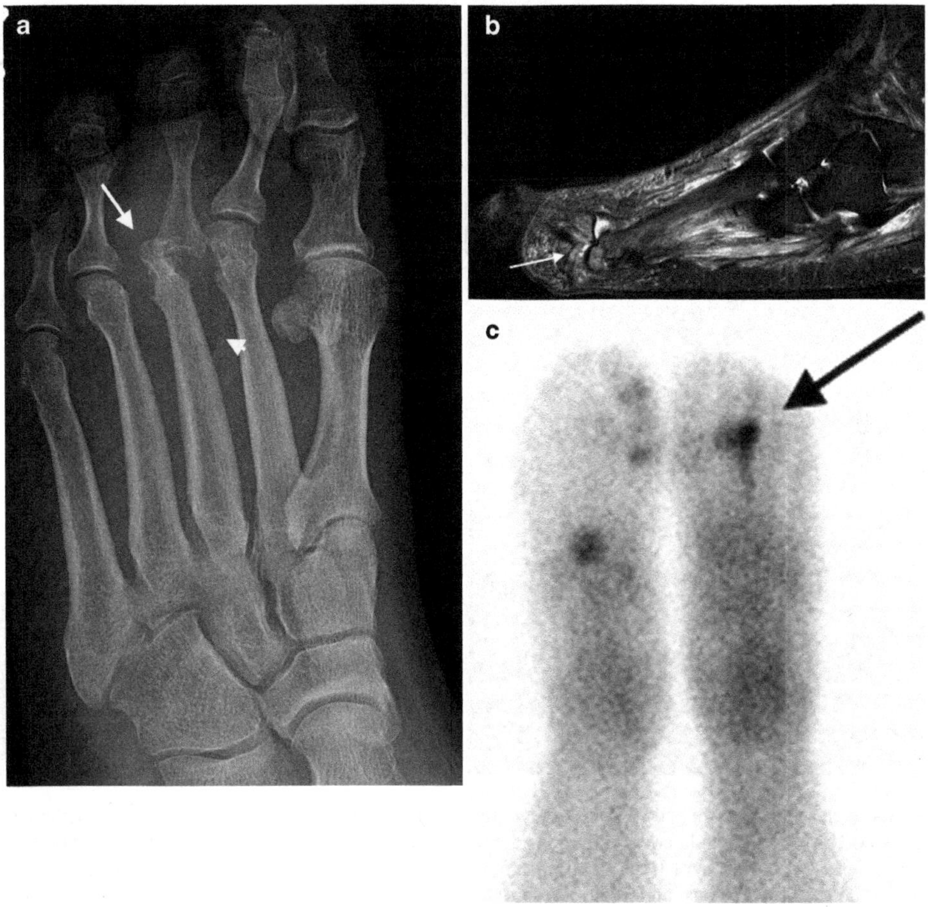

Fig. 14.6 Septic arthritis of the 3rd MTPJ in a 43-year-old male diabetic. (**a**) Oblique radiograph of the left foot demonstrates dislocation at the 3rd MTPJ (*arrow*) with erosions of the metatarsal head and diffuse soft tissue oedema. Note the mild vascular calcification (*arrowhead*). (**b**) Sag T1FS post-gadolinium in the same patient demonstrating enhancement within the joint and pericapsular and periarticular bone marrow oedema enhancement. (**c**) Delayed image from a bone scan, plantar view, demonstrating increased uptake at 3rd MTPJ (*arrow*) (also increased on flow and blood pool phases, not shown)

suggests ulceration. The underlying bone should be carefully assessed. There may be atrophy of the soft tissues at the site of ulceration. Gas produced from anaerobic infections can be appreciated in the tissues on radiographs. Periosteal reaction on the surface of bones may also be a helpful clue to osteomyelitis, particularly if soft tissue changes as described above are

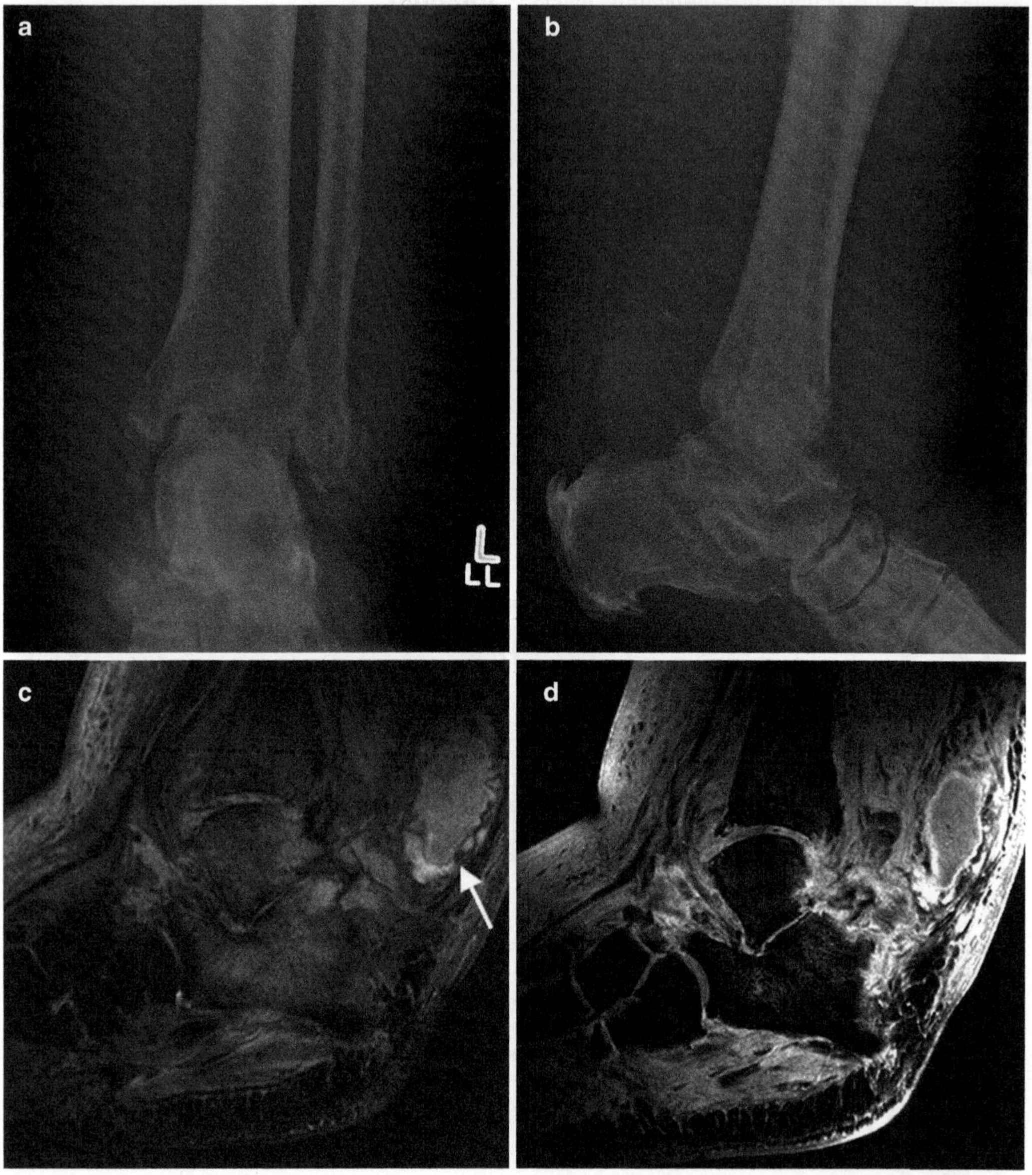

Fig. 14.7 A 61-year-old male diabetic with osteomyelitis of the left ankle. (**a**) AP and (**b**) lateral radiographs demonstrate joint effusion, diffuse soft tissue swelling, joint space loss with central erosions and multiple chronic (well corticated) avulsed bone fragments. (**c**) Mid-Sag T2FS MRI with extensive bone marrow oedema in the tibia, talus and calcaneus and ankle joint effusion communicating with a large collection in Kager's fat pad (*arrow*). (**d**) Sag T1FS post-gadolinium demonstrating diffuse soft tissue and ankle joint enhancement with rim enhancement collection posteriorly. (**e**) Lateral Sag T1FS PG demonstrating similar enhancement as in (**d**) but also demonstrates extensive erosions of the fibula (*arrowhead*) and infective tenosynovitis adjacent to the peroneal tendon sheaths with tendinosis. (**f**) Delayed bone scan image, AP view, with marked uptake at ankle joint

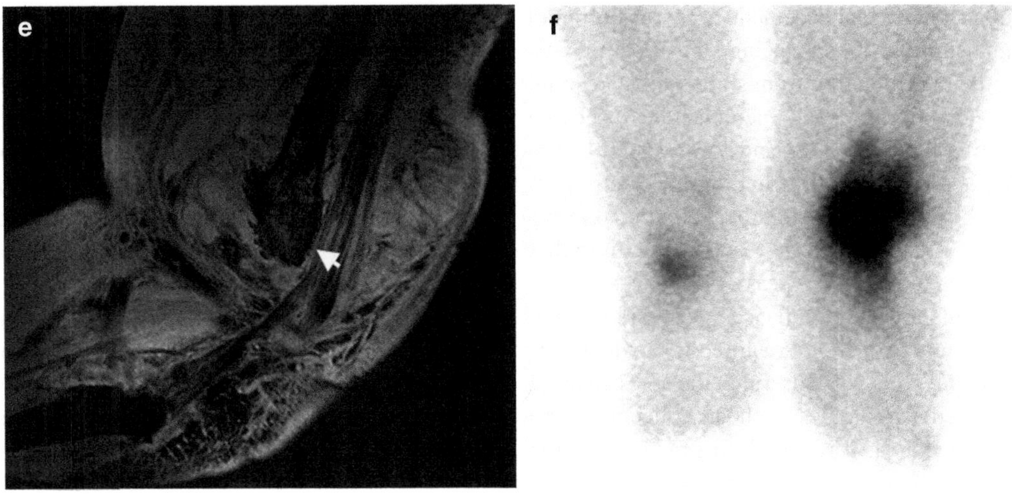

Fig. 14.7 (continued)

present. Overall the sensitivity and specificity for plain radiographs in diabetic foot infections is low (~50 and ~75 %, respectively); however their availability and low cost means that they are generally still the first modality used in the evaluation of the diabetic foot.

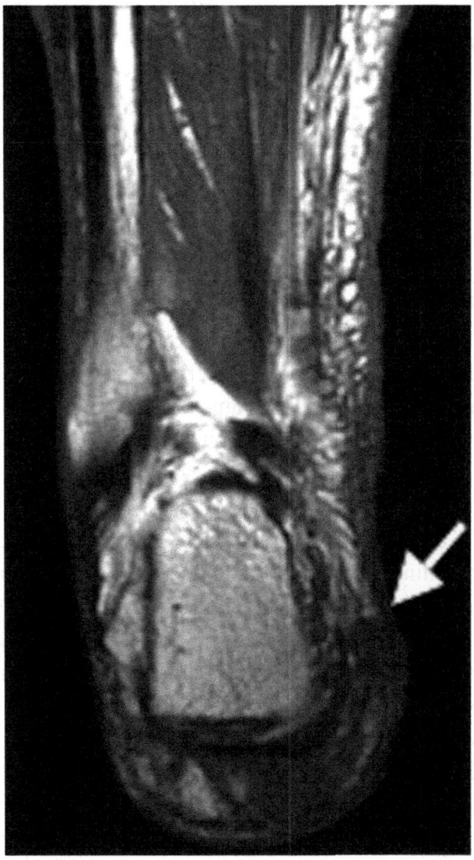

Fig. 14.8 An 86-year-old with DM, chronic renal failure and foot ulcer over medial calcaneus (*arrow*) extending to deep soft tissues. Note the normal underlying marrow SI on T1 indicating no imaging features of osteomyelitis

MRI (Figs. 14.6, 14.7, and 14.8)

Identification of osteomyelitis in diabetic foot infections and differentiating it from reactive bone marrow oedema seen in a neuropathic joint are best accomplished with MRI. Given that osteomyelitis typically occurs via contiguous spread from a surface ulcer, the common sites of osteomyelitis correspond to the most common sites of cutaneous ulceration: the areas distal to the tarsometatarsal joints, the calcaneus as well as the malleoli of the ankle. Midfoot areas can develop osteomyelitis particularly in the setting of a neuropathic arthropathy where an ulcer develops over a pressure area created by the abnormal configuration of the rocker-bottom foot.

Evidence of a soft tissue infection overlying the area of bone marrow oedema strongly suggests osteomyelitis. Ulcers can be appreciated on MRI as an area of focal skin interruption with raised edges and associated soft tissue defect in the centre. The ulcer base is often hyperintense on T2W imaging due to the presence of granulation tissue with a high water content and demonstrates enhancement post-gadolinium administration. An enhancing sinus tract may be identifiable extending from skin to bone or joint. The underlying bone demonstrates oedema which is high SI on T2 and low SI on T1. The latter is a more sensitive finding for osteomyelitis. If bone marrow is high on T2 but not clearly low on T1, this suggests reactive osteitis rather than osteomyelitis. Areas of bone marrow involvement may enhance post-gadolinium. Gadolinium is often not required in the diagnosis of osteomyelitis but is useful in the assessment of associated pathologies such as collections and devitalized areas if required. Restricted diffusion may be present on diffusion-weighted imaging.

Differentiation between septic arthritis and neuropathic joint follows some of the principles outlined above and can be very challenging. The findings of a contiguous soft tissue infection or sinus tract are highly suggestive of septic arthritis. Typically, septic arthritis is associated with complex joint effusions with intense synovial enhancement. Reactive marrow changes, or more significant changes with low intensity on T1W images indicating osteomyelitis, may be seen in the adjacent bone.

Ultrasound

Ultrasound can be helpful for the appreciation of abscesses, soft tissue collections and joint effusions which are also amenable to ultrasound-guided drainage (see section "Abscess" Chap. 13).

CT

CT can be helpful to better assess bony changes, including fragmentation and erosive change, and is the most sensitive modality for determining the presence of gas in the tissues. It is limited in the assessment of soft tissue pathology and cannot assess bone marrow oedema.

Nuclear Medicine (Figs. 14.6 and 14.7)

Osteomyelitis can be seen on bone scan as abnormal uptake in the affected area, particularly in phase 1 and 2 of scanning. Unfortunately, a neuropathic joint will often demonstrate the same abnormalities. There is some benefit to following a positive bone scan with an indium-labelled white blood cell scan, which will reveal areas of active inflammation or infection, as white blood cells will migrate to these areas. Early on in the acute phase of neuropathic arthropathy, a white blood cell scan may be positive and thus may appear identical to osteomyelitis; however once the arthropathy has become more chronic, the vigorous migration of white blood cells into the bone ceases, giving a negative result. A negative finding white blood cell scan would argue against the presence of osteomyelitis.

PET

Positron emission tomography (PET) is a modality whereby ^{18}F-fluorodeoxy-D2-labelled glucose (FDG) molecules accumulate in states of high cellular metabolism and cell turnover and thus accumulate at sites of infection. It has been observed that in patients with diabetic foot, FDG accumulates significantly more in patients with osteomyelitis than in those with neuropathic arthropathy. In addition, PET can be coupled with CT scanning to better delineate the anatomy. This modality continues to be under investigation and is not readily available in many centres; thus it is not typically used as a first-line investigation in diabetic foot.

Further Reading

1. Chantelau E, Poll L. Evaluation of the diabetic Charcot foot by MR imaging or plain radiography – an observational study. Exp Clin Endocrinol Diabetes. 2006;114:428–31.
2. Donovan A, Schweitzer M. Current concepts in imaging diabetic pedal osteomyelitis. Radiol Clin North Am. 2008;46:1105–24.
3. Sanverdi S, Ergen F, Oznur A. Current challenges in imaging of the diabetic foot. Diabet Foot Ankle. 2012;3. doi:10.3402/dfa.v3i0.18754.
4. Toledano T, Fatone E, Weis A, Cotten A, Beltran J. MRI evaluation of bone marrow changes in the diabetic foot: a practical approach. Semin Musculoskelet Radiol. 2011;15:257–68.

Spine

15

John O'Neill

Degenerative Disease of the Spine

Overview

Degenerative disc disease (DDD), intervertebral osteochondrosis, is one of the commonest causes of low back pain. Low back pain is a leading disability and may be related to multiple factors (Table 15.1). Predisposing factors include age, genetics, and axial loading. DDD may impact upon the adjacent nerves and be a source of symptoms. However, DDD may also cause low back pain from the release of cytokines and stimulate nociceptors. There may also be related facet joint disease. DDD is present in the majority of imaged middle-aged and older patients and may or may not be a source of symptoms, and close clinical correlation is required.

Table 15.1 Common etiologies of low back pain

Mechanical	Degenerative disc Degenerative joint disease Vertebral fracture Spondylosis Muscle strain
Neurogenic	Herniated disc Spinal stenosis
Rheumatologic	Inflammatory spondylitis DISH Fibromyalgia
Neoplastic/infiltrative	Benign/Malignant, metastatic
Infection	Spondylodiscitis Osteomyelitis
Referred visceral pain	AAA, pancreatitis
Miscellaneous	Depression Malingering

Clinical Presentation

Patients with DDD may be asymptomatic, have acute or chronic low back pain, or present with neurologic sequelae. Symptoms and clinical evaluation will help separate those with and without mechanical etiologies. LBP is a leading cause of disability and can be difficult to treat. Chronic LBP is present if symptoms last more than 3 months. Care should be taken to identify red flags, which require urgent investigation (Table 15.2).

J. O'Neill, MB, BAO, BCh, MRCPI, MSc, FRCR
Associate Professor, Musculoskeletal Imaging,
Diagnostic Imaging, McMaster University/
St Joseph's Healthcare,
Hamilton, ON L8N4A6, Canada
e-mail: joneill2@me.com

Imaging

Radiographs

Radiographs are limited in the assessment of DDD. Degenerative changes are common and nonspecific. Radiographs can be acquired in

J. O'Neill (ed.), *Essential Imaging in Rheumatology*,
DOI 10.1007/978-1-4939-1673-3_15, © Springer Science+Business Media New York 2015

Table 15.2 Red flags in patients with back pain

Onset <20 or >55 years
Sphincter or gait disturbance
Saddle anesthesia
Severe or progressive motor loss
Widespread neurologic deficit
Previous carcinoma
Systemic unwellness
HIV
Weight loss
IV drug abuse
Steroids
Structural deformity

patients with red flags as the initial line of investigation to help localize pathology for a more detailed cross-sectional imaging study. Vertebral body number, height, and intervertebral disc space height should be assessed (Fig. 15.1). In DDD, there is a loss of intervertebral disc space height, associated reactive vertebral endplate sclerosis, and multidirectional endplate osteophytes. Vacuum phenomena are collections of gas, predominantly nitrogen, and occur in sites of negative pressure within the nucleus pulposus (Fig. 15.2). Vacuum phenomena are a good indicator of

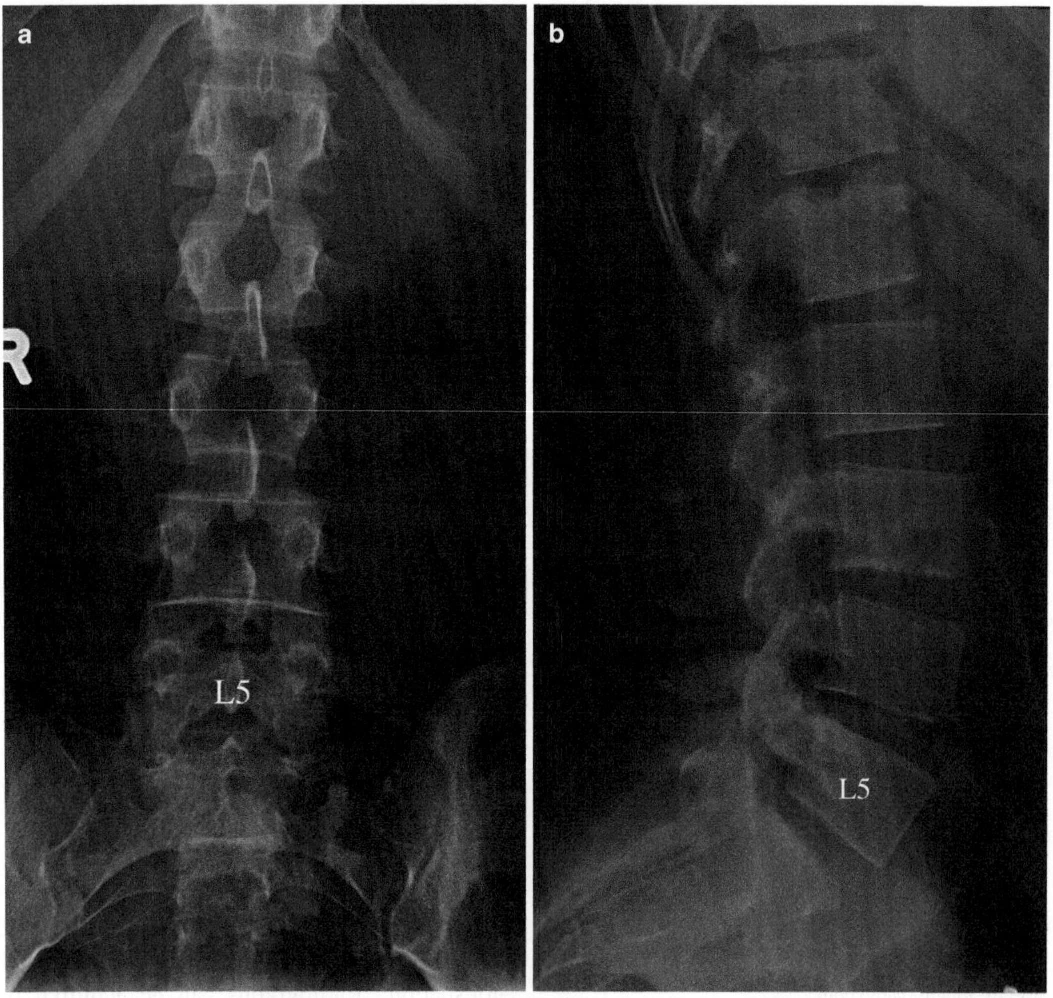

Fig. 15.1 Normal (**a**) AP and (**b**) lateral lumbar spine. *L5* indicates the fifth lumbar vertebra. Note the excellent demonstration of the sacroiliac joints on a well-positioned AP study

DDD and may be circular or linear in appearance. They increase in extension related to the increased distraction of the degenerative disc. Small foci confined to the annulus may occur in spondylosis deformans. In cases of endplate disruption such as Schmorl's nodes, gas may track into the vertebrae with a vertical branching pattern.

Cross-Sectional Imaging

We will adopt the accepted nomenclature from the combined taskforce developed to standardize description of discs (Table 15.3). This is a morphologically based definition and classification model.

MRI

MRI is the noninvasive gold imaging standard in the imaging of DDD with excellent anatomical detail, soft tissue contrast, and lack of radiation. MRI can assess the internal characteristic of the disc. The normal bright nucleus pulposus on T2 losses signal as it desiccates (Fig. 15.3). Vertebral body height, alignment, and disc space height are assessed. CT is more sensitive in the assessment of osteophytes, but MRI can demonstrate Modic endplate changes which, other than sclerosis, may not be visible on CT (Table 15.3). The high signal intensity of CSF on T2-weighted sequences allows for an excellent contrast with the intermediate to low signal intensity disc.

Facet joint degeneration includes joint space loss, and subchondral sclerosis can be readily assessed. Related osteophytosis may extend anteriorly and encroach upon the neuroforamina. With the loss of intervertebral disc height, the ligamentum flavum also decreases in height, is less stretched, and hence can form more mass effect upon the thecal sac (see Fig. 15.20c). In patients with prior disc surgery, intravenous contrast may be required to help differentiate recurrent disc disease from postoperative fibrosis. Postoperative residual disc may enhance up to 6 months postsurgery after which time only epidural fibrosis typically enhances (Fig. 15.8).

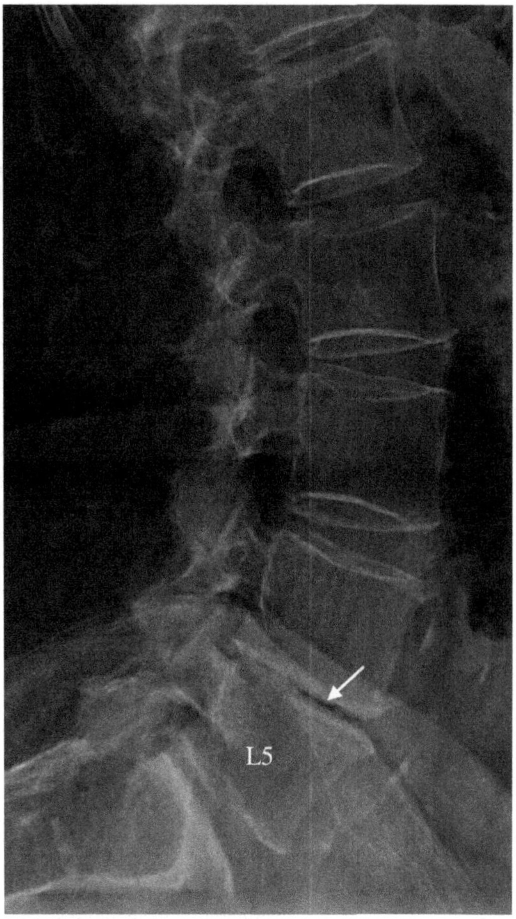

Fig. 15.2 Lateral radiograph lumbar spine in an 80-year-old female with L4–5 and L5–S1 degenerative disc disease demonstrating loss of intervertebral disc space height, vacuum phenomenon (*arrow* L4–5), minor endplate sclerosis, and minimal osteophytic lipping. Note moderate osteopenia

Table 15.3 Nomenclature and classification of lumbar disc pathology

Normal (Fig. 15.3)	Disc is fully and normally developed and free of disease, trauma, or aging
Annular tear/fissure (Fig. 15.4)	Loss integrity annulus, radial/transverse/concentric in shape
Degenerative disc	Aging and pathologic degenerative changes. Changes in a disc characterized by desiccation, fibrosis and cleft formation in the nucleus, fissuring and mucinous degeneration of the annulus, defects and sclerosis of endplates, and/or osteophytes at the vertebral apophyses
Degenerative disc disease	A clinical syndrome characterized by manifestations of disc degeneration and symptoms thought to be related to those changes
Herniated disc (Fig. 15.5)	Localized (less than 50 %/180°) of the circumference of the disc displacement of nucleus, cartilage, fragmented apophyseal bone, or fragmented annular tissue beyond the intervertebral disc space (disc space, interspace). The interspace is defined, cranial and caudal, by the vertebral body endplates and, peripherally, by the edges of the vertebral ring apophyses, exclusive of osteophytic formations
Chronic disc herniation	Disc herniation with the presence of calcification, ossification, or gas accumulation within the displaced disc material, suggesting that the herniation is not of recent origin
Protrusion (Fig. 15.6)	A disc is "protruded," if the greatest distance, in any plane, between the edges of the disc material beyond the disc space is less than the distance between the edges of the base in the same plane. The term "protrusion" is only appropriate in describing herniated disc material. Protrusions with a base less than 25 % (90°) of the circumference of the disc are "focal." If disc material is herniated so that the protrusion encompasses 25–50 % of the circumference of the disc, it is considered "broad-based protrusion"
Extruded disc (Fig. 15.7)	A herniated disc in which, in at least one plane, any one distance between the edges of the disc material beyond the disc space is greater than the distance between the edges of the base in the same plane, or when no continuity exists between the disc material beyond the disc space and that within the disc space. Extruded discs in which all continuity with the disc of origin is lost may be further characterized as *sequestrated*. Disc material displaced away from the site of extrusion may be characterized as *migrated*
Bulging disc	A disc in which the contour of the outer annulus extends, or appears to extend, in the horizontal (axial) plane beyond the edges of the disc space, over greater than 50 % (180°) of the circumference of the disc and usually less than 3 mm beyond the edges of the vertebral body apophyses. This is not a form of herniation
Radial annular tear/ fissure (Fig. 15.4)	Disruption of annular fibers extending from the nucleus outward toward the periphery of the annulus, usually in the vertical (craniocaudal) plane, with occasional horizontal (transverse) components
Spondylosis deformans	Degenerative process of the spine involving essentially the annulus fibrosus and characterized by anterior and lateral marginal osteophytes arising from the vertebral body apophyses, while the intervertebral disc height is normal or only slightly decreased
Modic changes	Reactive vertebral body modifications associated with disc inflammation and degenerative disc disease, as seen on MR images. Type 1 refers to decreased signal intensity on T1-weighted/increased signal intensity on T2-weighted images, indicating bone marrow edema associated with acute or subacute inflammatory changes. Types 2 and 3 indicate chronic changes. Type 2 refers to increased signal intensity on T1-weighted images/ isointense or increased signal intensity on T2-weighted images, indicating replacement of the normal bone marrow by fat. Type 3 refers to decreased signal intensity on both T1- and T2-weighted images, indicating reactive osteosclerosis

Adapted with permission from Lippincott Williams and Wilkins/Wolters Kluwer Health: *Spine* 2001, 26:E93–113, Fardon, DF, et al, Nomenclature and classification of lumbar disc pathology. Recommendations of the Combined task Forces of the North American Spine Society, American Society of Spine Radiology, and American Society of Neuroradiology, copyright 2001

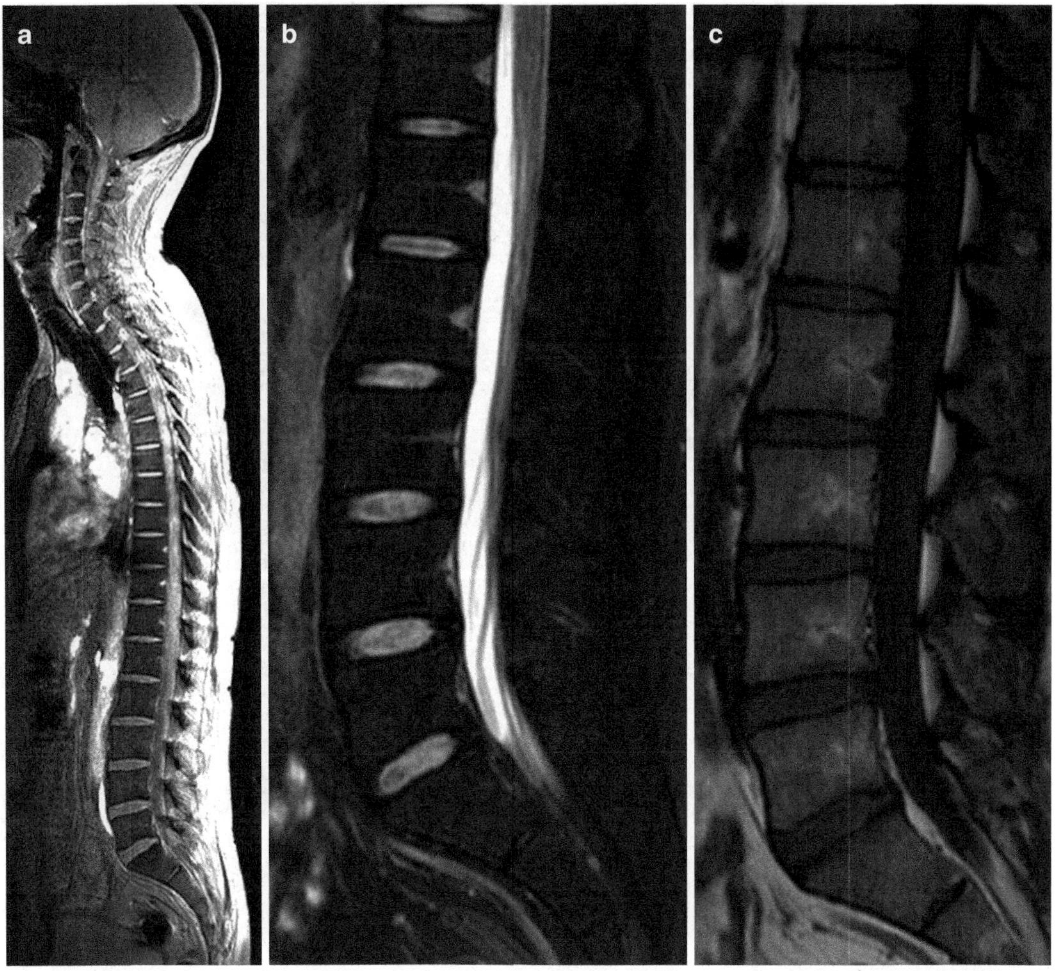

Fig. 15.3 Normal MRI lumbar spine: (**a**) localizer midsagittal image allows for correct counting lumbar vertebrae, (**b**) Sag T2FS demonstrating uniform fat-suppressed marrow SI, central high and peripheral low SI disc and high SI CSF, (**c**) Sag T1 normal morrow SI, low SI CSF, (**d**) Sag T1 through neural foramina demonstrating exciting neural roots and perineural fat, (**e**) axial T2FS at disc level demonstrating the thecal sac with high SI CSF and low SI *dots* representing the cauda equina/nerve roots, and (**f**) inferior to (**e**) at level lateral recesses (*arrows*)

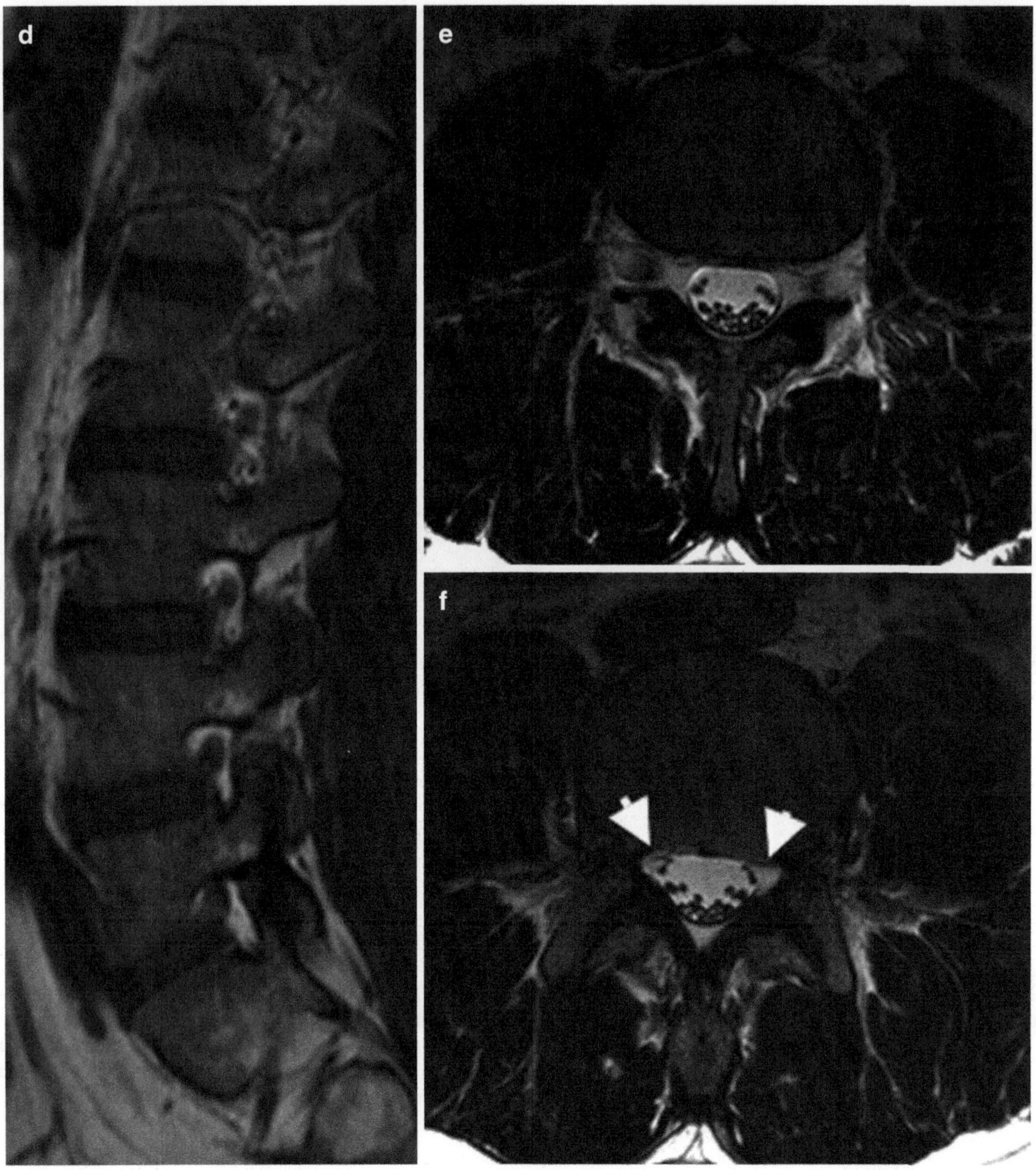

Fig. 15.3 (continued)

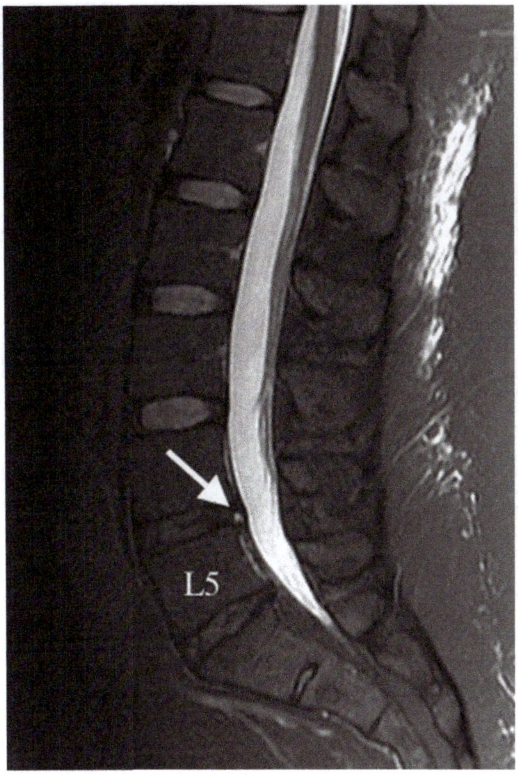

Fig. 15.4 Annular tear shown as a high signal intensity zone (*arrow*) in posterior L4–5 degenerative disc (loss normal signal intensity and height, also present at L5–S1) in a 31 F on midsagittal T2FS

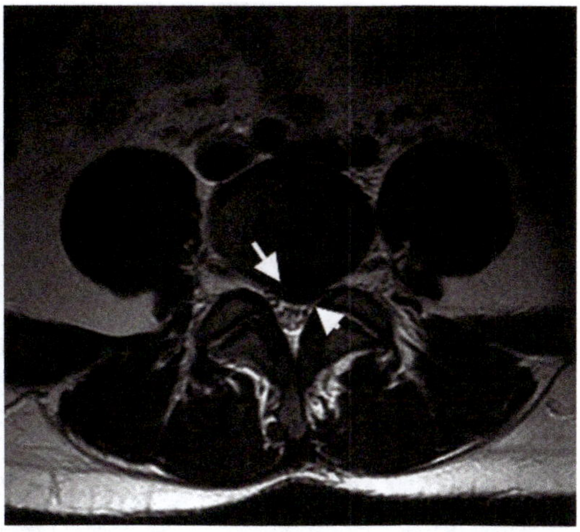

Fig. 15.6 Axial T2FS at L4–5 demonstrating a focal protrusion, base disc herniation wider than AP extension and involving less than 25 % disc circumference, indenting the thecal sac, impinging the left L5 nerve root (*arrowhead*), and abutting without impinging the right L5 nerve root

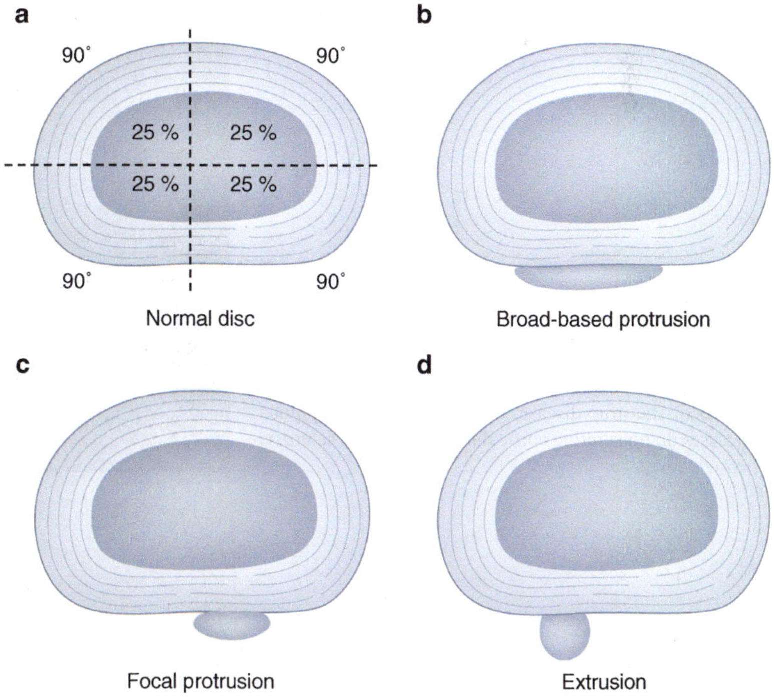

Fig. 15.5 Illustration herniated disc types: (**a**) normal disc divided into four quadrants, (**b**) broad-based protrusion with >25 % disc circumference involved, (**c**) focal protrusion involving less than 25 % disc circumference, and (**d**) extruded disc

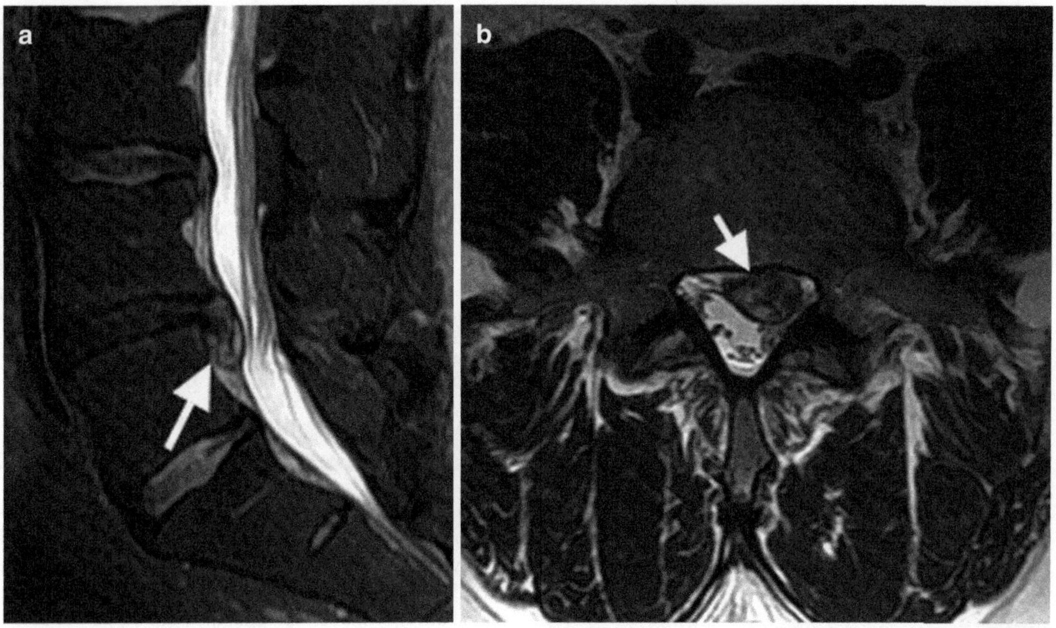

Fig. 15.7 Extruded disc (*arrow*) with inferior migration, without sequestration, at L4–5 extending into the left lateral recess and impinging the left L5 and upper sacral nerve roots (**a**) Sag and (**b**) axial T2FS

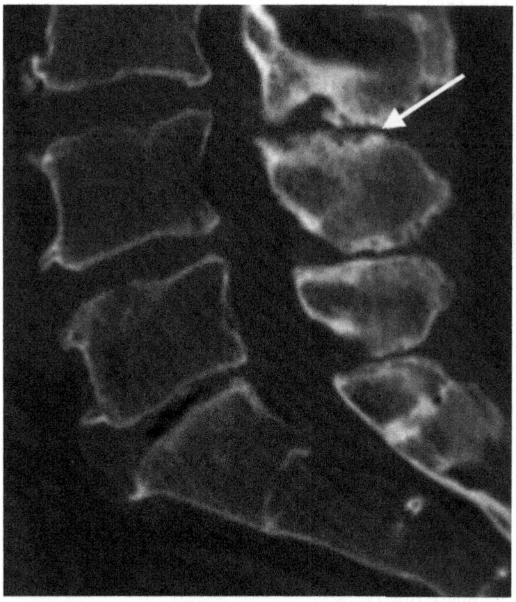

Fig. 15.8 Degenerative disc disease on reformatted Sag CT, bone windows, demonstrating loss of disc height, vacuum phenomenon, minor endplate osteophytosis L5–S1. Less pronounced degeneration at L4–5. Note imaging features of Baastrup disease, contacting adjacent spinous processes demonstrating cortical irregularity and sclerosis (*arrow*)

CT

CT assessment of DDD, particularly of the lumbar spine, is decreasing due to the radiation dose related to CT, increased availability, and higher soft tissue resolution of MRI. CT is not indicated in the assessment of cervical or thoracic DDD due to the limited resolution of the intervertebral disc in these regions unless MRI is unavailable or contraindicated. CT is acquired axially through the intervertebral disc, and alignment can be adjusted for variable lumbar lordosis. Images can then be reformatted in axial and saggital planes and occasionally in the coronal plane.

Intervertebral disc space height, vacuum phenomena, vertebral endplate osteophytes, erosions, and sclerosis are assessed (Fig. 15.9). Disc irregularity, disc bulge, and herniation, as defined in Table 15.3, are assessed in axial and saggital planes. In chronic disc herniation, vacuum phenomena may be presented in the herniated disc. Neuroforaminal/spinal canal narrowing or stenosis can be readily assessed. Saggital images are optimal for assessing the neuroforamina. Neural abutment, disc touches nerve, or impingement, disc adjusts the normal course of the nerve, should be noted. Imaging studies are acquired with the patient in a supine position; however, some changes, such as neural abutment, may only become evident in the erect or flexed positions. DDD is not assessed as a single entity, and associated degenerative changes of the facet joints, ligamentum flavum, and congenital abnormalities such as congenital canal stenosis are reviewed to form a comprehensive assessment of pathology.

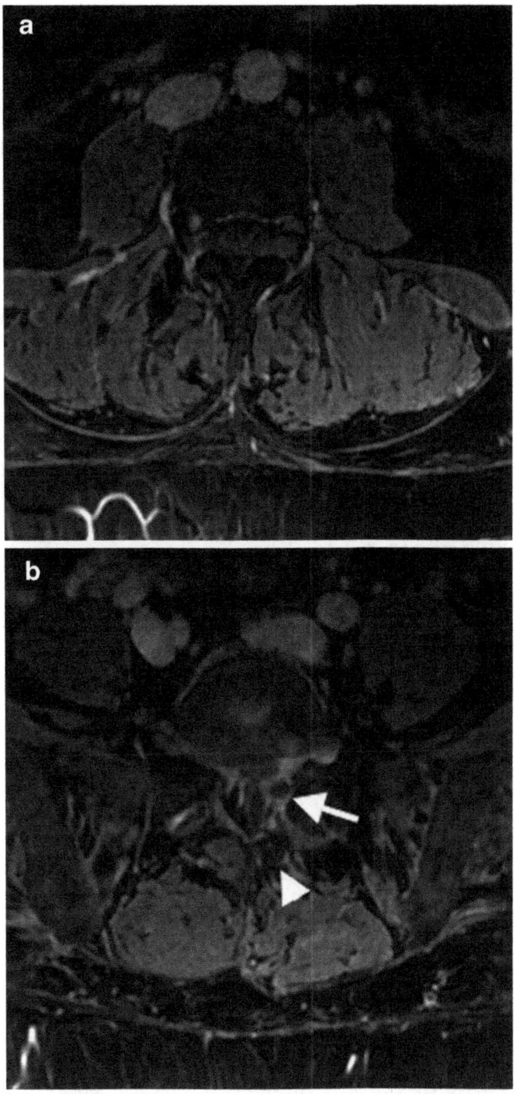

Fig. 15.9 Axial T1FS images (**a**) pre- and (**b**) post contrast demonstrating enhancing soft tissue (*arrow*) surrounding an enlarged left S1 nerve root in keeping with epidural fibrosis in a 58-year-old male patient 1-year post left L5 laminectomy (*arrowhead*)

Ultrasound

Ultrasound currently has no role in the assessment degenerative disc disease.

Nuclear Medicine

Nuclear medicine has a limited role. It may be useful as a skeletal assessment in patients with history of carcinoma in the assessment of metastatic disease.

Cervical and Thoracic Degenerative Disc Disease

The cervical spine has the greatest range of motion and is the second commonest spinal site of DDD after the lumbar spine, usually occuring at the C5–6 and C6–7 levels (Fig. 15.10). In the cervical spine, exiting nerve roots are one level above their disc level, i.e., C6 nerve exits at C5–6. This continues to C8, below which nerves exit below disc level, i.e., L4 exits at L4–5. Uncovertebral joints, joints of Luschka, are present only within the posterolateral aspects of the five lowermost cervical vertebrae. Osteophytes related to degeneration of these joints extend posteriorly into the cervical spinal canal and posterolaterally into the neuroforamina. These joints are best appreciated on the frontal and oblique radiographs of the cervical spine (Fig. 15.11).

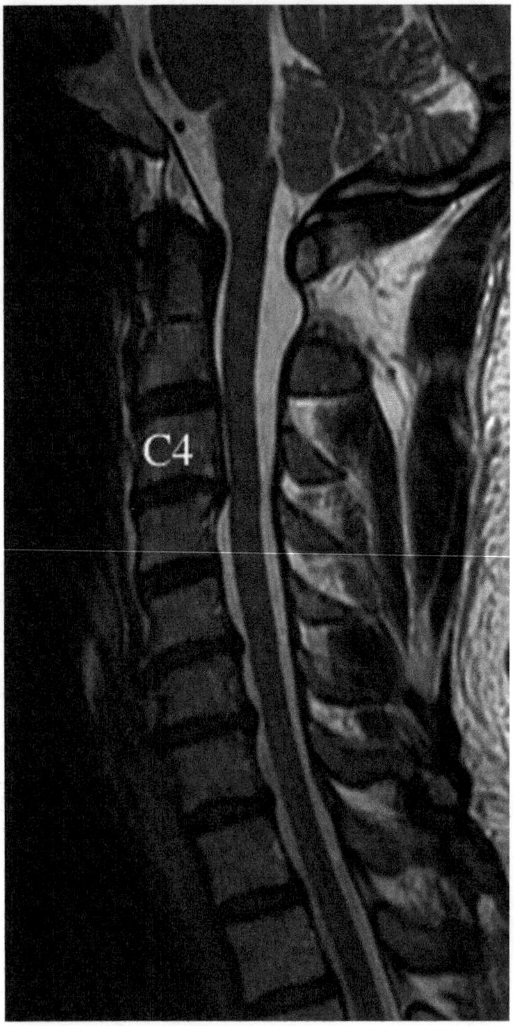

Fig. 15.10 Sag T2FS MRI cervical spine with multilevel mild degenerative disc disease

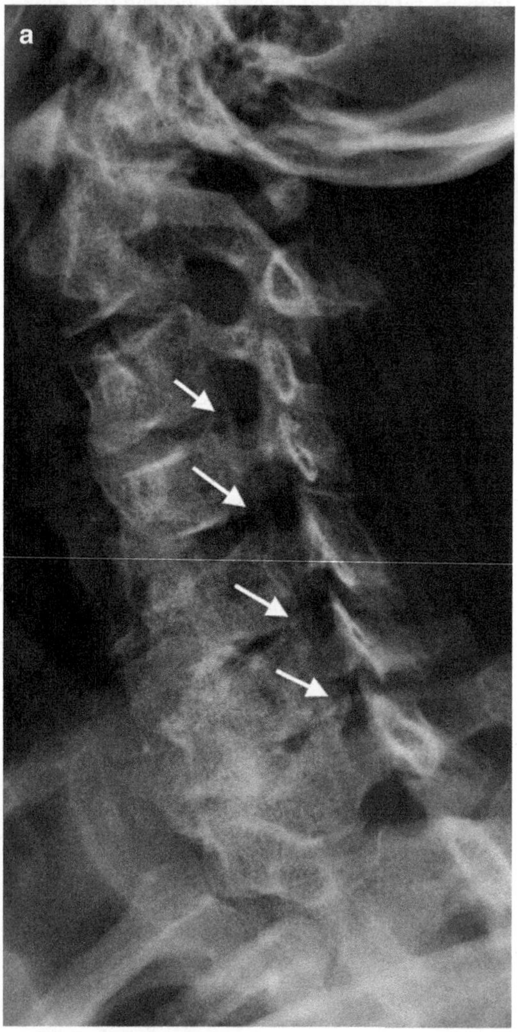

Fig. 15.11 Oblique radiographs cervical spine demonstrating (**a**) left neural foramina with mild to moderate stenosis, gradual worsening as one extending inferiorly, secondary to uncovertebral and degenerative disc disease with loss of height and endplate osteophytes (*arrows*) and (**b**) normal left oblique for comparison

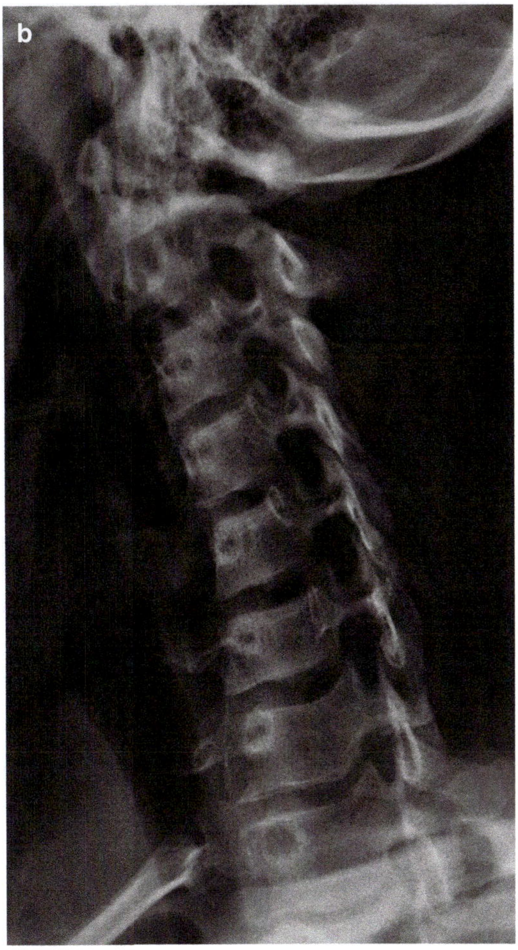

Fig. 15.11 (continued)

It is common to find uncovertebral degeneration at the same level as DDD.

The thoracic spine is least involved by DDD due to limited range of motion and ribcage support.

Transitional Vertebra

Transitional vertebrae at the lumbosacral junction are a common congenital anomaly (Figs. 15.12 and 15.13). The upper sacral segment can become lumbarized, and likewise the lowermost lumbar segment can become sacralized. They may be associated with LBP, Bertolotti syndrome (Fig. 15.14). Symptoms are more common in Castellvi types 2 and 4 (Table 15.4).

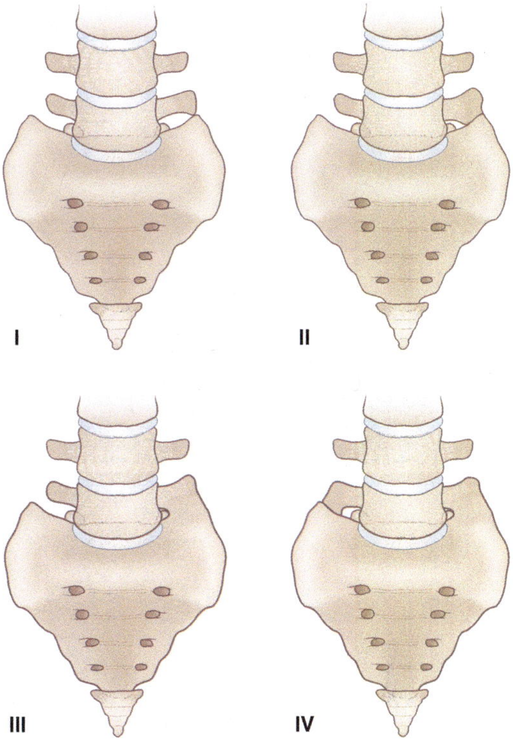

Fig. 15.12 Illustration of Castellvi classification lumbosacral transitional vertebrae (types 1–3 may be unilateral or bilateral)

In sacralization of the lowermost lumbar vertebrae, an elongated unilateral or bilateral transverse process is present which may or may not articulate with the sacrum or occasionally the ilium. This joint may also be fused. There is increased degenerative changes noted in the opposite facet joint and increased risk of DDD at the level above due to decreased range of motion at the level below. In the case of lumbarization of S1, the S1 vertebra is more square in appearance, and there may be a fully formed disc and usually has facet joints instead of the normal fusion at S1–2. Identification of transitional vertebrae is important particularly in surgical patients so correct nomenclature is employed and surgery is performed at the correct level. CT is more sensitive in identifying transitional vertebrae due to wider field of view and ability to differentiate hypoplastic 12th ribs from prominent transverse processes. Identification of the iliolumbar ligament arises from the transverse process of L5 and is a useful landmark.

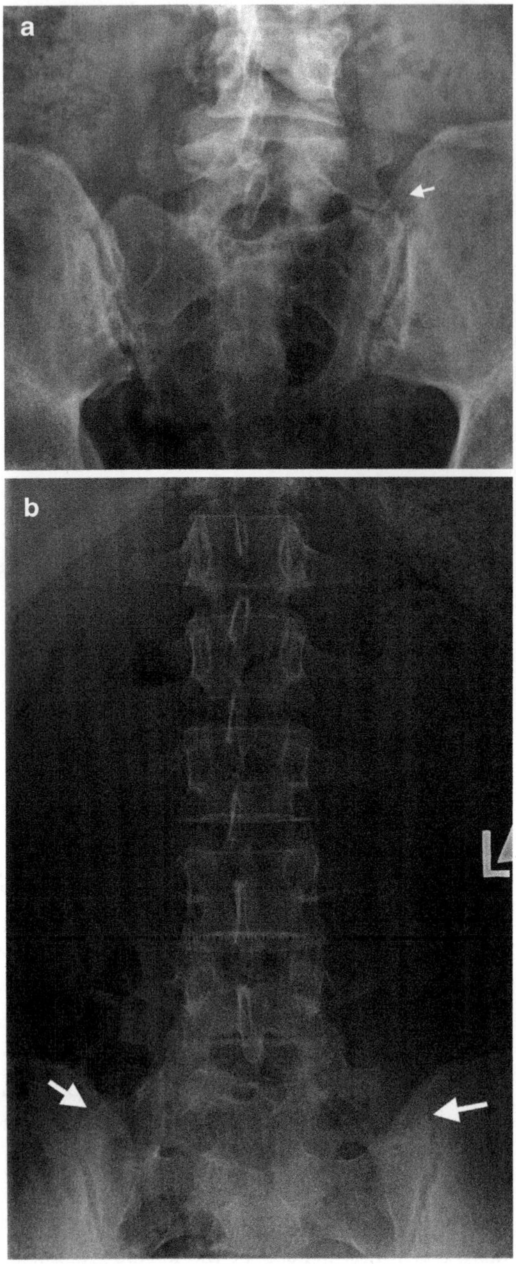

Fig. 15.13 AP radiographs transitional L5 vertebra: (**a**) type 2A, left synchondrosis (*arrow*) and (**b**) type 4, left synchondrosis and right-sided fusion transverse process L5 and sacrum (*arrows*)

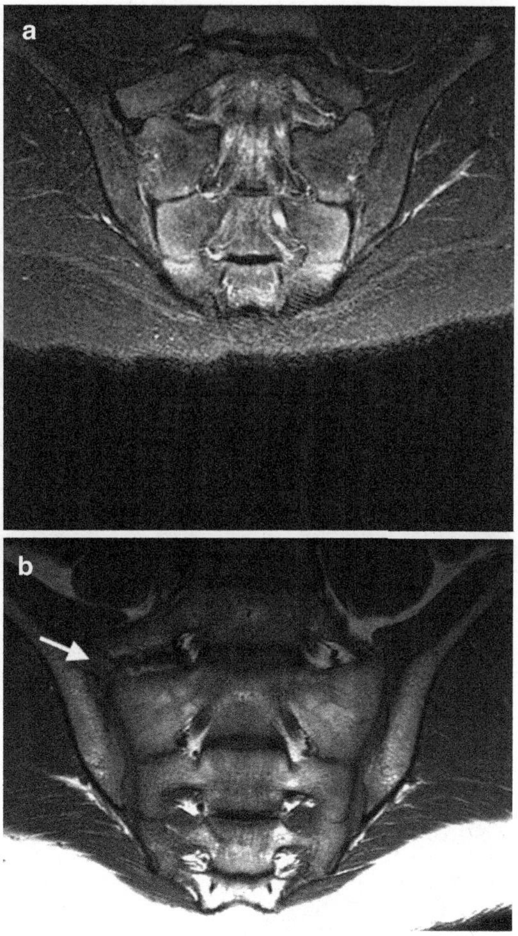

Fig. 15.14 MRI transitional vertebra type 2 b in a symptomatic 15-year-old female elite gymnast with Bertolotti syndrome: (**a**) no osteitis demonstrated on Cor T2FS; (**b**) Cor T1 does demonstrate cortical irregularity and post-inflammatory fat accentuation at right synchondrosis (*arrow*)

Table 15.4 Castellvi classification lumbosacral transitional vertebrae

Type 1 – forme fruste, dysplastic transverse process, >19 mm height
Type 2 – incomplete, enlarged transverse process with pseudoarthrosis with the adjacent sacral ala
Type 3 – complete, enlarged transverse process with complete fusion with the adjacent sacral ala
Type 4 – mixed, type 2 and type 3 on alternate sides

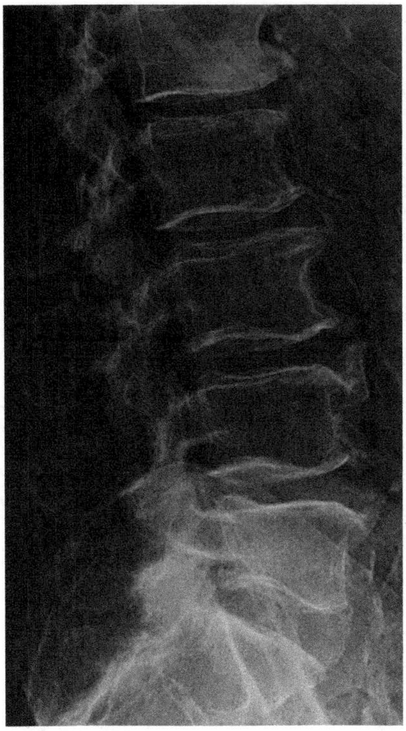

Fig. 15.15 Lateral radiograph lumbar spine demonstrating endplate osteophytosis with maintenance intervertebral disc space height

Spondylosis Deformans

Degenerative process of the spine involves essentially the annulus fibrosus and is characterized by the anterior and lateral marginal osteophytes arising from the vertebral body apophyses, while the intervertebral disc height is normal or only slightly decreased (Fig. 15.15). Occasionally, foci of gas are identified in the peripheral annulus fibrosus of the disc. Osteophytes are usually anterior and lateral with increasing prevalence after 40 years of age.

Spondylolisthesis and Spondylolysis

Spondylolisthesis, from the Greek "a vertebra that slips," indicates anterior or posterior translation, slippage, of a vertebra upon a vertebra above or below it. Spondylolisthesis occurs in up to 4 % of the population, the commonest at the two lowermost lumbar levels. It is divided into open or closed arch. In open arch, there is bilateral spondylolysis, a defect in the pars interarticularis, i.e., that portion of the bone between the superior and inferior articular facets (Fig. 15.16). This is

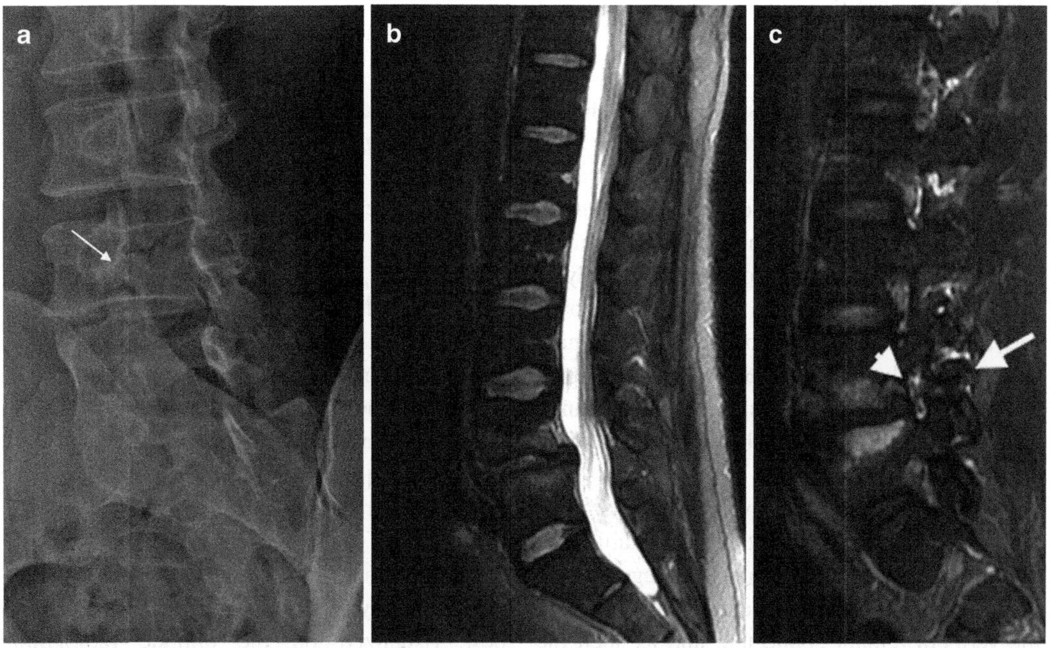

Fig. 15.16 Bilateral spondylolysis and spondylolisthesis of L4 on L5: (**a**) oblique radiograph demonstrating spondylolysis (*arrow*) and (**b**) Sag T2FS same patient presenting 10 years later with right L4 neural impingement having developed grade 1 spondylolisthesis and (**c**) Sag T2FS at the neuroforamina with secondary bilateral foraminal stenosis (*arrowhead*) secondary to uncovered disc, (**d**) Axial T2FS uncovered disc occupying right foramina (*arrow*), (**e**) Sag CT with L4 pars defect (*arrow*) in a different patient

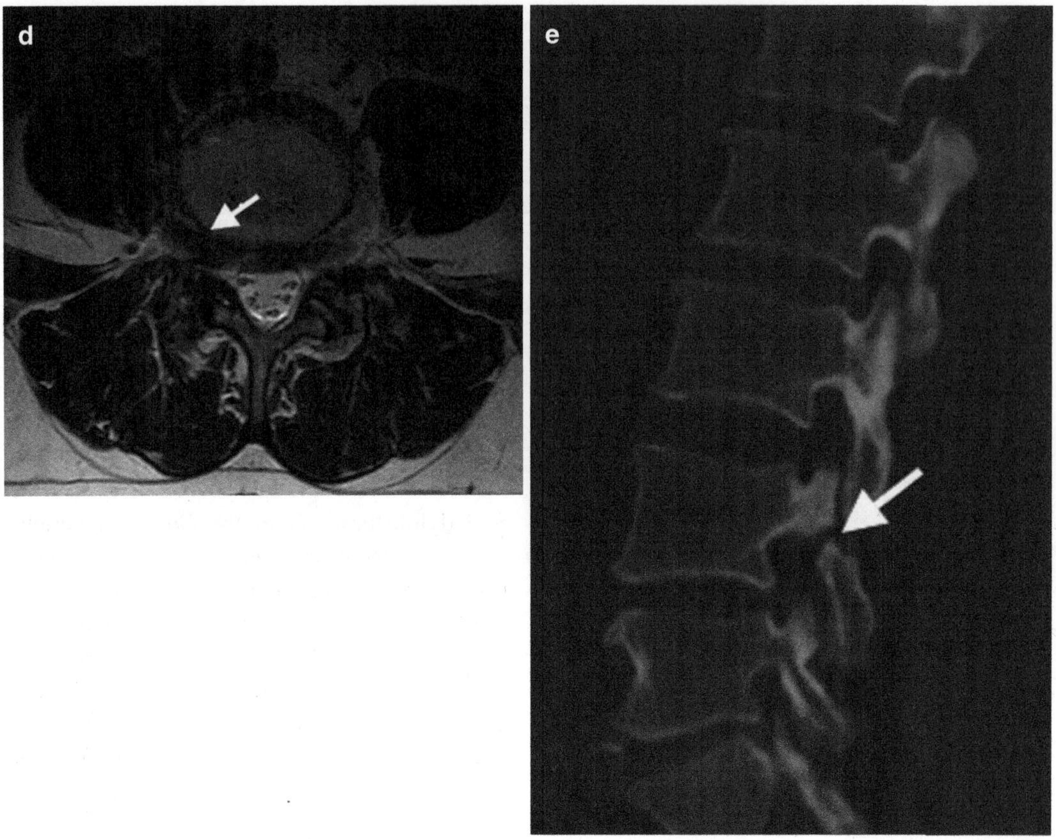

Fig. 15.16 (continued)

usually secondary to a stress fracture related to recurrent microtrauma rather than a single traumatic event. Hypoplasia of the pars may predispose patients to stress fracture. It is more common in adolescent active males and symptomatic in up to 50 % of cases. It will predispose to spondylolisthesis if bilateral. While the vertebra moves forward, the posterior vertebral elements remain in alignment with the adjacent vertebral processes and do not encroach upon the spinal canal. The intervertebral disc may be degenerative with related disc bulge.

In closed arch, degenerative spondylolisthesis, the pars is intact; however, there is instability at the facet joint usually related to degenerative change. The anterior and posterior elements of the vertebra remain connected, and as such the posterior elements move forward and encroach upon the spinal canal and may cause a spinal canal and foraminal stenosis. Retrolisthesis, posterior slippage, may occur, although less common, related to DDD. The cervical and lumbar spines are the most frequently involved.

Radiography

The lateral radiograph best demonstrates the spondylolisthesis. The degree of spondylolisthesis can be measured or graded, grades 1–4 with each grade equivalent to 25 % of the AP diameter of the vertebra, i.e., grade 2 equates to 26–50 % (Fig. 15.17). Anterior slippage of the posterior elements occurs in degenerative spondylolisthesis. In spondylosis, a bony defect in the pars is best visualized on the oblique radiograph. Instability can be assessed with flexion and extension views.

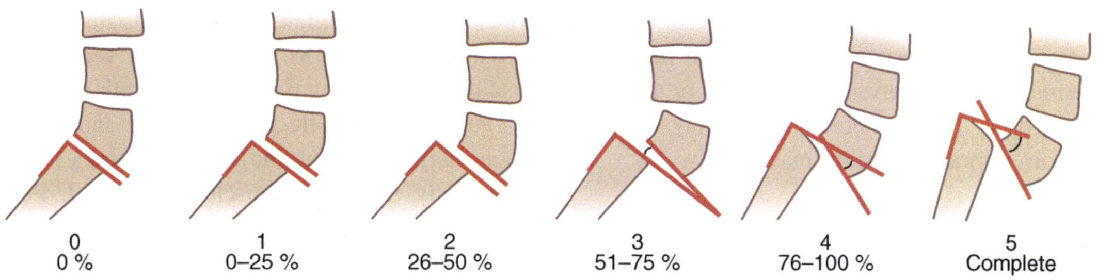

Fig. 15.17 Illustration grades 0–5 spondylolisthesis

CT

CT demonstrates excellent bony detail of the pars (Fig. 15.16e) and the facet joints. It can also assess any associated intervertebral disc disease.

MRI

MRI is less sensitive in assessing pars defect than CT. MRI is excellent and however is assessing associated degenerative disc disease and neuroforaminal/canal stenosis. MRI can also demonstrate Modic endplate type 1 changes, which may relate to instability (Fig. 15.16b–d).

Ultrasound and Nuclear Medicine

Ultrasound has no role to play in diagnosis. Nuclear medicine may localize osteoblastic activity to the involved level but is not routinely indicated given the associated radiation dose and the availability of CT and MRI.

Spondylodiscitis

Overview

Spondylodiscitis is infection of the vertebra and intervertebral disc. Infection can spread via three routes, hematogenous (the commonest), direct external, and contiguous tissue. The lumbar, thoracic, and cervical spine are affected in decreasing order of frequency. There is a bimodal age distribution, <20 and >50 years with males more commonly affected. In children, vascular supply to the disc is present and infection often commences in the disc. In adults, the disc is relatively avascular, and infection begins in the vertebral body and spreads to the disc. Infection can spread into the adjacent soft tissues as a paravertebral collection including psoas and epidural abscesses. Infection may be bacterial, myobacterial, and rarely fungal or parasitic. Common pathogens include *Staph aureus*, *E. Coli*, *Pseudomonas* (drug addicts), and TB.

Clinical Presentation

Presentation is often delayed, as often there is nonspecific back pain. Localized tenderness may be present with limited or no systemic symptoms. With the development of an iliopsoas abscess, there may be secondary hip contracture.

Imaging

Radiographs

Radiographs have low sensitivity early in the course of infection. Infection begins in the vertebral body and spreads to the adjacent disc. Disc space height is decreased, and the vertebral endplates become irregular and ill-defined with increasing osteolysis. Infection spreads into the adjacent vertebra. Endplate irregularity is the most sensitive indicator early in the course of disease. As disease progresses, reactive changes occur in the vertebrae with increasing sclerosis. Paravertebral collections are usually not assessable on radiographs. Occasionally, the psoas soft tissue outline will become enlarged on the affected side. In tuberculous spondylitis (Pott disease), infection spreads not via the disc to adjacent vertebra but via subligamentous spread.

The disc space height is thus preserved. The anterior vertebral margins on the lateral radiograph demonstrate osteolysis with limited or no related sclerosis. The vertebral body may collapse. Paravertebral collections may calcify.

MRI

MRI is the gold imaging standard in the assessment of spondylodiscitis. It provides excellent assessment of the extent of bone and soft tissue involvement. The involved vertebral body is of decreased signal intensity on T1, and this may be secondary to edema with or without sclerosis. T2 high signal intensity confirms the extent of edema, and sclerosis will be low signal intensity on T1 and T2. Focal bone destruction, osteolysis, can be identified but is best appreciated on CT. The intervertebral disc demonstrates loss of height and central fluid signal intensity. The endplates demonstrate multifocal erosions (Fig. 15.18). The adjacent vertebra is usually involved by time of presentation.

Paravertebral collections, abscess and phlegmon, may extend into adjacent soft tissues, and classically the psoas muscle is involved. Posterior extension of phlegmon or abscess may occur into the neuroforamina or spinal canal. Phlegmon will be intermediate to high signal on T2 and low on T1 and demonstrates diffuse increased intensity on T1 post contrast, whereas abscess post contrast will demonstrate peripheral enhancement only. Abscesses may also show restricted diffusion.

CT

CT provides excellent assessment bony architecture, destruction and osteolysis, endplate erosions, loss of intervertebral disc space height, and

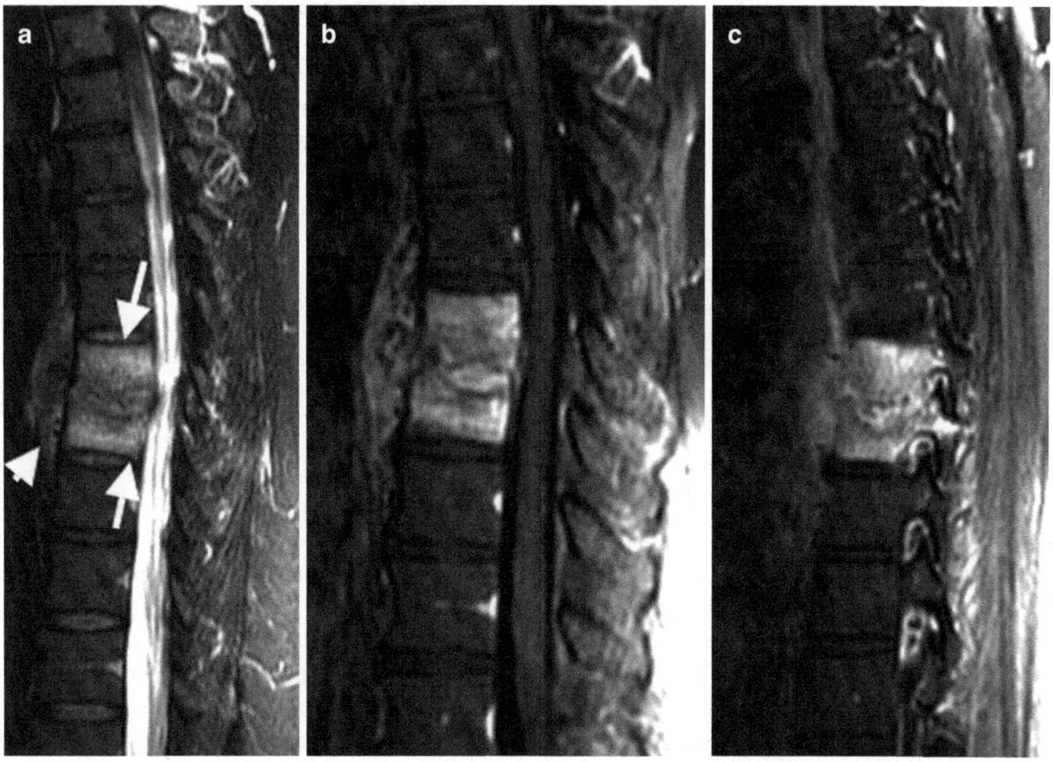

Fig. 15.18 Spondylodiscitis in a 58-year-old male secondary to a *Staph aureus* septicemia: (**a**) Sag T2FS thoracic spine demonstrating osteomyelitis (*arrows*) with high T2 SI in both T8 and T9 vertebral bodies intervening discitis and anterior paravertebral abscess (*arrowheads*). Note the endplate erosions (**b**) Sag T1FS post gadolinium (PG) demonstrating enhancement involved vertebral bodies, disc, and abscess and (**c**) Sag T1FS PG with narrowing neural foramina secondary to extension of paravertebral collection

paravertebral collections. The latter demonstrates enhancement patterns as described above. CT is not as sensitive as MRI in assessing soft tissue or epidural involvement.

Ultrasound

Ultrasound has no role in direct imaging of spondylodiscitis. Occasionally, a posterior paravertebral collection will develop, more common in postsurgical patients, and ultrasound can be used as image guidance for a diagnostic aspiration and therapeutic drainage.

Nuclear Medicine

Scintigraphy, three-phase study will demonstrate areas of increased osteoblastic activity at the site of infection; however, it is nonspecific. It can be helpful to exclude infection, but radiation dose should be considered. Indium- or technetium-labeled leukocytes can be used. Positron emission tomography with F18 FDG (PET) is sensitive in demonstrating increased metabolic activity as hot spots. Malignancy may however have a similar appearance.

Spinal Tumors

Hemangiomas are the commonest benign tumors, and the majority are incidental. They are rounded foci with well-defined margins and of increased signal intensity on both T1 and T2 with areas of signal loss on T2 fat-saturated sequences due to their internal fat component (Fig. 15.19). Atypical hemangiomas have little or no fat and may appear low signal on T1 and can be difficult to separate from more aggressive lesions such as a metastatic lesion. The latter however would be unlikely if only a single lesion was present in the absence of history of malignancy. Occasionally, CT can be performed to confirm atypical hemangioma, which demonstrates a focal lucency with intact thickened internal trabeculae. Large hemangiomas extending to both superior and inferior

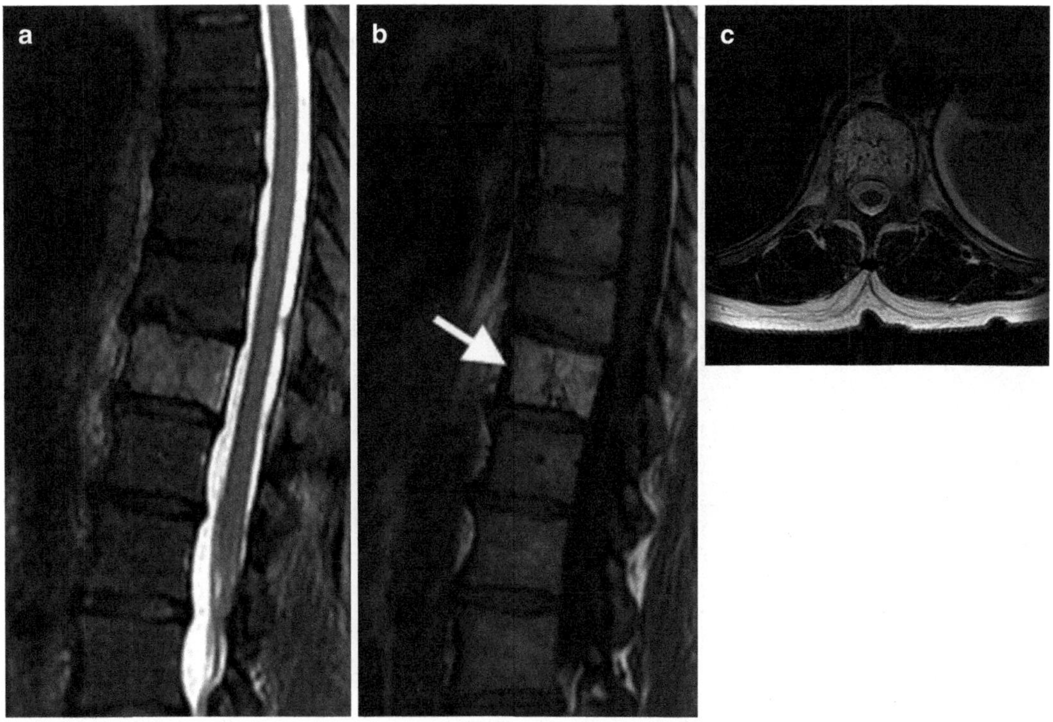

Fig. 15.19 Hemangioma T11, incidental finding: (**a**) Sag T2FS, (**b**) Sag T1, (**c**) axial T1 demonstrating high SI (*arrow in b*) lesion on all sequences occupying all the vertebral body with sparing posterior elements, no associated vertebral collapse. Note the low SI dots on axial T1 due to residual thickened trabeculae

endplates vertebrae predispose to vertebral collapse. Other benign lesions include osteoid osteoma, osteoblastoma, and aneursymal bone cyst. Their description is beyond the scope of this text.

Metastatic lesions are the commonest malignancy of the spine (Fig. 15.20). Multiple focal lesions of low signal intensity on T1, high on T2 if lytic, and low signal on T1 and T2 if sclerotic. Myeloma can have multiple imaging presentations including having a normal marrow appearance. Other varieties include a metastatic like, variegated, and diffuse. Lymphomas, primary or secondary involvement, sarcomas, and chordomas all affect the spine.

Diffuse Idiopathic Skeletal Hyperostosis

Overview

Diffuse idiopathic skeletal hyperostosis (DISH), also commonly known as Forestier disease, is a common idiopathic skeletal disorder producing hyperostosis within the axial and appendicular skeleton. It usually begins in middle age and is almost twice as common in men. Diagnosis requires spinal involvement with anterior flowing ossification of the anterior longitudinal ligament over four contiguous vertebrae and not associated with degenerative disc disease at these levels and absent ankylosis of apophyseal or sacroiliac joints. The latter helps to excludes spondyloarthropathy. There is increased prevalence in type 2 diabetics, and the process is influenced by hyperglycemia, insulin resistance, and growth hormone. There is increased bone proliferation at sites of prior surgery. Atypical imaging features may occur in patients with rheumatoid arthritis such as a lack of associated osteoporosis normally seen in RhA and bone proliferation around erosions. Common areas of involvement are at sites of ligamentous or tendons insertions where excessive new bone formation is present.

Clinical Presentation

DISH is often incidentally diagnosed on radiographs taken for alternate reasons, e.g., lateral chest radiograph. It is slowly progressive, and

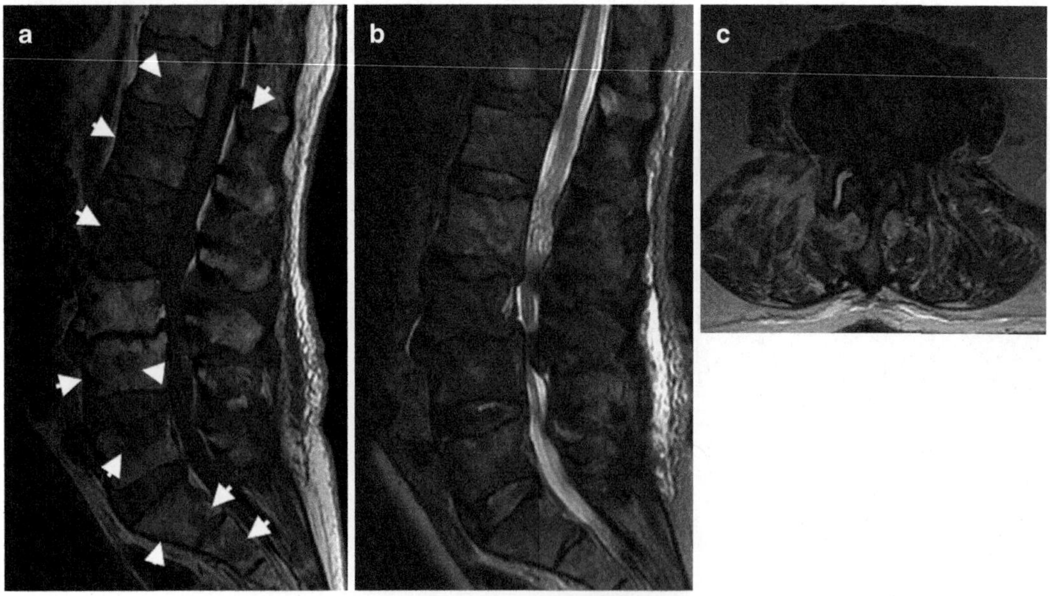

Fig. 15.20 A 74-year-old female with diffuse metastatic breast disease to the lumbar spine superimposed on advanced degenerative disc disease and spinal stenosis: (**a**) Sag T1 with diffuse (*arrowheads*) ill-defined low SI lesions within anterior and posterior elements. (**b**) Sag T2FS lesions are heterogeneous and of intermediate to high SI. (**c**) Axial T2FS L3–4 disc level with severe spinal canal stenosis due to a combination of moderate disc bulge, facet joint degeneration with secondary anterolisthesis, and ligamentum flavum hypertrophy

minor changes may be identified in middle age, which becomes more obvious as the patient ages. The patient is often asymptomatic but may complain of stiffness and spinal restricted range of motion. Peripherally, tendinopathy at tendinous insertion may be present. Rarely, ossification of the posterior longitudinal ligament within the cervical spine and/or ligamentum flavum will produce a secondary spinal canal stenosis with related symptoms.

Imaging

Radiographs

DISH is most commonly diagnosed within the mid- to lower thoracic spine, followed by the lower cervical spine. Ossification or calcification of the anterior longitudinal ligament and paraspinal connective tissue occurs over at least four contiguous vertebrae; this is usually central or right lateral due to the inhibiting effect of pulsations from the thoracic aorta (Fig. 15.21). There may be subtle radioloucency between the band of ossification and the underlying anterior margin vertebral body and intervertebral disc. Anterior osteophytes may be present at the level of the disc, noting that disc space height is maintained. There is no ankylosis of apophyseal joints. There may be related hyperostosis of the adjacent posterior ribs. Ossification of the posterior longitudinal ligament may occur within the cervical spine. This may encroach upon the spinal canal producing spinal canal stenosis. Occasionally, the ligamentum flavum may also calcify/ossify. Similar changes can be seen within the supraspinous and interspinous ligaments. Hyperostosis at the atlantoaxial joint may occur.

Degenerative disc disease may be seen within the lumbar and may be incidental to DISH. The

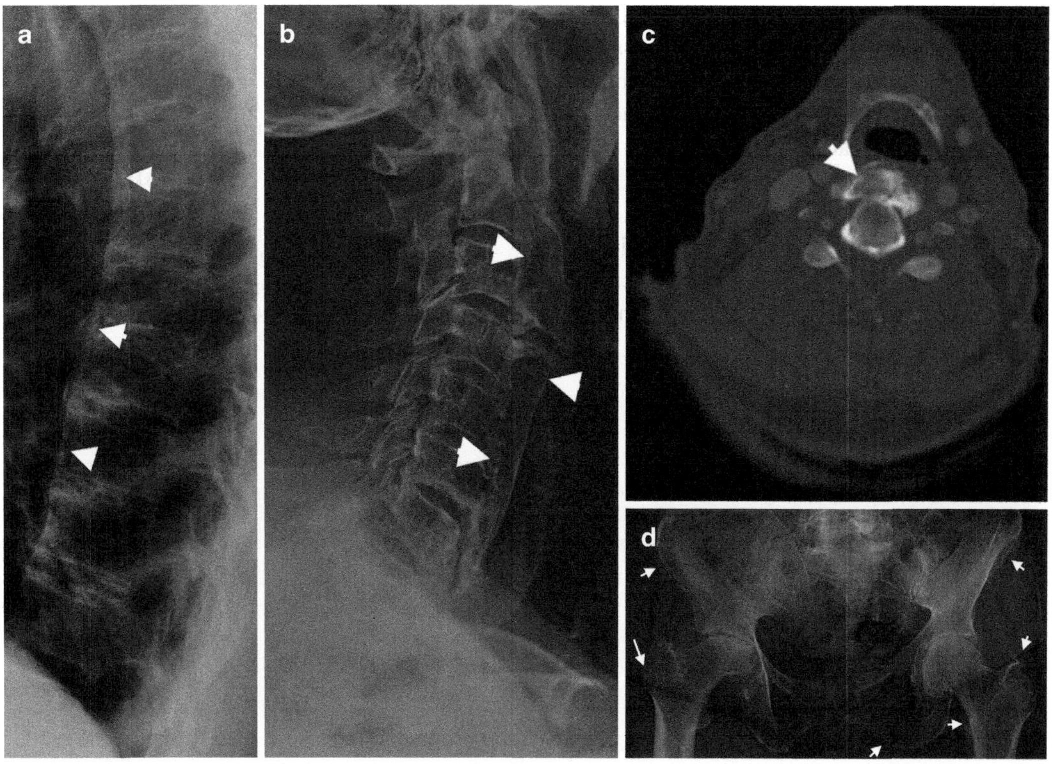

Fig. 15.21 DISH lateral radiograph: (**a**) thoracic and (**b**) cervical spine demonstrating thin ossification thoracic and thick ossification anterior longitudinal ligament (*arrowheads*) in two different patients. (**c**) Axial CT same patient as (**b**) with cervical anterior longitudinal ligament ossification. AP pelvis (**d**) demonstrating prominent enthesophytes (*arrows*) at multiple sites tendon insertion in patient with DISH. Note collapsing femoral head, Postel's coxarthropathy (see Chap. 10)

sacroiliac joints may demonstrate prominent anterior bridging osteophytosis without joint ankylosis or erosions. There is an increased risk of fracture in patients with long-standing DISH related in part to the decreased range of motion secondary to new bone formation. Typical fracture sites are at the junction of a long fused segment and normal spine, and through the mid-vertebral body where the anterior ossification is the thinnest.

Extraspinal disease is common demonstrating new bone formation at ligamentous and tendon attachments. In the pelvis, involvement of the iliac crest and ischial tuberosities is common; femur, greater trochanters; knee, patella/tibial tuberosity; foot, Achilles insertion/base fifth metatarsal; and elbow, olecranon process.

MRI

MRI is usually not performed for the diagnosis of DISH but is occasionally used when complications occur. In acute spinal fractures, as described above, MRI will demonstrate any intraspinal/neural involvement. In patients with associated ossification of the posterior longitudinal ligament or ligamentum flavum, MRI is excellent at assessing related spinal canal stenosis.

CT

CT is required for the same indications for MRI. CT will demonstrate bony detail, calcification, and ossification in better detail; however, MRI is the gold standard for assessing any neural-related symptoms (Fig. 15.21c).

Ultrasound/Nuclear Medicine

Not indicated.

Further Reading

1. Bogduk N. Degenerative joint disease of the spine. Radiol Clin North Am. 2012;50(4):613–28.
2. Burke CJ, Shah D, Saha S, Houghton R. Spondylolisthesis: a pictorial review. Br J Hosp Med (Lond). 2012;73(12):691–5.
3. Del Grande F, Maus TP, Carrino JA. Imaging the intervertebral disk: age-related changes, herniations, and radicular pain. Radiol Clin North Am. 2012;50(4):629–49.
4. Diehn FE. Imaging of spine infection. Radiol Clin North Am. 2012;50(4):777–98.
5. Fardon DF. Nomenclature and classification of lumbar disk pathology. Recommendations of the combined task forces of the North American Spine Society Radiology and the American Society of Neuroradiology. Spine. 2001;26:E93–113.
6. Konin GP, Walz DM. Lumbosacral transitional vertebrae: classification, imaging findings, and clinical relevance. AJNR Am J Neuroradiol. 2010;31(10):1778–86.
7. Olivieri I, D'Angelo S, Palazzi C. Diffuse idiopathic skeletal hyperostosis: differentiation from ankylosing spondylitis. Curr Rheumatol Rep. 2009;11(5):321–8.
8. Taljanovic MS, Hunter TB, Wisneski RJ. Imaging characteristics of diffuse idiopathic skeletal hyperostosis with an emphasis on acute spinal fractures: review. AJR Am J Roentgenol. 2009;193(3 Suppl):S10–9.
9. Wald JT. Imaging of spine neoplasm. Radiol Clin North Am. 2012;50(4):749–76.

Soft Tissue Calcifications

16

Raja S. Bobba and John O'Neill

Overview

Soft tissue calcifications are a relatively common finding on radiographs. Knowledge of the different patterns and locations can lead to accurate diagnosis of various disease processes. This chapter will focus on soft-tissue calcification commonly encountered in rheumatology.

Soft tissue calcification permeates many diseases, and their pathophysiology and clinical implications can vary just like their appearance in radiological evaluation. There is no universally accepted classification; however, the etiology of soft tissue calcification is commonly divided into dystrophic, metastatic, and idiopathic. Dystrophic calcification is by far the most common cause of soft tissue calcification and is present in damaged tissue such as in areas of trauma, inflammation, and devitalized tissue and in neoplasms. Connective tissue disease, hydroxyapatite, and calcium pyrophosphate deposition are included in this subdivision. The *VINDICATE* acronym provides a more extensive differential for dystrophic calcification (*V*ascular, *I*nfectious, *N*eoplastic, *D*rug, *A*utoimmune, *T*rauma, and *E*xtravascular findings).

Metastatic calcifications occurs in the setting of raised calcium and/or phosphorus, with subsequent deposition of calcium salts within normal soft tissue and includes: hyperparathyroidism, hypoparathyroidism, renal osteodystrophy with secondary hyperparathyroidism, milk alkali syndrome, sarcoidosis, hypervitaminosis D, and conditions with extensive bone destruction as can occur in leukemia and myeloma. Idiopathic calcinosis occurs in tumoral calcinosis. Soft tissue ossification should be differentiated from calcification. New bone formation within soft tissues is commonly posttraumatic, physical or thermal injuries (heterotopic ossification), secondary to neurologic disease, or related to benign or malignant tumors. Soft tissue ossification demonstrates an internal trabecular pattern and when fully formed has a corticated rim, both of which are absent in calcification, and thus allows for easy differentiation. The following is an overview of the most commonly encountered soft tissue calcification in clinical practice.

R.S. Bobba, MD, Msc (✉)
Assistant Professor, Department of Medicine,
McMaster University, Hamilton,
ON L8N 1Y2, Canada
e-mail: bobbars@gmail.com

J. O'Neill, MB, BAO, BCh, MRCPI, MSc, FRCR
Associate Professor, Musculoskeletal Imaging
Diagnostic Imaging, McMaster University
/St Joseph's Healthcare,
Hamilton, ON L8N4A6, Canada
e-mail: joneill2@me.com

J. O'Neill (ed.), *Essential Imaging in Rheumatology*,
DOI 10.1007/978-1-4939-1673-3_16, © Springer Science+Business Media New York 2015

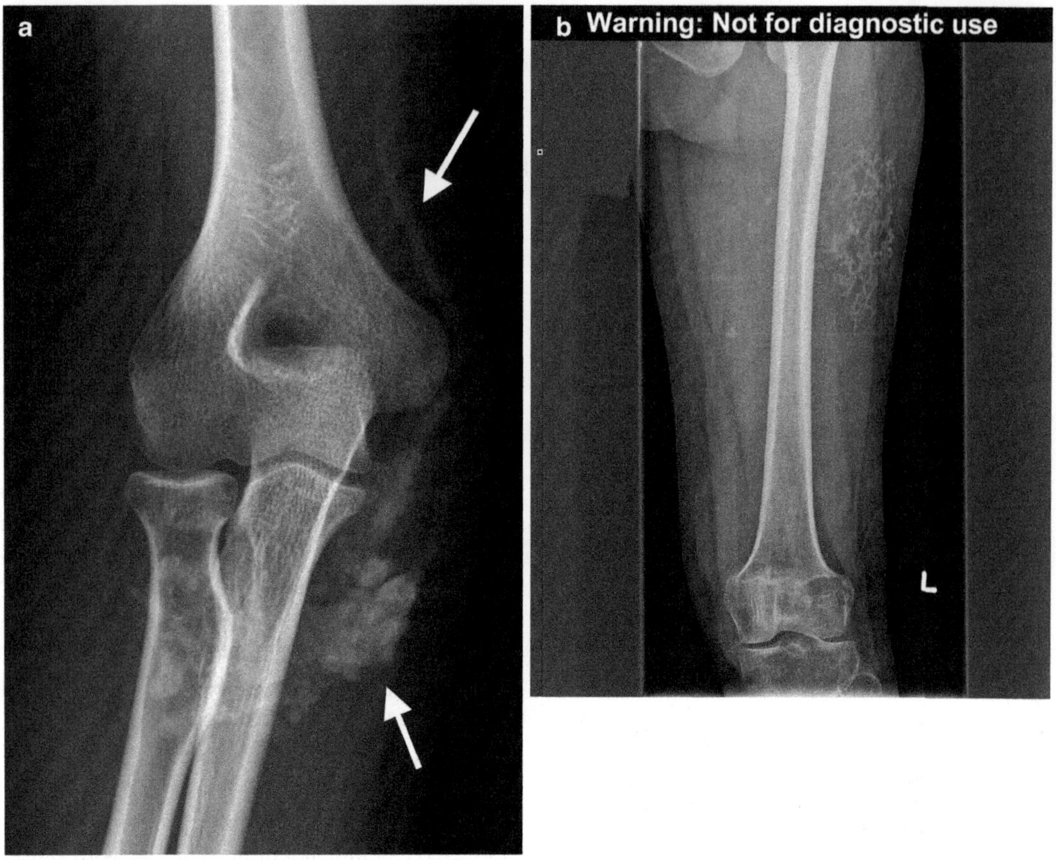

Fig. 16.1 (**a**) Periarticular soft-tissue calcification in a 16-year-old female with scleroderma. (**b**) Sheetlike soft-tissue calcification in a different patient with scleroderma

Connective Tissue Disease

Scleroderma and *CREST* syndrome (calcinosis, Raynaud's, esophageal dysmotility, sclerodactyly, and telangiectasia) can present with soft tissue calcification (Fig. 16.1). On radiographic evaluation, the lesions are present in the hands and feet as well as areas of the extremities such as the elbow that frequently rub or experience other forms of mild trauma. Hydroxyapatite crystals are frequently present. The soft-tissue calcifications of scleroderma may be either focal or diffuse. A cobblestone appearance is often noted, similar to ESRD or tumoral calcinosis. Calcifications are homogenously dense without associated septa or calcium-fluid level. Another key diagnostic feature of scleroderma-related soft-tissue calcifications are their unique predilection for the hands, being seen in over 50 % of afflicted individuals.

Systemic lupus erythematosus patients may develop periarticular or soft tissue calcification (Fig. 16.2). Calcification can occasionally ulcerate and become secondarily infected.

Other connective tissue diseases which contribute to soft tissue calcification include *dermatomyositis* and *polymyositis*. Fascial calcifications are almost invariably secondary to the closely

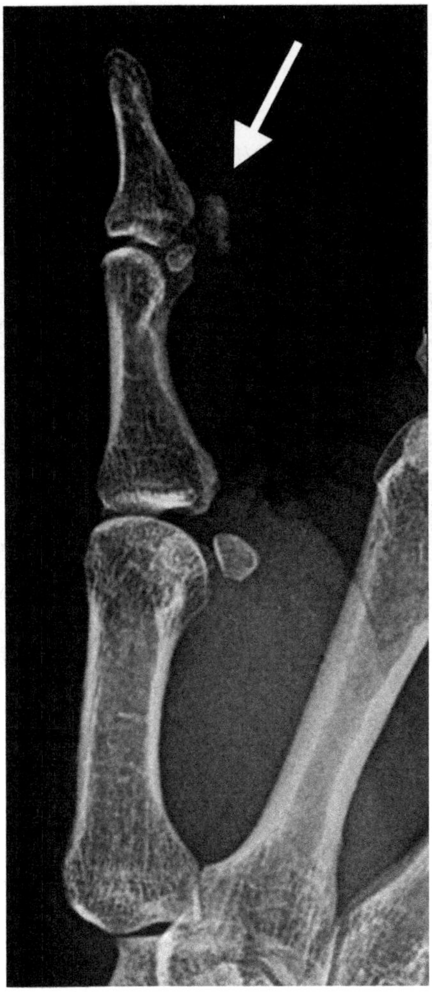

Fig. 16.2 Periarticular calcification within the volar soft tissues, calcinosis cutis, overlying the distal phalanx thumb in a 27-year-old female patient with SLE

related diseases of dermatomyositis and polymyositis. Each of these entities is an uncommon idiopathic inflammatory myopathy. During healing from episodes of myositis, calcifications develop in areas of necrosis (granulomatous changes incorporating calcium) involving the fascial planes and sometimes the subcutaneous tissues. Calcification develops with recurrent myositis. Radiographically, this manifests as numerous small densities in the appendicular skeleton that go on to coalesce and become sheetlike in appearance along ligaments, tendons, and fascial planes and is termed calcinosis universalis (Fig. 16.3).

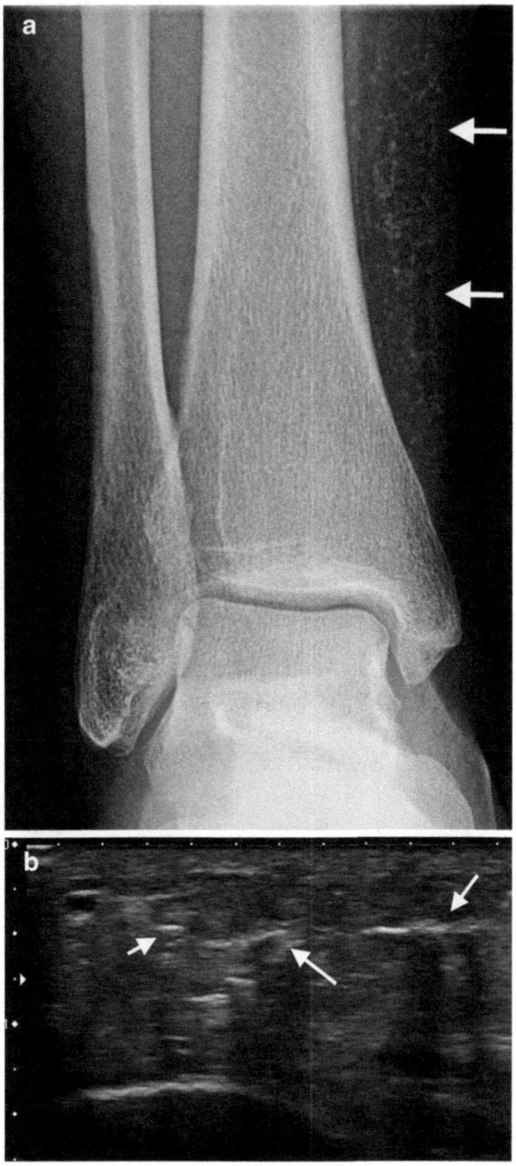

Fig. 16.3 Dermatomyositis with sheetlike subcutaneous calcification (*arrows*) over the medial margin distal tibia in a 57-year-old male patient on (**a**) radiograph and (**b**) ultrasound demonstrating calcification as linear hyperechoic bands

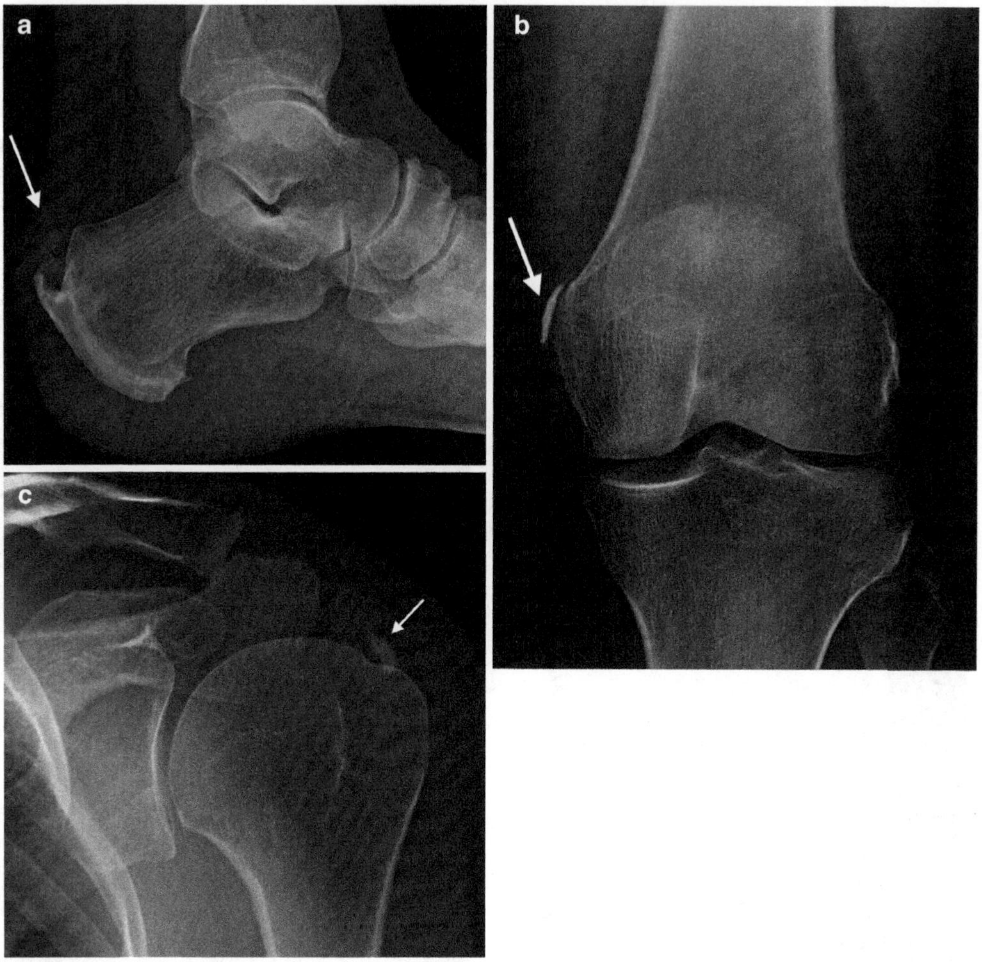

Fig. 16.4 (**a**) Thickened tendonotic distal Achilles with intratendinous calcification (*arrows*). (**b**) 50-year-old female patient with Pellegrini-Stieda lesion (calcification within dystrophic medial collateral ligament posttrauma) and (**c**) supraspinatus tendon calcification

Crystal Depositional Diseases

Calcium pyrophosphate depositional disease (CPPD), hydroxyapatite depositional disease (HADD), and gout are reviewed in detail in Chap. 8. Calcific tendinosis is most commonly related to the deposition of hydroxyapatite calcific deposits in dystrophic tendons (Fig. 16.4). This is commonly seen around the shoulder, hip, elbow, and wrist. CPPD crystal deposition can occur in hyaline and fibrocartilage. Classically involved areas include the wrist (triangular fibrocartilage), pubic symphysis, knee (hyaline cartilage and meniscus), hip, and shoulder (Fig. 16.5). Calcification can also occur in the rotator cuff muscle secondary to pyrophosphate crystals.

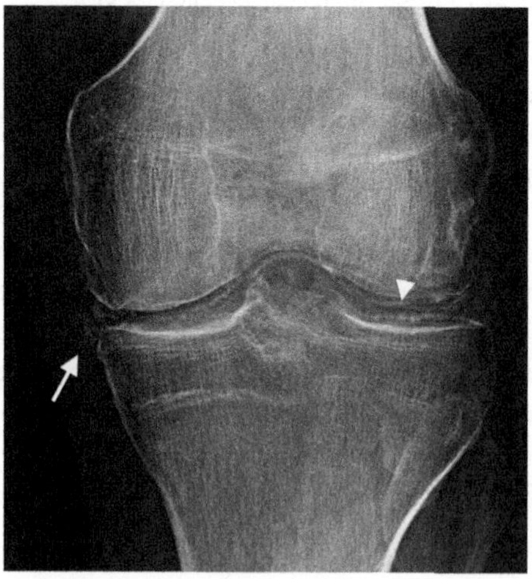

Fig. 16.5 Chondrocalcinosis with calcification of an extruded medial meniscus (*arrow*) and calcification articular cartilage (*arrowhead*)

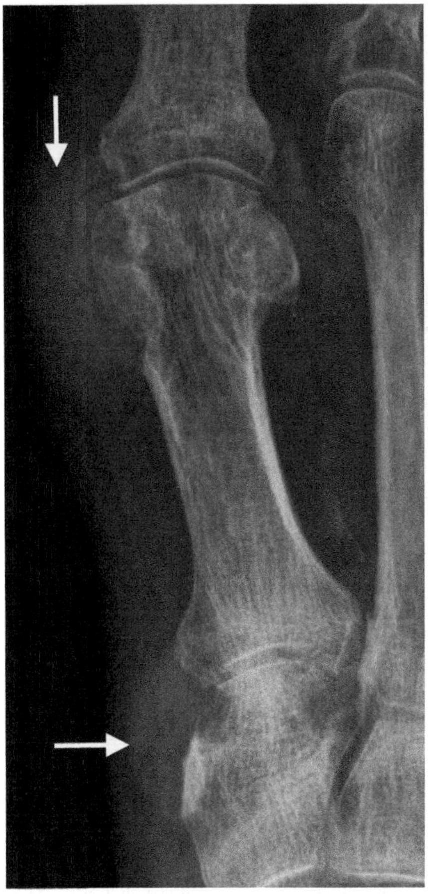

Fig. 16.6 An 87-year-old male with polyarticular gout demonstrating high attenuation gout tophi on the medial margin first TMTJ and MTPJ (*arrows*)

Calcified tophi in gout appear as periarticular soft tissue calcification of variable density (Fig. 16.6).

Tumoral Calcinosis

Tumoral calcinosis is an uncommon familial entity characterized by the presence of large lobulated masses of calcifications located in the subcutaneous juxta-articular soft tissues and extensor aspect of the extremities (Fig. 16.7).

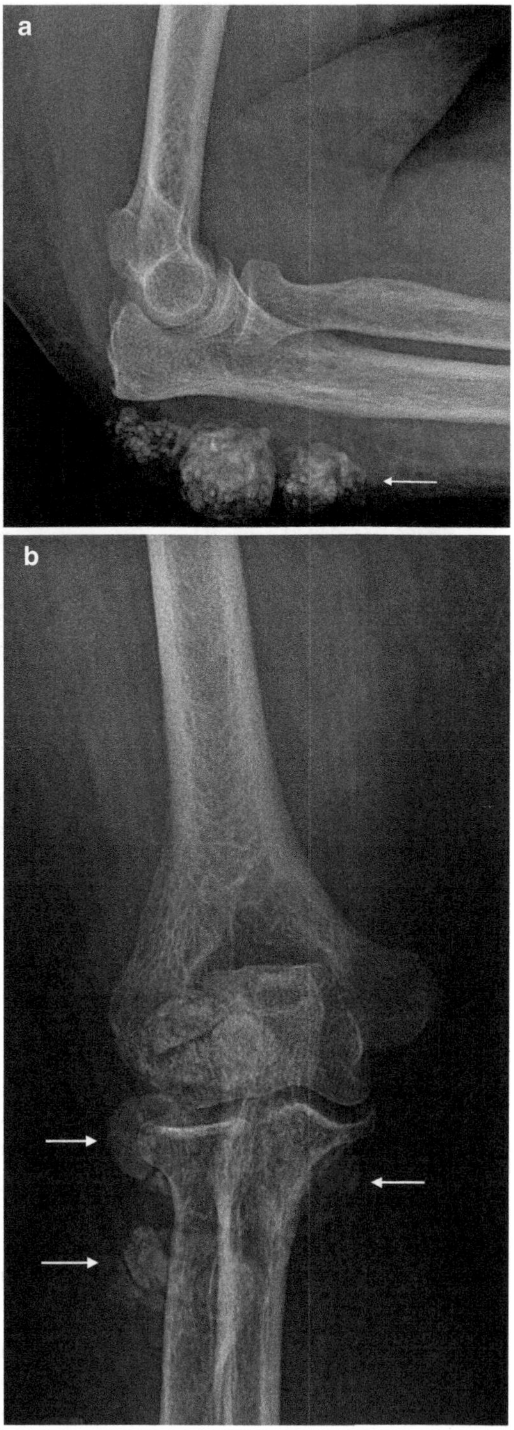

Fig. 16.7 Tumoral calcinosis with dense calcification within enlarged olecranon bursa. (**a**) Lateral and (**b**) AP radiographs

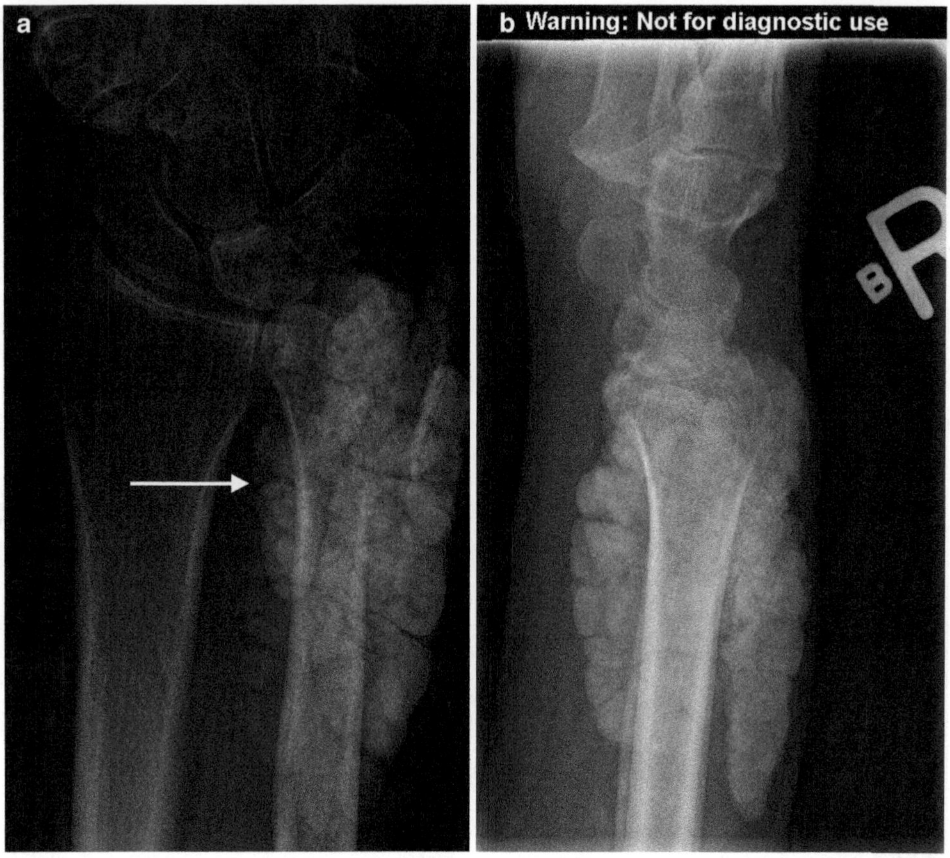

Fig. 16.8 A 53-year-old male patient with end-stage renal disease with enlarging hard juxta-articular soft tissue mass (*arrow*) distal forearm and wrist on (**a**) AP and (**b**) lateral radiographs demonstrating dense calcification of the soft tissues

While the majority of individuals are asymptomatic, diminished range of motion is a known complication from large juxta-articular masses as well as neuropathic symptoms due to compression of nearby nerves. Lesions develop in the first two decades, commonly in the locations of known bursae around the hip, elbow, and shoulder. Deposits are often cystic and are composed primarily of calcium hydroxyapatite crystals. Calcium levels are normal, and there is often a mild hyperphosphatemia. Patients may develop associated periosteal reaction, a CPPD-like arthropathy and dental abnormalities. Tumoral calcinosis mimics include the many etiologies of metastatic calcifications, most commonly chronic renal failure.

Chronic Renal Disease

Soft tissue calcification in end-stage renal disease is a manifestation of secondary and tertiary hyperparathyroidism. Primary hyperparathyroidism may frequently manifest as soft-tissue calcification independent of renal disease. Such manifestations of primary hyperparathyroidism occur quite frequently. With continued advances in hemodialysis and transplantation, leading to improved survival, the radiographic findings of this disease are encountered with increasing frequency. It is an inappropriately high level of calcium and phosphorus that result in the soft-tissue calcifications commonly seen in these individuals (Fig. 16.8).

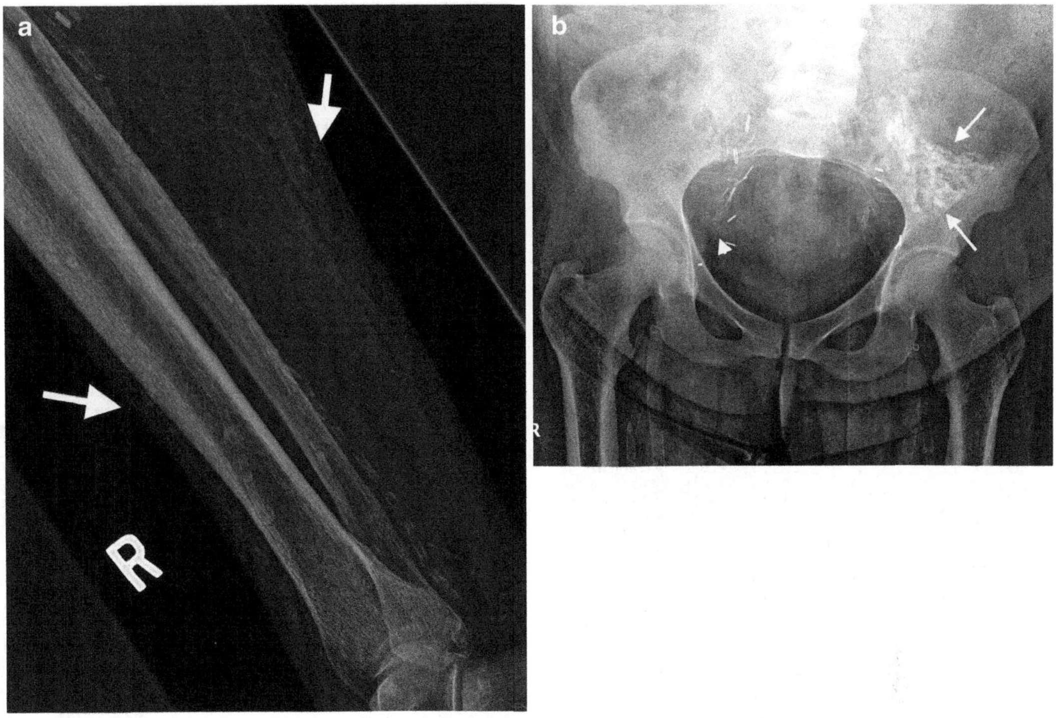

Fig. 16.9 (**a**) Radiograph in a patient with chronic renal failure with heavy vascular calcification and early calciphylaxis. (**b**) Calcified failed renal transplant left iliac fossa (*arrows*) and heavy vascular calcification

Another cutaneous manifestation of soft-tissue calcification is calciphylaxis which occurs in end-stage renal disease and renal transplant patients (Fig. 16.9). Calciphylaxis occurs due to calcium deposition in arterioles, which leads to ischemic ulceration of overlying skin. Calciphylaxis is most common in hyperparathyroidism secondary to chronic renal impairment and rarely occurs in the setting of normal renal function.

Benign and Malignant Tumors

Malignancy can also manifest as soft-tissue calcification or ossification within a mass (Fig. 16.10). Malignancies include hemangioma, synovial sarcoma, leiomyosarcoma, giant cell tumor, chondrosarcoma, and osteosarcoma. Calcification of muscle tissue can have manifestations that originate in sarcomatous origins. Radiographs of hemangiomas demonstrate a soft-tissue mass containing phleboliths (as described with arterial/venous calcification), which are seen as round densities ranging from 2 to 8 mm in size with a characteristic central lucency.

Leiomyoma and leiomyosarcoma are benign and malignant neoplasms of mesodermal etiology with smooth muscle differentiation. Recurrent rapid growth can lead to deposition of calcific tissue. Histologically, mineralization in leiomyosarcoma appears to be caused by either nonneoplastic ossification or dystrophic mineralization in the tumor. This feature can cause leiomyosarcomas to be confused with other neoplasms. Extraskeletal chondrosarcoma may present as either a noncalcified or a calcified soft-tissue mass. Calcified masses are common findings in extraskeletal chondrosarcoma, often showing stippled and ring- or arc-like calcifications.

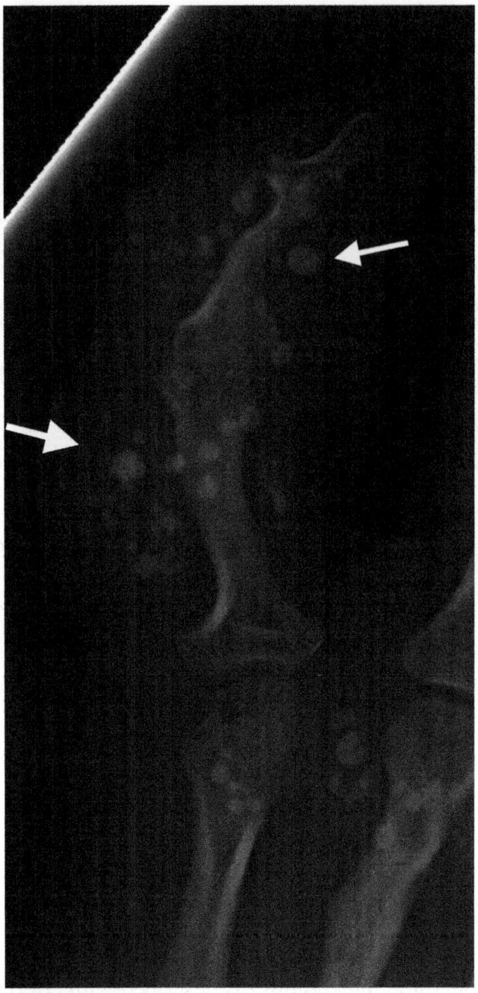

Fig. 16.10 Calcifications (phleboliths) within a low flow venous malformation of the hand

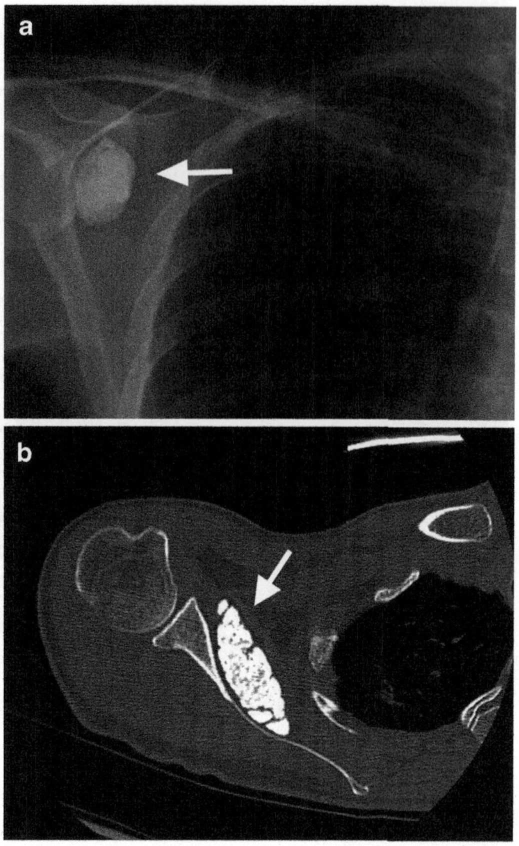

Fig. 16.11 A 43-year-old female with incidental soft tissue calcified mass over the right scapula (a) on CXR and (b) CT. Imaging in keeping with an intracapsular chondroma within the subscapularis recess

Vascular Calcification

Atherosclerotic vascular disease is a disease of the arterial intima that arises from the abnormal deposition of fatty substances, cholesterol, and calcium. It typically involves the large- and medium-sized arteries. A primary manifestation of vascular disease is arterial calcification. They present as patchy, irregular, plaquelike or even tubular densities of variable shape and size distributed along the path of large- and medium-sized arteries (Fig. 16.11).

Venous insufficiency in the extremities is generally seen in the superficial venous system and therefore mostly limited to the subcutaneous compartment. Their development occurs in the presence of long-standing varicosities and/or thrombus formation. Any partial occlusions can result in vascular turbulence and calcific deposition. These factors result in venous stasis, which in turn leads to calcium deposition along the venous intimal layer. On radiographs of the extremities, venous insufficiency calcification most frequently appears as phleboliths in the subcutaneous tissue. Phleboliths have a ring or oval shape with a central lucency that represents a focus of calcified thrombus. Associated evidence of chronic venous stasis may be present such as soft-tissue edema or in chronic cases adjacent periosteal reaction.

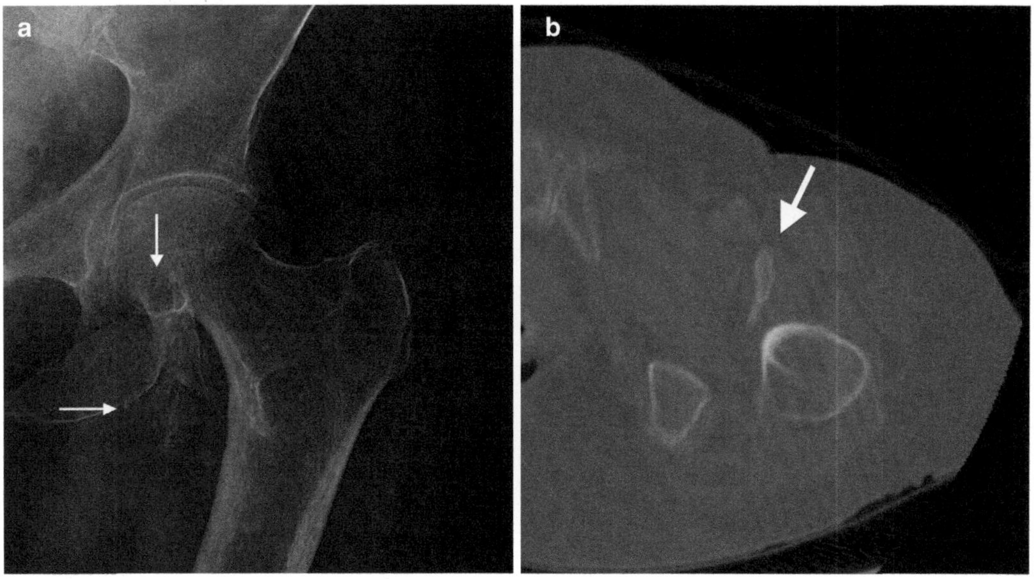

Fig. 16.12 Posttraumatic heterotopic ossification of the left iliopsoas in an 81-year-old female on (**a**) radiograph (*arrows*) and (**b**) CT (bone windows)

Heterotopic Ossification

Heterotopic ossification is the pathological development of ossification within soft tissue (Fig. 16.12). It is usually related to direct trauma to the affected musculoskeletal tissue or may be neurogenic in origin, e.g., spinal cord injury. Occasionally no precipitating factor is identified. Mechanical traumas include high-voltage electric injury, burns, post joint arthroplasties, and soft-tissue hematomas. The involved area may become swollen, tender, and erythematosus with associated fever with loss of adjacent joint function and diminished mobility although in the majority of cases there are limited symptoms. Radiographically there is a peripheral rim of calcification that proceeds to ossify with initially a lucent center and gradual centripetal advancement of ossification. In addition there is a non-ossified cleft between the ossification and adjacent cortical bone. These two findings are important to help differentiate heterotopic ossification from a more aggressive lesion such as an osteosarcoma.

Further Reading

1. Abedin M, Tintut Y, Demer LL. Vascular calcification: mechanisms and clinical ramifications. Arterioscler Thromb Vasc Biol. 2004;24(7):1161–70.
2. Banks KP, Bui-Mansfield LT, Chew FS, Collinson F. A compartmental approach to the radiographic evaluation of soft-tissue calcifications. Semin Roentgenol. 2005;40(4):391–407.
3. Boulman N, Slobodin G, Rozenbaum M, Rosner I. Calcinosis in rheumatic diseases. Semin Arthritis Rheum. 2005;34(6):805–12.
4. Olsen KM, Chew FS. Tumoral calcinosis: pearls, polemics, and alternative possibilities. Radiographics. 2006;26(3):871–85.
5. Vanden Bossche L, Vanderstraeten G. Heterotopic ossification: a review. J Rehabil Med. 2005;37(3):129–36.

Bone and Synovial Tumors

17

Sanjay Dixit and John O'Neill

Bone Tumors

Unsuspected bone tumors occasionally present to the rheumatologist. Tumors may be detected incidentally on imaging performed for alternate indications, or patients may be referred for investigation of nonspecific musculoskeletal symptoms, which are secondary to a bone or joint neoplasm. As such, the rheumatologist should have an understanding of the common imaging appearance of the bone and joint neoplasms.

Primary malignant bone tumors are very rare with an estimated incidence of 0.9/100,000 people. To place this in perspective, consider the incidence of lung cancer, which approaches 63/100,000 people. Primary musculoskeletal malignancies account for less than 1 % of all cancers. Because of its rare occurrence, a systematic approach is imperative for the clinician to adequately evaluate a bony lesion. The major challenge is to differentiate between a benign and malignant lesion as this directly influences further evaluation, treatment, and prognosis. Useful information includes patient history, physical, and radiographic appearance.

S. Dixit, MBBS, MS, MD, ABIM, FRCPC (✉)
Assistant Clinical Professor, Department of Medicine and Rheumatology, McMaster University, Hamilton, ON L8N3Z5, Canada
e-mail: sanjay.dixit@medportal.ca

J. O'Neill, MB, BAO, BCh, MRCPI, MSc, FRCR
Associate Professor. Musculoskeletal Imaging Diagnostic Imaging, McMaster University/ St Joseph's Healthcare,
Hamilton, ON L8N4A6, Canada
e-mail: joneill2@me.com

Clinical History and Physical

Clinical history is incredibly useful in helping to guide differentiation of benign and malignant bony lesions. Key information includes age and gender, symptoms, and family or personal history of cancer. Certain tumors have a predilection for age (Table 17.1). Common malignant tumors in children and young adults include osteosarcoma and Ewing sarcoma. Conversely in an adult, over the age of 40 years, the more common lesions are metastatic lesions and myeloma. Most primary tumors have a male predominance, with the exception of parosteal osteosarcoma, giant cell tumor, aneurysmal bone cyst, and hemangioma, which favor women slightly.

Presenting symptoms may include pain, swelling, or even pathologic fracture. Although there certainly is overlap, benign tumors tend more to be incidental findings. Some benign tumors however can mimic malignant behavior with mass affect or pathologic fracture such as a giant cell tumor. Malignant lesions tend to cause bone destruction leading to localized findings, rest or night pain, and systemic symptoms such as fevers

J. O'Neill (ed.), *Essential Imaging in Rheumatology*,
DOI 10.1007/978-1-4939-1673-3_17, © Springer Science+Business Media New York 2015

Table 17.1 Common primary malignant bone tumors by age

0–9 years	10–19 years	20–29 years	30+ years
Ewing sarcoma	Osteosarcoma	Osteosarcoma	Myeloma
Osteosarcoma	Ewing sarcoma	Chondrosarcoma	Chondrosarcoma
Primary lymphoma	Primary lymphoma	Ewing sarcoma	Osteosarcoma
	Primary lymphoma	Primary lymphoma	
		MFH/fibrosarcoma	Chordoma
			MFH/fibrosarcoma

Reprinted from Chew FS: *Skeletal Radiology: The Bare Bones* (3rd ed). Philadelphia, PA: Lippincott Williams & Wilkins, 2010
For each age range, the tumor types are listed in order of frequency and account for over 90 % of the primary tumors
MFH malignant fibrous histiocytoma

and weight loss. Pain may occasionally be an important distinguishing feature. For example, a benign enchondroma usually does not present with pain unless fractured, whereas a similarly appearing low-grade chondrosarcoma maybe painful. Other pertinent symptoms include a history of trauma or infection. Family history may suggest a heritable condition such as multiple hereditary exostoses. Likewise, personal history of cancer such as the breast or colon may suggest possible metastases.

Physical exam includes local inspection (i.e., swelling), lymph node assessment, and systemic observation (i.e., weight loss).

Imaging

Radiographs

The radiograph is the first line of imaging for initial evaluation of a bone lesion. This imaging modality is easy to access and inexpensive and provides a wealth of information that is essential to narrowing the differential diagnosis of most primary bone tumors. The entire bone should be imaged. Often a diagnosis is made with radiographs, and if benign, no further workup may be required. Further imaging with MRI, CT, or bone scan may be required if radiographic features are nonspecific. The selection of further imaging options should be discussed with your radiologist. Occasionally, radiography can fail to show an abnormality, such as a lytic lesion, which may only become detectable when it has resulted in 30–50 % loss of mineralization. In cases where there is a high clinical suspicion of underlying pathology with normal initial imaging, further modalities should be employed.

The key to radiographic assessment of bone tumors is the concept that their appearance reflects their underlying pathology. Crucial characteristics to evaluate include lesion location, growth rate, margin, matrix, periosteal reaction, and cortical involvement (Fig. 17.1). Although there is a significant overlap, tumors have common sites of involvement, for example, primary bone lymphoma preferentially involves the femur and pelvis. Multiple lesions are suspicious for metastasis although there are benign exceptions such as multiple hereditary exostoses and hemangiomas.

Very slow-growing or unchanged lesions over time usually suggest a benign process. The growth pattern reflects the balance between bone destruction and proliferation. A sclerotic rim indicates that the lesion's growth rate is slow enough to allow new bone to form at the periphery. If the lesion grows too rapidly, new bone is unable to form around the lesion. An important consideration is the lesion's impact on the structural integrity of the bone and adjacent structures. Aggressive features include periosteal reaction at the lesion's edge indicating it has breached the cortex. An exception to this is a fracture through a benign lesion with secondary benign periosteal reaction. There are various subtypes of periosteal reaction based on appearance including laminated, hair-on-end, sunburst, or Codman triangle

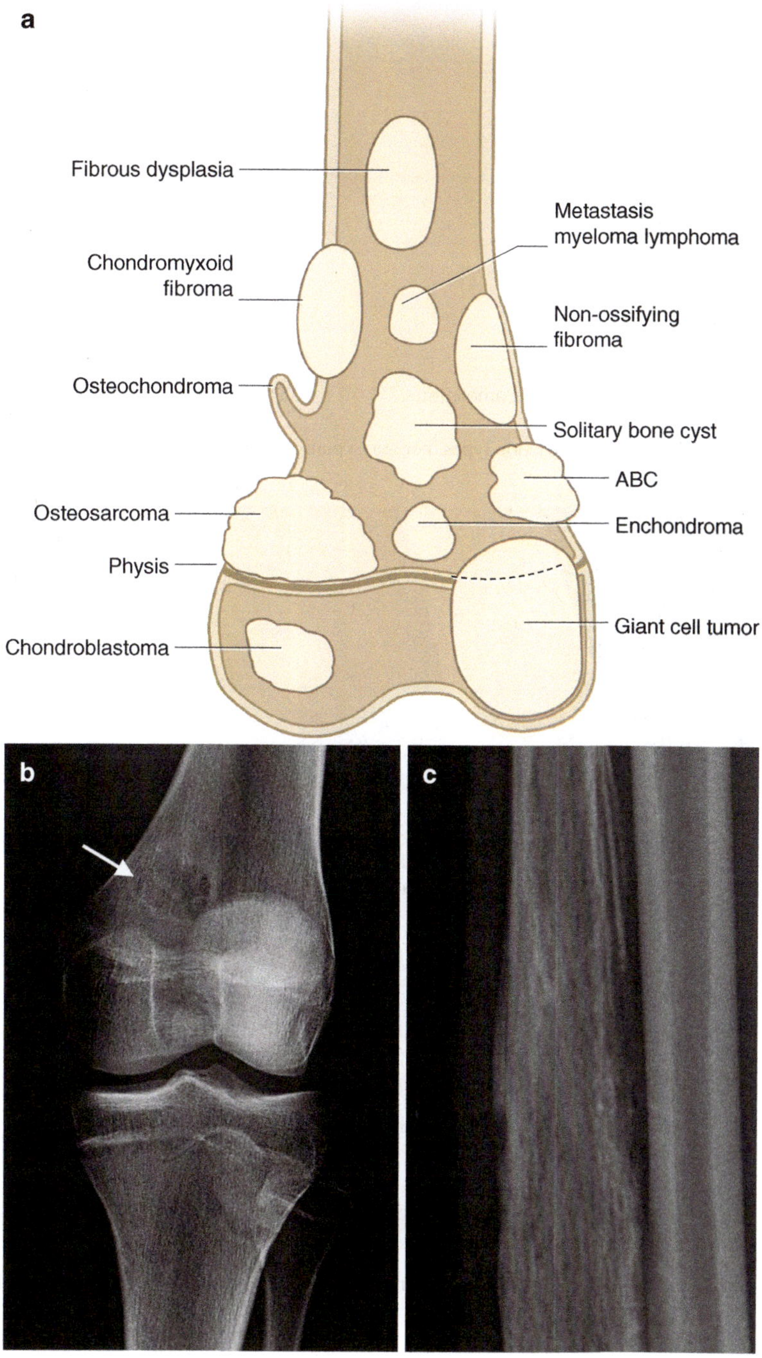

Fig. 17.1 (**a**) Common locations of bone tumors, (**b**) typical features of a benign bone lesion (*arrow*) with a well-defined margin, thin sclerotic rim, no cortical destruction, soft tissue mass or periosteal reaction and exhibited stability over time, lesion is typical for fibrous cortical defect when viewed in conjunction with lateral radiograph (not shown); (**c**) malignant lesion, Ewing sarcoma, with moth-eaten bone destruction, aggressive periosteal reaction and cortical breach

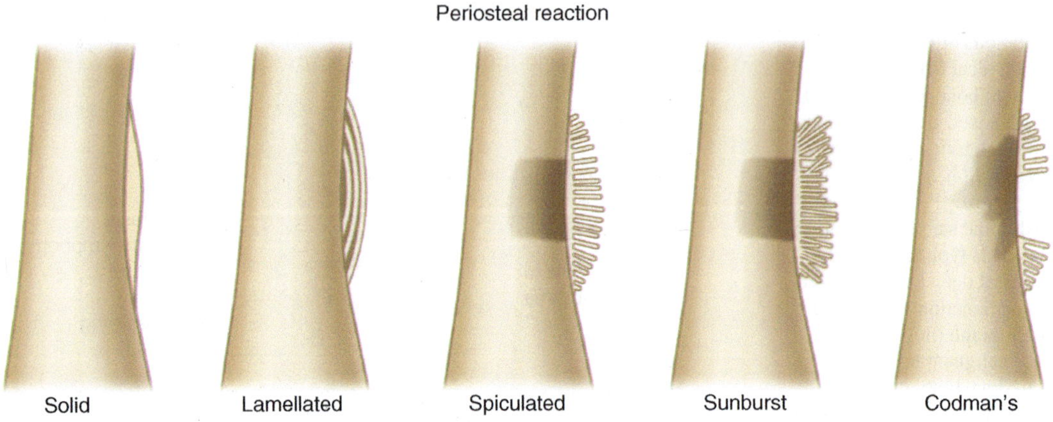

Fig. 17.2 Periosteal reaction types, benign to malignant (*left to right*)

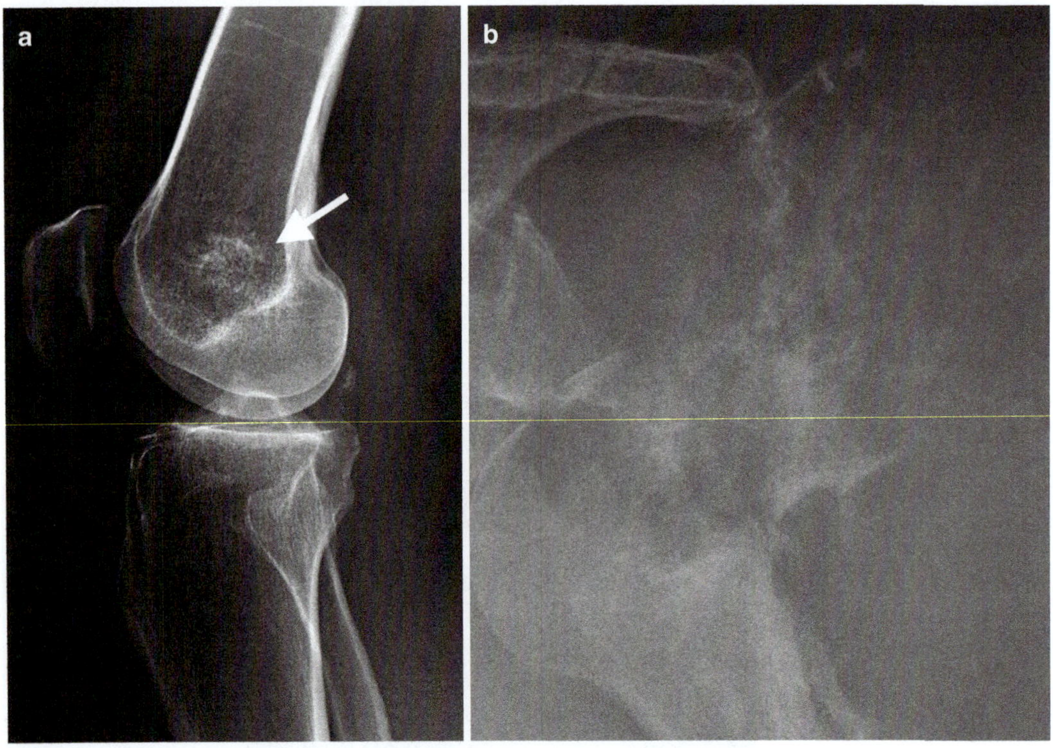

Fig. 17.3 Chondroid matrix in a benign enchondroma (*arrow*) (**a**) and a malignant chondrosarcoma (**b**)

(Fig. 17.2). Soft tissue reactions represent tumor extension and are concerning. MRI is the most sensitive modality for assessing this although CT can be useful. Finally, many bone tumors have an internal matrix mineralization pattern that can suggest the underlying etiology. For example, chondroid matrix can appear as calcified rings and arcs. This pattern can be seen in both benign and malignant chondroid lesions and result from calcification at the periphery of multiple cartilaginous lobules (Fig. 17.3).

Radiographic features suggesting a benign etiology include stability over time, narrow zone of transition, thin sclerotic rim, and without a cortical breach, soft tissue mass, or periosteal new bone. Conversely, cortical destruction, a wide zone of transition, and associated soft tissue mass and aggressive periosteal reaction are concerning features of malignancy.

MRI and CT

MR is excellent in evaluating the marrow signal intensity and soft tissue extension and can provide information not available with other imaging modalities. In general, the entire bone should be scanned to evaluate for skip lesions. MRI is the most sensitive technique for detecting marrow-based lesions. The MR imaging protocol for tumor evaluation depends on the location and radiographic features of the lesion. In certain cases, CT is preferable to MR imaging for tumor evaluation. CT is very useful to assess suspected intralesional mineralization, i.e., matrix. It is also excellent at demonstrating cortically based lesions, such as the central nidus of osteoid osteoma, and for evaluating subtle cortical erosion or penetration. In patients who cannot undergo MRI, CT with multiplanar capability is a reasonable substitute.

Bone scans may be helpful in assessing activity of a lesion and multiplicity, e.g., metastatic disease. In general, benign lesions demonstrate no or mild uptake and malignant lesions increased uptake on bone scans secondary to the osteoblastic response induced by the lesion. Bone scans carry a significant radiation burden, and discussion with your radiologist on the optimal imaging algorithm for your patient is advised in all cases.

The following is a brief overview of common tumors.

Benign Bone Tumors

Osteoma (Fig. 17.4)

Osteoma is a slow-growing tumor and usually presents as an incidental finding. There is no gender or age association. This lesion is made of both woven and dense bone originating from the skull and occasionally in the long bones. All imaging modalities show a characteristic sharply defined bony surface lesion originating from the cortex.

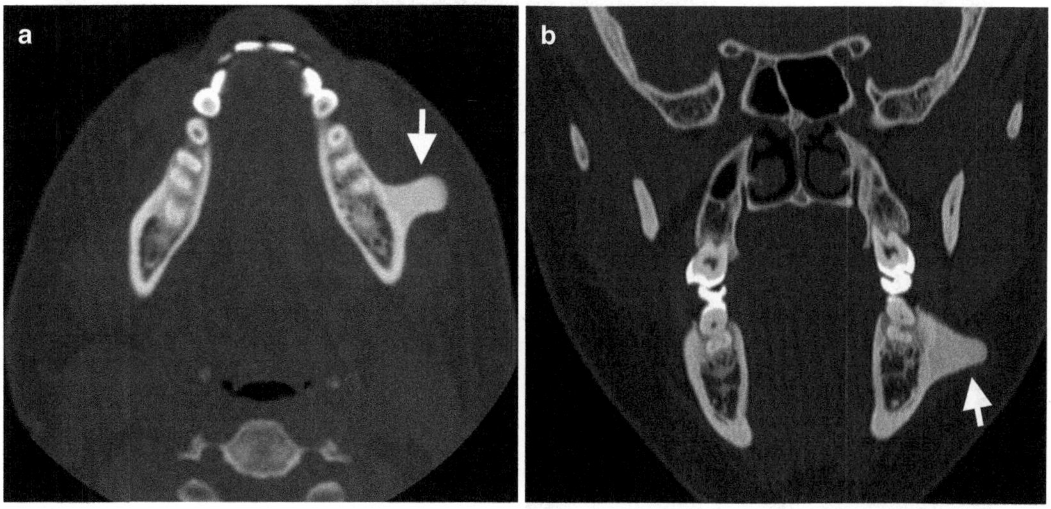

Fig. 17.4 Osteoma in an adult male patient presenting with a slow-growing mass left body mandible. (**a**) Axial and (**b**) coronal CT demonstrate a well-demarcated dense "ivory"-like bony lesion attached to an intact cortex

Osteoblastoma

This is a rare osteoid-producing tumor that histologically is indistinguishable from an osteoid osteoma. A tumor size of 2 cm or larger is the main differentiating criterion. There are a variety of appearances depending on location. Spinal osteoblastomas tend to be expansile with a mineralized matrix and have a narrow zone of transition. In contrast in long bones, they may appear aggressive with prominent bone expansion, partial cortical destruction, with soft tissue infiltration.

Osteochrondroma (Fig. 17.5)

These are cartilage-forming tumors and are relatively common. They are composed of lamellar bone covered by a cartilage cap. There is a male predominance and usually occurs in patients younger than 20 years. Imaging demonstrates cortical and medullary continuity, and it can be sessile or pedunculated in appearance. CT and MRI demonstrate a cartilage cap. After skeletal maturity, the cap should not be thicker than 2 cm. Increased thickness suggests possible transformation to chondrosarcoma.

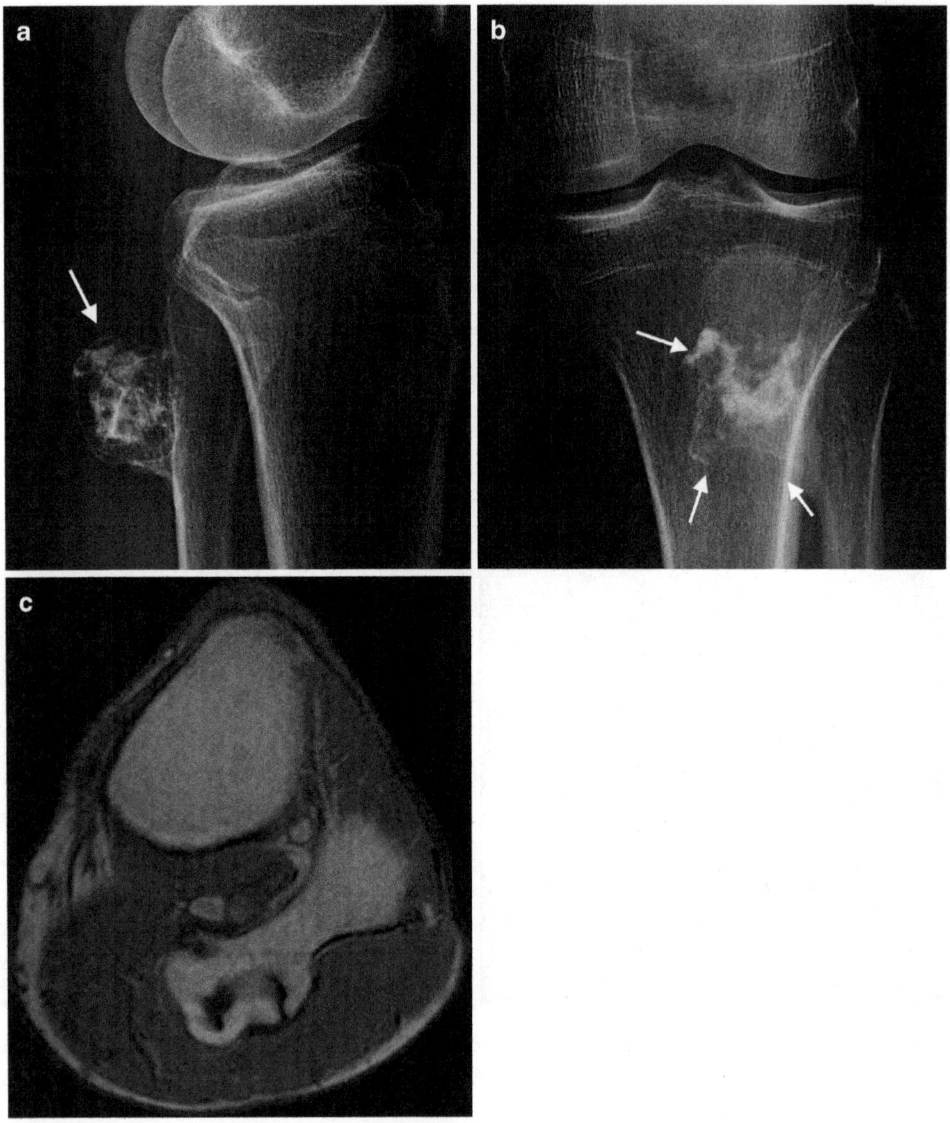

Fig. 17.5 Osteochondroma in a 15-year-old male presenting with knee discomfort postexercise. (**a**) Lateral and (**b**) AP radiographs demonstrate a well-defined lesion arising from a broad base and in continuity with the cortex of the proximal fibular diametaphysis with internal calcified matrix. (**c**) Axial T1 demonstrates no significant cartilage cap to lesion which extends along the posterior margin tibial neurovascular bundle and demonstrates continuity with underlying cortex (*arrows*)

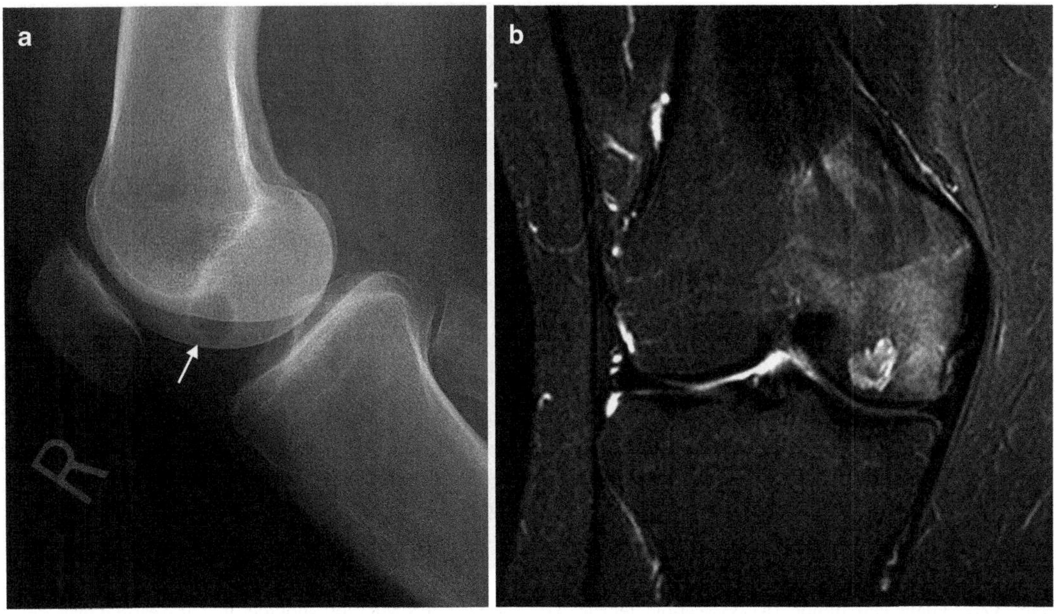

Fig. 17.6 Chondroblastoma in an 18-year-old male presenting with knee pain. (**a**) Lateral radiograph knee demonstrates a well-defined lytic lesion with thin sclerotic rim in the epiphysis medial femoral condyle (*arrow*). (**b**) Coronal T2FS MRI demonstrates the same lesion as well defined with internal heterogenous increased signal intensity on T2, thin low SI rim, and extensive surrounding bone marrow edema which is typical for this lesion

Chrondroblastoma (Fig. 17.6)

This is a rare lesion comprising less than 2 % of benign bone lesions. It occurs close to joints and therefore can present with some loss of joint function. It is twice as common in males as females, and most cases occur in children and young adults. Histologically, it is comprised of chondroblasts, occasional giant cells, and abundant chondroid matrix. It is most commonly seen in the proximal femur. Radiographs show a lucent lesion within the epiphysis with a thin sclerotic rim. The subtle chondroid matrix is better seen on CT, along with the adjacent periosteal reaction. The hallmark of this cartilaginous lesion is demonstrated on MR imaging and shows a typical low-to-intermediate signal of the tumor on fluid sensitive with extensive surrounding reactive marrow edema.

Giant Cell Tumor (Fig. 17.7)

This tumor comprises 10 % of all primary bone tumors, occurs slightly more often in females, and affects people after skeletal maturity with a peak incidence in the third decade. Histology reveals multinucleated giant cells on a background of mononuclear cells. Radiography shows a characteristic expansile lytic lesion at the end of the bone with a narrow zone of transition. CT can show a partially sclerotic zone of transition and confirms a lack of matrix mineralization. On MR imaging, the T1- and T2-weighted sequences are low-to-intermediate signal. The lower T2 signal, compared with other lesions, maybe caused by hemosiderin deposits or increased cellularity.

Primary Malignant Bone Tumors

Within the malignant bone tumor differential, there are only a few common primary etiologies (Table 17.2). They are classified based on their cellular origin. The most frequent will be discussed below.

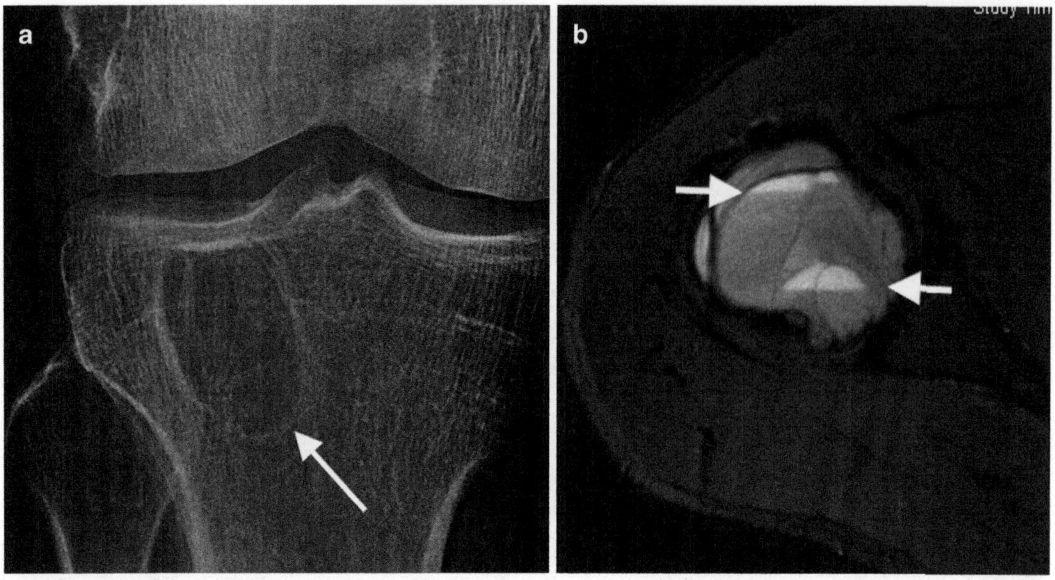

Fig. 17.7 Giant cell tumor. (**a**) 33-year-old female AP knee demonstrates a well-defined lytic lesion with thin sclerotic rim extending to subchondral plate (*arrow*). (**b**) Axial T2FS MRI left shoulder in a 38-year-old male demonstrating a well-defined lytic lesion in the humeral head with typical internal fluid–fluid levels (*arrows*)

Table 17.2 Relative frequencies of common primary malignant tumors

Tumors	Frequency
Osteosarcoma	35.1
Chondrosarcoma	25.8
Ewing sarcoma	16
Chordoma	8.4
Malignant fibrous histiocytoma	5.7
Angiosarcoma	1.4
Unspecified	1.2
Others	6.4

Osteosarcoma (Fig. 17.8)

This is the most common primary malignant tumor of the bone and the most common bone malignancy in children. There is a predilection for males. Approximately 50 % occur around the bones of the knee joint. The composition can vary from osteoid to chondroid and fibroid. The radiographic picture is therefore variable. Characteristic radiographic findings include aggressive tumor pattern with a large lesion and osteoid matrix (90 %) with a pattern of fluffy opacities that destroy the cortex causing cortical breach and periosteal reaction. There usually is a wide zone of

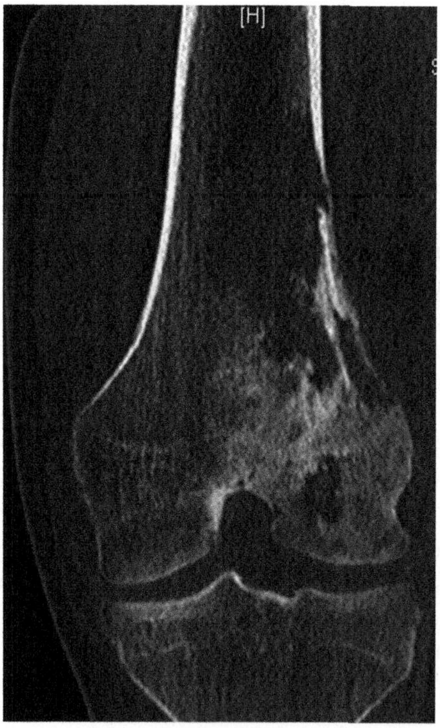

Fig. 17.8 Osteosarcoma: 19-year-old male distal femoral lesion extending from diaphysis to epiphysis. Mixed lytic sclerotic lesion with poorly defined margins and cortical destruction. Limited periosteal reaction

transition with a soft tissue mass. A Codman angle with elevation of the periosteum is common.

Chondrosarcoma (Fig. 17.9)

These account for 25 % of primary bone tumors. They usually occur in the pelvis and proximal femur of adults, more men than women and usually in their fifth decade.

Imaging depends on the grade of the lesion. This can vary from a well-defined lucent lesion with a chondroid matrix to popcorn calcification and aggressive features such as ill-defined margins, cortical expansion, and erosion. MRI can show associated tissue edema and soft tissue expansion. Central chondroma has a low T1 signal and high T2 signal because of the high water content of the cartilage. This tumor also demonstrates a "rings and arcs" pattern of enhancement. CT can help identify matrix calcification and subtle cortical erosion.

Ewing Sarcoma (Fig. 17.10)

These represent 10 % of primary bone tumors. They usually occur in children and young adults with a slight predilection for males. They tend to arise in the diaphysis or metaphyseal–diaphyseal part of long bones, pelvis, and ribs. They can also occur in soft tissues without bone involvement. Histologically, these tumors are of neuroendoectodermal origin. Imaging typically shows ill-defined, moth-eaten bone destruction. There usually is lytic bone destruction with a wide zone of transition, and typical "onion skin" multilayered periosteal reaction is seen in half the tumors. Metastatic disease occurs early to the lungs, bone, and bone marrow. Findings of cortical permeation and destruction are seen in over a third of patients.

Chordoma

These are very rare tumor comprising 2–4 % of primary bone tumors. They typically occur in the sacrum and intracranially. These are found in patients in the fifth and sixth decades and more common in men than women. They are characterized by slow growth, local destruction of bone, and extension into adjacent soft tissue. Sclerotic margin and narrow transition zone may be present because of slow growth.

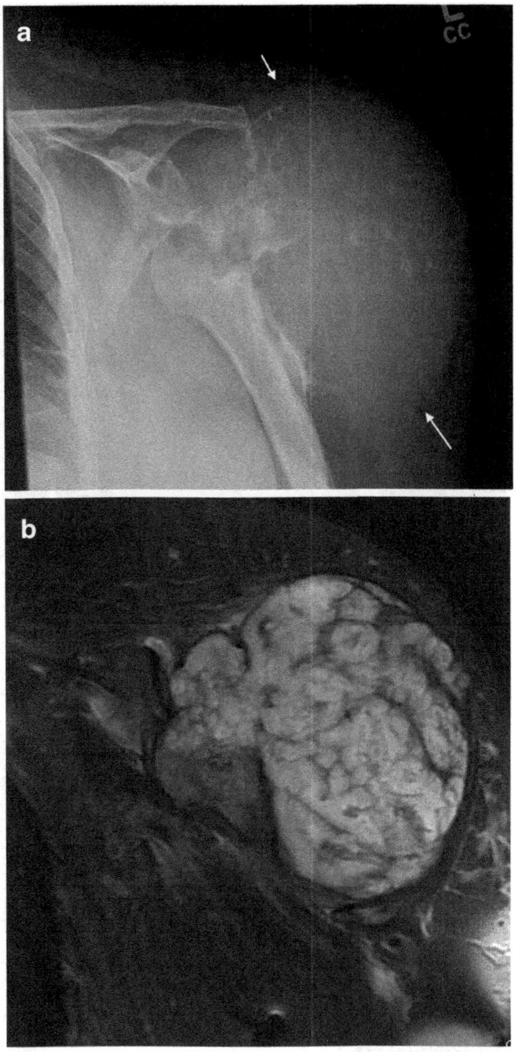

Fig. 17.9 Chondrosarcoma: 86-year-old female presenting with enlarging left shoulder mass and decreased range of motion. (**a**) AP radiograph demonstrates a large soft tissue mass originating from the left humeral greater tuberosity with significant bone destruction, poorly defined bone margins, and a large soft tissue mass which defined margins and heterogenous internal calcification (*arrows*). (**b**) Coronal T2 MR image same patient demonstrating heterogenous high signal intensity of the chondroid matrix

Malignant Fibrous Histiocytoma

This accounts for 2–5 % of primary bone tumors. It is slightly more common in males and seen in the fifth to seventh decades. Radiographs show an eccentric aggressive lytic lesion and soft tissue invasion. Periosteal reaction is rarely seen.

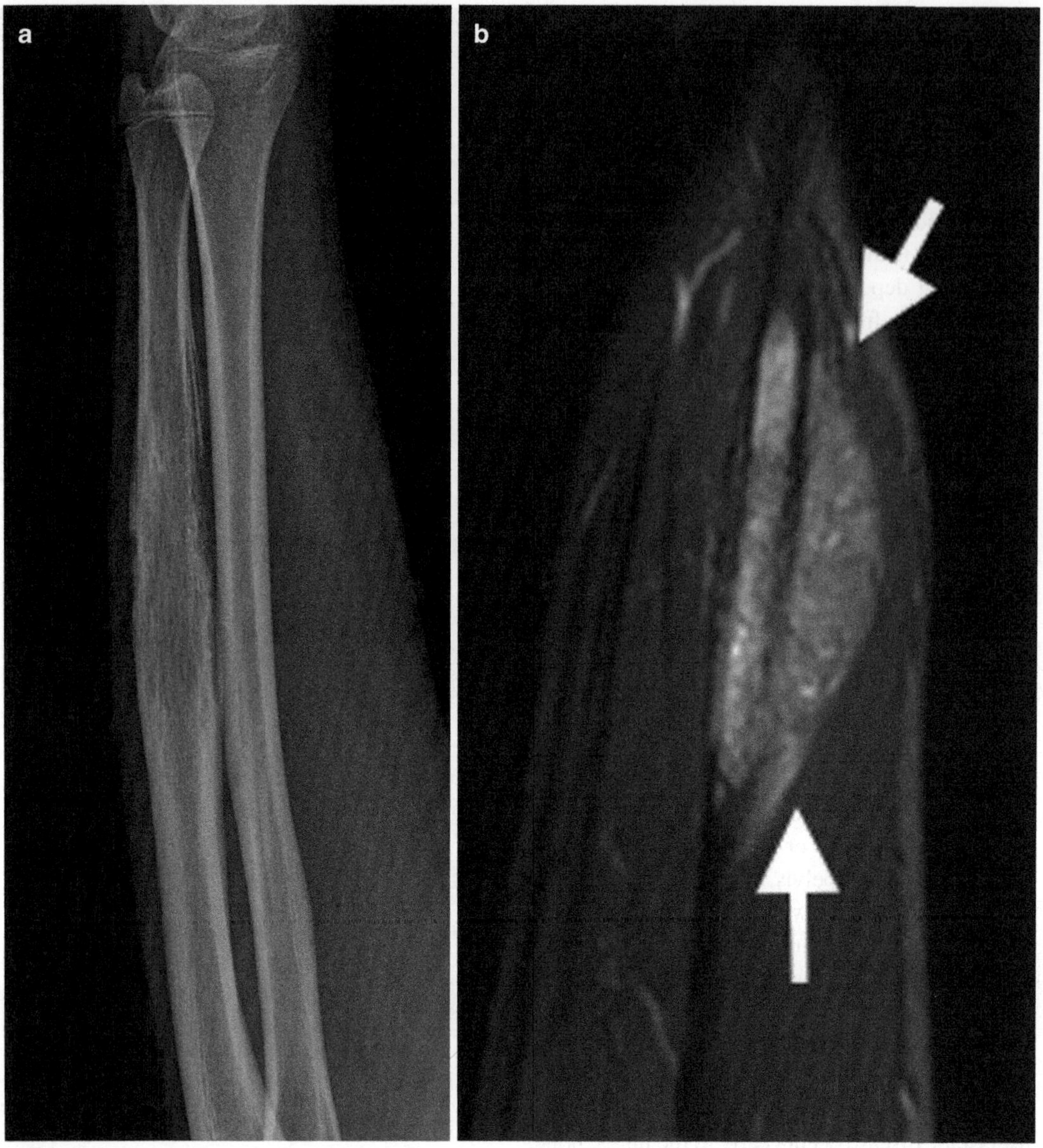

Fig. 17.10 Ewing sarcoma, a 13-year-old male presenting with forearm pain. (**a**) Radiograph demonstrates an aggressive bony lesion with moth-eaten pattern, poorly defined margins, cortical destruction, and aggressive periosteal reaction but underestimates the extent of soft tissue involvement as seen in (**b**) saggital T2FS MRI (*arrows*)

Synovial Tumors

Synovial Chondromatosis

Synovial chondromatosis or synovial osteochondromatosis is an uncommon benign disorder (Fig. 17.11). It is distinguished by metaplastic proliferation of multiple cartilaginous nodules in the synovial membrane of the joints, bursae, or tendon sheaths. Usually monoarticular but may also rarely present with polyarticular involvement. It can be categorized into primary or secondary. Primary disease occurs where cartilaginous tissue arising directly from metaplastic synovial tissue. In secondary disease, loose bodies arise from displaced hyaline cartilage or bone from degenerative joint disease, trauma, or neuropathic arthropathy. In 1977, Milgram described synovial chondromatosis as occurring in three stages: early, transitional, and

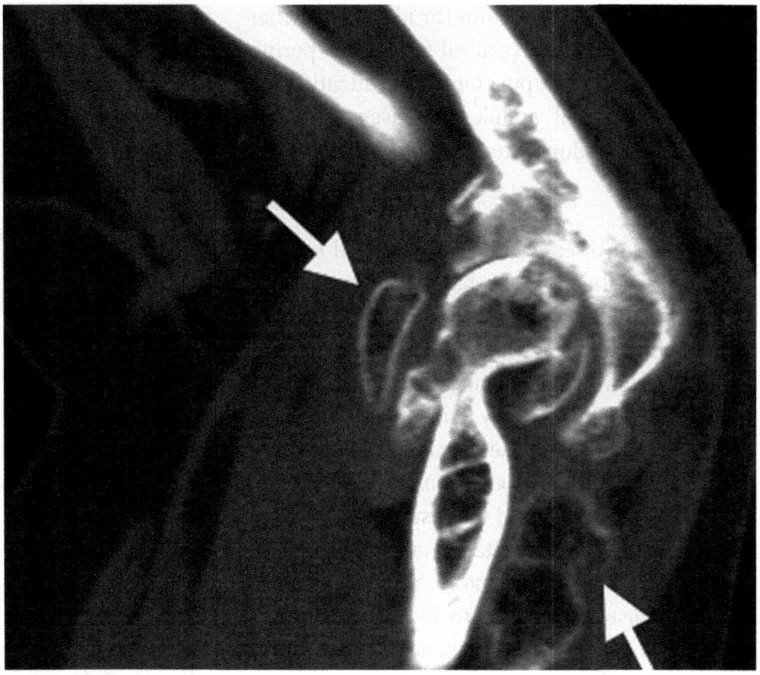

Fig. 17.11 Synovial osteochondromatosis, saggital reconstructed CT image elbow demonstrating secondary posttraumatic degenerative disease with multiple intra-articular loose ossified bodies (*arrows*)

late. Phase 1, or early disease, is defined by active intrasynovial disease on histology with no loose bodies; phase 2, or transitional stage, has active disease and loose bodies; and phase 3, or late stage disease, shows multiple loose bodies with no intrasynovial disease.

Clinical Presentation

It has a male to female ratio of 2:1. It is usually discovered between the third and fifth decades of life. The knee is the most common site of involvement, with the hip, shoulder, elbow, and ankle accounting for most of the remaining cases. Patients often notice pain and swelling. On examination, the presence of a soft tissue mass, limitation in range of motion, tenderness, and joint effusion are often present.

Imaging

Radiographs

Soft tissue masses are commonly seen resulting from a combination of non-mineralized cartilaginous bodies, hyperplastic synovium, and associated joint effusion. Calcifications are seen in 70–95 % of cases; multiple calcified bodies, typically smooth, round, and of similar size scattered throughout the joint are diagnostic. These calcifications frequently show a pathognomonic appearance of being numerous and homogenous in appearance. The degree of mineralization ranges from small areas of calcification to large ossified bodies containing central radiolucent fatty bone marrow surrounded by dense cortical bone. Secondary degenerative changes such as joint space narrowing, periarticular sclerosis, and osteophyte formation are found in the late stages of the disease, but periarticular osteoporosis is seldom a feature unless related to disuse. In addition, secondary synovial chondromatosis often shows several rings of calcification compared with a single ring seen in primary disease. Radiographic findings are normal in 5–30 % of primary intra-articular synovial chondomatosis.

CT

CT is the optimal modality to detect calcified bodies. It can show a key diagnostic finding: multiple nodules enclosed by the joint capsule, finely stippled, and confluent tending to form a soft tissue mass of water density that elevates the capsule. CT will also clarify adjacent subchondral bone changes as areas of pressure erosion rather than aggressive destruction and can establish whether a calcified mass on plain film is intra-articular, although this latter feature can also be well seen on MRI.

CT is particularly helpful for identifying characteristic ring and arc (central focus with peripheral calcification) or punctate mineralization and the multiplicity of nodules in cases for which radiographic findings are normal or equivocal.

MRI

The extent of disease is best appreciated on MRI due to its superior musculoskeletal anatomical definition. Although both CT and MRI can show early erosive changes, MRI will detect bone marrow infiltration (a sign of malignant transformation). This modality is helpful not only in identifying the chondromatosis but also in detecting synovitis, joint erosion, and extracapsular extension.

Kramer has described three subtypes based on the MR signal of the osteochondromal nodules. Pattern A is a lobulated, intra-articular mass with signal intensity isointense to hypointense to the muscle on T1-weighted sequences and hyperintense to the muscle on T2-weighted sequences. This pattern occurs in 17 % of cases and corresponds to cases where there is no calcification on plain x-rays. The B subtype accounts for the majority of cases (75 %). These osteochondromal nodules are of low signal intensity on all sequences due to calcification of cartilaginous nodules. Other features are similar to pattern A. Pattern C, corresponding to cases with both calcification and ossification on plain x-rays, is found in about 10 % of cases and shows features of both patterns A and B as well as ossified bodies with a peripheral low signal (dense calcification) and central high signal (fatty marrow). This pattern corresponds to foci of endochondral ossification on x-rays or CT.

Pigmented Villonodular Synovitis

Pigmented villonodular synovitis (PVNS) is a benign, neoplastic disease of unknown etiology with significant synovial proliferation (Fig. 17.12). This rare disease has an incidence of 1.8 cases per million people per year. The most commonly affected joint is the knee joint followed by the hip, ankle, and shoulder. The synovium shows villous and/or nodular changes. PVNS can be locally aggressive, but does not metastasize. It occurs most often in patients between the ages of 30 and 50 years, and there is no gender bias.

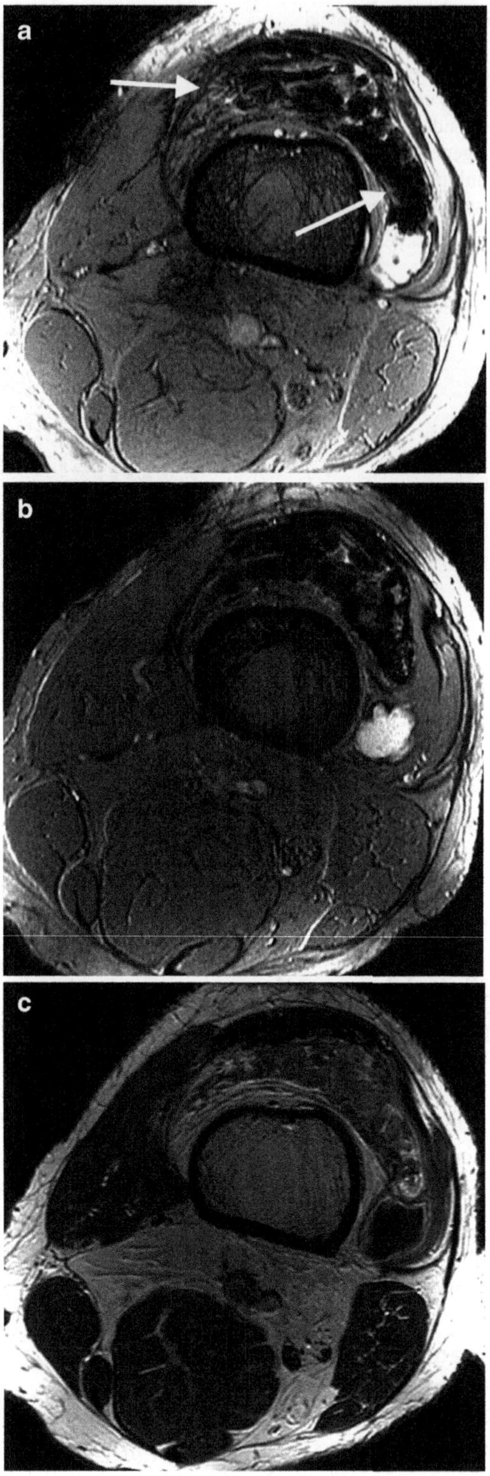

Fig. 17.12 PVNS knee in a 57-year-old female with recurrent hemarthrosis and joint pain. (**a**) Axial T2 with marked regions of low signal intensity in the suprapatellar recess (*arrows*). (**b**) Axial GRE exaggerates low signal intensity due to blooming artifact from hemosiderin. (**c**) Axial T1 post gadolinium enhancement demonstrating enhancing soft tissue

Clinical Presentation

Pain and swelling of the affected joint along with locking and decreased range of motion is a common presenting symptom. Localized PVNS usually presents as a painless slow-growing mass. Physical exam includes swelling and tenderness to palpation. According to Jaffe et al. who first described PVNS in 1941, it is caused by an inflammatory response with hyperplasia of undifferentiated connective tissue cells of the synovial membrane. They concluded that various PVNS lesions with differing gross morphologies are variants of the same disorder. Based on their observation, the present classification includes:

1. Localized pigmented nodular synovitis: Localized discrete nodular lesions that may be intra- or extra-articular. Extra-articular lesions can involve tendon sheaths, also known as giant cell tumor of the tendon sheath. It is seen usually in older females in the fifth or sixth decade. It usually affects digits of the hands or feet. In the hand, it usually involves the palmar aspect of the digit and is the second most common soft tissue tumor of the hand.
2. Diffuse PVNS: Entire synovial membrane of a joint or bursa is affected. It usually presents in the knee joint with more predilection for the patellofemoral joint.

Imaging

Radiographs

Localized PVNS may not show any abnormalities on x-rays. The most common finding on plain radiographs of PVNS is soft tissue or joint swelling. Radiography is insensitive to differentiate effusion from synovial thickening and proliferation. Some may show juxta-articular osteoporosis or scalloped cortical erosion with sclerotic margin usually due to pressure effect.

CT Scan

CT is usually not indicated as MRI is the gold imaging standard. CT scans without contrast may show increased attenuation coefficient due to hemosiderin content in the soft tissues. With contrast, synovial proliferation can be identified. This modality is also useful in delineating bone cyst formation and erosions.

MRI

MRI is the gold imaging standard and is highly accurate in defining the extent of disease. This modality has superior tissue contrast, suitable for identifying synovial proliferation, joint effusion, and bone erosion. The MRI findings reflect the histologic composition of the tissues comprising the lesion. The appearance depends on the relative proportions of lipid, hemosiderin, fibrous stromal fluid, and cellular elements. Hemosiderin is a magnetic material and alters the MRI signal. Although these deposits can be seen in hematomas, giant cell tumors, and pseudoaneurysms as a result of hemorrhage, the combination of these deposits with villonodular soft tissue masses and/or multiple bone erosion is highly sensitive for PVNS. The most characteristic finding is nodular intra-articular masses of low signal intensity on T1-, T2-, and proton density-weighted sequences: the low signal intensity is a result of the hemosiderin deposition. Multinodular, intra-articular lesions with patchy area of hemosiderin and fat are diagnostic of PVNS.

Synovial Hemangioma

Rare benign condition involving primarily the anterior compartment of the knee joint may also be found in the elbow, wrist, and ankle joint. It usually occurs in children and adolescents. It is often associated with skin or subcutaneous hemangioma and hence often classified as intra-articular, juxta-articular, or intermediate. Patients usually present with recurrent joint swelling and limitation in range of motion.

Radiographs are usually normal but rarely may show erosions. MRI is the ideal modality. It detects a soft tissue mass with an intermediate signal intensity on T1-weighted sequences, isointense with or slightly brighter than the muscle but less bright than fat. On fat suppression, the lesion shows thin, often serpentine low-intensity septa within it. Hemangiomas enhance post-gadolinium.

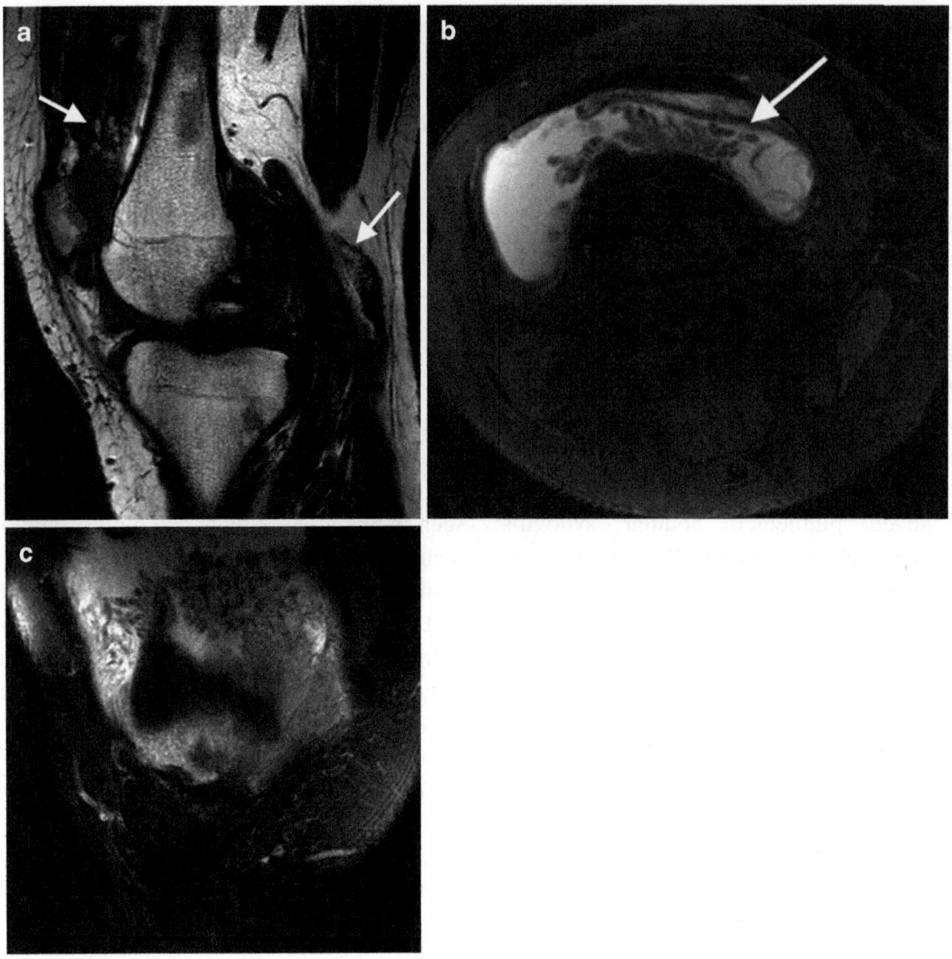

Fig. 17.13 Lipoma arborescens, 51-year-old female with recurrent knee effusions. (**a**) Saggital T1 MRI demonstrating fat fronds with the suprapatellar recess and within a Baker's cyst (*arrows*). (**b**) Axial T2FS fronds are low signal on fat-saturated sequences and surrounded by high SI joint fluid. (**c**) Coronal T2FS demonstrating similar findings as in part (**b**)

Lipoma Arborescens

Lipoma arborescens is an uncommon intra-articular lipoma-like lesion characterized by fatty proliferation of the subsynovial connective tissue (Fig. 17.13). It is also referred to as villous lipomatous proliferation of the synovial membrane, diffuse lipoma of the joint, or diffuse synovial lipoma. It is considered to be one of the rarest of synovial proliferative lesions, which presents in the fifth to seventh decades. Often associated with a joint effusion. It is most common within the suprapatellar recess. Radiographs usually demonstrate a joint effusion. Ultrasound demonstrates an effusion with capsular thickening demonstrating frond like projections into the joint recesses. Similar findings are noted on CT, which can also show the fronds as low attending fat fronds. MRI is the gold imaging standard with fat fronds as high signal intensity on T1, which demonstrate the loss of SI on fat saturation. A mild metaplasia of the subsynovial tissue may occur in degenerative disease and develop a low-grade lipoma arborescens.

Further Reading

1. Balach T, Stacy S, Peabody TD. The clinical evaluation of bone tumors. Radiol Clin N Am. 2011;49:1079–93.
2. Cheng XG, You YH, Liu W. MRI features of pigmented villonodular synovitis (PVNS). Clin Rheumatol. 2004;23:31–4.
3. Dorwart RH, Genanat HK, Johnston WH, Morris JM. Pigmented villonodular synovitis of synovial joints: clinical, pathologic and radiologic features. AJR. 1984;143:877–85.
4. Garner HW, Besti JM. Benign synovial tumors and proliferative processes. Semin Musculoskelet Radiol. 2013;17:177–88.
5. Jaganathan S MD, Goyal A, Gadodia A, Rastogi S, Mittal R, Gamanagatti S. Spectrum of synovial pathologies: a pictorial assay. Curr Probl Diagn Radiol. 2012;41:30–42.
6. McKenzie G, Raby N, Ritchie D. A pictorial review of primary synovial osteochondromatosis. Eur Radiol. 2008;18:2662–9.
7. Miller SL, Hoffer FA. Malignant and benign bone tumors. Radiol Clin N Am. 2001;39(4):673.
8. Motamedi K, Seeger LL. Benign bone tumors. Radiol Clin N Am. 2011;49:1115–34.
9. Narvaez JA, Narvaez J, Aguilera C, De Lama E, Portabella F. MR imaging of synovial tumors and tumor-like lesions. Eur Radiol. 2001;11:2549–60.
10. Pommersheim WJ, Chew FS. Imaging, diagnosis, and staging of bone tumors: a primer. Semin Roentgenol. 2004;39(3):361–72.
11. Rajiah P, Ilaslan H, Sundaram M. Imaging of primary malignant bone tumors (nonhematological). Radiol Clin N Am. 2011;49:1135–61.
12. Sulabha Masih, Alon Antebi. Imaging of pigmented villonodular synovitis. Semin Musculoskelet Radiol. 2003;7(3):205–16.
13. Wittkop B, Davies AM, Mangham DC. Primary synovial chondromatosis, and synovial chondrosarcoma. Eur Radiol. 2002;12:2112–9.

Appendix: Image Scoring Methods in Arthritis

Raj Carmona

Radiographic Scoring in Rheumatoid Arthritis (RA)

Radiographic progression, as determined by plain radiographs, continues to be a major outcome measure in rheumatoid arthritis. In clinical practice, assessment is typically descriptive. In contrast, recognised scoring systems are utilised in clinical trials. The results of these trials are highly dependent on joint positioning and technical quality of the radiographs. For radiographs of the hands and feet, most investigators opt for postero-anterior views. The first quantification of radiographic damage was proposed by *Steinbrocker* in 1949 [1]. This provided a global damage score for the hands and wrists on a four-point scale and was determined by the worst joint. The narrow scale, ranging from I (minimal damage) to IV (severe damage), precluded the ability to assess change in status. In similar fashion, the *Kellgren* method provided a global grade representing the overall abnormalities for all joints in both hands and wrists [2]. Currently, the most widely used systems are based on the work of A. Larsen and J. T. Sharp and provide a continuous quantitative scale that is a summation of scores at individual joints.

The Larsen Method

The Larsen method, developed in 1974, includes both erosions and joint space narrowing in each joint as a single score from 0 to 5 according to reference radiographs [3]. Several modifications have been published, including revisions by Larsen himself in 1995 [4]. The main differences from the original are deletion of scores for the thumbs and first metatarsophalangeal (MTP) joint, subdivision of the wrist into four quadrants, deletion of soft-tissue swelling and periarticular osteopenia and distinction between erosions of different sizes. The included joints are therefore the 2nd–5th proximal interphalangeal (PIP) joints and the 2nd–5th metacarpophalangeal (MCP) joints in each hand, four quadrants in each wrist, and the 2nd–5th MTP joints in each foot (see Fig. A1). The score therefore ranges from 0 to 160 (Table A1).

The Sharp Method

Sharp et al. originally proposed a method for scoring the hands and wrists (only) in 1971 [5]. Twenty-nine areas in each hand and wrist were considered for erosions using a scale of 0–5, resulting in a total erosion score of 0–290. Twenty-seven joints were considered for joint space narrowing (JSN) in each hand with a scale of 0–4, resulting in a total JSN score of 0–216. This original version is no longer used.

A modification proposed in 1985 is now considered the standard Sharp method (see Fig. A2) [6]. This modification includes 17 areas for erosion (5 PIPs, 5 MCPs, first metacarpal base, multangular as one unit, navicular, lunate, triquetrum (and pisiform), radius, ulnar bone for each hand and wrist). Each erosion scores 1 point, with a maximum of 5 points for each area (reflecting

R. Carmona, MBBS, FRCPC
Assistant Professor, Department of Medicine, McMaster University, Hamilton, ON L8N1Y2, Canada

J. O'Neill (ed.), *Essential Imaging in Rheumatology*,
DOI 10.1007/978-1-4939-1673-3, © Springer Science+Business Media New York 2015

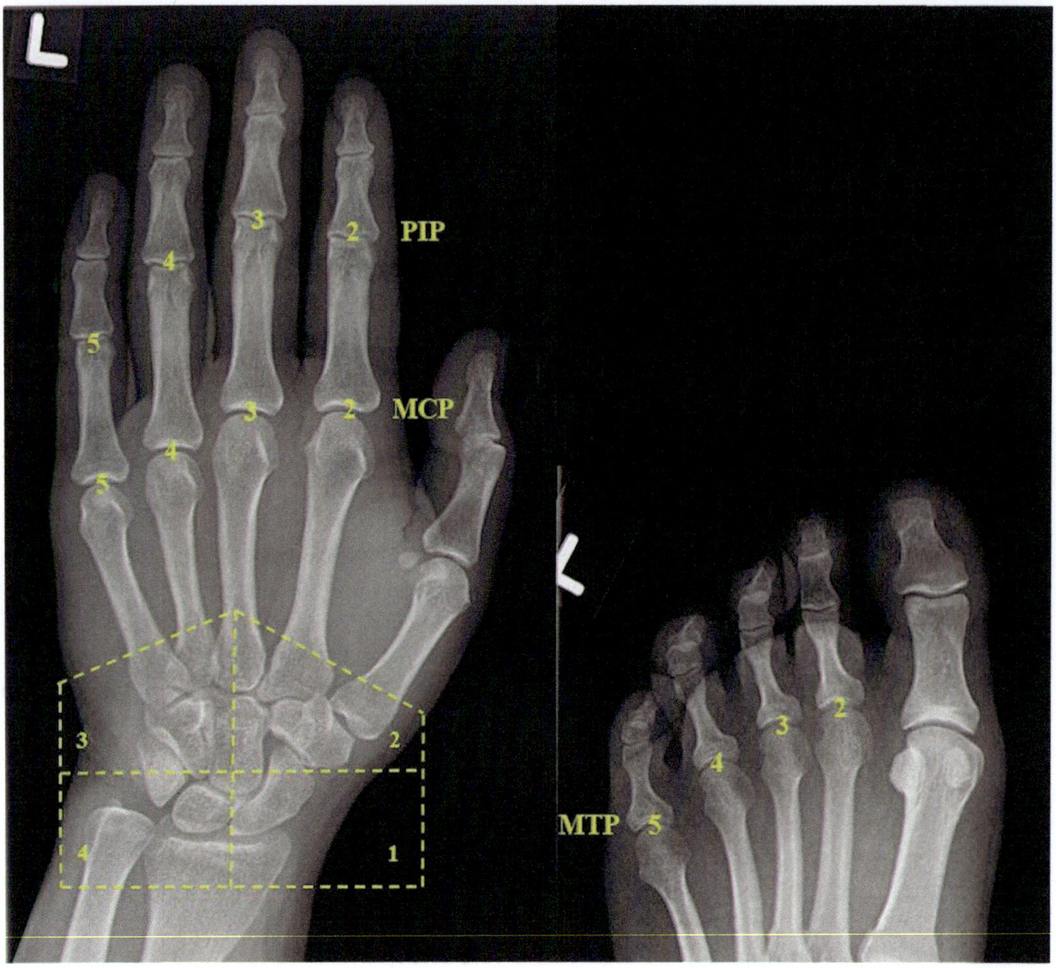

Fig. A1 Larsen's scoring method. There are 32 areas for radiographic evaluation in a single patient – eight areas in each hand (2nd–5th MCPs and PIPs), four areas in each wrist (quadrants), and four areas in each foot (2nd–5th MTPs)

a loss of more than 50 % of either articular bone) and thus a total score of 0–170. The Sharp method also considers 18 areas for JSN (5 PIPs, 5 MCPs, 3rd–5th carpometacarpal (CMC) joints, multangular-navicular, lunate-triquetrum, capitate-navicular-lunate, radiocarpal, radioulnar joints for each hand and wrist). One point is scored for focal narrowing, two points for diffuse narrowing <50 % of the original space and three points if reduction is more than half of the original joint space. Ankylosis is scored as four points. JSN therefore ranges from 0 to 144.

van der Heijde Modification of the Sharp Score (SvHS)

In the SvHS, the number and selection of joints in the Sharp score evolved from having only the hands and wrists to including the feet as well (see Fig. A3) [7]. In the final SvHS (Table A1), 16 areas from each hand and wrist are included in the erosion score with range 0–5. Six areas in each foot (the 5 MTPs and the interphalangeal joint of the great toe) are assessed. The maximum erosion score is 160 for the hands and wrists and 120 for the feet.

Table A1 Radiographic scoring methods in rheumatoid arthritis

	Larsen scoring [3]	van der Heijde modification of Sharp scoring (SvHS) [7]	Simple erosion narrowing score (SENS) [8]
Joints assessed	*Both hands* PIP 2–5; MCP 2–5; 4 quadrants in the wrist; MTP 2–5	*Both hands* All MCPs, 1st IP, all PIPs, scapho-radial, lunate-radial, distal ulna, trapeziometacarpal *Both feet* All MTPJs, 1st IPJ	Same as SvHS
Joint space narrowing		0 = normal 1 = focal narrowing 2 = reduction of less than 50 % of the joint space 3 = reduction of greater than 50 % of the joint space 4 = ankylosis	0 = absent 1 = present
Erosions		0 = normal 1 = discrete erosions 2–3 = larger erosions according to surface area involved 4 = erosions extending over middle of the bone, and 5 = complete collapse	0 = absent 1 = present
Composite of JSN and erosions	0 = intact bony outlines and normal joint space 1 = erosion <1 mm diameter or joint space narrowing 2 = one or several small erosions, diameter >1 mm 3 = marked erosions 4 = severe erosions, where there is usually no joint space left, and the original bony outlines are partly preserved 5 = mutilating changes, where the original bony outlines have been destroyed		
Total maximum score	160	448	86
Smallest detectable difference (SDD)	5.8	5	
Minimal clinically significant difference	Approx. 1 % of total score	Approx. 1 % of total score	

SvHS joint space narrowing (JSN) is assessed at 15 areas from each hand and wrist and 6 areas from each foot, scored as per the original Sharp method above. The maximum JSN score is 120 for the hands and wrists and 48 for the feet. Therefore, the total SvHS score ranges from 0 to 448. Studies have shown that this method has greater precision and sensitivity to change, and it has become the most widely used in clinical trials.

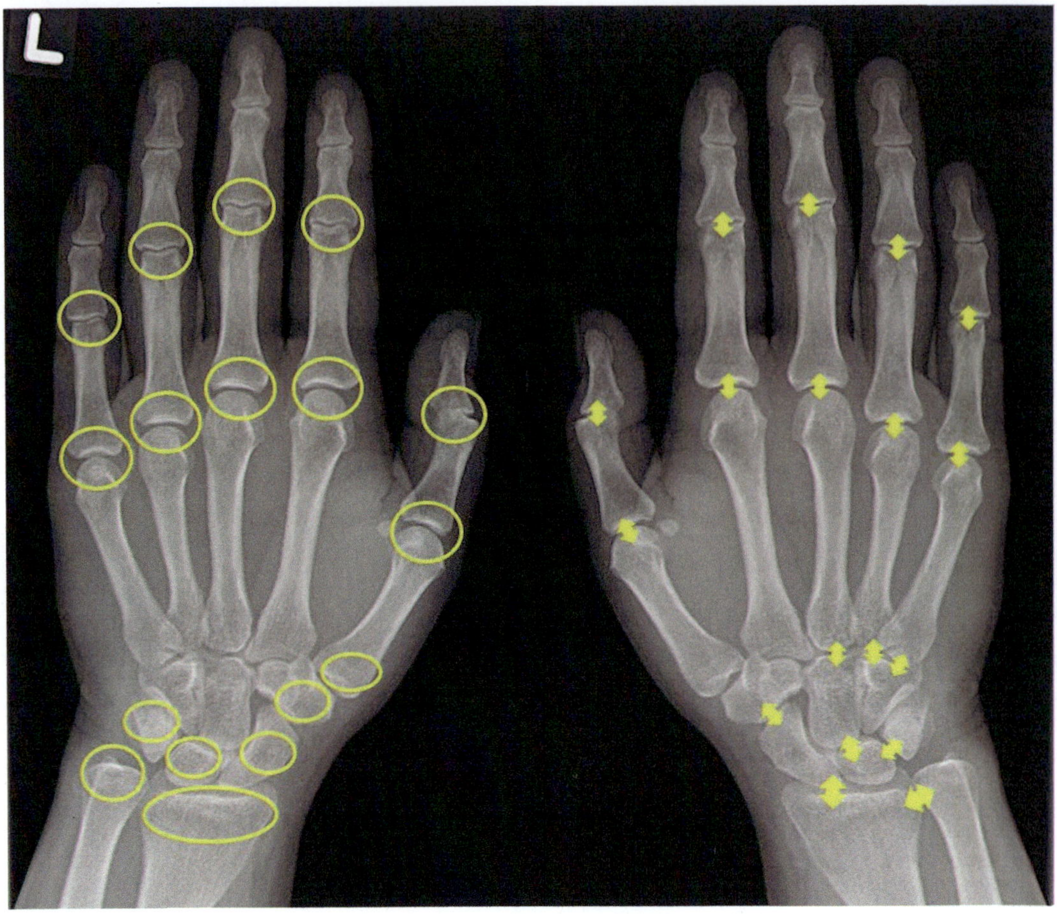

Fig. A2 The Sharp method. Seventeen areas in each hand (marked with *dots*) are scored for erosion. Eighteen areas in each hand (marked with *parallel lines*) are scored for joint space narrowing

SENS Method

van der Heijde described the SENS method in 1999 [8]. It is a simplified method that assesses the same joints as the SvHS system. It foregoes the grading of joints and instead simply sums the number of joints with erosions and with JSN. Erosion is scored in 32 joints in the hand and 12 in the feet and JSN in 30 and 12 joints, respectively. The total SENS score ranges from 0 to 86. With its relative simplicity, this method can be used in clinical trials and in clinical practice.

Ultrasound Scoring in Rheumatoid Arthritis

Multiple studies have demonstrated that ultrasound scan (US) is more sensitive than clinical assessment for the detection of joint swelling. Standardised definitions of US abnormalities in patients with inflammatory arthritis were proposed at the Seventh OMERACT Conference (Table A2).

US assessment in clinical practice is typically descriptive or semi-quantitative at best. The

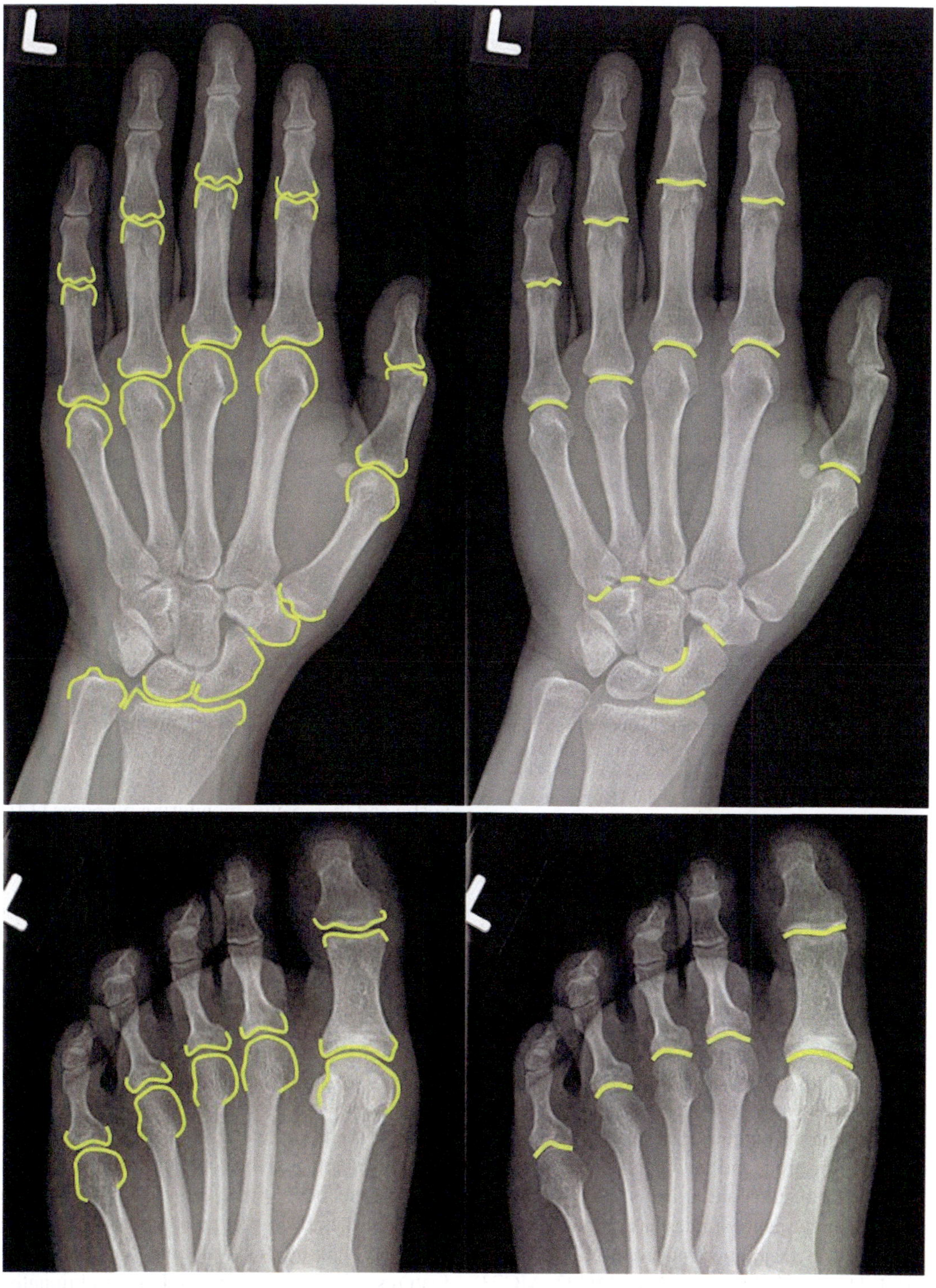

Fig. A3 The van der Heijde modification of the Sharp score. The *left* panels show the joints and surfaces assessed for erosions. The *right* panels show the joints assessed for joint space narrowing

Table A2 Definitions of USS pathology according to Seventh OMERACT Conference (Wakefield et al. [9])

Synovial fluid	Abnormal hypoechoic or anechoic (relative to subdermal fat, but sometimes may be isoechoic or hyperechoic) intraarticular material that is displaceable and compressible but does not exhibit Doppler signal
Synovial hypertrophy	Abnormal hypoechoic (relative to subdermal fat, but sometimes may be isoechoic or hyperechoic) intraarticular tissue that is non-displaceable and poorly compressible and which may exhibit Doppler signal
Bone erosions	An intraarticular discontinuity of the bone surface that is visible in two perpendicular planes
Tenosynovitis	Hypoechoic or anechoic thickened tissue with or without fluid within the tendon sheath, which is seen in two perpendicular planes and which may exhibit Doppler signal
Enthesopathy	Abnormally hypoechoic (loss of normal fibrillar architecture) and/or thickened tendon or ligament at its bony attachment (may occasionally contain hyperechoic foci consistent with calcification) seen in two perpendicular planes that may exhibit Doppler signal and/or bony changes including enthesophytes, erosions or irregularity

development of scoring systems for use in clinical trials continues to be an area of active research. In most studies, semi-quantitative scoring systems are used for both grey-scale and power Doppler findings (Table A3).

Research goals include the standardisation of examination techniques, the image acquisition and the location and number of joints to be assessed in rheumatoid arthritis. The number of joints in high-quality studies has ranged from 5 to 60 [11]. The 12-joint count proposed by Naredo et al. [12] (including the wrist, MCP2, MCP3, knee, ankle and elbow, evaluated bilaterally) and the 7-joint count proposed by Backhaus et al. [13] (wrist, MCP2, MCP3, PIP2, PIP3, MTP2 and MTP5) showed good reliability and sensitivity to change. The OMERACT Ultrasound Task Force is currently developing a global synovitis score (GLOSS), a standardized scoring system for synovitis in RA at the patient level that is applicable to all joints [11]. It is still unclear whether different indices will be needed for diagnostic and therapeutic monitoring purposes [14].

Table A3 Grading of US findings in RA (Dougados et al. [10])

Synovial hypertrophy	0 = no thickening 1 = mild 2 = moderate 3 = marked
Power Doppler signal	0 = no signal 1 = mild: 1–2 vessels signal (including 1 confluent vessel) for small joints or 2–3 signals for large joints (including two confluent vessels) 2 = moderate: confluent vessels > grade 1 and <50 % of normal area 3 = marked – vessels signal in >50 % of the synovial area
Erosions	0 = no erosion 1 = very small (<1 mm) 2 = small (1–2 mm) 3 = moderate (2–4 mm) 4 = large (>4 mm)

Magnetic Resonance Imaging (MRI) Scoring in Rheumatoid Arthritis

OMERACT (Outcome Measures in Rheumatology Clinical Trials) RAMRIS (Rheumatoid Arthritis MRI Scoring System)

Multiple methodological and observational studies have established the construct validity of MRI depiction of bone erosions and cartilage loss in RA. MRI has been proven to be more sensitive than radiography for detecting these standard features of joint damage in RA. Additionally, MRI is uniquely able to identify the upstream processes of synovitis and osteitis. In contrast to radiographs, randomised control trials demonstrate that it is possible to discriminate therapeutic

Table A4 MRI scoring in rheumatoid arthritis (OMERACT RAMRIS)

Synovitis	Assesses 3 wrist regions (distal radioulnar joint, radiocarpal joint, intercarpal and carpometacarpal joints) and each MCP joint. The first carpometacarpal and first MCP joints are not scored
	Scale: 0–3 in increments of 33 % of the synovial compartment
Bone erosions	Each bone (wrists – carpal bones, distal radius, distal uln a, metacarpal bases; MCP joints – metacarpal heads, phalangeal heads) is scored separately
	Scale: 0–10 in increments of 10 % of articular bone loss
Osteitis	Each bone is scored separately (as for erosions)
	Scale: 0–3 in increments of 33 % of bone oedema

efficacy of different structure-modifying therapies with MRI in less than 6 months, and less than 3 months in some cases [15].

Studies utilise the validated semi-quantitative OMERACT RAMRIS. This scores the wrists and MCP joints of the hands for synovitis, erosions and osteitis (Table A4) [16]. The original definition relies on the use of a contrast agent, but subsequent sequences using fast spin echo, Short Tau Inversion Recovery (STIR) and T2-weighted images with fat saturation without contrast have good concordance [17].

- *Synovitis* is defined as an area of increased gadolinium enhancement, within a joint, of a width greater than that of the normal synovium.
- *Erosion* is a sharply marginated bone lesion visible in two planes with a clear cortical break visible in at least one plane.
- *Bone oedema* is an ill-defined lesion of high signal intensity (on T2) within the trabecular bone.

Radiographic Scoring in Psoriatic Arthritis

The radiographic scoring methods for psoriatic arthritis (PsA) have their basis in scoring methods for rheumatoid arthritis. There are two global methods and two detailed scoring methods.

Modified Steinbrocker [18]

The original Steinbrocker classification (for RA) scored a patient according to their worst joint. In this modified method, each joint is scored on a scale of 0–4 (below) [18]. This includes all the joints of the hands (with the wrist considered as one joint), all metatarsophalangeal joints (MTPS) and the interphalangeal joint of the great toe. This results in 40 joints altogether, with a score range of 0–160. The interobserver and intraobserver intraclass correlation coefficients (ICC) are similar to the Larsen method.

0	Normal
1	Juxtaarticular osteopenia or soft-tissue swelling
2	Presence of erosions
3	Presence of erosion and joint space narrowing
4	Total joint destruction (osteolysis or ankylosis)

Psoriatic Arthritis Ratingen Score (PARS) [19]

This method includes 40 joints of the hands and feet, with each scored separately for destruction and proliferation (Table A5). The destruction score ranges from 0 to 5. The proliferation score captures any kind of bony proliferation that is typical for PsA and ranges from 0 to 4. The total destruction score (0–200) and the proliferation score (0–160) are summed to give a total score (0–360).

PsA Scoring Method Based on Sharp's Scoring Method for RA [20]

The erosion scale ranges from 0 to 5 and is applied to 21 joints in each hand and to 6 joints in each foot, resulting in a range of 0–210 for the hands and 0–60 for the feet (Table A6). This scale was expanded to include the scores of 6 and 7 to accommodate the more extensive bone destruction seen in psoriatic arthritis (such as

Table A5 Psoriatic arthritis Ratingen score (PARS)

PARS scale	Destruction	Proliferation
0	Normal	Normal
1	One or more definite erosions with interruption of the cortical plate >1 mm but <10 % of the joint surface destroyed	Bony proliferation of 1–2 mm measured from the original bone surface or not exceeding 25 % of the original diameter of the bone
2	Destruction of 11–25 % of the joint surface	Bony proliferation of 2–3 mm or bone growth of 25–50 %
3	Destruction of 25–50 % of the joint surface	Bony proliferation of >3 mm or bone growth of >50 %
4	Destruction of 51–75 % of the joint surface	Bony ankylosis
5	Destruction of >75 % of the joint surface	–

gross osteolysis or pencil-in-cup). However, the scores of 6 and 7 are not added but instead are noted separately. The scoring of joint space narrowing is on a scale of 0–4, as is used in RA, with the addition of widening which is automatically scored when gross osteolysis is present. The score for widening is also not added but rather noted separately. Joint space narrowing is scored in 20 joints in each hand and 5 joints in each foot, leading to a range of 0–160 for the hands and 0–40 for the feet.

Sharp-van der Heijde (SvH)-Modified Scoring Method for PsA [20]

This is similar to the scoring system in RA. The same joints are assessed for erosions and joint space narrowing, with the addition of the eight DIPs for erosions and the eight DIPS and two IPs of the thumbs for joint space narrowing (Table A7). The maximum score for erosions is five in the joints of the hands, and ten for each joint of the feet (maximum of five for each side). Gross osteolysis and pencil-in-cup are scored separately. In the final summary score, joints with one of these abnormalities get the maximum erosion and JSN score. The total range for erosions is 0–200 for the hands and 0–120 for the feet, while the total range for JSN is 0–160 for the hands and 0–48 for the feet. Thus, the maximum total erosion score is 320 and the maximum joint space narrowing score is 208, for a grand total of 528.

Table A6 PsA scoring method based on Sharp's scoring method for RA

Sharp PsA scale	Erosion	Joint space narrowing
0	No erosion	Normal
1	1 Discrete erosion or <21 % of the joint area affected	Asymmetrical and/or minimal narrowing
2	2 Discreet erosions or 21–40 % of the joint area affected	Definite narrowing with loss of up to 50 % of the joint space
3	3 Discreet erosions or involvement of 41–60 % of the joint area affected	Definite narrowing with 51–99 % loss of joint space or subluxation
4	4 Discreet erosions or 61–80 % of the joint area affected	Absence of joint space, presumptive evidence of ankylosis
5	Extensive destruction involving >80 % of the joint	[a]Widening
6, 7	[a]Extensive destruction such as gross osteolysis or pencil-in-cup deformity	

[a]Score not added (noted separately)

Table A7 Sharp-van der Heijde modified scoring method for PsA

SvH scale for PsA	Erosion	Joint space narrowing
0	Normal	Normal
1	Discreet erosion	Asymmetrical or minimal narrowing up to 25 % of the joint space
2	Large erosion not passing the midline	Definite narrowing with loss of up to 50 % of the joint space
3	Large erosion passing the midline	Definite narrowing with 50–99 % loss of the joint space or subluxation
4	–	Absence of joint space, presumptive evidence of ankylosis or complete luxation

Table A8 Psoriatic arthritis MRI scoring system (PsAMRIS)

	Scoring	Joints
Synovitis	0–3	MCP, PIP, DIP
Erosion	0–10	Proximal and distal segments of MCP, PIP and DIP
Bone marrow oedema	0–3	Proximal and distal segments of MCP, PIP and DIP
Tenosynovitis	0–3	MCP, PIP, DIP
Periarticular inflammation	0/1	MCP, PIP, DIP palmar and dorsal
Bone proliferation	0/1	MCP, PIP, DIP

Psoriatic Arthritis MRI Scoring System (PsAMRIS)

The PsAMRIS, initially developed in 2004 by an OMERACT MRI working group, assesses fingers 2–5 [21]. Each finger is divided into six segments or joint regions by transverse lines through the joint spaces (MCP, PIP, DIP) and across the midpoint of the metacarpals and proximal and middle phalanges. Each joint is scored for synovitis and each segment for erosions and bone oedema (Table A8). Tenosynovitis is scored at each joint region in each of the four flexor tendons on a scale of 0–3. Periarticular inflammation is scored as present or absent adjacent to each joint region on the dorsal and palmar aspect of the finger. Bone formation is also scored in each joint region. Validation exercises have shown good reliability and sensitivity to change in synovitis, tenosynovitis and periarticular inflammation. However, sensitivity to change for bone marrow oedema, erosions and bone proliferation was poor, likely due to slow progression of patients on treatment over the 12-month period between sequential scans [22].

Axial Spondyloarthritis

Plain Radiography: Assessment of the Spine

Plain radiography is the traditional imaging method for diagnostic evaluation and classification of SpA. However, it is widely recognised that radiographic changes are a late development, and radiography has limited sensitivity particularly in earlier stages of the disease.

Three methods have been described for scoring abnormalities in the spine and are outlined below. A comparison of these methods concluded that intra-rater and inter-rater rater reliabilities for status scores are all good to very good [23]. However, mSASSS was rated as the preferred method by the OMERACT consensus conference in 2004, based on superior reproducibility and sensitivity to change (which is a major focus of clinical trials).

Bath Ankylosing Spondylitis Radiology Index (BASRI)

This is a global grading of the lateral cervical spine, the anterior and lateral lumbar spine combined and the sacroiliac joints (SIJs) [24]. Each site is scored from 0 (normal) to 4 (fusion involving at least three vertebrae). The sum of the sites gives the BASRI-spine (BASRI-s), which ranges from 0 to 12. A similar grading is described for the hips (0–4) which, when added to the spine score, results in the BASRI-total (BASRI-t) with a maximum score of 16. This system is plagued by ceiling effects, poor reproducibility and poor sensitivity to change with only 20 % demonstrating change after 2 years.

Stoke Ankylosing Spondylitis Spine Score (SASSS)

This assesses abnormalities in the anterior and posterior corners of each lumbar vertebra [25]. It does not include the cervical or thoracic spine. Each corner is scored for the presence of squaring, sclerosis, erosions, syndesmophytes and bridging syndesmophytes. The SASSS is also limited by poor sensitivity to change.

Modified Ankylosing Spondylitis Spine Score (mSASSS)

In this method, a total of 24 sites are scored on lateral cervical and lumbar spine radiographs on a scale of 0–3 (below) [26]. These comprise the anterior corners of the vertebrae from the lower border of C2 to the upper border of T1 inclusive and from the lower border of T12 to the upper border of S1 inclusive. It does not include the thoracic spine which is frequently affected but difficult to evaluate because of overlapping structures. Each corner is scored from 0 to 3, resulting in a range from 0 to 72 for the total mSASSS.

0	Normal
1	Sclerosis, squaring or erosion
2	Syndesmophyte
3	Bony bridge

Progression, defined as "change greater than zero", is useful in assessing patients after a follow-up of 2 years [23]. The methodologically more appropriate "smallest detectable difference" provides a cut-off level that is too insensitive for many patients [27].

Plain Radiography: Assessment of the Sacroiliac Joint

Although many centres perform dedicated views of the sacroiliac joints (SIJs), one study of 445 patients showed that a single anteroposterior pelvic radiograph is sufficient for evaluation of the SIJs [28]. The SIJs are graded as below (Table A9) [29]. It should be noted that this is used for staging SIJ involvement, particularly for diagnosis according to the modified New York Criteria and not as a scoring system to follow progression in clinical trials.

Magnetic Resonance Imaging: Scoring of the Sacroiliac Joints

An adequate MRI of the sacroiliac joints (SIJs) must include at least a T1w sequence without fat saturation and STIR sequences in a semicoronal plane (parallel to the axis of the sacral bone). The need for further sequences depends on the goal of the examination. MRI assessment of activity in the SIJs is described below. Methods for assessment of damage in the SIJs have been proposed, but validation of these methods is limited and the clinical value above radiography is uncertain.

Table A9 Modified New York criteria radiographic assessment sacroiliitis

Grade 0	Normal
Grade 1	Suspicious changes
Grade 2	Minimal abnormality – small localised areas with erosion or sclerosis, without alteration in the joint width
Grade 3	Unequivocal abnormality – moderate or advanced sacroiliitis with one or more of erosions, evidence of sclerosis, widening, narrowing or partial ankylosis
Grade 4	Severe abnormality – total ankylosis

MRI Assessment for Activity in the Sacroiliac Joints

In general, the presence and extent of bone marrow oedema in the cartilaginous portion of the joint is the primary MRI feature that is scored. Some methods also score inflammation in the joint space and/or ligamentous portion of the joint (Table A10).

The *Spondyloarthritis Research Consortium of Canada (SPARCC) scoring method* focuses on the cartilaginous portion with six consecutive semicoronal slices. On each slice, both SIJs are divided into quadrants according to a vertical axis drawn through the joint cavity and a horizontal axis bisecting this line at its midpoint. The presence of bone marrow oedema in each quadrant is scored on a dichotomous basis (present = 1, absent = 0), with additional weighing for intensity and depth. In a multi-reader exercise, agreement between readers and sensitivity to change was found to be better for the SPARCC method [30].

Two other scoring systems provide global grading of bone marrow oedema in each quadrant. The *Leeds scoring system* applies scores from 0 to 3 (0, normal; 1, <25 %; 2, 25–75 %; 3, >75 % of quadrant), while the *Berlin method* has grades 0–4 (0, normal; 1, in joint space/erosions

Table A10 MRI assessment for activity in the sacroiliac joints

	SPARCC [31]	Berlin [32]	Leeds [33]
Images	Semicoronal STIR	Semicoronal STIR, T1w and T1w FS and post-Gd T1w FS	Semicoronal T1w, STIR and post-Gd T1w FS
Features	Bone marrow oedema	Joint space oedema/enhancement (grade 1), bone marrow oedema/enhancement (grades 2–4)	Bone marrow oedema, bone marrow enhancement
Grades	In each of 6 semicoronal slices: 0–1 per quadrant, +1 per joint for depth >1 cm and +1 per joint for high signal intensity	Grades 0–4 per quadrant	A, global status: 0–3 per quadrant and B, global change between scans (–3 to +3)
Total score range (per patient)	0–72	0–32	0–24

Modified from Ostergaard et al. [50], Copyright 2010 with permission from Elsevier

Table A11 MRI assessment for activity in the spine

	SPARCC [31]	ASspiMRI-a [34]	Berlin modification of the ASspiMRI-a score [35]
Images	Sagittal STIR	Sagittal STIR and post-Gd T1w FS	Sagittal STIR and sagittal post-Gd t1w FS
Area	6 most affected DVUs	All 23 DVUs	All 23 DVUs
Features	Bone marrow oedema	Bone marrow oedema/enhancement in combination with bone erosion	Bone marrow oedema/enhancement
Grades	0–1 per DVU quadrant, +1 per joint for depth ≥1 cm, +1 per joint for high signal intensity of lesion	0–6 per DVU	0–3 per DVU
Total score range (per patient)	0–108	0–138	0–69

Modified from Ostergaard et al. [50], Copyright 2010 with permission from Elsevier

only; 2, <33 % of bone quadrant area with bone marrow oedema; 3, 33–66 %; 4, >66 %).

Magnetic Resonance Imaging: Scoring of the Spine

In general, adequate MRI of the spine for spondyloarthritis must include a sagittal T1w sequence without fat saturation and a sagittal STIR sequence. Images should extend sufficiently laterally that the facet and costovertebral joints are covered. The two primary scoring methods are based on assessment of the discovertebral unit (DVU) – the area between two horizontal lines drawn through the middle of two adjacent vertebral bodies.

MRI Assessment for Activity in the Spine (Table A11)

Ankylosing Spondylitis Spine MRI: Activity (ASspiMRI-a) Index [34]

This scores the severity of bone oedema and erosions at all 23 DVUs in a single sagittal plane of view. Each DVU is scored along a range of 0–6, with the higher scores assigned to the presence of erosions. Grade 0 is normal, whereas grades 1–3 represent bone marrow oedema or post-contrast enhancement in ≤25 %, 25–50 % and >50 % of the DVU, and grades 4–6 represent erosion in ≤25 %, 25–50 % and >50 % of the DVU coexisting with some degree of oedema / enhancement.

Table A12 MRI assessment for structural lesions in the spine

	ASspiMRI-c [34]	Canada-Denmark [38]	Aarhus-Madsen [39]
Images	Sagittal T1w and STIR	Sagittal T1w and STIR	Sagittal T1w and STIR
Area	All 23 DVUs	All 46 vertebral endplates (at all 23 spinal levels from C2/3 to L5/S1) and facet joints	All 23 DVUs
Features	Sclerosis, squaring, bone erosion, syndesmophytes, bridging/fusion	Bone erosion, fat infiltration, bone spurs, ankylosis	Bone erosion, fatty deposition, syndesmophytes/ankylosis
Grades	Global: 0–6 per DVU	Each feature: 0–1 at each of the various locations per DVU	Each feature: 0–3 per DVU
Total score range (per patient)	0–138		0–207

Modified from Ostergaard et al. [50], Copyright 2010 with permission from Elsevier

Berlin Modification of the ASspiMRI-a Score [35]

This Berlin modification of the ASspiMRI-a score omitted grades 4–6 and therefore grades activity 0–3 in each of the 23 DVUs.

Spondyloarthritis Research Consortium of Canada (SPARCC) Scoring Method [31]

This is a more detailed system that evaluates the six most severely affected DVUs in three consecutive sagittal slices. Limiting the assessment to the six most severely affected DVUs has been shown to be at least as reliable as assessing all 23 DVUs and was actually more discriminatory [36]. Each of the six DVUs is divided into quadrants, and bone oedema (increased T2 signal) is scored dichotomously (0 = absent, 1 = present). This is repeated for each of the three consecutive slices giving a maximum score of 12 per DVU. Additionally, weighting is applied for intensity and depth. On each slice, the presence of a lesion exhibiting intense signal in any quadrant is given an additional score of 1. Similarly, the presence of a lesion exhibiting a depth of ≥ 1 cm in any quadrant was given an additional score of 1, resulting in a maximum additional score of 6 for that level and bringing the total score to 18 per DVU. In an ASAS-OMERACT multi-reader exercise, the SPARCC method had the highest sensitivity to change, as judged by Guyatt's effect size, and the highest reliability as judged by the inter-reader intra-class correlation coefficient [37].

MRI Assessment for Structural Lesions in the Spine

Ankylosing Spondylitis Spine MRI: Chronicity (ASspiMRI-c) Index [34]

The *ASspiMRI-c* assesses each DVU with a score of 0–6 based on an overall assessment of sclerosis, squaring of vertebrae, syndesmophytes and ankylosis [34]. Unfortunately, the reliability has been shown to be poor, and in a comparative study, this MRI system was not superior to radiography for detection of new bone formation.

The *Canada-Denmark system* [38] uses an anatomy-based set of definitions and an assessment system for structural spine lesions in SpA by which bone erosions, fat infiltration, bone spurs and ankylosis are assessed separately at various anatomic locations in each DVU. This system needs further validation. Another system (Table A12) scores bone erosions, fatty deposition and syndesmophytes/ankylosis separately (each 0–3) in each DVU [39].

Radiographic Scoring in Osteoarthritis (OA)

Despite the advent of more advanced imaging techniques such as MRI, radiography continues to be the most commonly used imaging modality for OA. Articular cartilage damage is indirectly assessed by evaluating joint space narrowing (JSN), as well as other distinguishing features of

OA including subchondral sclerosis, subchondral cysts and osteophytes.

The Kellgren-Lawrence (KL) Scale [40]

The KL scale is commonly used to define OA radiographically for epidemiological study purposes (Table A13). It provides a global grading of osteoarthritis severity and was initially applied to the knee. The major criticism of this scale is the requirement for osteophytes. An increase in the severity of other radiological features cannot be registered in the absence of osteophytes. Another deficiency is the inability to grade individual radiological features. Notwithstanding these deficiencies, one study showed good interobserver and intraobserver reliability and sensitivity to change when compared to other scoring methods (see below) [41].

The Kallman Scale [42]

In the Kallman radiographic scale, individual joints of the hands are scored for six radiographical features according to a semi-numerical scale: osteophytes (0–3), JSN (0–3), subchondral sclerosis (0–1), subchondral cysts (0–1), lateral bony deviation (≥15°; 0–1) and cortical collapse (0–1). Twenty-two joints are assessed consisting of the distal interphalangeal joints (DIPs), proximal interphalangeal joints (PIPs), interphalangeal joint of the thumb (IP), first carpometacarpal joint (CMC1) and trapezioscaphoid joint (TS). The score ranges from 0 to 208.

The Verbruggen Scoring System [43]

This is a numerical scoring system for the anatomical evolution of OA of the finger joints. The included joints are the metacarpophalangeal joints (MCPs), PIPs, DIPs and IP of the thumb. The TS and CMC1 are not included in this score. The score ranges from 0 to 218.

Table A13 Kellgren-Lawrence grading of osteoarthritis

Grade	Description
0: Normal	
1: Questionable	Doubtful narrowing of the joint space and possible osteophytic lipping
2: Mild	Definite osteophytes and possible narrowing of the joint space
3: Moderate	Moderate multiple osteophytes, definite narrowing of the joint space and some sclerosis and possible deformity of bone ends
4: Severe	Large osteophytes, marked narrowing of the joint space, severe sclerosis and definite deformity of bone ends

Comparison of Scoring Methods

The Kellgren-Lawrence, Kallman and Verbruggen systems were tested for reproducibility and sensitivity to change in a study of osteoarthritis of the hand [41]. All scales performed well with respect to interobserver and intraobserver reliability and sensitivity to change over 1 year. The Verbruggen and Kallman scales performed better with respect to reliability, while the Kallman method was slightly more sensitive to change.

MRI of Osteoarthritis

Although radiographic bony findings are common in OA, radiography cannot directly visualise the surrounding soft-tissue structures. In contrast, MRI can visualise most components of the joint including the bone marrow, bone, subchondral cysts, articular cartilage, menisci, intraarticular ligaments, synovium and other periarticular and intraarticular lesions. The current status of MRI in the assessment of osteoarthritis, including challenges of definition and quantification, is well outlined in a 2012 review by Hayashi et al. [44]. There is currently little standardisation of MRI interpretation, likely because of the absence of criteria for MRI OA structural diagnosis. MRI-based definitions of OS were only recently published in 2011 [45].

Several semi-quantitative scoring systems for knee OA have been introduced. These include the whole-organ magnetic resonance system (WORMS) [46], the Knee Osteoarthritis Scoring System (KOSS) [47], the Boston Leeds Osteoarthritis Knee Score (BLOKS) [48] and the MRI Knee OA Score (MOAKS) [49]. It is beyond the scope of this appendix to provide a detailed description of these complex systems; further details can be obtained via the provided references. Each system assesses a number of features essential to the functional integrity of the knee or to the pathophysiology of OA. These features include articular hyaline cartilage integrity, bone marrow abnormalities, subchondral cysts, subarticular bone attrition, osteophytes, meniscal integrity and extrusion, synovitis and effusion, intraarticular loose bodies, periarticular cysts and bursitidies. Whole-organ semi-quantitative MRI assessment has shown adequate reliability, sensitivity and specificity, as well as ability to follow the progression of lesions.

References

1. Steinbrocker O, Traeger C, Batterman R. Therapeutic criteria in rheumatoid arthritis. JAMA. 1949;140:659–62.
2. Kellgren J, Bier F. Radiological signs of rheumatoid arthritis: a study of observer differences in the reading of hand films. Ann Rheum Dis. 1956;15:55–60.
3. Larsen A. A radiological method for grading the severity of rheumatoid arthritis. Academic dissertation. Helsinki: University of Helsinki; 1974.
4. Larsen A. How to apply Larsen score in evaluating radiographs of rheumatoid arthritis in long-term studies. J Rheumatol. 1995;22:1974–5.
5. Sharp JT, Lidsky MD, Collins SC, Moreland J. Methods of scoring the progression of radiological changes in rheumatoid arthritis. Correlation of radiologic, clinical and laboratory abnormalities. Arthritis Rheum. 1971;14:706–20.
6. Sharp JT, Young DY, Bluhm GB, et al. How many joints in the hands and wrists should be included in a score of radiologic abnormalities used to assess rheumatoid arthritis? Arthritis Rheum. 1985;28:1326–35.
7. Van der Heijde D, van Riel PL, Nuver-Zwart IH, et al. Effects of hydroxychloroquine and sulfasalazine on progression of joint damage in rheumatoid arthritis. Lancet. 1989;i:1036–8.
8. Van der Heijde D, Dankert T, Nieman F, et al. Reliability and sensitivity to change of a simplification of the Sharp/van der Heijde radiological assessment in rheumatoid arthritis. Rheumatology (Oxford). 1999;38:941–7.
9. Wakefield RJ, Balint PV, Szkudlarek M, OMERACT 7 Special Interest Group, et al. Musculoskeletal ultrasound including definitions for ultrasonographic pathology. J Rheumatol. 2005;32:2485–7.
10. Dougados M, Jousse-Joulin S, Mistretta F, et al. Evaluation of several ultrasonography scoring systems for synovitis and comparison to clinical examination: results from a prospective multicentre study of rheumatoid arthritis. Ann Rheum Dis. 2010;69(5):828–33.
11. Mandl P, Naredo E, Wakefield RJ, OMERACT Ultrasound Task Force, et al. A systematic literature review analysis of ultrasound joint count and scoring systems to assess synovitis in rheumatoid arthritis according to the OMERACT filter. J Rheumatol. 2011;38:2055–62.
12. Naredo C, Rodriguez M, Campos C, et al. Validity, reproducibility, and responsiveness of a 12-joint simplified power Doppler ultrasonographic assessment of joint inflammation in rheumatoid arthritis. Arthritis Rheum. 2008;59:515–22.
13. Backhaus M, Ohrndorf S, Kellner H, et al. Evaluation of a novel 7-joint ultrasound score in daily rheumatologic practice: a pilot project. Arthritis Rheum. 2009;61:1194–201.
14. Epis O, Paoletti F, d'Errico, et al. Ultrasonography in the diagnosis and management of patients with inflammatory arthritides. Eur J Intern Med. 2013. http://dx.doi.org/10.1016/j.ejim.2013.08.700
15. Peterfy C, Ostergaard M, Conaghan P. MRI comes of age in RA clinical trials. Ann Rheum Dis. 2013;72:794–6.
16. Ostergaard M, Edmonds J, McQueen F. An introduction to the EULAR-OMERACT rheumatoid arthritis MRI reference image atlas. Ann Rheum Dis. 2005;64(Suppl I):i3–7.
17. Ostergaard M, Conaghan PG, O'Connor P, et al. Reducing invasiveness, duration, and cost of magnetic resonance imaging in rheumatoid arthritis by omitting intravenous contrast injection – Does it change the assessment of inflammatory and destructive joint changes by the OMERACT RAMRIS? J Rheumatol. 2009;36(8):1806–10.
18. Rahman P, Gladman DD, Cook RJ, et al. Radiological assessment in psoriatic arthritis. Br J Rheumatol. 1998;37:760–5.
19. Wassenberg S, Fischer-Kahle V, Herborn G, et al. A method to score radiographic change in psoriatic arthritis. J Rheumatol. 2001;60:156–66.
20. van der Heijde D. Quantification of radiological damage in inflammatory arthritis: rheumatoid arthritis, psoriatic arthritis and ankylosing spondylitis. Best Prac Res Clin Rheum. 2004;18:847–60.
21. Ostergaard M, McQueen F, Wiell C, et al. The OMERACT psoriatic arthritis magnetic resonance imaging scoring system (PsAMRIS): definitions of key pathologies, suggested MRI sequences, and preliminary scoring system for PsA hands. J Rheumatol. 2009;36:1816–24.
22. Boyesen P, McQueen F, Gandjbakhch F, et al. The OMERACT psoriatic arthritis magnetic resonance imaging score (PsAMRIS) is reliable and sensitive to

change: results from an OMERACT workshop. J Rheumatol. 2011;38:2034–8.
23. Wanders AJ, Landewe RB, Spoorenberg A, et al. What is the most appropriate radiologic scoring method in ankylosing spondylitis? A comparison of the available methods based on the outcome measures in rheumatology clinical trials filter. Arthritis Rheum. 2004;50:2622–32.
24. MacKay K, Mack C, Brophy S, et al. The Bath Ankylosing Spondylitis Radiology Index (BASRI): a new, validated approach to disease management. Arthritis Rheum. 1998;41:2263–70.
25. Averns HL, Oxtoby J, Taylor H, et al. Radiological outcome in ankylosing spondylitis: use of the stoke ankylosing spondylitis spine score (SASSS). Br J Rheumatol. 1996;35:373–6.
26. Creemers MC, Franssen MJ, vant Hof MA, et al. Assessment of outcome in ankylosing spondylitis: an extended radiographic scoring system. Ann Rheum Dis. 2005;64:127–9.
27. Spoorenberg A, de Vlam K, van der Linden S, et al. Radiological scoring methods in ankylosing spondylitis. Reliability and change over 1 and 2 years. J Rheumatol. 2004;31:125–32.
28. van der Linden S, Valkenburg HA, Cats A. Evaluation of diagnostic criteria for ankylosing spondylitis. A proposal for modification of the New York criteria. Arthritis Rheum. 1984;27:361–8.
29. Bennett P, Burch T. Population studies of the rheumatic diseases. Amsterdam: Excerpta Medica Foundation; 1968. p. 456–7.
30. Landewe R, Hermann KG, van der Heijde, et al. Scoring sacroiliac joints by magnetic resonance imaging. A multiple-reader reliability experiment. J Rheumatol. 2005;32:2050–5.
31. Maksymowych WP, Inman RD, Salonen D, et al. Spondyloarthritis Research Consortium of Canada magnetic resonance imaging index for assessment of sacroiliac joint inflammation in ankylosing spondylitis. Arthritis Rheum. 2005;53(5):703–9.
32. Herman KG, Braun J, Fischer T, et al. Magnetic resonance tomography of sacroiliitis: anatomy, histological pathology, MR-morphology, and grading. Radiology. 2004;44(3):217–28.
33. Marzo-Ortega H, McGonagle D, O'Connor P, et al. Efficacy of etanercept in the treatment of the entheseal pathology in resistant spondyloarthropathy: a clinical and magnetic resonance imaging study. Arthritis Rheum. 2001;44(9):2112–7.
34. Braun J, Baraliakos X, Golder W, et al. Magnetic resonance imaging examinations of the spine in patients with ankylosing spondylitis, before and after successful therapy with infliximab: evaluation of a new scoring system. Arthritis Rheum. 2003;48(4):l 1126–36.
35. Haibel H, Rudwaleit M, Brandt HC, et al. Adalimumab reduces spinal symptoms in active ankylosing spondylitis: clinical and magnetic resonance imaging results of a fifty-two-week open-label trial. Arthritis Rheum. 2006;54(2):678–81.
36. Maksymowych WP, Dhillon SS, Park R, et al. Validation of the Spondyloarthritis Research Consortium of Canada (SPARCC) MRI Spinal Inflammation Index: is it necessary to score the entire spine? Arthritis Rheum. 2007;57:501–7.
37. Lukas C, Braun J, van der Heijde D, et al. Scoring inflammatory activity of the spine by magnetic resonance imaging in ankylosing spondylitis: a multireader experiment. J Rheumatol. 2007;34(4):862–70.
38. Ostergaard M, Maksymowych WP, Pedersen SJ, et al. Structural lesions detected by magnetic resonance imaging in the spine of patients with spondyloarthritis – Definitions, assessment system and reference image set. J Rheumatol. 2009;36 Suppl 84:18–34.
39. Madsen KB, Jurik AG. MRI grading method for active and chronic spinal changes in spondyloarthritis. Clin Radiol. 2010;65(1):6–14.
40. Kellgren JH, Lawrence JS. Radiological assessment of osteoarthrosis. Ann Rheum Dis. 1957;16(4):494–502.
41. Maheu M, Cadet C, Gueneugues S, et al. Reproducibility and sensitivity to change of four scoring methods for the radiological assessment of osteoarthritis of the hand. Ann Rheum Dis. 2007;66:464–9.
42. Kallman DA, Wigley FM, Scott WW, et al. New radiographic grading scales for osteoarthritis of the hand. Arthritis Rheum. 1989;32:1584–91.
43. Verbruggen G, Veys EM. Numerical scoring systems for the anatomic evolution of osteoarthritis of the finger joints. Arthritis Rheum. 1996;39:308–20.
44. Hayashi D, Guermazi A, Roemer F. MRI of osteoarthritis: the challenges of definition and quantification. Semin Musculoskelet Radiol. 2012;16:419–30.
45. Hunter DJ, Arden N, Conaghan PG, OARSI OA Imaging Working Group, et al. Definition of osteoarthritis on MRO: results of a Delphi exercise. Osteoarthritis Cartilage. 2011;198:963–9.
46. Peterfy CG, Guermazi A, Zaim S, et al. Whole Organ Magnetic Resonance Imaging Score (WORMS) of the knee in osteoarthritis. Osteoarthritis Cartilage. 2004; 12(3):177–90.
47. Kornaat PR, Ceulemans RY, Kroon HM, et al. MRI assessment of knee osteoarthritis: Knee Osteoarthritis Scoring System (KOSS) – inter-observer and intra-observer reproducibility of a compartment-based scoring system. Skeletal Radiol. 2005;34(2): 95–102.
48. Hunter DJ, Lo GH, Gale D, et al. The reliability of a new scoring system for knee osteoarthritis on MRI and the validity of bone marrow lesion assessment: BLOKS (Boston Leeds Osteoarthritis Knee Score). Ann Rheum Dis. 2008;67(2):206–11.
49. Hunter DJ, Guermazi A, Lo GH, et al. Evolution of semi-quantitative whole joint knee assessment of knee OA: MOAKS (MRI Osteoarthritis Knee Score). Osteoarthritis Cartilage. 2011;19(8):990–1002.
50. Ostergaard M, Poggenborg RP, Axelsen MB, Pedersen SJ. Magnetic resonance imaging in spondyloarthritis – how to quantify findings and measure response. Best Pract Res Clin Rheumatol. 2010; 24(5):637–57.

Index

J. O'Neill (ed.), *Essential Imaging in Rheumatology*,
DOI 10.1007/978-1-4939-1673-3, © Springer Science+Business Media New York 2015

O

R

S

9781493916726